Oxford Textbook of

Cancer in Children

Oxford Textbook of

Cancer in Children

SEVENTH EDITION

EDITED BY

Hubert N. Caron

Professor of Paediatric Oncology, Emma Children's Hospital AMC,
University of Amsterdam, Amsterdam, The Netherlands
Group Medical Director for Pediatric Oncology, Hoffmann-La Roche, Basel, Switzerland

Andrea Biondi

Professor of Pediatrics, University of Milano-Bicocca, and Director, Department of Pediatrics,
Fondazione MBBM/Hospital San Gerardo, Monza, Italy

Tom Boterberg

Associate Professor, Department of Radiation Oncology,
Ghent University Hospital, Ghent, Belgium

François Doz

Professor of Pediatrics, School of Medicine, University Paris Descartes,
and Pediatric Oncologist, SIREDO Center, Institut Curie, Paris, France

OXFORD
UNIVERSITY PRESS

OXFORD
UNIVERSITY PRESS

Great Clarendon Street, Oxford, OX2 6DP,
United Kingdom

Oxford University Press is a department of the University of Oxford.
It furthers the University's objective of excellence in research, scholarship, and education by publishing worldwide. Oxford is a registered trade mark of Oxford University Press in the UK and in certain other countries

First Edition published 1975
Second Edition published 1986
Third Edition published 1992
Fourth Edition published 1998
Fifth Edition published 2005
Sixth Edition published 2012
Seventh Edition published 2020

Impression: 1

Published in the United States of America by Oxford University Press
198 Madison Avenue, New York, NY 10016, United States of America

British Library Cataloguing in Publication Data
Data available

Library of Congress Control Number: 2020935774

ISBN 978–0–19–879721–0

Printed in Great Britain by
Bell & Bain Ltd., Glasgow

Preface

This is the seventh edition of *Cancer in Children*, first published in 1975. The outlook for children with cancer has greatly improved since then, mainly due to strong international collaboration between clinicians of various relevant specialties as well as preclinical researchers. Still, we are not able to cure all children with cancer, and cure comes at a cost, with many survivors of childhood cancer facing significant health problems later in life. However, the last decades have brought an explosion of biological knowledge and genomic data. Translating these into clinically useful tests and therapies remains a challenge. Also, incorporating the emerging new cancer immunotherapies in paediatric oncology requires innovation and collaboration.

We think that this book will offer readers a clear understanding of what is now possible and what is still needed to take things forward into the future.

We would like to thank the contributors to this edition, our colleagues and collaborators, and all others who have helped with the preparation of this book. We would also like to thank the many members of the International Society of Paediatric Oncology (SIOP) who contributed to this work and appreciate SIOP's continued efforts on behalf of children with cancer in all countries.

Hubert N. Caron
Andrea Biondi
Tom Boterberg
François Doz

Acknowledgement

We thank the many SIOP members who contributed to this work and appreciate SIOP's continued efforts on behalf of children with cancer.

Contents

Abbreviations

6-MP	6-mercaptopurine
6-TG	6-thioguanine
A	actinomycin D
AAPCOB	American Academy of Pediatrics Committee on Bioethics
ABVD	doxorubicin, bleomycin, vinblastine, dacarbazine
aCPP	atypical choroid plexus papilloma
ACTH	adrenocorticotropic hormone
ADC	apparent diffusion coefficient
ADCC	antibody-dependent cellular cytotoxicity
ADV	adenovirus
AER	absolute excess risk
AF	aggressive fibromatosis
AFP	alpha fetoprotein
AJCC	American Joint Committee on Cancer
ALCL	anaplastic large-cell lymphoma
ALK	anaplastic lymphoma kinase
ALL	acute lymphoblastic leukaemia
ALT	alternate lengthening of telomeres
AMKL	acute megakaryoblastic leukaemia
AML	acute myeloid leukaemia
AMPK	activation of AMP-activated protein kinase
APL	acute promyelocytic leukaemia
APO	adriamycin (doxorubicin), prednisone, and vincristine
A-RMS	alveolar rhabdomyosarcoma
ASPS	alveolar soft-part sarcoma
ASR	age-standardized rate
ATO	arsenic trioxide
ATRA	all-*trans* retinoic acid
ATRT	atypical teratoid rhabdoid tumour
AYA	adolescent and young adult
BCD	bleomycin, cyclophosphamide, and actinomycin D
BCH	benign cephalic histiocytosis
BCNU	bis-chlorethylnitrosourea
BCR	B-cell receptor
BCRP	breast cancer resistance protein
BEACOPP	bleomycin, etoposide, doxorubicin, cyclophosphamide, vincristine, prednisolone and procarbazine
BEAM	BCNU, etoposide, cytarabine, and melphalan
BEP	cisplatin, etoposide, and bleomycin
BFM	Berlin–Frankfurt–Munster
BITE	bispecific T-cell engaging
BL	Burkitt lymphoma
BM	bone marrow
BMD	bone mineral density
BOIN	Bayesian optimal interval
BSA	body surface area
Bu	bulsulfan
BV	brentuximab vedotin
BW	body weight
BWS	Beckwith–Wiedemann syndrome
C	cyclophosphamide
CAR	chimeric antigen receptor
CB	cord blood
CBTRUS	Central Brain Tumor Registry of the United States
CBV	cyclophosphamide, BCNU, and etoposide
CCC	Cochrane Childhood Cancer
CCG	Children's Cancer Group
CCNU	procarbazine, 6-thioguanine, dibromodulcitol, and lomustine
CCS	childhood cancer survivor
CCSK	clear-cell sarcoma
CCSS	Childhood Cancer Survivor Study
CDS	complement-dependent cytotoxicity
CEUS	contrast-enhanced ultrasound
CEVAIE	carboplatin, epirubicin, vincristine, actinomycin D, ifosfamide, and etoposide
CHC	choriocarcinoma
CHOP	cyclophosphamide, doxorubicin, vincristine, and prednisone
CHL	classical variant of Hodgkin lymphoma
CHS	Chédiak–Higashi syndrome
CI	confidence interval
CIR	cumulative incidence of relapse
CKD	chronic kidney disease
CML	chronic myelogenous/myeloid leukaemia
CMML	chronic myelomonocytic leukaemia
CMN	congenital mesoblastic nephroma
CMV	cytomegalovirus
CNS	central nervous system
COG	Children's Oncology Group
COJEC	cisplatin, vincristine, carboplatin, etoposide, and cyclophosphamide
COMP	cyclophosphamide, vincristine, methotrexate, and prednisone
COPAD	cyclophosphamide, vincristine, prednisone, and doxorubicin

COPDAC	vincristine, cyclophosphamide, dacarbazine, and prednisone
COPP	vincristine, cyclophosphamide, procarbazine, and prednisone
COSS	Cooperative Osteosarcoma Study
CPC	choroid plexus carcinoma
CPG	clinical practice guideline
CPP	choroid plexus papilloma
CPT	choroid plexus tumour
CR	complete remission
CRM	continual reassessment method
CRS	cytokine release syndrome
CRT	cranial/conformal radiotherapy
CsA	cyclosporine A
CSC	cancer stem cell
CSF	cerebrospinal fluid
CSI	craniospinal irradiation
CT	computed tomography
ctDNA	circulating tumour DNA
CTL	cytotoxic lymphocyte
CTR	clinical trial regulation
CTV	clinical target volume
CWS	German Soft Tissue Sarcoma Cooperative Group
CXR	chest X-ray
D	doxorubicin
DC	dyskeratosis congenital
DC	dendritic cell
DDS	Denys–Drash syndrome
DEXA	dual X-ray absorptiometry
DFP	dermatofibrosarcoma protuberans
DFS	disease-free survival
DHAP	dexamethasone, high-dose cytarabine, and cisplatin
DI	diabetes insipidus
DIA/DIG	desmoplastic infantile astrocytoma/ganglioglioma
DIPG	diffuse intrinsic pontine glioma
DLBCL	diffuse large B-cell lymphoma
DLI	donor lymphocyte infusion
DLT	dose-limiting toxicity
DNT	dysembryoplastic neuroepithelial tumour
DS	Down syndrome
DSRCT	desmoplastic small round-cell tumour
DVH	dose volume histogram
DWI	diffusion-weighted imaging
DXA	dual X-ray absorptiometry
E	etoposide
eIPV	enhanced inactivated polio vaccine
E-RMS	embryonal rhabdomyosarcoma
EBM	evidence-based medicine
EBMT	European Group for Blood and Marrow Transplantation
EBRT	external-beam radiotherapy
EBV	Epstein–Barr virus
EC	embryonal carcinoma
ECG	electrocardiogram
EFS	event-free survival
EGF	epidermal growth factor
EGFR	epidermal growth factor receptor
EICNHL	European Intergroup for Childhood Non-Hodgkin Lymphoma
EMA	European Medical Agency
EMT	epithelial-mesenchymal transition
ENTYAC	European Network for Teenagers and Young Adults with Cancer
EpSSG	European paediatric Soft-tissue sarcoma Study Group
ES	Ewing sarcoma
ESR	erythrocyte sedimentation rate
EtD	evidence to decision
ETV	endoscopic third ventriculostomy
EU CTD	EU Clinical Trials Directive
FA	fibrillary astrocytoma
FAB	French–American–British
FAP	familial adenomatous polyposis
FDA	Federal Drug Agency
FDG	18-fluorodeoxyglucose
FHL	familial haemophagocytic lymphohistiocytosis
FISH	fluorescent *in situ* hybridization
FL	follicular lymphoma
FN	febrile neutropenia
FSH	follicle-stimulating hormone
G-CSF	granulocyte colony-stimulating growth factor
GA	general anaesthetic
GBM	glioblastoma multiforme
GCB	germinal centre B-cell
GCT	germ-cell tumour
GFR	glomerular filtration rate
GG	ganglioglioma
GH	growth hormone
GIST	gastrointestinal stromal tumour
GM-CSF	granulocyte macrophage colony-stimulating growth factor
GNB	ganglioneuroblastoma
GO	gemtuzumab ozogamicin
GP	general practitioner
GPOH	German Society for Paediatric Oncology and Haematology
GRADE	grading of recommendations, assessment, development, and evaluation
GSII	Griscelli syndrome type II
GTV	gross tumour volume
GvH	graft-versus-host
GvL	graft-versus-leukaemia
GvT	graft-versus-tumour
GWS	genome-wide association
HART	hyperfractionated accelerated radiotherapy
HbF	fetal haemoglobin
HBV	hepatitis B virus
HC	haemorrhagic cystitis
HCG	β-human chorionic gonadotropin
HCV	hepatitis C virus
HD	high-dose
HDAC	histone deacetylase
HDCT	high-dose chemotherapy
HER2	human epidermal growth factor receptor 2
hFLMPC	human fetal liver multipotent progenitor cell

HGG	high-grade glioma
HHV8	human herpesvirus 8
HIC	high-income countries
HIPEC	hyperthermic intraperitoneal chemotherapy
HIV	human immunodeficiency virus
HL	Hodgkin lymphoma
HLA	human leukocyte antigen
HLH	haemophagocytic lymphohistiocytosis
HPA	hypothalamic pituitary axis
HPF	high-power field
HPV	human papilloma virus
HR	hypophosphataemic rickets
HR	hazard ratio
HRS	Hodgkin/Reed Sternberg
HSC	haematopoietic stem cell
HSCR	haematopoietic stem-cell rescue
HSCT	haematopoietic stem-cell transplantation
HSV	herpes simplex virus
HVA	homovanillic acid
HvG	host-versus-graft
I	ifosfamide
IBMFD	inherited bone-marrow failure disorder
IBMTR	International Bone Marrow Transplant Registry
ICCC-3	International Classification of Childhood Cancer, Third Edition
ICD-O	International Classification of Diseases for Oncology
ICE	ifosfamide, carboplatin, and etoposide
ICG	Italian Cooperative Group
ICP	intracranial pressure
ICU	intensive-care unit
IDRF	image-defined risk factor
IEP	ifosfamide, etoposide, and prednisolone
IESS	Intergroup Ewing Sarcoma
IFS	infantile fibrosarcoma
IGEV	gemcitabine, prednisone, ifosfamide, and vinorelbine
IGF	insulin-like growth factor
IGHG	International Guideline Harmonization Group
IGRT	image-guided radiotherapy
IMAT	intensity-modulated arc therapy
IMC	immunohistochemistry
IMRT	intensity-modulated radiotherapy
IMT	inflammatory myofibroblastic tumour
INPC	International Neuroblastoma Pathology Classification
INRG	International Neuroblastoma Risk Group
INRGSS	International Neuroblastoma Risk Group Staging System
INSS	International Neuroblastoma Staging System
IPSS	International Prognostic Scoring System
IR	intervention radiology
IRSS	International Retinoblastoma Staging System
IT	intrathecal
ITCC	Innovative Therapies for Children with Cancer
ITD	internal tandem duplication
ITT	insulin tolerance test
IV	intravenous
IVAD	ifosfamide, vincristine, actinomycin D, and doxorubicin
JCML	juvenile chronic myeloid leukaemia
JEB	carboplatin, etoposide, and bleomycin
JMML	juvenile myelomonocytic leukaemia
JNBSG	Japanese Neuroblastoma Study Group
JPA	juvenile pilocytic astrocytoma
JXG	juvenile xanthogranuloma
KIR	killer-cell immunoglobulin-like receptor
LAE	late adverse event
LAIP	leukaemia-associated immunophenotype
LC	large-cell
LCH	Langerhans cell histiocytosis
LD-PCR	long-distance polymerase chain reaction
LDH	lactate dehydrogenase
LFS	leukaemia-free survival
LFS	Li–Fraumeni syndrome
LGA	low-grade astrocytoma
LGG	low-grade glioma
LGGNT	low-grade glial-neuronal tumour
LH	luteinizing hormone
LL	lymphoblastic lymphoma
LMIC	low- and middle-income countries
LN	lymph node
LOH	loss of heterozygosity
LOI	loss of imprinting
LRP	lung resistance-related protein
LSC	leukaemic stem cell
LTFU	long-term follow-up
LyP	lymphoid papulosis
MALT	mucosa-associated tissue lymphoma
MA	myeloablative
mAb	monoclonal antibody
MAPK	mitogen-activated protein kinase
MAS	macrophage activation syndrome
MBEN	medulloblastoma with extensive nodularity
M-CSF	macrophage-colony stimulating factor
MCV	mean corpuscular volume
MD	matched donor
MDD	minimal disseminated disease
MDP	methylene-diphosphonate
MDR	multidrug resistance
MDS	myelodysplastic syndrome
MDS-EB	myelodysplastic syndrome with excess blasts
MDT	multidisciplinary team
MFD	matched family donor
MGCT	malignant germ-cell tumour
MHC	major histocompatibility complex
MIBG	metaiodobenzylguanidine
miRNA	microRNA
ML-DS	myeloid leukaemia of Down syndrome
MMAE	monomethyl auristatin E
MMD	mismatched donor
MMR	measles, mumps, rubella
MoAb	monoclonal antibody
MPNST	malignant peripheral nerve sheath tumour
MPO	myeloperoxidase
MRC	Medical Research Council
MRD	minimal residual disease
MRI	magnetic resonance imaging

MRP	multidrug resistance protein
MRT	malignant rhabdoid tumour
MS	metabolic syndrome
MS	multisystem
MSD	matched sibling donor
MSKCC	Memorial Sloan-Kettering Cancer Center
MSTS	Musculoskeletal Tumor Society
MTD	maximum tolerated dose
MTPI	modified toxicity probability interval
mTOR	mammalian target of rapamycin
MTP-PE	muramyl tripeptide
MTX	methotrexate
MUD	matched unrelated donor
MZL	marginal zone lymphoma
NBL	neuroblastoma
NCI	National Cancer Institute
ND	neurodegeneration
NDI	nephrogenic diabetes insipidus
NF1	neurofibromatosis
NGGCT	non-germinomatous germ-cell tumour
NGS	next-generation sequencing
NHL	non-Hodgkin lymphoma
NICE	National Institute of Clinical Excellence
NK	natural killer
NLPHL	nodular lymphocyte predominant Hodgkin lymphoma
NMDA	N-methyl-D-aspartate
NMSC	non-melanomatous skin cancer
NMZL	nodal marginal-zone lymphoma
NOPHO	Nordic Society of Paediatric Haematology and Oncology
NOS	not otherwise specified
NPM	nucleophosmin
NRM	non-relapse mortality
NRSTS	non-rhabdomyomatous soft-tissue sarcoma
NS	Noonan syndrome
NSAID	non-steroidal anti-inflammatory drug
NSCLC	non-small-cell lung cancer
NSE	neuron-specific enolase
NTV	neuroendoscopic third ventriculostomy
OEPA	vincristine, etoposide, prednisone, and adriamycin
OMS	opsoclonus-myoclonus syndrome
ORR	objective response rate
OS	overall survival
OS	osteosarcoma
PA	pilocytic astrocytoma
PAS	periodic-acid-Schiff
PB	peripheral blood
PBSC	peripheral blood stem cells
PCP	pneumocystis pneumonia
PCR	polymerase chain reaction
PCU	paediatric cancer unit
PDGF	platelet-derived growth factor
PDGFR	platelet-derived growth factor receptor
PD-L1	programmed death ligand 1
PEI	ifosfamide, cisplatin, and etoposide
PET	positron emission tomography
PF	posterior fossa
PFS	progression-free survival
PFT	pulmonary function test
PGC	primordial germ cell
PHPV	persistent hyperplastic primary vitreous
PIP	paediatric investigational plan
PIS	patient information sheet
PLAP	placental alkaline phosphatase
PMBL	primary mediastinal large B-cell lymphoma
PNET	primitive neuro-ectodermal tumour
pNT	peripheral neuroblastic tumour
POG	Paediatric Oncology Group
PPB	peuropulmonary blastoma
(p)PNET	(peripheral) primitive neuroectodermal tumour
PPR	prednisone poor response
PR	partial remission
PRETEXT	pre-treatment extent
PTC	principal treatment centre
PTCL	peripheral T-cell lymphoma
PT-Cy	post-transplant cyclophosphamide
PTSD	post-traumatic stress disorder
PTV	planning target volume
PVB	cisplatin, vinblastine, and bleomycin
PXA	pleomorphic xanthoastrocytoma
RA	refractory anaemia
RAEB	refractory anaemia with excessive blasts
RAEB-t	refractory anaemia with excessive blasts in transformation
RARS	refractory anaemia with ringed sideroblasts
RC	refractory cytopenia
RCC	refractory cytopenia of childhood
RCC	renal-cell carcinoma
RCT	randomized controlled clinical trial
RDD	Rosai–Dorfman disease
REAL	Revised European–American Lymphoma Classification of HL
RECIST	response evaluation criteria in solid tumours
RFS	relapse-free survival
RIC	reduced-intensity conditioning
RMS	rhabdomyosarcoma
RR	relative risk
RR	relapsed and refractory
RT	radiotherapy
RTA	renal tubular acidosis
RTK	rhabdoid tumour of the kidney
RTK	receptor tyrosine kinase
RT-PCR	reverse transcriptase polymerase chain reaction
SC	sclerosing cholarigitis
SC	stem cell
SCF	stemcell factor
SCT	stem-cell transplantation
SCN	severe congenital neutropenia
SDD	selective decontamination of the digestive tract
SDS	Shwachman–Diamond syndrome
SE	subependymoma
SEER	surveillance, epidemiology, and end results
SEGA	subependymal giant-cell astrocytoma
SEN	subependymal nodule
SHH	sonic hedgehog

SHML	sinus histiocytosis with massive lymphadenopathy
sIg	suface immunoglobin
SIOP	International Society of Paediatric Oncology
SIOPEL	International Childhood Liver Tumor Strategy Group
SMN	secondary malignant neoplasm
SMR	standardized mortality ratio
SNP	single nucleotide polymorphism
SOS	sinusoidal obstructive syndrome
SP	spine
SS	synovial sarcoma
ST	supratentorial
STS	soft-tissue sarcoma
STS	sodium thiosulfate
STSC	Soft Tissue Sarcoma Committee
SVC	superior vena cava
TAM	transient abnormal myelopoiesis
TBI	total body irradiation
TCR	T-cell receptor
TDI	total diagnostic interval
TDM	therapeutic drug monitoring
TdT	terminal deoxynucleotidyl transferase
TKI	tyrosine kinase inhibitor
TLCT	transitional liver cell tumour
TLP	traumatic lumbar puncture
TLS	tumour lysis syndrome
TMP/SMZ	trimethoprim/sulfamethoxazole
TMZ	temozolomide
TN	tenascin
TNFR	tumour necrosis factor receptor
TNM	tumour-node-metastasis
TPMT	thiopurine methyltransferase
TRH	thyrotropin-releasing hormone
TRM	transplant-related mortality
TSC	tuberous sclerosis complex
TSH	thyroid-stimulating hormone
TTL	target toxicity level
UCH	uncommon histiocytosis
UNCRC	UN Convention of the Rights of the Child
URD	unrelated donor
US	ultrasound
UV	ultraviolet
V	vincristine
VAC	vincristine, actinomycin, and cyclophosphamide
VDC-IE	vincristine, doxorubicin, cyclophosphamide, ifosfamide, and etoposide
VEGF	vascular endothelial growth factor
VIP	vinblastine, ifosfamide, and cisplatin
VHR	very high risk
VMA	vanillylmandelic acid
VOD	veno-occlusive disease
VP	ventriculo-peritoneal
VTC	topotecan, cyclophosphamide, and vincristine
VZV	varicella zoster virus
WAGR	Wilms tumour, aniridia, genital deformity, retardation
WBC	white blood cell
WCC	World Child Cancer
WGS	whole-genome sequencing
WHO	World Health Organization
WT	Wilms tumour
WVI	whole ventricular irradiation
XLP	X-linked lymphoproliferative syndrome
YST	yolk sac tumour

Contributors

Femke Aarsen Pediatric Clinical Neuropsychologist, Princess Máxima Center for Pediatric Oncology, Utrecht, The Netherlands

Maurizio Aricò Coordinator of Rare Pediatric Diseases Center, Meyer University Hospital, Florence, Italy

Adriana Balduzzi Pediatric Clinic University of Milan Bicocca, MBBM Foundation, San Gerardo Hospital, Monza, Italy

Christophe Bergeron Paediatric Oncologist, Institute of Hematology and Pediatric Oncology (IHOPE), Centre Léon Bérard, Lyon, France

Stefan Bielack Medical Director, Department of Pediatric Oncology, Hematology and Immunology, Stuttgart Cancer Center, Stuttgart Hospital—Olgahospital, Stuttgart, Germany

Andrea Biondi Professor of Pediatrics, University of Milano-Bicocca, and Director, Department of Pediatrics, Fondazione MBBM/Hospital San Gerardo, Monza, Italy

Gianni Bisogno Associate Professor, Department of Women's and Children's Health, University of Padua, Padua, Italy

Tom Boterberg Associate Professor, Department of Radiation Oncology, Ghent University Hospital, Ghent, Belgium

Eric Bouffet Garron Family Chair in Childhood Cancer Research, Director, Paediatric Neuro-Oncology Program, and Professor of Paediatrics, Hospital for Sick Children, Toronto, Canada

Garrett M. Brodeur Director of the Cancer Predisposition Program, Children's Hospital of Philadelphia, and Perelman School of Medicine, University of Pennsylvania, Pennsylvania, USA

Gabriele Calaminus Department of Pediatric Hematology and Oncology, Bonn University Children's Hospital, Bonn, Germany

Hubert N. Caron Professor of Paediatric Oncology, Emma Children's Hospital AMC, University of Amsterdam, Amsterdam, The Netherlands

Guillermo Chantada Head of Precision Medicine, JP Garrahan Hospital, and Principal Researcher, CONICET, Buenos Aires, Argentina; Associated Member, Hospital Sant Joan de Deu, Barcelona, Spain

Cecile Faure Conter Pediatric Oncologist, Institute of Pediatric Hematology and Oncology (IHOPe), Lyon, France

Finella Craig Consultant in Paediatric Palliative Medicine, Great Ormond Street Hospital for Children, London, UK

Jean-Hugues Dalle Head of HSCT Pediatric Unit, Hematology and Immunology Department, Robert-Debre Hospital, Assistance Publique, Hopitaux de Paris and University of Paris, Paris, France

Gianpietro Dotti Professor, Department of Microbiology and Immunology, University of North Carolina, Chapel Hill, USA

François Doz Professor of Pediatrics, School of Medicine, University Paris Descartes, and Pediatric Oncologist, SIREDO Center, Institut Curie, Paris, France

Angelika Eggert Director, Department of Pediatrics, Division of Oncology and Hematology, Charité University Medical Center Berlin, Berlin, Germany

Andrea Ferrari Pediatric Oncology Unit, Fondazione IRCCS Istituto Nazionale dei Tumori, Milan, Italy

Didier Frappaz Pediatric Oncologist, Institute of Pediatric Hematology and Oncology (IHOPE), Lyon, France

Stefania Galimberti Professor of Medical Statistics, School of Medicine and Surgery, University of Milano-Bicocca, Milan, Italy

Maria Luisa Garrè Department of Neuro-Oncology, IRCCS Istituto Giannina Gaslini, Genova, Italy

Gemma Gatta Evaluative Epidemiology Unit, Fondazione IRCCS Istituto Nazionale dei Tumori, Milan, Italy

Mark Gaze Consultant Clinical Oncologist, University College London Hospitals and Great Ormond Street Hospital for Children, London, UK

Norbert Graf Department of Pediatric Oncology and Hematology, Saarland University, Homburg, Germany

Martha Grootenhuis Princess Máxima Center for Pediatric Oncology, Utrecht, The Netherlands

Rupert Handgretinger Chair, Department of Hematology/Oncology, Children's University Hospital, University of Tuebingen, Tuebingen, Germany

Darren Hargrave Haematology and Oncology Department, Great Ormond Street Hospital for Children, London, UK

Henrik Hasle Professor, Pediatrics and Adolescent Medicine, Aarhus University Hospital, Aarhus, Denmark

Riccardo Haupt Epidemiology and Biostatistics Unit, DOPO Clinic, IRCCS Istituto Giannina Gaslini, Genova, Italy

Lee Helman Attending Physician, Children's Center for Cancer and Blood Diseases, Children's Hospital Los Angeles, Los Angeles, USA

Koichi Hirabayashi Lineberger Comprehensive Cancer Center, University of North Carolina, Chapel Hill, USA

Lars Hjorth Paediatric Oncology and Haematology, Department of Paediatrics, Skåne University Hospital, Clinical Sciences, Lund University, Sweden

Scott C. Howard Professor and Associate Dean for Research in the College of Nursing, University of Tennessee College of Health Sciences, Memphis, USA

Thierry A.G.M. Huisman Radiologist-in-Chief, Texas Children's Hospital, Houston, USA

Trijn Israels Pediatric Oncologist, Coordinator Clinical Research Sub-Saharan Africa, Outreach Programme, Princess Máxima Center for Pediatric Oncology, Utrecht, The Netherlands

Momcilo Jankovic Pediatric Hemato-Oncologist, Pediatric Clinic University of Milano-Bicocca, Foundation MBBM, Monza, Italy

Lucy J.W. Jones Medical Oncology Registrar, St James's University Hospital, Leeds, UK

David T.W. Jones Group Leader, Pediatric Glioma Research Group, Hopp Children's Cancer Center Heidelberg (KiTZ), and German Cancer Research Center (DKFZ), Heidelberg, Germany

Gertjan Kaspers Director of the Academy, Princess Máxima Center for Pediatric Oncology, Utrecht, and Professor of Pediatric Oncology, Amsterdam UMC/Vumc, The Netherlands

Pamela Kearns Professor of Clinical Paediatric Oncology, Institute of Cancer and Genomic Sciences, University of Birmingham, and Honorary Consultant, Birmingham Children's Hospital, Birmingham, UK

Michelle Koh Paediatric Palliative Care Consultant, University Hospital Southampton NHS Foundation Trust, Southampton, UK

Leontien C.M. Kremer Department of Pediatrics, Amsterdam UMC, Amsterdam, The Netherlands; Princess Máxima Center for Pediatric Oncology, Utrecht, The Netherlands

Judith Landman-Parker Pediatric Hematology and Oncology Department, Armand Trousseau Hospital, Paris, France

Erik A.H. Loeffen Pediatrician-in-training, Beatrix Children's Hospital, University Medical Center Groningen, Groningen, The Netherlands

Mignon Loh Professor of Clinical Pediatrics, Division of Hematology Oncology, Helen Diller Family Comprehensive Cancer Center, University of California San Francisco, San Francisco, USA

Giovanna Lucchini BMT Department, Great Ormond Street Hospital for Children, London, UK

Maura Massimino Pediatric Unit Director, Fondazione IRCCS Istituto Nazionale dei Tumori, Milan, Italy

Kieran McHugh Consultant Paediatric Radiologist, Great Ormond Street Hospital for Children, London, UK

Hans Merks Pediatric Oncologist, Princess Máxima Center for Pediatric Oncology, Utrecht, The Netherlands

Gisela Michel Department of Health Sciences and Medicine, University of Lucerne, Lucerne, Switzerland

Véronique Minard-Colin Department of Pediatric and Adolescent Oncology, Gustave Roussy, Université Paris-Saclay, Villejuif, France

Elizabeth Molyneux Honorary Professor of Paediatrics and Child Health, University of Malawi College of Medicine, Malawi, and Strategic Advisor for East and West Africa, Royal College of Paediatrics and Child Health, London, UK

Françoise Montravers Head of the Nuclear Medicine Department, Assistance Publique Hôpitaux de Paris, Paris, France

Lucas Moreno Clinical Director, Paediatric Oncology and Haematology Division, Vall d'Hebron Hospital, Barcelona, Spain

James C. Nicholson Department of Paediatric Oncology, Cambridge University Hospitals NHS Foundation Trust, Cambridge, UK

Charlotte M. Niemeyer Professor, Division of Pediatric Hematology and Oncology, Department of Pediatrics and Adolescent Medicine, Medical Center, Faculty of Medicine, University of Freiburg, Freiburg, Germany

Kristian W. Pajtler Hopp-Children's Cancer Center Heidelberg (KiTZ); Division of Pediatric Neurooncology, German Cancer Research Center (DKFZ); Department of Pediatric Hematology and Oncology, Heidelberg University Hospital, Heidelberg, Germany

Catherine Patte Department of Pediatrics, Institut Gustave Roussy, Paris, France

Michael Paulussen Medical Director, Datteln Children's Hospital, Datteln, and Chair of Pediatrics, Witten/Herdecke University, Witten, Germany

Giorgio Perilongo Department of Women's and Children's Health, University of Padua, Padua, Italy

Stefan M. Pfister Hopp-Children's Cancer Center Heidelberg (KiTZ); Division of Pediatric Neurooncology, German Cancer Research Center (DKFZ); Department of Pediatric Hematology and Oncology, Heidelberg University Hospital, Heidelberg, Germany

Robert S. Phillips Centre for Reviews and Dissemination, University of York, York, UK, and Leeds Children's Hospital, Leeds Teaching Hospitals NHS Trust, Leeds, UK

Rob Pieters Pediatric Oncologist, Board of Directors, and Chief Medical Officer, Princess Máxima Center for Pediatric Oncology, Utrecht, The Netherlands

Vijay Ramaswamy Assistant Professor, Division of Haematology and Oncology, Hospital for Sick Children, Toronto, Canada

Dirk Reinhardt Director, Pediatrics III and Department of Pediatric Oncology, Hematology, Pneumology, Stem Cell Therapy, Cardiology, and Rheumatology, University Hospital Essen, Essen, Germany

Carlos Rodríguez-Galindo Executive Vice-President, Chair of the Department of Global Pediatric Medicine, and Director of St Jude Global, St Jude Children's Research Hospital, Memphis, USA

Emmanouil Saloustros Department of Oncology, University Hospital of Larissa, Larissa, Greece

Barbara Savoldo Lineberger Comprehensive Cancer Center, University of North Carolina, Chapel Hill, USA

Denis Schewe Christian-Albrechts University Kiel and University Medical Center Schleswig-Holstein, Kiel, Germany

Gudrun Schleiermacher SIREDO Care, Innovation and Research for Children, Adolescents and Young Adults with Cancer, Pediatric Oncology Center; Deputy Director for Translational Research; Team Leader, SiRIC RTOP Translational Research in Pediatric Oncology, INSERM U830 PARIS, France

Martin Schrappe Chair of Pediatrics, Christian-Albrechts University Kiel and University Medical Center Schleswig-Holstein, Kiel, Germany

Rod Skinner Department of Paediatric and Adolescent Haematology and Oncology, Great North Children's Hospital, and Newcastle University Centre for Cancer, Newcastle University, Newcastle, UK

Dan Stark Associate Professor of Cancer Medicine and Honorary Consultant in Medical Oncology, Leeds Institute for Medical Research and Leeds Teaching Hospitals NHS Trust, Leeds, UK

Charles A. Stiller Lead on Childhood Cancer, National Cancer Registration and Analysis Service, Public Health England, UK

Dominik Sturm Physician Scientist, Pediatric Glioma Research Group, Hopp Children's Cancer Center Heidelberg (KiTZ), Clinic for Pediatric Oncology, Hematology, and Immunology, University Hospital Heidelberg, and German Cancer Research Center (DKFZ), Heidelberg, Germany

Maria Grazia Valsecchi Professor of Medical Statistics, School of Medicine and Surgery, University of Milano-Bicocca, Milan, Italy

Marianne van de Wetering Pediatric Oncologist, Princess Máxima Center for Pediatric Oncology, Utrecht, The Netherlands

Esther van den Bergh Clinical Psychologist, Princess Máxima Center for Pediatric Oncology, Utrecht, The Netherlands

Cor van den Bos Pediatric Oncologist, Princess Máxima Center for Pediatric Oncology, Utrecht, The Netherlands

Dannis van Vuurden Pediatric Neuro-Oncologist, VU University Medical Center, Amsterdam, The Netherlands

Gareth J. Veal Professor of Cancer Pharmacology, Newcastle University Centre for Cancer, Newcastle upon Tyne, UK

David Walker Professor of Paediatric Oncology, Children's Brain Tumour Research Centre, University of Nottingham, Nottingham, UK

Sheila Weitzman Pediatric Oncologist, The Hospital for Sick Children, Toronto, Canada

Shaarna Whitton Children's Brain Tumour Research Centre, University of Nottingham, Nottingham, UK

Joanne Wolfe Director, Pediatric Palliative Care, Boston Children's Hospital, and Division Chief, Pediatric Palliative Care Service, Department of Psychosocial Oncology and Palliative Care, Dana-Farber, Cancer Institute, Boston, USA

Michel Zerah Head of the Department of Pediatric Neurosurgery, Hôpital des Enfants Malades, Paris, France

József Zsiros Pediatric Oncologist, Princess Máxima Center for Pediatric Oncology, Utrecht, The Netherlands

C. Michel Zwaan Professor of Paediatric Oncology, Princess Máxima Center for Pediatric Oncology, Utrecht, and Erasmus MC, Rotterdam, The Netherlands

1

The Epidemiology of Cancer in Children and Adolescents

Charles A. Stiller and Gemma Gatta

Introduction

Childhood and adolescent cancers account for less than 2% of all cancers in industrialized countries, but the young age at which they occur means that they account for a much larger proportion of total population life years potentially lost to cancer. We consider here the classification of childhood and adolescent cancer, incidence and survival rates, late effects, and aetiology.

Classification

The current standard classification for those under the age of 15 years is the *International Classification of Childhood Cancer, Third Edition* (ICCC-3), with groups defined by the codes for morphology and topography in the third edition of the *International Classification of Diseases for Oncology* (ICD-O). Most of these groups are limited to malignant neoplasms, but benign and unspecified intracranial and intraspinal tumours are also included, since it is hard to distinguish between malignant and non-malignant tumours and they are recorded by many cancer registries.

In the most recent version of the standard classification for cancers of adolescents and young adults (15–24 years), diagnostic groups are defined by morphology and topography codes in the second edition of ICD-O. The grouping of diagnoses is more logical than ICCC-3 for cancers affecting adolescents and young adults especially at age 20–24 years, but some comparability with data on childhood cancer is thereby sacrificed.

Incidence

Incidence in England

Table 1.1 gives numbers of cases and incidence rates for the main groups and principal subgroups of ICCC-3 among children aged 0–14 years in England during 2003–2012. The pattern of incidence is typical of that found among mainly white populations of industrialized countries. The total age-standardized rate (ASR) was 156.5 per million children, giving a cumulative risk of 1 in 438 of developing cancer during the first 15 years of life.

Overall, incidence is almost 15% higher in boys than in girls. The male excess is greatest for lymphomas. Extracranial germ-cell tumours, melanomas, and carcinomas of several sites are markedly more frequent in girls than in boys. Within childhood, total incidence of cancer is highest in the first five years of life. There are also marked early age peaks for acute lymphoblastic leukaemia (ALL) and for all the distinctive embryonal tumours. In contrast, Hodgkin lymphoma and bone sarcomas are virtually never seen before the age of two years, and their incidence increases steeply throughout childhood. Gonadal germ-cell tumours are most frequent among boys in early childhood, whereas they are rare among girls until the postpubertal increase, which begins earlier than among boys.

Table 1.2 gives numbers of cases and incidence rates for the main groups and subgroups of the Birch classification among adolescents aged 15–19 years in England during 2003–2012. The total annual incidence was 200 per million. About 23% of all adolescent cancers are lymphomas, predominantly Hodgkin lymphoma. Leukaemias, central nervous system tumours, and carcinomas each account for 14–16% of all cancers, and germ-cell tumours for 11%.

International variations

Total incidence of cancer in children and adolescents tends to be higher in industrialized countries and in parts of tropical Africa, and lower in developing countries elsewhere. The relative frequencies of different types of cancer also vary considerably between world regions and between ethnic groups in the same country.

Leukaemias

In the industrialized countries of all continents, leukaemias form the largest diagnostic group of childhood cancer, with an ASR of 40–60 per million, and often account for one third of all malignancies. Incidence is lower in less industrialized countries of Asia and Africa, and among black children in the United States. ALL is the most commonly occurring leukaemia, and variation in the magnitude of the early childhood peak accounts for much of the international variation in total incidence.

Table 1.1 Childhood cancer in England, 2003–2012: numbers of registrations, age-specific and age-standardized (World Standard Population) incidence rates, and sex ratio of age-standardized rates (not calculated for groups with fewer than 20 registrations)

Diagnostic group	Total registrations	Annual rate per million by age group			Age-standardized rate per million	Sex ratio (M/F)
		0–4 years	5–9 years	10–14 years		
All cancers	14,113	207.4	116.1	133.4	156.5	1.1
Leukaemias, myeloproliferative and myelodysplastic diseases	4,219	74.1	36.0	26.7	48.1	1.2
Lymphoid leukaemias	3,277	59.5	29.0	17.8	37.6	1.2
Acute myeloid leukaemias	698	10.6	5.3	6.7	7.8	1.1
Chronic myeloproliferative diseases	63	0.2	0.4	1.4	0.6	0.9
Myelodysplastic syndrome and other myeloproliferative diseases	115	2.4	0.8	0.5	1.3	1.3
Lymphomas and reticuloendothelial neoplasms	1,513	8.8	14.3	25.7	15.5	2.1
Hodgkin lymphomas	620	1.3	4.4	14.2	6.0	1.7
Non-Hodgkin lymphomas including Burkitt lymphoma	776	5.3	9.0	10.9	8.1	2.6
Central nervous system and miscellaneous intracranial and intraspinal neoplasms	3,510	42.7	37.4	33.8	38.4	1.1
Ependymomas and choroid plexus tumours	347	6.4	2.9	2.0	4.0	1.1
Astrocytomas	1,466	17.8	16.2	13.6	16.1	1.0
Embryonal tumours	638	9.2	7.0	4.6	7.1	1.4
Other gliomas	378	3.6	4.6	4.1	4.1	1.1
Other specified	533	3.7	5.5	8.1	5.5	1.0
Unspecified	148	2.1	1.2	1.4	1.6	1.1
Neuroblastoma and other peripheral nervous cell tumours	836	23.0	3.1	0.9	10.2	1.0
Neuroblastoma and ganglioneuroblastoma	830	23.0	3.1	0.8	10.1	1.0
Retinoblastoma	371	11.4	0.4	0.1	4.6	0.9
Renal tumours	793	19.4	4.9	1.5	9.5	0.8
Wilms tumour and other non-epithelial renal tumours	771	19.2	4.8	1.0	9.3	0.9
Hepatic tumours	176	4.4	0.5	0.8	2.1	1.1
Hepatoblastoma	144	4.1	0.4	0.2	1.8	1.3
Malignant bone tumours	605	1.3	5.5	12.7	6.0	1.1
Osteosarcomas	334	0.3	2.8	7.6	3.2	1.1
Ewing tumour and related bone sarcomas	225	0.7	2.3	4.3	2.3	1.1
Soft-tissue and other extraosseous sarcomas	928	11.8	7.9	10.3	10.1	1.3
Rhabdomyosarcomas	461	7.2	4.6	3.1	5.2	1.5
Fibrosarcomas, peripheral nerve sheath tumours, and other fibrous neoplasms	93	1.1	0.5	1.4	1.0	1.3
Other specified soft-tissue sarcomas	298	2.9	2.1	4.6	3.1	1.1
Germ-cell tumours, trophoblastic tumours, and neoplasms of gonads	506	7.1	2.0	7.1	5.5	0.7
Intracranial and intraspinal germ-cell tumours	164	1.4	1.0	2.9	1.7	1.4
Malignant extracranial and extragonadal germ-cell tumours	130	3.7	0.2	0.3	1.6	0.6
Malignant gonadal germ-cell tumours	191	2.0	0.7	3.4	2.0	0.6
Other malignant epithelial neoplasms and malignant melanomas	544	1.5	3.2	12.7	5.3	0.7
Thyroid carcinomas	106	0.3	0.6	2.6	1.0	0.4
Malignant melanomas	97	0.4	0.7	2.0	1.0	0.6
Skin carcinomas	111	0.3	0.8	2.5	1.1	0.8
Other and unspecified carcinomas	187	0.3	1.0	4.7	1.8	0.8
Other and unspecified malignant neoplasms	112	1.7	0.8	1.1	1.2	1.0

Source: data from National Cancer Registration and Analysis Service (NCRAS), Public Health England.

Table 1.2 Adolescent cancer in England, 2003–2012: numbers of registrations, age-specific incidence rates, and sex ratio of rates (not calculated for groups with fewer than 20 registrations)

Diagnostic group	Total registrations	Annual rate per million, 15–19 years	Sex ratio (M/F)
All cancers	6,596	200.4	1.2
Leukaemias	894	27.2	1.5
Acute lymphoblastic leukaemia	420	12.8	2.1
Acute myeloid leukaemia	258	7.8	1.1
Chronic myeloid leukaemia	76	2.3	1.1
Myelodysplastic syndrome and other myeloproliferative diseases	93	2.8	0.9
Lymphomas	1,533	46.6	1.2
Non-Hodgkin lymphoma	451	13.7	1.9
Hodgkin lymphoma	1,082	32.9	1.0
Central nervous system and other intracranial and intraspinal neoplasms	1,065	32.4	1.3
Astrocytoma	343	10.4	1.6
Other glioma	163	5.0	1.4
Ependymoma	54	1.6	2.1
Embryonal tumours	71	2.2	1.6
Other specified	362	11.0	0.9
Unspecified	72	2.2	1.2
Bone tumours	484	14.7	1.6
Osteosarcoma	245	7.4	2.0
Ewing sarcoma	178	5.4	1.3
Soft-tissue sarcomas	307	9.0	1.1
Rhabdomyosarcoma	97	2.9	1.9
Other specified soft-tissue sarcomas*	136	4.0	0.8
Germ-cell tumours	720	21.2	4.7
Gonadal	638	18.8	4.6
Non-gonadal	82	2.4	5.6
Melanoma	467	13.8	0.6
Carcinomas	971	28.6	0.5
Thyroid	292	8.6	0.3
Other head and neck carcinomas	138	4.1	0.8
Genito-urinary tract	183	5.4	0.1
Gastro-intestinal tract	268	7.9	1.0
Miscellaneous, specified	77	2.3	0.6
Unspecified	78	2.3	1.0

* Except fibrosarcoma

Source: data from National Cancer Registration and Analysis Service (NCRAS), Public Health England.

Incidence of leukaemia among adolescents is generally between 20 and 35 per million, and international variations are again mostly attributable to ALL. Incidence of acute myeloid leukaemia (AML), the second most frequent subtype in children and adolescents, varies relatively little.

Lymphomas

The ASR of lymphomas in childhood is as high as 30–60 per million in parts of tropical Africa, 20–25 per million in Mediterranean regions, and 12–16 per million in most other populations. They account for 15–25% of all childhood cancers in Africa and the Middle East, 10–13% in Europe, the Americas, and Oceania, and 8–10% in Eastern and South-Eastern Asia. The most common subtype in countries with the highest incidence is Burkitt lymphoma. Hodgkin lymphoma is rare among children in tropical Africa and Eastern and South-Eastern Asia. In developing countries, the incidence of Hodgkin lymphoma sometimes peaks at 5–9 years, whereas in industrialized countries it increases more steeply at the onset of adolescence.

In adolescence, incidence of lymphomas is highest in Southern Europe and lowest in India, South-Eastern Asia, and among Native

Americans. Hodgkin lymphoma is more common than non-Hodgkin lymphoma (NHL) in most world regions, but NHL predominates in sub-Saharan Africa and in Eastern and South-Eastern Asia. Hodgkin lymphoma is around twice as frequent among boys under 15 years of age as it is among girls, but at age 15–19 years incidence among females is usually at least as high as among males. NHL is nearly everywhere more frequent among males than females throughout childhood and adolescence.

Brain and spinal tumours

Brain and spinal tumours are the second most frequent childhood cancer in industrialized countries, accounting for 20–25% of all cases. They also occur in substantial numbers in adolescence. Incidence in the United States, in both children and adolescents, is considerably higher in non-Hispanic whites than in other ethnic groups. Recorded incidence is consistently lower in developing countries, where under-diagnosis is likely to be a factor.

Neuroblastoma

Neuroblastoma occurs most frequently in infancy. Its incidence is higher in industrialized countries than in developing countries, probably in large part because of a higher rate of diagnosis of asymptomatic tumours. Higher incidence among infants has been found in several industrialized countries compared with the UK, possibly because of increased detection of otherwise silent tumours at routine health checks. Mass screening proved to be ineffective, resulting in especially high incidence in infants, but without lowering the incidence of advanced stage neuroblastoma at older ages.

Retinoblastoma

Retinoblastoma has relatively constant incidence worldwide, although it tends to account for a higher proportion of all childhood cancers in developing countries.

Wilms tumour

Incidence of Wilms tumour tends to depend on ethnicity rather than geographical area. Incidence is highest in black populations, with an ASR of 9–12 per million, and lowest in those of Asian origin, with an ASR often under five per million.

Liver tumours

Hepatoblastoma has an ASR of under three per million children in all world regions. The incidence of hepatocellular carcinoma in young people is highest in regions where there is a high proportion of chronic carriers of hepatitis B in the population, namely East Asia, Melanesia, and sub-Saharan Africa.

Bone tumours

Incidence of malignant bone tumours increases with age, reaching a peak in late adolescence. The two most common subtypes in children and adolescents are osteosarcoma and Ewing sarcoma. Osteosarcoma has fairly constant incidence worldwide, whereas Ewing sarcoma is rare in East Asian and black populations.

Soft-tissue sarcomas

In parts of East and Central Africa with high levels of human herpesvirus 8 (HHV8) infection, Kaposi sarcoma is the most frequent cancer in young people, with incidence sometimes above 40 per million in children and adolescents. Elsewhere, incidence of soft-tissue sarcomas in childhood rarely exceeds 11 per million and rhabdomyosarcoma is the most frequent type. Children of Asian origin have a lower incidence of soft-tissue sarcoma.

Germ-cell tumours

Childhood germ-cell tumours are most frequent in East Asia. In adolescence, testicular cancer has an incidence of 25–30 per million in Europe, North America, and Oceania, and less than 10 per million in most other populations. Ovarian germ-cell tumours have an incidence of 5–10 per million at age 15–19 years and are one of the very few types of cancer whose peak incidence occurs in this age group. Intracranial and intraspinal germ-cell tumours have an incidence of five per million among adolescents in Eastern Asia and below three per million elsewhere.

Trends in incidence

The best-documented trend concerns ALL, the most common childhood cancer in all developed countries. The early childhood peak emerged in mortality data in England and Wales in the 1930s, and was well established among white children in the USA by the early 1940s. Incidence continued to rise, particularly in early childhood, in some western countries until at least the end of the twentieth century. Small increases have also been observed in western populations for many other childhood cancers, but part of these increases may be attributed to changes in diagnostic and registration practice rather than in underlying risk.

Survival rates in Europe

Survival of European children and adolescents diagnosed with cancer between 1978 and 2007 has been analysed in the EUROCARE project. The population-based data reported here are from the EUROCARE-5 database and include 29 European countries covered by 74 cancer registries. About 78,000 European children and adolescents diagnosed with cancer between 2000 and 2007, and followed up to the end of 2008, were considered in this analysis.

Survival of children and adolescents by cancer type

In children, five-year survival was high for lymphoid leukaemia (86%), Burkitt lymphoma and other NHL (83% for both), and Hodgkin lymphoma (95%), but only 61% for AML. Five-year survival for CNS cancers was modest (57%), with limited variation in relation to morphology. Five-year survival for retinoblastoma was very high at 98%. Survival was also good (89%) for nephroblastoma and chondrosarcoma, but lower for neuroblastoma (71%), osteosarcoma, Ewing sarcoma, and rhabdomyosarcoma (all 67%) (Table 1.3).

In adolescents, five-year survival was above 90% for Hodgkin lymphoma, gonadal germ-cell cancer, and skin melanoma, intermediate for NHL (78%), and relatively low for lymphoid leukaemia (62%) and AML (52%).

Poorer survival in adolescents than in children was statistically significant for ALL, AML, NHL, astrocytomas, osteosarcoma, Ewing sarcoma, rhabdomyosarcoma, fibrosarcomas, and gonadal germ-cell tumours. For Hodgkin lymphoma and skin melanoma, however, survival figures were similar between children and adolescents,

Table 1.3 Comparison of five-year relative survival (RS) with standard error (SE) by major diagnostic category for the European pool of children and adolescents with cancer diagnosed in the period 2000–2007

Diagnostic group (ICCC-3)	0–14 years		15–19 years		p value 15–19 vs 0–14
	N	RS (SE)	N	RS (SE)	
Lymphoid leukaemias	15,089	85.8 (0.4)	1378	62.2 (1.6)	<0.0001
Acute myeloid leukaemias	2,944	60.5 (1.0)	704	52.2 (2.2)	0.0007
Hodgkin lymphomas	2,995	95.1 (0.5)	3,541	94.3 (0.5)	0.21
Non-Hodgkin lymphomas (except Burkitt lymphoma)	2,407	83.0 (0.9)	1,217	78.0 (1.4)	0.0023
CNS and miscellaneous intracranial and intraspinal neoplasms	8,856	57.2 (0.6)	1,464	61.8 (1.5)	0.0090
Astrocytoma	2,584	61.9 (1.1)	604	50.8 (2.5)	0.0003
Intracranial and intraspinal embryonal neoplasms	2,951	56.3 (1.1)	233	67.0 (3.8)	0.0074
Medulloblastomas	2,156	63.2 (1.3)	158	72.8 (4.5)	0.041
Retinoblastoma	1,627	96% (0.5)	-	-	-
Nephroblastoma and other non-epithelial renal tumours	3,554	89% (0.6)	-	-	-
Neuroblastoma and ganglioneuroblastoma	4,588	71% (0.8)	-	-	-
Osteosarcomas	1,430	66·8 (1·5)	765	60.3 (2.2)	0.012
Chondrosarcomas	66	89.4 (3.4)	140	80.7 (3.8)	0.092
Ewing tumour and related sarcomas of bone	1,322	66.6 (1.5)	448	51.1 (2.7)	<0.0001
Soft-tissue and other extraosseous sarcomas (excluding Kaposi)	3,871	69.3 (0.9)	1,185	63.0 (1.6)	0.0007
Rhabdomyosarcomas	2,124	66.6 (1.3)	280	39.6 (3.4)	<0.0001
Fibrosarcomas	209	83.8 (3.6)	47	72.8 (9.8)	0.29
Germ-cell tumours, trophoblastic tumours, and neoplasms of gonads	1,805	91.5 (0.8)	2,238	92.2 (0.7)	0.55
Intracranial and intraspinal germ-cell tumours	466	85.9 (2.2)	158	79.5 (4.2)	0.18
Malignant gonadal germ-cell tumours	821	96.8 (0.8)	2,011	93.6 (0.7)	0.0015
Malignant skin melanoma	394	92.2 (1.6)	1,248	91.2 (1.2)	0.64

Adapted with permission from Trama, A. et al. 'Survival of European adolescents and young adults diagnosed with cancer in 2000–07: population-based data from EUROCARE-5', *The Lancet Oncology*, Volume 17, Issue 7, pp. 896–906. Copyright © 2016 Elsevier Ltd. DOI: https://doi.org/10.1016/S1470-2045(16)00162-5

and adolescents had significantly higher survival for intraspinal and intracranial embryonal tumours including medulloblastoma. Poorer survival in adolescents has been attributed to various factors including no or few clinical trials conducted in adolescents, dearth of specific treatment guidelines, differences in cancer biology, variations in the pharmacokinetics of chemotherapeutic agents, and delays in diagnosis and treatment. Adolescents with cancer are, in many ways, neglected by both paediatric and adult oncologists, yet effective disease management necessitates a multi-professional approach incorporating expertise from both specialties.

Survival in children by age

Infants younger than one year old had the lowest five-year survival for several cancers, particularly ALL, AML, NHL, ependymoma, embryonal CNS cancers, and all CNS cancers. By contrast, children younger than age one year with neuroblastoma had good survival (91%), whereas less than 60% of older children survived for five years. Five-year survival was worst for children aged 10–14 years with astrocytomas, nephroblastoma, and Ewing sarcoma (**Table 1.4**).

Several factors may explain poor outcome in infants, including increased risk of metastatic disease at presentation, characteristic genetic mutation, increased rate of subtotal resection, not receiving radiation therapy, and increased risk of death from toxic effects mostly due to infection.

European geographical variation

Because countries varied widely in how they attributed malignancy of CNS tumours and how data for non-malignant CNS tumours were collected by population-based registries, five-year survival by country is presented for all childhood cancers, except CNS tumours. For most countries, five-year survival ranged between 80% and 85%, but all eastern European countries (except Poland) had lower survival (60–77%) (**Figure 1.1**). Many factors could explain the poor survival in Eastern Europe. These countries have a lower gross domestic product (GDP) than countries in other European regions, and this is likely to have several effects. Drugs might be unavailable, or supplies might run out so that treatment has to be halted before completion. Specialized centres for childhood cancers might not have enough beds or resources to treat all patients in their catchment areas, and poorer countries might be unable to afford the multidisciplinary teams typical of paediatric oncology units in richer countries. Treatment could be delayed because diagnosis is delayed, or patients might die of drug toxicity because modern equipment is not available to accurately measure serum drug concentrations.

Table 1.4 Country-weighted five-year survival (%) by ICCC-3 diagnostic category and age, with 95% confidence intervals (95% CI), for children in Europe with cancer diagnosed in the period 2000–2007

Diagnostic group	N	Age <1 year		Age 1–4 years		Age 5–9 years		Age 10–14 years	
		5-yr survival	95% CI	5-yr survival	95% CI	5-yr survival	95% CI	5-yr survival	95% CI
All cancers combined	57,956	77.9	76.4-79.4	79.3	78.4-80.0	77.6	76.6-78.5	76.6	75.7-77.5
I(a) Lymphoid leukaemias	15,860	61.8	56.0-67.1	90.6	89.5-91.7	88.1	86.8-89.3	77.7	75.5-79.7
I(b) Acute myeloid leukaemias	3,094	53.5	47.0-59.6	65.1	61.4-68.5	67.9	63.5-71.9	59.5	55.1-63.5
II(a) Hodgkin lymphomas	3,142	-	-	95.5	91.1-97.8	94.1	89.9-96.6	95.8	94.5-96.8
II(b) Non-Hodgkin lymphomas (except Burkitt lymphoma)	2,544	63.3	49.8-74.0	78.1	72.7-82.5	87.0	83.8-89.6	85.4	82.7-87.8
II(c) Burkitt lymphoma	1,443	-	-	89.3	85.3-92.3	91.1	88.8-93.0	87.2	84.0-89.8
III CNS and miscellaneous intracranial and intraspinal neoplasms	9,277	48.3	43.8-52.7	57.4	55.0-59.8	57.0	54.6-59.3	60.3	57.8-62.7
III(a) Ependymomas and choroid plexus tumours	1,233	42.4	30.0-54.3	55.3	50.6-59.8	74.7	66.5-81.1	76.2	68.6-82.2
III(b) Astrocytomas	2,714	64.1	56.3-70.9	79.4	75.6-82.7	55.6	51.1-60.0	49.3	45.0-53.5
III(c) Intracranial and intraspinal embryonal tumours	3,119	33.3	26.6-40.2	46.5	42.3-50.5	67.3	63.3-71.0	67.3	62.2-71.9
IV(a) Neuroblastoma and ganglioneuroblastoma	4,588	91.1	89.6-92.5	58.7	54.8-62.5	52.1	45.8-58.0	55.7	45.5-64.6
V Retinoblastoma	1,627	98.3	96.6-99.1	94.6	89.9-97.2	96.4	79.9-99.4	-	-
VI(a) Nephroblastoma and other nonepithelial renal tumours	3,554	84.3	80.2-87.6	91.4	89.7-92.9	88.2	85.4-90.4	76.7	66.0-84.5
VIII(a) Osteosarcomas	1,500	-	-	59.8	47.6-70.1	72.1	66.7-76.8	68.5	64.9-71.9
VIII(c) Ewing tumour and related sarcomas of bone	1,397	70.6	58.8-79.6	73.7	64.6-80.7	76.3	71.5-80.4	62.1	57.1-66.6
IX(a) Rhabdomyosarcomas	2,197	61.0	49.7-70.5	71.2	66.2-75.5	70.6	65.5-75.2	62.3	56.6-67.5

- No cases

Adapted with permission from Gatta, G. et al. 'Childhood cancer survival in Europe 1999–2007: results of EUROCARE-5—a population-based study', *The Lancet Oncology*, Volume 15, Issue 1, pp. 35–47. Copyright © 2013 Elsevier Ltd. DOI: https://doi.org/10.1016/S1470-2045(13)70548-5

Survival trends 1999–2007

Figure 1.2 shows trends in five-year survival among children and adolescents for all malignancies together, the major haematological tumours, CNS tumours, and skin melanoma. Five-year survival during the period 1999–2007 improved by 2% and 3% per year in children and adolescents, respectively. Despite faster improvement for adolescents during the study period, survival remained significantly worse than in children for several cancers (Table 1.3). Significant progress was reported in ALL and NHL for both children and adolescents, and for AML and soft-tissue sarcomas (not shown in Figure 1.2) in children only. No significant progress was observed for CNS tumours or melanoma. Among children, survival also did not improve for Hodgkin lymphoma, neuroblastoma, nephroblastoma, Ewing sarcoma, and osteosarcoma. The absence of substantial survival increases for several cancers during 1999–2007 may confirm the beliefs of some paediatric oncologists and researchers that optimization of present treatments has reached its limits. New research approaches are therefore needed to improve survival further, especially for high-risk groups. New approaches to trial design and greater international collaboration are needed to recruit enough participants for studies of small and homogeneous subgroups of patients.

To improve outcomes for adolescents, various initiatives—including promoting collaboration between paediatric and adult oncologists, developing national policies for managing adolescents with cancer, and setting up specific treatment units—have been implemented in several European countries and worldwide. For cancers in adolescents that also affect children, it has been suggested that adolescents should be treated in an integrated paediatric–adult multidisciplinary setting. This change should increase the likelihood of adolescents being included in clinical trials, and improve family and social support. The present situation could be improved by intensifying international collaboration with twinning programmes and by motivating politicians to create and develop sustainable infrastructure, recognizing the specific needs of children with cancer.

The rarity of most childhood cancers creates particular difficulties for small countries, since good results for these cancers are usually obtained only when treatment is centralized in high-volume centres of excellence. Collaborative programmes in which all patients are sent to a single centre could be a solution, through the implementation and extension of the European directive on cross-border healthcare, particularly to small countries that lack the resources and infrastructure to treat these diseases and are unlikely to develop such infrastructure because of the very small numbers of children with cancer.

A strength of these studies was that outcomes were evaluated in a large population-based database of children and adolescents, archived by European cancer registries. In the future, data provided by these registries will be vital to assess whether changes in management policies have had the desired effect of improving survival in European children and adolescents who develop cancer.

Follow-up

Continuing improvement in survival from childhood cancer has led to a great increase in long-term survivors, including substantial numbers of adults. For childhood cancer overall, excess mortality continues beyond 25 years from diagnosis, principally due to second primary cancers and circulatory diseases. The risk of developing a second primary cancer is about six times that in the general population, but it varies according to type of first cancer and treatment given. The risk is highest in those who received radiotherapy and among survivors of heritable retinoblastoma.

Survivors of childhood and adolescent cancer are at increased risk of a range of chronic diseases, which are discussed in other chapters.

Aetiology of cancer in children and adolescents

The short latency of childhood cancers suggests that events affecting *in utero* life and/or exposures affecting parents may be aetiologically important. Intensive investigation since the mid twentieth century

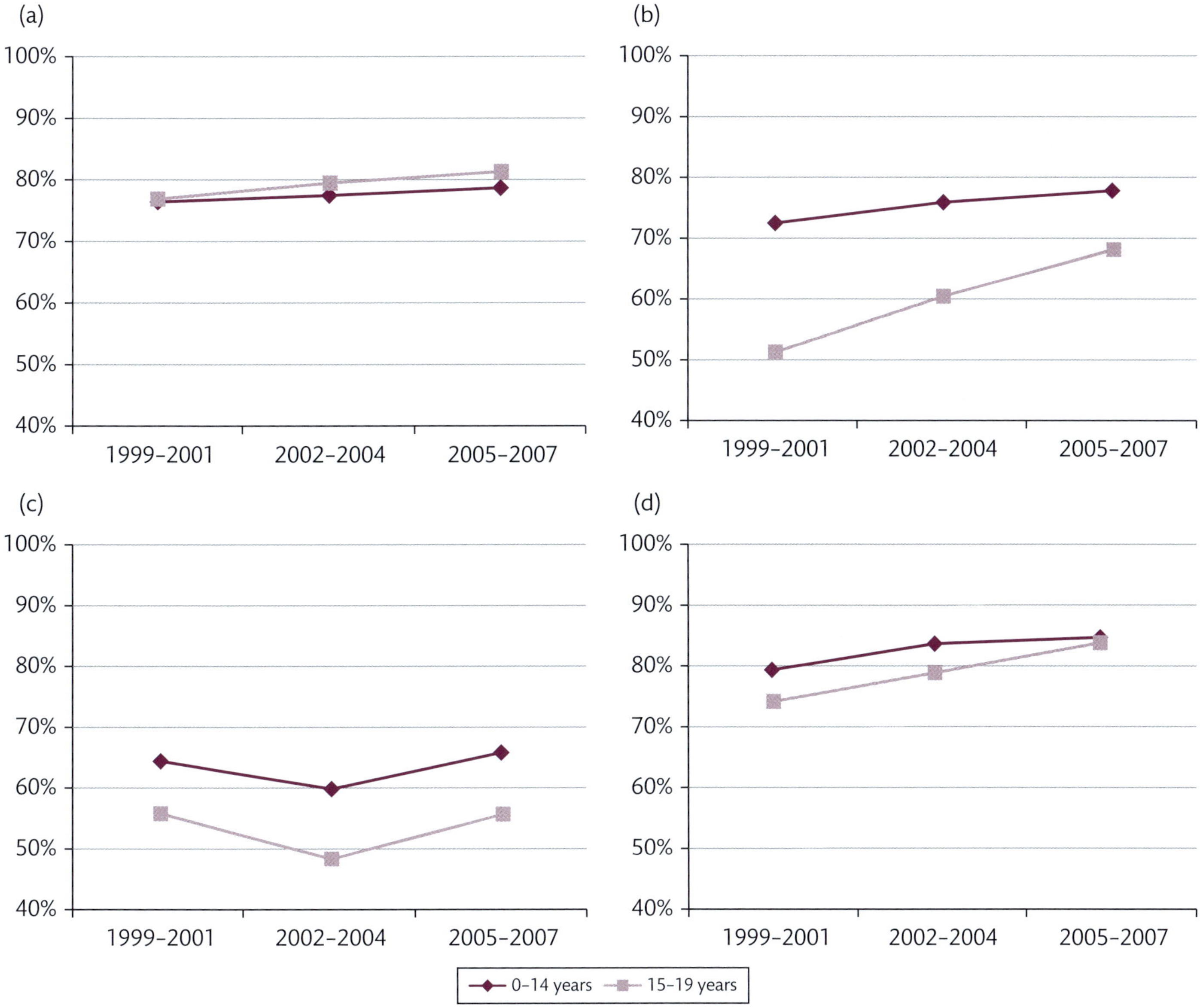

Figure 1.1 Five-year relative survival for children and adolescents with cancer in Europe in 1999–2001, 2002–2004, and 2005–2007: (a) all tumours; (b) acute lymphoid leukaemia; (c) acute myeloid leukaemia; (d) non-Hodgkin lymphoma; (e) central nervous system; (f) malignant melanoma; (g) Hodgkin lymphoma; (h) malignant gonadal germ-cell tumours; (i) Ewing tumour and related sarcomas of bone.

* indicates a statistically significant survival trend

Adapted with permission from Trama, A. et al. 'Survival of European adolescents and young adults diagnosed with cancer in 2000-07: population-based data from EUROCARE-5', *The Lancet Oncology*, Volume 17, Issue 7, pp. 896–906. Copyright © 2016 Elsevier Ltd. DOI: https://doi.org/10.1016/S1470-2045(16)00162-5

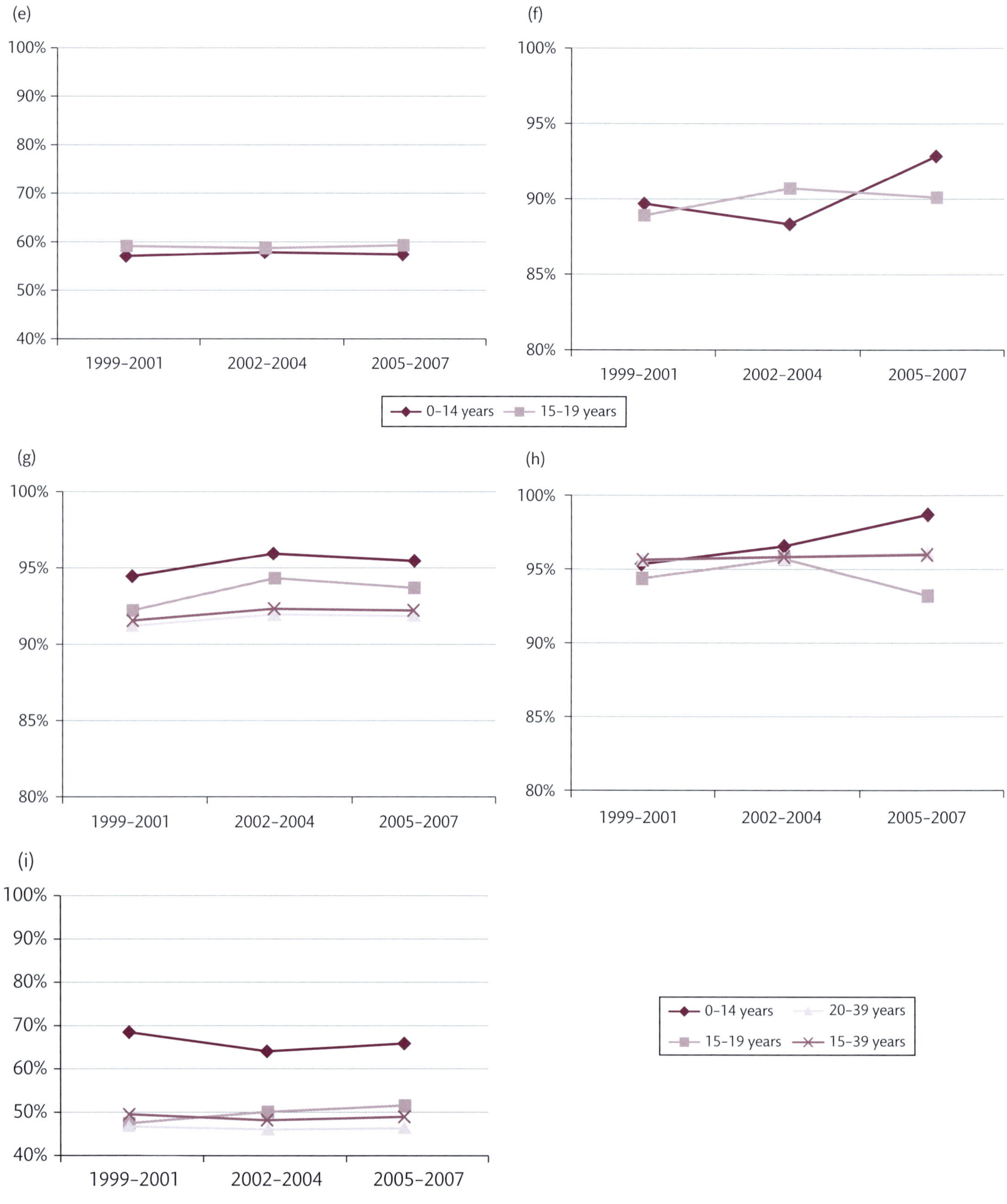

Figure 1.1 Continued

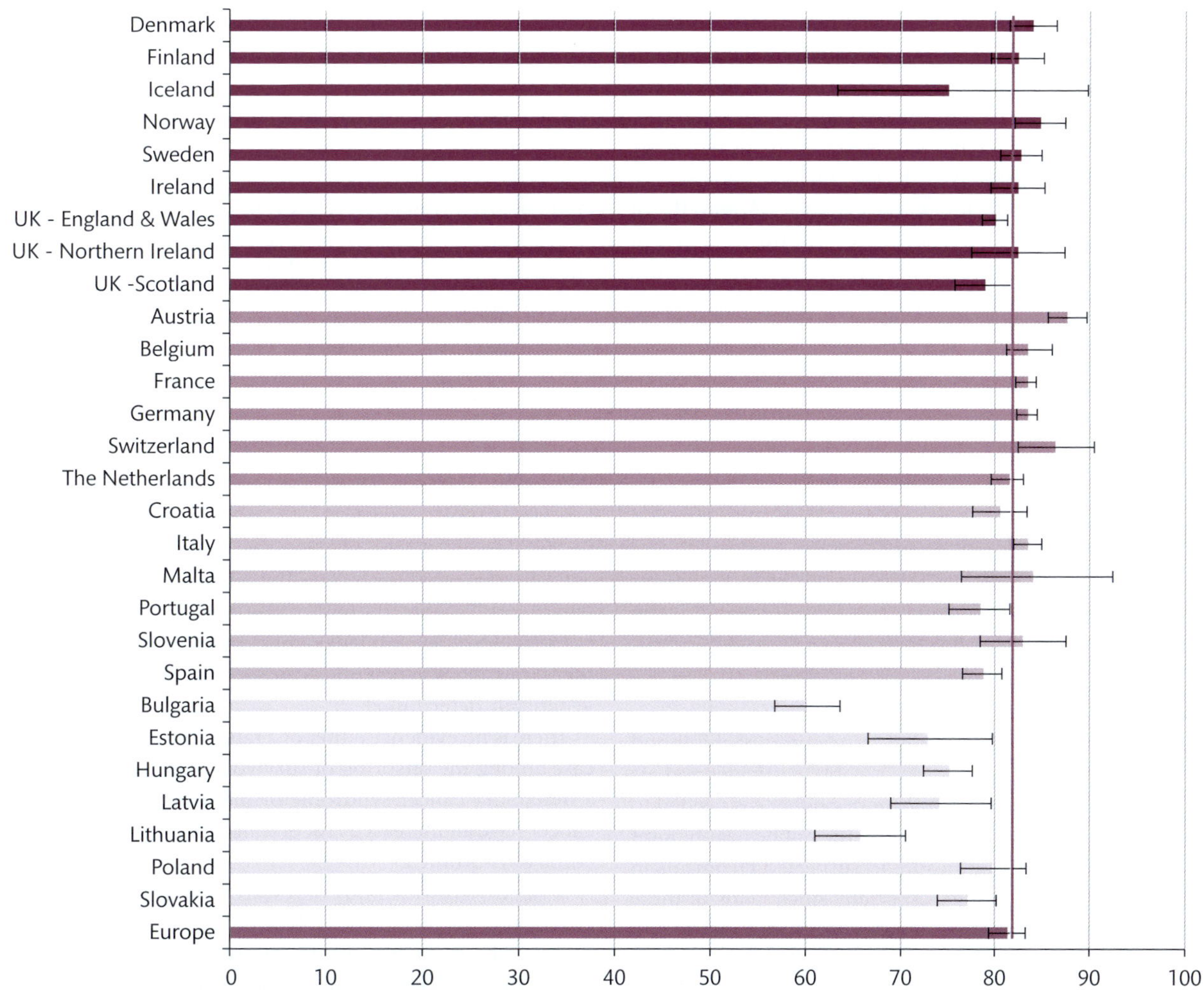

Figure 1.2 Five-year survival (%) for all cancers combined (CNS tumours excluded) diagnosed in 2000–2007, in European children (age 0–14 years) by country. Data adjusted for age, sex, case mix, and period of diagnosis.

Adapted with permission from Gatta, G. et al. 'Childhood cancer survival in Europe 1999-2007: results of EUROCARE-5—a population-based study'. *The Lancet Oncology*, Volume 15, Issue 1, pp. 35-47. Copyright © 2013 Elsevier Ltd. DOI:https://doi.org/10.1016/S1470-2045(13)70548-5

has indicated the complexity of mechanisms underlying the occurrence of cancer in children, but the causes of the great majority of cases remain unknown. Nevertheless, the knowledge accumulated is sufficient to inform public health plans aiming to reduce cancer incidence. Furthermore, risk factors for cancer in children and adolescents are also involved in other diseases affecting these age groups.

Environmental factors

Ionizing radiation

Exposure to ionizing radiation is one of the few factors generally accepted to increase the risk that a child will develop cancer. Recent studies do not themselves show an association with antenatal diagnostic X-ray exposure but are consistent with earlier, more powerful studies that do. In the past, antenatal radiography probably caused at most about 5% of childhood cancers, even when it was more widely used and doses were higher than they are now. The much higher doses of radiation given during radiotherapy are also carcinogenic but can only account for a tiny proportion of all childhood cancers. Naturally occurring background radiation is largely unavoidable and 15% of childhood leukaemia in Britain may be attributable to this source of exposure.

Non-ionizing radiation

Ultraviolet radiation from sunlight can cause melanoma and other skin cancers. There is no evidence of raised risk of childhood leukaemia with exposure to power-frequency electromagnetic fields at the levels experienced by more than 95% of children in western countries. A doubling of risk has been consistently found at the very highest exposure levels but the explanation is unknown, and only a tiny fraction of childhood leukaemia cases could be attributable to electromagnetic fields.

Infections

Worldwide, the most frequent virus-associated cancers among children and adolescents are Burkitt lymphoma, Hodgkin lymphoma and nasopharyngeal carcinoma (Epstein–Barr virus), liver carcinoma (hepatitis B), Kaposi sarcoma (HHV8 and human immunodeficiency virus), and cervical carcinoma (human papilloma virus).

For Hodgkin lymphoma, 60% of cases in children of 0–14 years in developed countries and 80% of cases in children aged 0–14 in developing countries can be attributed to Epstein-Barr virus, compared to only 30% of cases in people aged 15–44.

It is likely that infection is sometimes involved in the aetiology of childhood leukaemia, especially ALL. Two main hypotheses are supported by substantial epidemiological evidence. About 1% of children are born with a premalignant clone with the potential to develop into precursor B-cell ALL. Under the 'delayed infection' hypothesis, if they are protected from exposure to infection in infancy then heightened immune response to infection later in childhood acts as a promoter of leukaemia. Evidence supporting this hypothesis includes consistent associations of breastfeeding and attendance at daycare in early childhood with a reduced risk of leukaemia, particularly common ALL.

Under the 'population mixing' hypothesis, childhood leukaemia is an unusual response to one or more specific but as yet unidentified infectious agents, with higher risk occurring when susceptible and infected people are brought together. This is supported by numerous studies in which childhood leukaemia rates have increased when people from different areas come together.

Chemical exposures

Many epidemiological studies have found associations of childhood cancer with various chemical exposures, notably pesticides and atmospheric pollution from traffic. While more evidence is needed to establish causality, it would be justified, from the public health point of view, to reduce or eliminate exposure to suspected chemicals in children and in young fertile adults, especially since many of these chemicals are also involved in other diseases affecting children and adolescents.

Other factors associated with pregnancy and birth

There is considerable evidence that high birthweight is associated with a raised risk of leukaemia and several other cancers in childhood, possibly as a result of increased antenatal growth rate. Children who are twins have a risk of cancer that is about 80% that in singletons.

Several studies have found increased risk of specific cancers among children born following assisted reproductive technology, but with little consistency with respect to cancer types, numbers of cases of specific types of cancer were usually low, and the associations could well have been due to confounding with other factors.

Genetic epidemiology

The most obvious example of a genetically determined cancer is retinoblastoma; about 40% of cases have the heritable form of this disease. The pattern of inheritance is autosomal dominant, but in fact the gene *RB1* is the first example of a tumour suppressor gene; about 90% of individuals who inherit the mutated form of this gene from a parent subsequently suffer a mutation of the wild-type (normal) allele, leading to loss of heterozygosity and the development of retinoblastoma. These individuals are also at increased risk of a variety of other cancers. Wilms tumour is associated with an especially wide range of syndromes and congenital anomalies, but the pattern of inheritance is more complicated and the proportion of clearly hereditary cases much smaller.

Up to 10% of children and adolescents with cancer may have germline mutations in cancer predisposition genes. Other heritable syndromes carrying an increased risk of childhood cancer include neurofibromatosis types 1 and 2, tuberous sclerosis complex, Fanconi anaemia, ataxia telangiectasia, Li-Fraumeni syndrome, constitutional mismatch repair deficiency, xeroderma pigmentosum, and Bloom syndrome. There are also well-documented associations with chromosomal abnormalities; the strongest association is with Down syndrome, which occurs in a small percentage of cases of childhood leukaemia.

If one child in a family has malignant disease, then, in the absence of any further information about the existence of genetic disease in that family, and excluding twins and retinoblastoma, that child's siblings have approximately double the risk of the general population for developing childhood cancer. However, this excess could well be entirely accounted for by familial syndromes. In up to 25% of cases where a child who is a monozygotic twin has leukaemia, their co-twin will also develop leukaemia. These cases are usually due to *in utero* transfer of leukaemic or pre-leukaemic cells rather than being genetically determined.

There is no evidence either of a raised risk of cancer or genetic disease among the offspring of survivors who do not themselves have a hereditary cancer syndrome or that the parents of children with cancer have an increased risk of cancer in the absence of known hereditary syndromes.

A rapidly growing body of research has found significantly raised or reduced risk of ALL, neuroblastoma, and other childhood cancers associated with polymorphic variants of certain genes, sometimes interacting with exogenous factors, though many of these findings remain to be replicated.

FURTHER READING

Barr RD, et al. (2006) Classification schemes for tumours diagnosed in adolescents and young adults. *Cancer* **106**, 1425–30.

Bearer CF, et al. (eds.) (2016) Opportunities for cancer prevention during early life. *Pediatrics* **138 Suppl 1**, S1–S100.

Colt JS, Blair A (1998) Parental occupational exposures and risk of childhood cancer. *Environ Health Perspect* **106**, 909–25.

Draper GJ, et al. (1992) Patterns of risk of hereditary retinoblastoma and applications to genetic counselling. *Br J Cancer* **66**, 211–19.

Fidler MM et al. (2016) Long-term cause-specific mortality among 34,489 five-year survivors of childhood cancer in Great Britain: population-based cohort study. *BMJ* **354**, i4351.

Gatta G et al. (2014) Childhood cancer survival in Europe 1999–2007: results of EUROCARE-5—a population-based study. *Lancet Oncol* **15**, 35–47.

Infante-Rivard C (2008) Chemical risk factors and childhood leukaemia: a review of recent studies. *Radiat Prot Dosimetry* **132**, 220–27.

Johnson KJ et al. (2014) Childhood brain tumor epidemiology: a Brain Tumor Epidemiology Consortium review. *Cancer Epidemiol Biomarkers Prev* **23**, 2716–36.

Kaatsch P, et al. (2006) Time trends of cancer incidence in European children (1978–1997): report from the Automated Childhood Cancer Information System project. *Eur J Cancer* **42**, 1961–71.

Linabery AM, Ross JA (2008) Childhood and adolescent cancer survival in the US by race and ethnicity for the diagnostic period 1975–1999. *Cancer* **113**, 2575–96.

Lindor NM, et al. (2008) Concise handbook of familial cancer susceptibility syndromes, second edition. *J Natl Cancer Inst Monogr* **38**, 1–93.

Little J (1999) *Epidemiology of Childhood Cancer*. Lyon: IARC.

Olsen JH, et al. (1995) Cancer in the parents of children with cancer. *N Engl J Med* **333**, 1594–9.

Reulen RC et al. (2011) Long-term risks of subsequent primary neoplasms among survivors of childhood cancer. *JAMA* **305**, 2311–19.

Sankila R et al. (1998) Risk of cancer among offspring of childhood-cancer survivors. *N Engl J Med* **338**, 1339–44.

Siegel DA, et al. (2014) Cancer incidence rates and trends among children and adolescents in the United States, 2001–2009. *Pediatrics* **134**, e945–55.

Steliarova-Foucher E, et al. (2005) International Classification of Childhood Cancer, third edition. *Cancer* **103**, 1457–67.

Steliarova-Foucher E et al. (2017) International incidence of childhood cancer, 2001–2010: a population-based study. *Lancet Oncol* **18**(6), 719–31.

Stiller C (ed.) (2007) *Childhood Cancer in Britain. Incidence, Survival, Mortality*. Oxford: Oxford University Press.

Stiller CA (2005) Constitutional chromosomal abnormalities and childhood cancer. *Ital J Pediatr* **31**, 347–53.

Trama A et al. (2016) Survival of European adolescents and young adults diagnosed with cancer in 2000–07: population-based data from EUROCARE-5. *Lancet Oncol* **17**, 896–906.

Wiemels J (2012) Perspectives on the causes of childhood leukemia. *Chem Biol Interact* **196**, 59–67.

Winther JF et al. (2001) Cancer in siblings of children with cancer in the Nordic countries: a population-based cohort study. *Lancet* **358**, 711–17.

Zhang J et al. (2015) Germline mutations in predisposition genes in childhood cancer. *N Engl J Med* **373**, 2336–46.

2

Imaging in Paediatric Oncology

Kieran McHugh and Thierry A.G.M. Huisman

Introduction

Some general principles apply with regard to the radiological approach to all mass lesions, despite the diverse range of pathologies seen in different body parts. Suspected abdominal and pelvic masses must be examined by ultrasound (US) first, and this may be all that is necessary to evaluate benign entities. Superficial lesions or palpable lumps should also be assessed by US initially. Lesion vascularity can be easily evaluated by Doppler interrogation, increased vascularity being an important finding with proliferating haemangiomas in infancy, for example, lesions that could otherwise mimic more sinister pathology. Further cross-sectional imaging, largely to determine lesion extent, will be guided by the US findings, tumour location, and local availability of magnetic resonance imaging (MRI). The reliable interpretation of imaging requires a radiologist with sufficient experience and expertise in paediatric oncology, particularly with the more advanced technologies such as X-ray computed tomography (CT), MRI, and positron emission tomography (PET).

Imaging modalities

Plain radiography

Plain films play a very limited role in the diagnostic work-up of new paediatric mass lesions. The major exception to this is with bone tumours, both benign processes and malignant lesions. In this setting, the plain X-ray probably has a bigger role in suggesting the proper diagnosis than other techniques. Bone lysis with ill-defined margins is highly suggestive of an aggressive process such as osteomyelitis or tumour, which may be indistinguishable on imaging, but often have very different clinical presentations. Sclerotic well-defined margins in an osseous mass suggest a benign process. The dilemma of benign versus malignant for bone tumours is usually relatively straightforward at plain radiography, and the role of MRI in this setting is largely to define the extent of the lesion, and to evaluate for a soft-tissue mass which is likely to be underestimated on plain radiographs.

Although the chest X-ray (CXR) is performed routinely and plays an important role in staging for metastatic disease at diagnosis, particular reliance is placed on chest CT to exclude pulmonary metastases in virtually all extra-cranial malignancies, with the exception of neuroblastoma. Posterior rib erosion and rib separation with an obvious chest mass are virtually pathognomic of a neurogenic tumour such as neuroblastoma. Another important role for the plain CXR, notably the lateral film, is assessing for airway compression from an anterior mediastinal mass. Follow-up during treatment and later surveillance for metastatic relapse is also performed with serial CXRs. The CXR is also useful in detecting secondary infection or other complications of treatment, such as rib osteochondromas secondary to irradiation, during follow-up.

Ultrasound

Ultrasound (US) entails no radiation burden and so can be done repeatedly without harm. Soft-tissue masses can be easily evaluated to assess their cystic or solid nature, and presence of calcification. US is a dynamic real-time examination. With large abdominal masses, invasion into other organs can be difficult to interpret on CT or MRI, but may be easily evaluated with US. Movement of the liver separate from a renal mass is a reliable sign of non-invasion of the liver by the mass. Similarly, movement of the mass separately from the psoas muscle means the mass is not adherent to the psoas. With additional Doppler assessments, the degree of vascularity of a mass lesion can be identified. US is the best technique for detecting and excluding tumour thrombus extension into the inferior vena cava from a renal or adrenal tumour. US is the most sensitive technique in the detection of early fungal infiltration of the liver or spleen in the immunocompromized, best evaluated with linear-array high-resolution transducers.

Most percutaneous imaging-guided biopsies are done simply with US guidance. Contrast-enhanced ultrasound (CEUS), with sonovue (Bracco), is not licenced for use in children at present in Europe, but is being increasingly used within paediatrics. Its major use in the oncology setting is in differentiating benign from malignant liver lesions.

Computed tomography

The size and extent of large masses are easily assessed with CT, but with that comes the added radiation burden of CT. The newer multidetector CT scanners are extremely fast at examining any body region, avoiding the need for sedation or anaesthesia in many circumstances. CT is the optimal method for assessing the lung parenchyma. Calcification in a mass, often not apparent on MRI, is easily detected with CT. For chest and abdominal scanning in children, non-contrast enhanced CT studies are usually of little help due to children's lack of mediastinal or retroperitoneal fat. Thus, for paediatric chest and abdominal CT, single-phase post contrast-enhanced images are all that is generally required to evaluate a mass lesion, including liver tumours (although the latter are better evaluated with MRI). Bone detail is very well demonstrated on CT such that, for example with skull base tumours, an MRI to assess soft-tissue extent and a CT to assess erosion of the skull base or facial bones may be necessary.

Magnetic resonance imaging

MRI is the ideal imaging modality because of its better characterization of tissues, multi-planar capabilities, and lack of ionizing radiation. Tumour extent is best assessed with MRI, although for large masses CT can be as accurate. As MRI is sensitive to oedema (seen as hyperintense or bright signal on T2-weighted sequences), it is generally impossible to differentiate tumour margins from oedema. In addition, at the end of treatment or after surgery, MRI often cannot distinguish residual fibrosis or benign residual tissue from residual tumour. Diffusion-weighted imaging with apparent diffusion coefficient (ADC) maps has an established role now in the assessment of tumours all over the body. Highly cellular tumours with restricted diffusion are generally malignant lesions and appear dark on ADC images. Tumour response after chemotherapy, with or without a change in tumour size, can be evident with a change in the diffusion pattern on follow-up. MRI studies generally take a minimum of 30 minutes, which means that most children less than six years of age need general anaesthesia or sedation for the MRI examination.

Nuclear medicine

Wilms tumours and hepatoblastoma seldom metastasize to bone and so do not merit routine bone scanning with technetium^{99}-MDP (methylene-diphosphonate). Suspected neuroblastoma metastases are best assessed with iodine^{123}-MIBG (metaiodobenzylguanidine) scans. If the primary tumour is not avid for MIBG, then a PET-CT scan with ^{18}fluorodeoxyglucose (FDG) is recommended to evaluate for skeletal and other metastases in this setting. Most sarcomas and other solid tumours historically required routine bone scans for staging at diagnosis; however, following paediatric sarcoma trials in both Europe and North America, PET-CT is now recommended for staging at diagnosis and also increasingly at follow-up to assess for tumour response.

Interventional radiology

Paediatric interventional radiology (IR) has developed remarkably in the past 20 years. All children's oncology centres should have access to IR services that provide common procedures such as tumour biopsy, line placement, angiography, gastrostomy insertion, and abscess drainage. More complicated procedures such as preoperative tumour embolization to reduce haemorrhage at surgery, radiofrequency ablation, and chemo-embolization techniques should also ideally be available in the bigger centres.

Tumours outside the central nervous system

The differential diagnosis of masses in childhood is largely influenced by the age of a child and the organ of origin or location of the lesion. Calcification in a neuroblastoma or fat plus calcium in a teratoma are useful in suggesting a diagnosis, but the imaging characteristics of the majority of tumours are in general relatively non-specific. Most tumours are, for example, hypovacular on contrast-enhanced CT with areas of low attenuation and heterogeneity. Homogeneous imaging appearances of a paediatric mass suggest a benign cause, such as haemangioma or fibromatosis in infancy. Tumours are typically of low or intermediate signal on T1-weighted (T1W) MRI sequences and high signal on T2W MRI, again with variable contrast enhancement after gadolinium administration. Calcification typically has no inherent signal at MRI scanning such that calcification in mass lesions is missed or underestimated at MRI. Some densely fibrotic lesions may be of low signal (hypointense) on both T1W and T2W MR images. Some of the most important issues to consider when imaging tumours beyond the central nervous system (CNS) will be addressed in this section.

Renal tumours

Ultrasound (US) should be utilized first to assess the origin of a potential renal tumour, tumour thrombus in the renal vein and/or inferior vena cava (IVC), the contralateral kidney, and liver. Dynamic real-time ultrasound is a very useful method for assessing tumour invasion of the liver or other organs, but tends to be under-utilized in this context. Abdominal CT should be performed only after intravenous contrast medium enhancement. Ipsilateral and contralateral small lesions or foci of nephroblastomatosis may be seen with Wilms tumour (nephroblastoma). A chest CT is required to detect or exclude pulmonary metastases. The diameter of pulmonary nodules should be measured on lung window settings, and these same settings should be used at follow-up. Ideally, MRI is preferred over CT in evaluating a primary renal tumour due to its superior contrast resolution and lack of radiation. Tumour extent is equally assessed by CT or MRI, but foci of nephroblastomatosis are much better visualized with MRI (**Figure 2.1**). All renal tumours in childhood have similar radiological appearances and age at presentation is the most important factor in the differential diagnosis. Clear cell sarcoma, because of its propensity for skeletal metastatic spread, merits routine radionuclide bone scanning for staging at diagnosis. Renal cell carcinoma, which usually manifests in adolescence, demonstrates calcification in approximately 25% of cases.

Neuroblastoma

Encasement of the aorta and upper abdominal arteries is the hallmark of the majority of abdominal neuroblastomas (**Figure 2.2**),

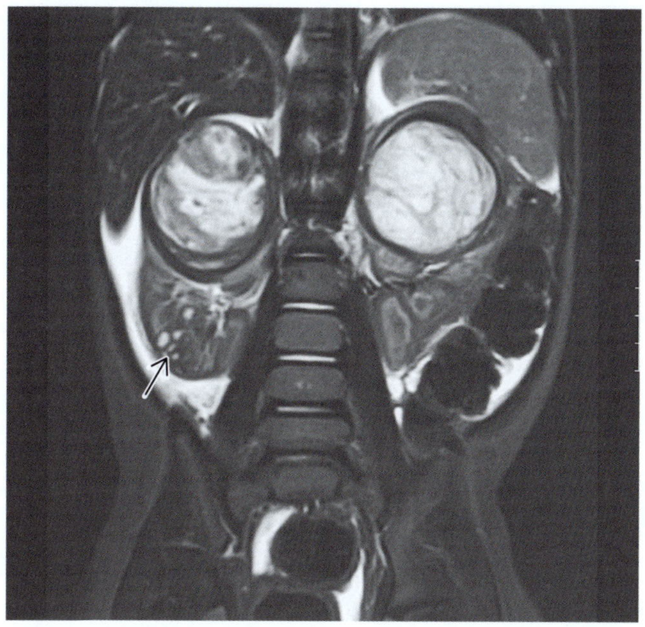

Figure 2.1 Nephroblastoma (Wilms tumour). Wilms tumours in the upper poles of both kidneys are seen as hyperintense heterogeneous round masses on coronal T2W MRI. A third possible tumour is seen in the right lower pole as a smaller cystic lesion (arrow).

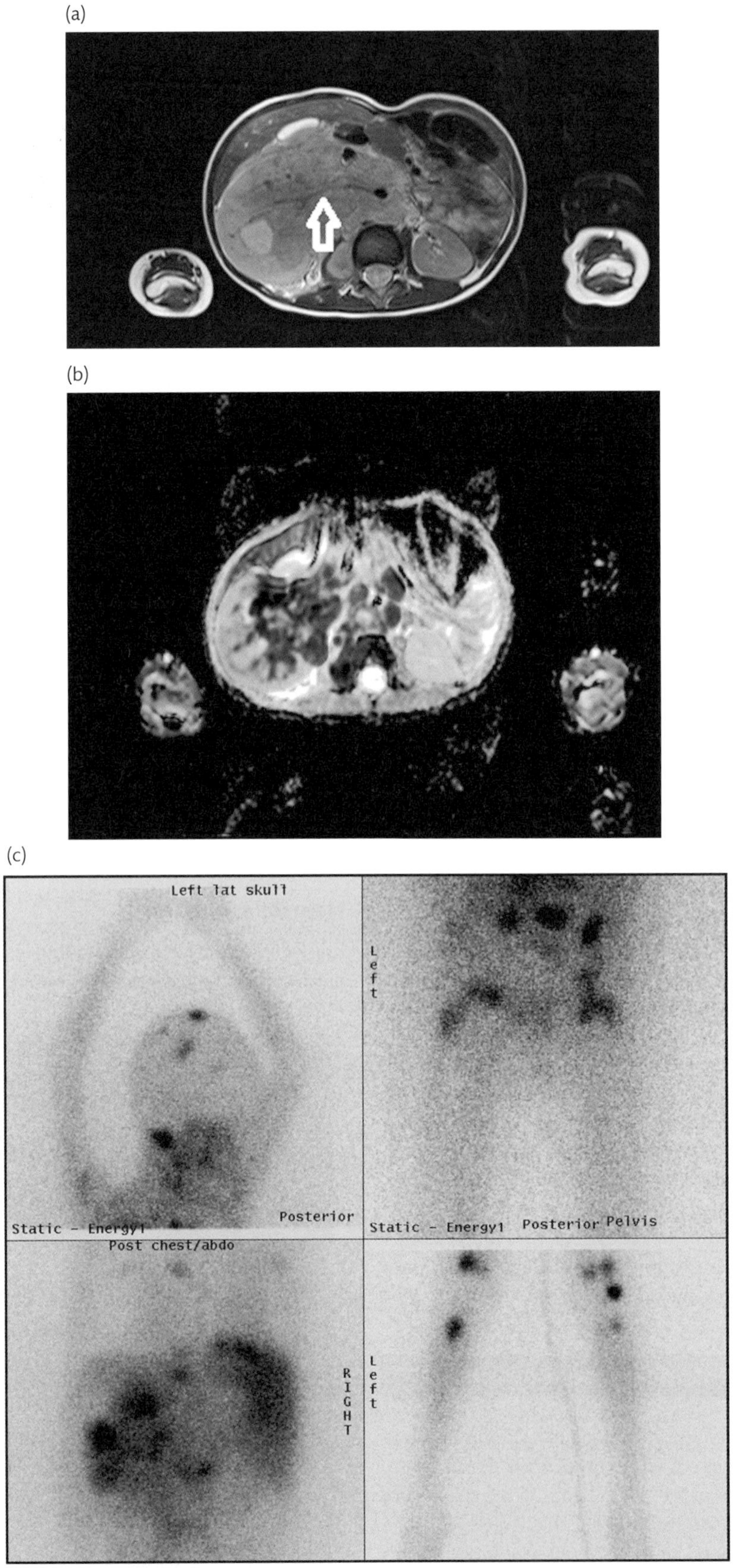

Figure 2.2 Neuroblastoma. (a) Axial T2W image showing a mass lesion in the right upper quadrant encasing the aorta and right renal artery (arrow). Encasement of more than 50% of the circumference of the aorta and tumour abutting the renal vessels are so-called imaging-defined risk factors. (b) Axial ADC map shows the mass lesion to be dark on this sequence, indicating restricted diffusion, in keeping with a highly cellular malignant lesion. (c) Planar images from a MIBG scan in another patient show uptake in the primary abdominal tumour and widespread skeletal metastases, stage M disease.

in contrast to renal tumours which tend to displace the aorta and IVC. Confinement to the suprarenal area and adrenal gland is more often seen in infants. MS (formerly 4S) disease causes hepatomegaly and diffuse hepatic infiltration by tumour. The infiltration may be subtle however, and only appreciated with a higher-resolution linear-array US transducer. MRI and CT are probably equivalent when assessing the primary tumour, but MRI is superior at evaluating for intraspinal disease and allows easier depiction of marrow metastases. Some surgeons prefer contrast-enhanced CT prior to surgery as CT tends to give a more reliable surgical roadmap of the vasculature, and more clearly demonstrates the extent of tumour calcification after chemotherapy. MIBG scanning is crucial for staging at diagnosis and for assessing response in patients with metastatic disease.

Rhabdomyosarcoma

Skull base tumours often need CT to assess the bony erosion and MR to evaluate the soft-tissue extent. MRI is also superior in demonstrating tumour involvement of the neural foramina and intracranial spread. Orbital tumours rarely have lymphatic loco-regional spread. US evaluation of the cervical chain of nodes is probably underutilized for head and neck tumours. Cervical lymph nodes metastases are often difficult to identify on all modalities and a low threshold for biopsy is advisable. MRI is the modality of choice for assessing genito-urinary primaries, after initial assessment with US (**Figure 2.3**). US of the liver should be performed in all patients to detect or exclude metastases. US of the retroperitoneal area should be performed in all patients with pelvic, paratesticular, or lower limb primaries. Limb primary tumours (leg or arm) should also have US of the inguinal region or axilla, and ideally the popliteal and epitrochlear areas too, to detect or exclude regional lymphadenopathy.

Liver tumours

Between 60% and 70% of all primary liver tumours in children are malignant, with hepatoblastoma and hepatocellular carcinoma constituting the vast majority of these malignancies. Haemangioendothelioma/haemangioma lesions and mesenchymal hamartoma account for nearly all the non-malignant tumours in children. The pre-treatment extent (PRETEXT) staging system used by the International Childhood Liver Tumor Strategy Group (SIOPEL) for hepatoblastoma has gained widespread acceptance. PRETEXT is used to describe tumour extent before any therapy, thus allowing comparison between studies conducted by different collaborative groups. PRETEXT staging is based on Couinaud's system of liver segmentation. The liver segments are grouped into four sections: segments 2 and 3 (left lateral section), segments 4a and 4b (left medial section), segments 5 and 8 (right anterior section), and segments 6 and 7 (right posterior section). Involvement of only one section by a hepatoblastoma mass is denoted as a PRETEXT I tumour; a tumour involving two, three, or all four sections is classified as PRETEXT II, III, or IV respectively. An increasing PRETEXT number gives, very roughly, an estimate of the difficulty of the planned surgical procedure.

US is particularly useful is assessing portal or hepatic venous, or biliary ductal, invasion by tumour. MRI is superior to CT in evaluating liver segmental involvement by tumour (**Figure 2.4**). Surveillance imaging after completion of therapy has recently been questioned as most relapses also result in a rise in serum alpha fetoprotein (AFP) levels. Hepatocellular carcinoma occurs in children older than five years, often against a background of pre-existing cirrhosis.

Germ-cell tumours

Midline germ-cell rests are thought to arise in arrested migration from the hind gut yolk sac to the genital ridge. Germ-cell tumours

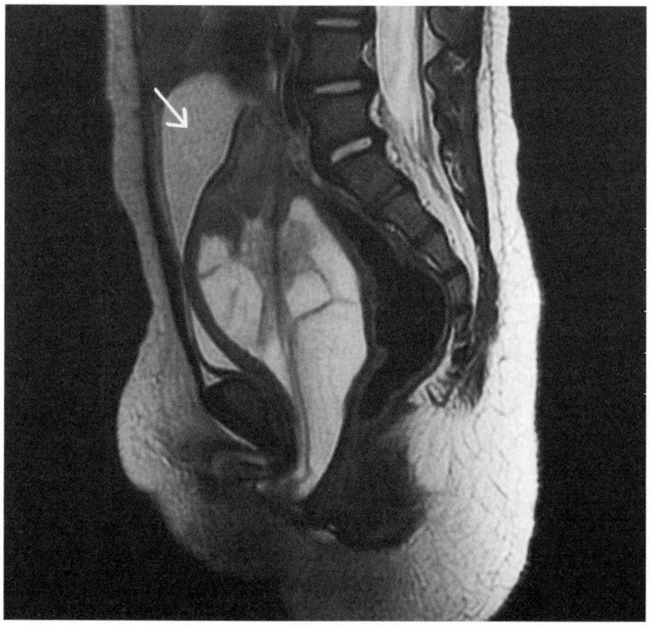

Figure 2.3 Rhabdomyosarcoma. Sagittal T2W midline pelvis image shows a cystic mass lesion with septations in the vagina distorting the cervix and uterus. The fluid-filled bladder is seen anteriorly (arrow). Gas in the rectum returns dark signal.

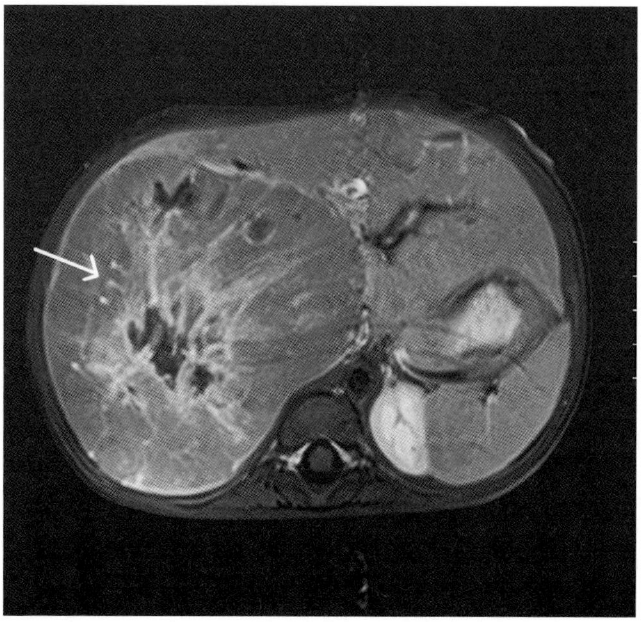

Figure 2.4 Hepatoblastoma. Right-lobe liver tumour (arrow) on a fat-suppressed T1-weighted MRI after gadolinium enhancement. Poor enhancement in the central tumour was due to necrosis. The middle and left hepatic veins were free of tumour which was classified as PRETEXT 2.

(GCTs) are thus commonly found in the pineal gland, neck, mediastinum, retroperitoneum, and sacrococcygeal area. All GCTs show mixed cystic and solid areas, often with foci of fatty attenuation and/or calcification. A mass lesion that contains both fatty tissues and calcification is virtually always a GCT. Fat, and calcification in particular, are easily evaluated with CT, but fat in a mass lesion is easily identified on MRI too; and CT or MRI is equally good at defining tumour extent. Rupture of a mediastinal teratoma may result in a pleural or pericardial effusion. Alternatively, pericardial invasion by tumour may cause a pericardial effusion. Radiology cannot differentiate a benign tumour from a malignant GCT. Of the malignant GCTs, dysgerminoma and yolk sac tumours are the most common, with elevated alpha fetoprotein (AFP) and human chorionic gonadotropin (HCG) levels. The latter tumour markers are so reliable that post-operative routine radiological surveillance is generally not required.

Lymphomas

In the abdomen, a non-Hodgkin lymphoma (NHL) may present as a mass or intussusception, usually identifiable by US. NHL in the mediastinum may cause airway compression such that CT in the supine position may be dangerous. Clinical airway assessment and a lateral chest X-ray to evaluate the trachea are warranted prior to a routine staging CT. NHL in Waldeyer's ring manifests as tonsillar enlargement and a nasopharyngeal mass. That mass tends to be associated with little if any adjacent osseous destruction, unlike rhabdomyosacoma in the nasopharynx which typically causes much skull base erosion.

At initial presentation, Hodgkin lymphoma merits high-resolution US to evaluate for splenic infiltration and a chest CT is necessary to evaluate the lung parenchyma. MRI of the neck and abdomen is as sensitive as CT for lymphadenopathy, and would reduce the radiation burden in young patients. PET-CT is now firmly established for staging of Hodgkin disease at diagnosis and for assessing response to therapy at follow-up.

Non-rhabdomyosarcomatous soft-tissue tumours

Approximately half of paediatric soft-tissue tumours are non-rhabdomyomatous soft-tissue sarcomas (NRSTSs). They are a heterogeneous group of tumours, all of mesenchymal origin, that share some biological characteristics but differ histologically. The most common NRSTSs are synovial cell sarcomas (17–42%), followed by fibrosarcomas (13–15%), malignant fibrous histiocytomas (12–13%), and malignant peripheral nerve sheath tumours (MPNSTs) (10%). The frequency of most of these tumours is age-dependent. Fibrosarcomas occur more commonly in children under one year of age, with synovial sarcomas and MPNSTs being more common in children aged over ten years. Many MPNSTs occur against a background of neurofibromatosis type 1. All these lesions generally have non-specific radiological findings of a soft-tissue mass. Like most paediatric tumours, they are hypovascular at Doppler US evaluation, and more usually solid than cystic in appearance. The lesions are isointense (similar signal intensity) to muscle on T1W MRI, hyperintense on T2W, and show variable enhancement after gadolinium administration. Locoregional adenopathy should be sought or excluded in all cases.

Bone tumours

Osteosarcomas mainly occur around the knee (in the metaphyses of the distal femur or proximal tibia) in adolescence. Radiation-induced sarcomas are rare in childhood. The Ewing's family of tumours, including primitive neuroectodermal tumours, tend to occur in children less than ten years of age in either a flat bone (pelvis, scapula) or in the diaphysis of a long bone. Plain films are more reliable than MRI in assessing the aggressive nature of a lytic bone lesion. MRI is best at depicting tumour extent, the associated soft-tissue mass, involvement of the neurovascular bundle, and spread of tumour across the growth plate into the epiphysis. Some centres report dynamic contrast enhanced MRI is useful at predicting percentage tumour necrosis after initial chemotherapy, but the technique is not widely used.

Tumours within the central nervous system

The frequently used phrase 'children are not small adults' is pertinent for paediatric radiology in general and paediatric neuroradiology in particular. Paediatric CNS tumours have multiple characteristic features that differ significantly from their adult counterparts (see Chapters 22 and 24).

Tumours of the paediatric central nervous system are typically diagnosed by emergent CT, followed by dedicated MRI. Correlating imaging findings (e.g. signal characteristics, primary tumour location, and contrast enhancement, perfusion, and diffusion characteristics) with the age and gender of the child allows to narrow down the differential diagnosis. Treatment options and outcome depend on multiple factors including histological subtype of the tumour. Until recently, most tumours were primarily classified based upon their histological features. In the past decade, correct tumour classification and, more importantly, subclassification, has progressively come to rely on molecular and genetic transcriptional data analysis. Histologically similar tumours may have different molecular characteristics linked to different outcomes. This advanced approach allows for a more reliable estimation of prognosis and survival rate, and consequently supports a tumour-specific, tailored treatment. These advances have significantly influenced posterior fossa medulloblastoma treatment options, preventing under- and overtreatment.

Each age group has typical tumours, and certain tumours are more frequent in boys than in girls, especially in the posterior fossa. The most frequent posterior fossa tumour is the pilocytic astrocytoma (PA), followed by the medulloblastoma, brainstem glioma, and ependymoma. These four tumours may be considered to be the 'big four'. If this 'frequency list' is combined with the age/gender of the patient, as well as the primary tumour location, the tumour type can frequently be predicted. In the supratentorial brain, the variety of tumours is significantly greater. Hemispheric astrocytomas/gliomas are the most frequent tumours, followed by craniopharyngeomas and hypothalamic/optic pathway gliomas.

The distribution of supra- versus infratentorial tumours also varies with age. In the first two years of life, supratentorial tumours are more frequent than infratentorial tumours; between two and ten years, infratentorial tumours outweigh supratentorial tumours, while in children aged ten years and older, supra- and infratentorial tumours are equally frequent.

Functional prognosis in children may be better because of the functional plasticity at a younger age. On the other hand, treatment options may be limited because the brain is more vulnerable for the potential deleterious effects of the various treatment options. For example, radiotherapy is frequently contraindicated in very young patients. In addition, radiotherapy may induce secondary neoplasm later in life, although it still plays an important role in the treatment of CNS tumours.

Infratentorial tumours

As mentioned earlier, the 'big four' posterior fossa tumours in children are the cerebellar astrocytomas, medulloblastomas, brainstem gliomas, and ependymomas. Of course many less frequent tumours may be found, including atypical teratoid/rhabdoid tumours (AT/RT), hemangioblastomas, cerebellar gangliocytomas. It would go beyond the scope of this chapter to discuss all these less frequent tumours.

Cerebellar astrocytomas

Cerebellar astrocytomas can be subdivided in the frequent pilocytic astrocytoma (PA) and the less common fibrillary astrocytoma. PA is a unique form of astrocytoma which is rather benign and has a good prognosis if the tumour is recognized early and completely resected. PAs may be seen associated with neurofibromatosis (NF1). The so-called 'epicentre' of the tumour is frequently within the cerebellar vermis, followed in frequency by the cerebellar hemisphere. Most children present with symptoms related to an obstructive hydrocephalus. PAs are usually well demarcated, have a solid, strongly contrast-enhancing tumour component, and a cystic component which shows no, or minimal, contrast enhancement (**Figure 2.5**). The cyst may be significantly larger than the solid tumour nodule. Calcifications are seen in approximately 20% of cases; vasogenic oedema is usually mild or minimal. The tumour typically compresses or displaces adjacent structures, including the brainstem and fourth ventricle, resulting in a supratentorial hydrocephalus. The imaging features may resemble hemangioblastomas. Hemangioblastomas are however significantly rarer, occurring usually as part of the von Hippel Lindau syndrome; tumour nodules are usually multiple, and dilated feeding and draining vessels may be seen.

Next to the 'benign' PAs, each grade of astrocytomas (WHO I–IV) may be encountered in the posterior fossa. Frequently, lesions start as lower-grade lesions with de-differentiation into higher-grade astrocytomas during disease progression. High-grade or anaplastic astrocytomas may show diffuse infiltrative, ill-defined tumour components and are, due to their close proximity to the fourth ventricle and subarachnoid space, at risk for leptomeningeal cerebrospinal fluid (CSF) seeding. Consequently, metastatic lesions should be searched for along the entire neuroaxis, including the most distal tip of the dural sack. Unfortunately, grade III and IV astrocytomas have a poor prognosis.

Medulloblastomas

Medulloblastomas are embryonal tumours of the posterior fossa that were, until recently, classified based upon their predominant histological features into four major types—classic; desmoplastic/nodular type; medulloblastoma with extensive nodularity (MBEN); large-cell anaplastic (LCA) medulloblastoma. Prognosis and late-term outcome showed a significant heterogeneity between and within the subtypes. As mentioned earlier, the recent merging of the histological and molecular/genetic transcriptional data has allowed a more prognostic-relevant subclassification. Based upon the molecular findings, medulloblastomas are now grouped as sonic hedgehog (SHH) activated, wingless (WNT) activated, group 3, and group 4. These tumours have very different behaviours, primary locations, and prognosis. Treatment options should consequently be tailored to maximize outcome while minimizing treatment-related collateral brain damage. WNT tumours have an excellent prognosis and arise from the lower rhombic lip in the dorsolateral brainstem in close proximity to cerebellopontine angle/foramen of Luschka. SHH medulloblastomas originate from the upper rhombic lip and are typically seen outside of the fourth ventricle within the cerebellar hemispheres, but may occasionally originate from the cerebellar vermis. Prognosis is good/intermediate depending on the age of the child. Group 3 and 4 include both classic and LCA histology subtypes, with a variable prognosis, being poor for group 3 and intermediate for group 4.

Most medulloblastomas are hyperdense on CT due to the high cellularity. On MR examination, the tumour is solid, predominantly T1-hypointense, and T2-iso-or hyperintense (**Figure 2.6**). Depending on the subtype, various degrees of contrast enhancement are noted. Exact identification of the epicentre of the tumour may allow differentiation of tumour subtype. In advanced stages, the tumour may invade the fourth ventricle making differentiation less reliable. If the fourth ventricle is invaded, CSF seeding of the neuroaxis must be excluded. Spinal imaging should preferably be done preoperatively, because a mild post-operative leptomeningeal enhancement may mimic tumour seeding.

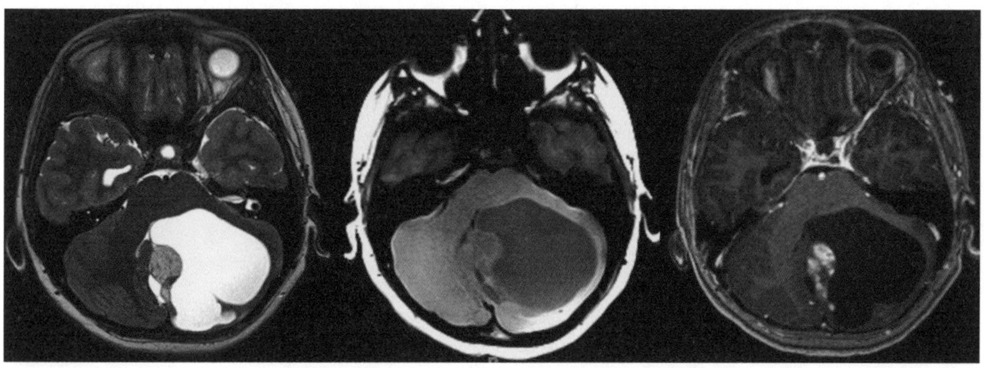

Figure 2.5 Axial T2-, T1-, and contrast-enhanced T1-weighted imaging of child with a partially solid, predominantly cystic pilocytic astrocytoma within the left cerebellar hemisphere and vermis. The fourth ventricle is compressed and displaced to the right.

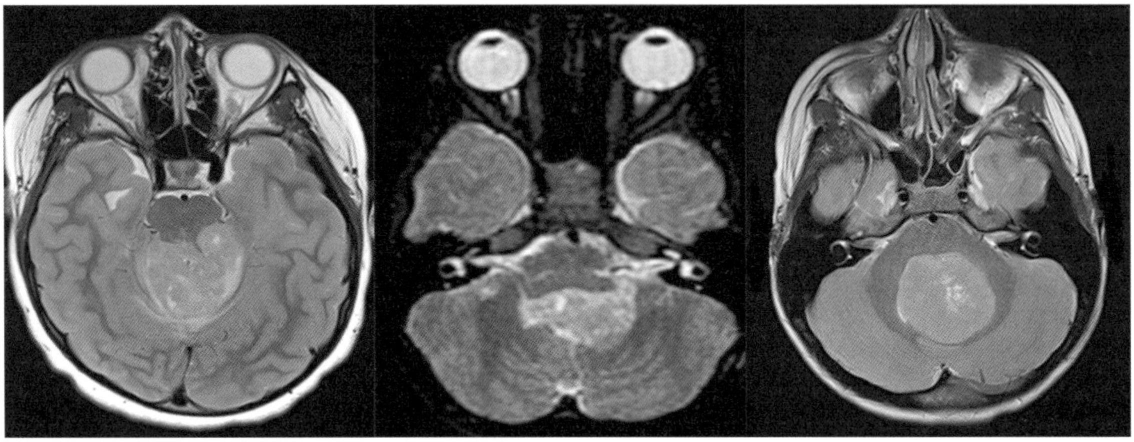

Figure 2.6 Axial T2-weighted MRI of three different children with a SHH (left), WNT (middle), and group 3 (right) medulloblastoma. The epicentre of the SHH subtype is midline and in a more cranial location (originating from the upper rhombic lip) compared to the WNT medulloblastoma (originating from the lower rhombic lip) which is consequently located in close proximity to the foramen of Luschka and CPA. The group 3 medulloblastoma is in a typical midline location.

Brainstem gliomas

Brainstem gliomas can be classified according to their primary location into (a) diffuse infiltrative brainstem glioma (also known as pontine glioma), (b) exophytic glioma of the medulla oblongata, and (c) tectal glioma. Clinical symptoms are determined by the primary location and degree of infiltration or compression of adjacent functional centres. Gliomas usually develop and grow slowly over a long time period before they become symptomatic. A sudden increase in size is usually an indication for a significant change in biological behaviour or malignancy grade. Patients may present with isolated or combined cranial nerve palsies as well as ataxia. Because these gliomas grow slowly, hydrocephalus is often encountered late in disease progression.

Most gliomas are recognized between three and ten years of age. Long-term prognosis of the diffuse infiltrative brainstem glioma remains poor. These brainstem gliomas have a low sensitivity for chemotherapy, and the young age of most patients, as well as the central location of the tumour, prevents high-dose radiotherapy or surgical exploration/resection. However, radiotherapy is still the most important treatment modality. The exophytic glioma of the medulla oblongata has a more favourable prognosis; histologically, they usually belong to the group of PAs and they are more accessible to surgical resection. Tectal gliomas have a good prognosis, may remain stable for many decades, and usually only require symptomatic treatment. The proximity to the Sylvian aqueduct usually results in an obstructive hydrocephalus which can be treated by a ventriculo-peritoneal shunt or a third ventriculostomy. Because of the stability of the lesions, several groups have discussed if a tectal glioma should be considered to be a variant hamartoma.

On MRI, most gliomas are T1-hypointense, T2-hyperintense, and show no or minimal contrast enhancement. Tectal gliomas are usually recognized as a 'thick/bulky' quadrigeminal plate. The exophytic glioma of the medulla oblongata is usually characterized by a large exophytic component attached to the medulla oblongata. The MR imaging features of the diffuse infiltrative brainstem glioma are considered to be sufficient to establish diagnosis. Typically, the lesion is centred in a diffuse enlarged pons, preserved fibre tracts may be seen as linear signal intensities within the lesion (seen especially well on T2-weighted imaging), the basilar artery is embraced, and, depending on the grade of malignancy, multifocal areas of contrast enhancement may be observed. These gliomas may extend into the lower brainstem as well as into the mesencephalon and diencephalon.

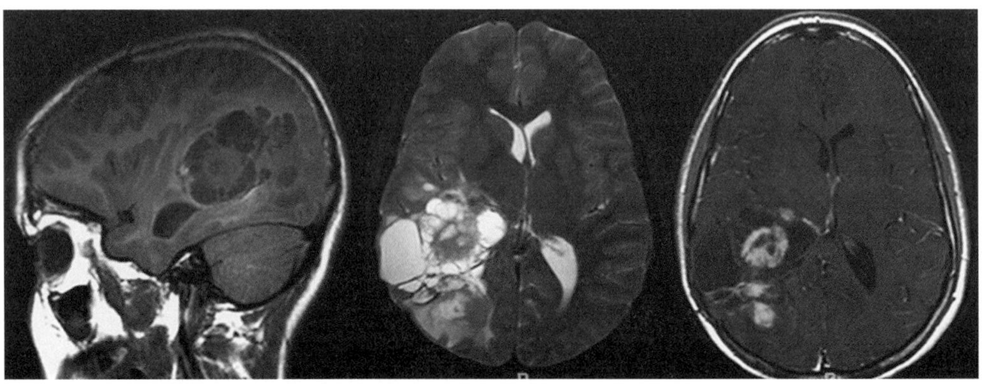

Figure 2.7 Sagittal T1-, axial T2-, and contrast-enhanced T1-weighted MRI of a child with a glioblastoma multiforme. A large, inhomogeneous, partially multicystic, partially solid, contrast-enhancing tumour is seen within the right parieto-occipital region.

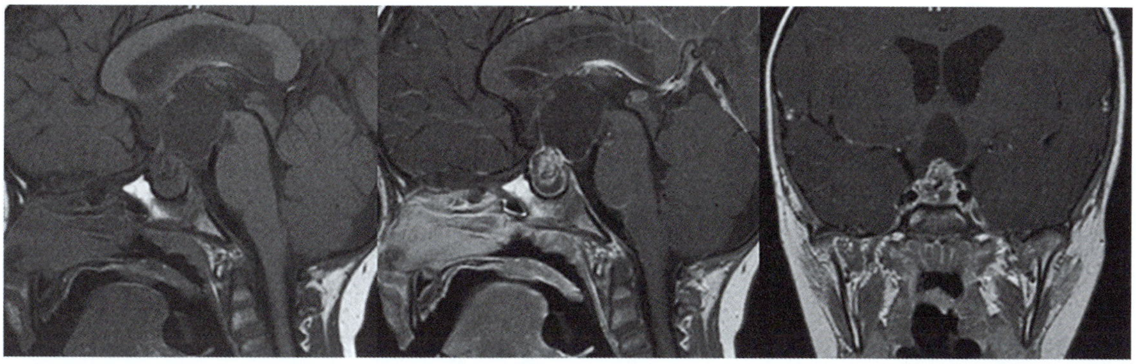

Figure 2.8 Sagittal T1, contrast-enhanced sagittal and coronal T1-weighted MRI of a child with a sellar/suprasellar craniopharyngeoma. The lesion shows inhomogeneous contrast enhancement with a large cyst protruding into the third ventricle. The optic chiasm is pushed anteriorly.

Ependymomas

Ependymomas typically originate from the ependymal lining of the fourth ventricle (60–70% of cases). In contrast to medulloblastomas, the 'epicentre' of ependymomas is within the fourth ventricle. Ependymomas rarely infiltrate the vermis, brainstem, or cerebellum. They typically respect the boundaries of the ventricular system and extend along the various outlet channels of the fourth ventricle (foramen of Luschka and Magendie), along the brainstem into basal cisterns and the spinal canal. CSF seeding may occur early due to the intraventricular location. Clinically, most children present with signs of an obstructive hydrocephalus or compression of the brainstem and cranial nerves. On imaging, ependymomas are solid, T1-iso-or hypointense, T2-iso-or hyperintense, with a variable degree of contrast enhancement. Calcifications are seen in 50%, cysts in 20%, and haemorrhage in 10% of cases.

Supratentorial tumours

In contrast to the posterior fossa, the variation of tumours is higher in the supratentorial region.

Astrocytomas

Astrocytomas (WHO I–IV) are the most frequent supratentorial tumours in children (30%). Clinical symptoms are determined by the primary location, degree of infiltration, and compression of functional centres. Focal functional deficits may be seen next to epileptic seizures and more general signs of increased intracranial pressure. Most paediatric astrocytomas are low-grade; however, in rare cases, grade IV glioblastoma multiforme occurs. PAs are much rarer in the supratentorial brain compared to the posterior fossa. Next to white-matter locations, astrocytomas may also be located within the thalami and basal ganglia. Depending on their WHO grade, the imaging appearance may differ on CT and MRI. Low-grade astrocytomas are T1-hypointense and T2-hyperintense, with no or minimal contrast enhancement or mass effect. High-grade gliomas typically show an intense, inhomogeneous contrast enhancement, with areas of necrosis within the centre of the tumour (Figure 2.7). Diffusion-weighted imaging may be helpful to differentiate between a necrotic tumour and an abscess.

Craniopharyngeomas

Craniopharyngeomas make up about 15% of CNS tumours in children. They are most frequently seen between 10 and 14 years of age and are typically located in the sellar/suprasellar region along the axis between the hypothalamus and pituitary gland. These tumours most likely originate from residual pluripotent cells after the development of the hypothalamus/pituitary gland. Clinical symptoms are related to compression of the optic chiasm/pathway, pituitary gland/hypothalamus, or infiltration of the connection between the hypothalamus and pituitary gland. Craniopharyngeomas are easily identified on CT and MRI. They are usually heterogeneous, with solid and cystic components, as well as variable degrees of calcification and contrast enhancement (Figure 2.8). The sellar may be enlarged.

Optic pathway gliomas

Optic pathway gliomas represent a separate group of astrocytomas and are frequently seen in NF1 patients. Histologically, they represent PAs. Non- or minimally enhancing optic nerve gliomas can be seen next to T2-hyperintense, strongly enhancing hypothalamic/chiasmatic tumours. These tumours may be stable for many years but typically present with slowly progressive blindness and pituitary/hypothalamic dysfunction.

Supratentorial ependymomas and atypical teratoid/rhabdoid tumours

Supratentorial ependymomas and AT/RTs are rare tumours in childhood. Of all ependymomas, only 20–40% are located within the supratentorial brain. Supratentorial ependymomas are most frequently located within the periventricular white matter; intraventricular ependymomas are much rarer. Local compression may result in trapped ventricles with asymmetrical hydrocephalus. Supratentorial AT/RTs are also rare. These tumours are usually large on initial presentation, heterogeneous, and may be located within the white matter as well as in the ventricles. Differentiation from other rare tumours like choroid plexus malignancies or intraventricular meningeomas may be challenging.

FURTHER READING

Abdel Razek AA, et al. (2009) Characterization of pediatric head and neck masses with diffusion-weighted MR imaging. *Eur Radiol* **19**, 201–8.

Arnold MA, et al. (2016) Histology, fusion status, and outcome in alveolar rhabdomyosarcoma with low-risk clinical features: a report from the Children's Oncology Group. *Pediatr Blood* Cancer **63**(4), 634–9. doi: 10.1002/pbc.25862

Bagatell R, et al. (2016) Assessment of primary site response in children with high-risk neuroblastoma: an international multicenter study. *J Clin Oncol* **34**(7), 740–6. doi: 10.1200/JCO.2015.63.2042

Brisse HJ, et al. (2011) Guidelines for imaging and staging of neuroblastic tumors: consensus report from the International Neuroblastoma Risk Group Project. Radiology **261**(1), 243–57. doi: 10.1148/radiol.11101352

Dome JS, et al. (2015) Advances in Wilms tumor treatment and biology: progress through international collaboration. *J Clin Oncol* **33**(27), 2999–3007. doi: 10.1200/JCO.2015.62.1888

Giraudo C, et al. (2016) 18F-fluorodeoxyglucose positron emission tomography/magnetic resonance in lymphoma: comparison with 18F-fluorodeoxyglucose positron emission tomography/computed tomography and with the addition of magnetic resonance diffusion-weighted imaging. *Invest Radiol* **51**(3), 163–9. doi: 10.1097/RLI.0000000000000218

Monclair T, et al. (2009) The International Neuroblastoma Risk Group (INRG) Staging System: an INRG task force report. *J Clin Oncol* **27**, 298–303.

Oberlin O, et al. (2015) Prognostic factors for outcome in localized extremity rhabdomyosarcoma. Pooled analysis from four international cooperative groups. Pediatr Blood Cancer **62**(12), 2125–31. doi: 10.1002/pbc.25684

Patay Z, et al. (2015) MR imaging characteristics of wingless-type-subgroup pediatric medulloblastoma. *Am J Neuroradiol* **36**, 2386–93.

Pearce MS, et al. (2012) Radiation exposure from CT scans in childhood and subsequent risk of leukaemia and brain tumours: a retrospective cohort study. Lancet **380**(9840), 499–505.

Roebuck DJ, Perilongo G (2006) Hepatoblastoma: an oncological review. *Pediatr Radiol* **36**, 183–6.

Rojas Y, et al. (2014) Relapse surveillance in AFP-positive hepatoblastoma: re-evaluating the role of imaging. *Pediatr Radiol* **44**(10), 1275–80. doi: 10.1007/s00247-014-3000-6

Taylor MD, et al. (2012) Molecular subgroups of medulloblastoma: the current consensus. *Acta Neuropathol* **123**, 465–72.

3

Chemotherapy and Other Anti-Cancer Drugs

Current Knowledge and New Perspectives

C. Michel Zwaan, Gareth J. Veal, and Lucas Moreno

Introduction

In contrast to many types of cancer arising in adults, the majority of those occurring in childhood are sensitive to cytotoxic chemotherapy. This is generally attributed to the high proliferation rate of childhood malignancies and the propensity of the malignant cells to undergo apoptosis—features that may be linked to the embryonal origin of many of these tumour types. Chemotherapy, therefore, has a major role in treatment and contributes significantly to the generally good outcome for most paediatric malignancies. The treatment of childhood acute lymphoblastic leukaemia (ALL) provides an excellent example in this respect, with survival in more than 90% of patients.

Chemotherapy is used either as the only treatment modality, or in combination with surgery and/or radiotherapy. However, some diseases remain or become refractory to chemotherapy, and evidence for the long-term toxicity of some chemotherapeutic compounds has emerged. Thus, there is a necessity to understand the mechanisms of both therapeutic failure and long-term toxicity. Taking into account biological and pathological differences between paediatric and adult cancer, it is clear that specific drug development programmes are needed to identify and test new drugs for children. Moreover, given the potential differences in drug metabolism at different ages, dosing may differ from adults. Young children may also need specific formulations (e.g. oral solutions). Fortunately, some of these challenges are now being addressed by specific regulations facilitating paediatric drug development both in the United States and Europe.

The first part of this chapter will summarize the current knowledge of conventional chemotherapeutic agents and their application. The second part will focus on the development of novel compounds, which is clearly needed as cancer remains the leading cause of death due to disease in children.

Conventional chemotherapeutic agents

Overview

Chemotherapy is a key element in the treatment of paediatric haematological malignancies. In ALL treatment consists of multiple agents given in combination for a total treatment duration of two to three years. Central to this is multi-agent induction treatment, followed by intrathecal and intravenous chemotherapy to avoid leukaemia relapse in the central nervous system (CNS). Further blocks of consolidation or reinduction therapy are introduced before the start of a prolonged phase of maintenance therapy that aims to eradicate minimal residual disease (MRD). In contrast, treatment duration is short in acute myeloid leukaemia (AML), with most protocols containing four or five blocks of intensive chemotherapy. In both diseases, many treatment optimization studies have been performed over several decades, fine-tuning the application of conventional chemotherapy. These have included studies implementing new analogues of existing compounds with greater potency or better pharmacological properties. Examples include asparaginase (*E. coli* derived asparaginase, PEGylated asparaginases, and, recently, recombinant asparaginase) and corticosteroids (prednisone being replaced by dexamethasone). Nevertheless, a small subset of patients still fail to achieve cure with current therapy and new agents are needed to improve outcomes for these individuals.

In paediatric solid tumours, chemotherapy is generally adapted to the diagnosis and stage of the malignancy. It is often used to obtain regression of the primary tumour in order to facilitate local tumour control by surgery and/or radiotherapy. Preoperative chemotherapy of this type, referred to as 'neoadjuvant' chemotherapy, also allows evaluation of the chemosensitivity of a particular tumour in a specific patient, which may influence the choice of postoperative treatment. Postoperative 'adjuvant' chemotherapy is used to treat presumed microscopic metastases or remaining viable tumour after incomplete local therapy. In other tumours, the primary approach is surgical removal of the localized primary tumour, after which adjuvant chemotherapy and/or radiotherapy is given in order to achieve optimal local and systemic control.

Chemotherapy regimens usually consist of combinations of two or more cytotoxic agents given as sequential courses in order to augment the probability of destroying the malignant cells. In most schedules, different classes of drugs with distinct mechanisms of action are used together in an attempt to achieve synergism and reduce the likelihood of chemoresistance. The choice of chemotherapy depends on several factors such as tumour type, preclinical evidence of *in vitro* cytotoxicity and *in vivo* activity of a specific drug, and on the expected toxicity of the proposed combination. Sometimes preclinical data provide evidence of synergy between two or more compounds, although most standard chemotherapy regimens utilized during the last three decades have been developed empirically.

Classification of chemotherapeutic agents

There are several classes of anti-cancer drugs that are defined by their mode of action. In general, drugs of different classes are chosen for combination regimens. The classification used for drugs most frequently used in paediatric oncology is summarized in Table 3.1.

Routes of administration

Most chemotherapy agents are given intravenously (IV), usually involving a central venous device. Some drugs are administered orally, either as tablets, capsules, or liquid preparations, with hospital pharmacies sometimes developing dose-adapted capsules or liquid preparations for those not commercially available. Nasogastric or enterostomy tubes may be utilized for drug administration in mainly younger children. Subcutaneous and intramuscular dosing is less acceptable in children due to the distress caused. Intrathecal administration of chemotherapy is used in leukaemia and most subtypes of non-Hodgkin lymphoma (NHL), and is sometimes also applied in treatment of brain tumours. Other specialized routes of administration which may be occasionally encountered include isolated limb perfusion for refractory sarcoma, or intra-arterial administration in hepatic tumours. A novel way of administration considered in brain tumours consists of intra-tumoural infusion via specifically developed catheters.

Toxicity of chemotherapy

Side effects of chemotherapy can be divided into acute and long-term toxicities. The latter become more relevant with increasing cure rates and because of the young age of most patients. Since most chemotherapeutics exert their mode of action on proliferating cells,

Table 3.1 Summary of chemotherapeutic drugs

Class	Mode of action	Examples
Alkylating agents	Form covalent bonds between alkyl groups and nucleotides in DNA	Mechlorethamine, cyclophosphamide, ifosfamide, melphalan, busulfan, thiotepa
	Alkylation alters DNA and its replication	Nitrosureas: carmustine (BCNU) and lomustine (CCNU)
	May induce mutations in DNA	Procarbazine and dacarbazine (DTIC)
		Temozolomide
Platinum compounds	Form covalent bonds between platinum atoms and DNA, resulting in intrastrand adducts or interstrand crosslinks, leading to DNA damage	Cisplatin, carboplatin, oxaliplatin
Anti-metabolites	Interfere with synthesis of DNA/RNA precursors	Purine analogues (mercaptopurine, thioguanine, fludarabine, clofarabine)
	Enzyme inhibition (e.g. dihydrofolate reductase or thymidylate synthetase)	Pyrimidine analogues (cytarabine, gemcitabine, 5-fluorouracil)
		Anti-folates (methotrexate, pemetrexed, trimetrexate)
Anti-microtubule compounds	Interfere with the formation of microtubules during cell division	Vinca alkaloids (vincristine, vinblastine, vinorelbine)
		Taxanes (paclitaxel, docetaxel)
		Ixabepilone
Topoisomerase I inhibitors	Inhibition of topoisomerase I	Irinotecan (CPT-11) and topotecan
Epipodophyllotoxins	Inhibition of topoisomerase II	Etoposide (VP16), teniposide (VM26)
Antibiotics: Anthracyclines Anthracenediones Others	Inhibition of topoisomerase II, but act also through DNA intercalation Oxidative DNA intercalation DNA binding drug and inhibitor of RNA and protein synthesis	Daunorubicin, doxorubicin, epirubicin, idarubicin Mitoxantrone Bleomycin, Dactinomycin
Miscellaneous		
Corticosteroids	Induction of apoptosis	Prednisolone, dexamethasone
Asparaginase	Inhibits asparagine synthetase and depletes intracellular asparagine levels	L-Asparaginase, erwinase, PEGylated-asparginase
Differentiation-inducing agents	Inhibitor of ribonucleotide reductase	Hydroxyurea
	Induces differentiation of promyeloctes or neuroblasts	All-*trans* retinoic acid, cis-retinoic acid, fenretinide

some normally dividing tissues are especially at risk of toxicity. These commonly include the bone marrow (aplasia), gastrointestinal mucosa (mucositis and diarrhoea), and hair follicles (alopecia), with most compounds causing transient toxicities on these organs. Some drugs may also have a specific toxicity on one or more organ functions, often with implications in the mid to long term. For example, the anthracyclines are well known for their potential cardiac toxicity, but this is rarely evident at the time of treatment. Cisplatin and, to a lesser extent, carboplatin may be ototoxic and/or nephrotoxic. Methotrexate may have acute renal, liver, or CNS toxicity, but this is generally not of long-term significance. The use of alkylating agents may result in secondary malignancy and fertility damage in the long term. Epipodophyllotoxins may induce secondary myelodysplasia and/or AML.

The risk of severe late effects may be avoided by reducing cumulative dose exposures, or by avoiding the use of compounds with unfavourable toxicity profiles. Such approaches are now being investigated, as exemplified by the current UK ALL 2011 study, which was designed with the primary objective to investigate the effect on serious treatment-related toxicity of receiving a higher dose but reduced number of days of dexamethasone treatment.

The common incidence of toxicity associated with the use of cytotoxic chemotherapy reinforces the need to develop drugs with novel mechanisms of action, directed against specific biological targets characteristic of a given cancer type (also referred to as targeted therapy). Targeted compounds may induce fewer side effects, although experience in children is still very limited and new toxicities may emerge. The toxicity profiles of various compounds commonly used in paediatric oncology are described in **Table 3.2**. The severity of chemotherapy-induced toxicity can be classified using the system of toxicity developed by the National Cancer Institute, the Common Terminology Criteria for Adverse Events.

Dose intensity

Chemotherapeutics are usually delivered at a maximum tolerated dose (MTD) in order to obtain the maximum anti-tumour effect, largely due to the exhibited dose–effect relationship and the narrow therapeutic window. The concept of dose intensity is defined as the amount of drug administered per unit of time. Strategies which incorporate high-dose intensity have proven beneficial in several paediatric tumours. For example, in Burkitt lymphoma more than 90% of the patients can now be cured by intensive multi-agent chemotherapy regimens of relatively short duration in combination with an anti-CD20 monoclonal antibody (rituximab). Dose-intensive regimens demand the shortest intervals possible between sequential courses of treatment and may cause severe toxicity. Improved supportive care protocols (e.g. anti-emetic therapy, haematopoietic growth factors, antibiotic and antifungal prophylaxis, transfusion support) have been developed, which has allowed further dose intensification without increasing treatment-related mortality.

More recently there has been increased interest in metronomic chemotherapy. This is based on the chronic administration of chemotherapeutic agents at relatively low, minimally toxic doses, and without prolonged drug-free breaks. The precise mechanism of action is uncertain and is likely to be multifactorial.

High-dose myeloablative chemotherapy

Several cytotoxic compounds have roughly linear dose–effect relationships and are suitable for administration at high doses, especially when the toxicity of these drugs is essentially haematological. The use of such high-dose (myeloablative) chemotherapy approaches requires autologous or allogeneic haematopoietic stem cell support, which assures reconstitution of haematopoiesis. Maximum therapeutic effect is obtained and non-haematological toxicity becomes the dose-limiting factor. High-dose chemotherapy strategies are mostly applied in very good partial or complete remission in chemotherapy-sensitive tumours with high risk of relapse. The most common examples of chemotherapeutics used for high-dose chemotherapy are the alkylating agents. In paediatric solid tumours, high-dose chemotherapy with autologous stem cell rescue is most often used in neuroblastoma (NBL), Ewing sarcoma, and, more recently, also in medulloblastoma. In relapsed or high-risk leukaemia, myeloablative regimens with allogeneic haematopoietic stem cell transplant may also include immunosuppressive drugs such as fludarabine, monoclonal antibodies directed against T cells, or total body irradiation. Where allogeneic stem cell support is used, a graft-versus-leukaemia effect may have an additional anti-tumour effect besides the cytotoxic effects of chemotherapy and/or TBI.

Drug resistance

There are several important mechanisms of drug resistance, of which the multidrug resistance (MDR) phenotype, commonly expressed by cancer cells, is the best characterized. This is caused by enhanced expression of drug-efflux pumps on the cancer cell membrane. Several proteins are implicated including P-glycoprotein, multidrug resistance proteins 1–8 (MRP), breast cancer resistance protein (BCRP), and the lung resistance-related protein (LRP). High expression of these membrane proteins in tumour cells has been correlated with poor outcome in some malignancies, although the value of such observations remains controversial. Various preclinical models have been developed to circumvent the MDR-related mechanism of drug resistance but clinical trials using MDR blocking agents (e.g. verapamil, ciclosporin A, PSC 833) have so far failed to demonstrate clear benefits. It is likely that other mechanisms are concurrently or sequentially involved in the development of drug resistance.

Dosing of drugs in paediatric oncology

Body surface area

The principle of using body surface area (BSA) for dosing chemotherapy results from pharmacological research studying drug absorption, distribution, metabolism, and excretion. Data show that the most reliable method of comparing physiological variables (e.g. kidney function (glomerular filtration rate), cardiac output, and basal metabolic rate) between species and across ages is by correcting for BSA. Use of body weight instead of BSA results in an unreliable interspecies correction of all mechanisms contributing to the exposure. Although the use of BSA is controversial in adult oncology, variability in weight and height is so great in children that prescriptions are almost always based on BSA. BSA can be calculated by formulas or the use of nomograms, with the 'gold standard' formula described by Dubois in 1916. Although very reliable, this formula is not easy to use and other formulas have since been validated, taking into account either weight and height/length or weight only (**Table 3.3**).

Table 3.2 Specific adverse effects of cytotoxic compounds categorized as short-term (days to weeks) and long-term (months to years) side effects. (General adverse effects such as bone marrow suppression, gastrointestinal toxicity, and alopecia are not included.)

Drug	Short-term side effects	Long-term side effects
Asparaginase	Clotting disorders, anaphylactic reactions, pancreatitis, hyperglycaemia	Sequelae from thrombosis/bleeding (CNS or elsewhere) or pancreatitis
Bleomycin	Fever, malaise, skin rash	Pulmonary fibrosis
Busulfan	Veno-occlusive disease (VOD), seizures, hyperpigmentation	Hyperpigmentation, pulmonary fibrosis, fertility disorders
Carboplatin	Ototoxicity, allergic reactions	Ototoxicity
Cisplatinum	Renal toxicity, ototoxicity, radio-sensitization	Renal toxicity, ototoxicity
Cyclophosphamide	Haemorrhagic cystitis	Fertility disorders, secondary leukaemia
Cytarabine	Mucositis, rash, conjunctivitis, fever, encephalopathy, seizures, pancreatitis	Encephalopathy
Dactinomycin	Jaundice, veno-occlusive disease, radio-sensitization	Unknown
Daunorubicin	Mucositis, cardiomyopathy, radio-sensitization	Cardiomyopathy, secondary leukaemia
Dexamethasone	Mood disorders, increased appetite, Cushingoid appearance, muscular atrophy, bone demineralization, skin disorders	Bone fractures, avascular femoral head necrosis, vertebral collapse, adrenal suppression, metabolic syndrome
Doxorubicin	Mucositis, cardiomyopathy, radio-sensitization	Cardiomyopathy, secondary leukaemia
Epirubicin	Mucositis, cardiomyopathy, radio-sensitization	Cardiomyopathy, secondary leukaemia
Etoposide (VP-16)	Allergic reactions, mucositis	Secondary leukaemia
Fludarabine	Mucositis, fever, pneumonitis, neurotoxicity, hepatitis	Unknown
Idarubicin	Mucositis, cardiomyopathy, radio-sensitization	Cardiomyopathy, secondary leukaemia
Ifosfamide	Haemorrhagic cystitis, tubulopathy, encephalopathy, seizures	Tubular and glomerular renal toxicity, fertility disorders
Irinotecan	Abdominal pain, diarrhoea, sweating, hyper lacrimation, salivary excess	Unknown
Melphalan	Mucositis, interstitial pneumonitis	Pulmonary fibrosis, fertility disorders
6-Mercaptopurine	Hepatitis	Unknown
Methotrexate	Hepatitis, mucositis, encephalopathy, renal toxicity	Liver fibrosis, encephalopathy
Mitoxantrone	Mucositis, cardiomyopathy	Cardiomyopathy
Prednisolone	Mood disorders, increased appetite, Cushingoid appearance, muscular atrophy, bone demineralization, skin disorders	Bone fractures, avascular femoral head necrosis, vertebral collapse, adrenal suppression, metabolic syndrome
Procarbazine	Allergic reactions, hepatic dysfunction, headache, paraesthesia, hallucinations	Fertility disorders
Temozolomide	Lymphocytopenia	Secondary malignancy
Teniposide (VM-26)	Allergic reactions, mucositis	Secondary leukaemia
6-Thioguanine	Hepatitis, VOD	Unknown
Thiotepa	Headache, encephalopathy, dizziness, allergic reactions, skin rash, fever	Fertility disorders
Topotecan	Mucositis, radio-sensitization	Unknown
Vinblastine	Paraesthesia, neuralgia, sensory disorders, hypertension, Raynaud's phenomenon	Raynaud's phenomenon
Vincristine	Paraesthesia, neuralgia, muscular weakness, sensory disorders, constipation, ileus, abdominal cramps, seizures, SIADH	Neurotoxicity

Table 3.3 Formulas for calculating body surface area (BSA), body mass index (BMI), and ideal body weight

Type	Formula
Dubois' formula	$BSA = W^{0.425} \times L^{0.725} \times 0.007184$
Mosteller's formula	$BSA = \sqrt{W \times L / 3600}$
Formula without using length	$BSA = (4W + 7)/(W + 90)$
Body mass index	$BMI\ (kg/m^2) = W/L^2$
Lawrence's formula	Ideal body weight (kg) = $[L-100]-[(L-150)/K]$

Key: BSA = body surface area in m^2; W = body weight in kg; L = body length in cm; K = 4 for males and 2 for females.

Chemotherapy in infants

Tolerance to chemotherapy at a given dose is generally poorer in infants when compared to older children and adults. Maturation of the physiological mechanisms that contribute to the pharmacokinetics of drug handling occurs during the first year of life. For example, the water content of the human body decreases from 75% at birth to 60% at age one and 55% in adults. The content of plasma proteins also changes during the first year of life and hepatic drug-metabolizing enzymes (cytochrome P450 isoenzymes, Uridine 5'-diphospho (UDP)-glucuronyltransferase, glutathione metabolizing enzymes) achieve their full physiological activity between six and twelve months of age. Glomerular filtration rate (GFR) attains values

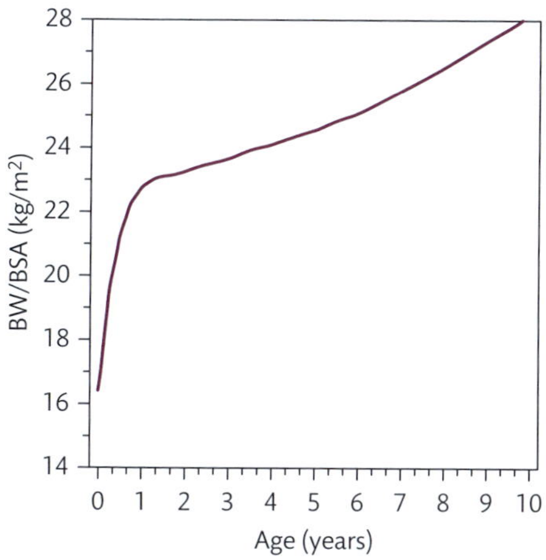

Figure 3.1 Development of body weight (BW) to body surface area (BSA) ratio during childhood.

comparable to those in adults at the age of five months. All these factors contribute to the poorer tolerance of infants to chemotherapy, and treatment doses should be reduced.

In general, chemotherapy in infants should be prescribed as mg/kg body weight instead of BSA, since the relationship between body weight and BSA is different in infants as compared to older children (**Figure 3.1**). A dose prescribed in mg/m^2 in an infant will lead to a higher dose than one prescribed in mg/kg (**Table 3.4**). In neonates and very young children (less than three months old), even greater caution is required and additional dose reductions are frequently applied, although many of these are empirical. It is important to appreciate the balance between avoiding drug exposures that are likely to lead to toxicity and ensuring that drug levels are achieved that will lead to effective anti-tumour activity.

In order to provide a more scientific rationale for the dosing of neonate and infant cancer patients, it is important that more clinical pharmacology studies are carried out in this population. An example is provided by the drug 13-cis-retinoic acid for NBL: pharmacokinetic studies highlighted a trend towards lower exposures being observed in children less than 12 kg, receiving a mg/kg dosing regimen, as compared to standard treatment in mg/m^2 in older children, resulting in removal of the mg/kg dosing recommendation. The study also highlighted the importance of the availability of appropriate drug formulations, as children unable to swallow isotretinoin capsules experienced lower drug exposures following extraction of the drug from capsules prior to administration. This again represents an area where more work needs to be done to facilitate the optimal treatment of childhood cancer.

Chemotherapy in obese patients

Obesity is associated with modifications in body composition that may change the pharmacokinetics of cytotoxic compounds, potentially resulting in either inadequate drug exposure or increased toxicity. Increased body fat mass will alter the distribution volume of a drug depending on its affinity for fatty tissues and plasma proteins. Fatty degeneration of liver tissue may also modify hepatic metabolizing capacity in obese patients.

The diagnosis of obesity is defined by the World Health Organization (WHO) as a body mass index (BMI) (**Table 3.3**) of more than 30 kg/m^2. For children up to five years of age, overweight and obesity are defined as more than two or three standard deviations above the median. For older children, this is defined as more than one or two standard deviations above the median.

For most cytotoxic compounds, no pharmacokinetic data are available in obese patients and, thus, it is recommended that chemotherapy is prescribed according to ideal body weight instead of actual body weight to avoid excessive toxicity. In adolescents and young adults, ideal body weight can be calculated according to the formula by Lawrence (**Table 3.3**). In younger children, the ideal body weight is best determined by the body weight corresponding to the centile of height.

For those drugs where clinical pharmacology studies have been carried out, clinically significant variations in pharmacokinetics have been observed in obese children for approximately two-thirds of drugs studied, with these differences resulting in marked differences in drug exposure in approximately one-third of cases. It is clear that more research needs to be carried out in this area, to achieve a consensus as to the most appropriate approach to dosing chemotherapy in obese children.

Prescribing chemotherapy in difficult situations

Some patients may require chemotherapy in an acute situation where organ failure (most typically hepatic or renal failure) limits the clearance of chemotherapy. In such situations, chemotherapy doses should be reduced, taking into account the type of drug and the mechanisms of clearance for that drug. In clinical situations where dialysis is used, consideration should be given to whether this contributes to the wash-out of the drug. In addition, the potential additional toxicity on the affected organ should be taken into account. Drugs which have been shown to exhibit marked differences in disposition in children receiving dialysis include platinum-based drugs and cyclophosphamide. Detailed recommendations about dose adaptations are available from other sources.

Table 3.4 Comparison between dose prescribed in mg/m^2 versus dose in mg/kg in children

Child's characteristics			Dose calculated as		Dose reduction from calculation using mg/kg compared to BSA
Age	Weight	BSA	100 mg/m^2	3.33 mg/kg	
10 years	30 kg	1 m^2	100 mg	100 mg	0%
1 year	10 kg	0.46 m^2	46 mg	33 mg	28%
3 months	6 kg	0.29 m^2	29 mg	20 mg	31%

Key: BSA = body surface area in m^2.

Intrathecal chemotherapy

It is important to recognize that, compared to adults, the CNS compartment in a child is proportionally larger than the rest of the body. For example, a child between four and six years of age has a CNS volume of 80–90% compared to the adult brain. This results in the prescription of intrathecal therapy in an absolute dose (mg), depending on the age of the patient, rather than in mg/m^2.

Pharmacogenetics and drug interactions

Intracellular metabolism contributes to the clearance of drugs by transforming them to metabolites in order to facilitate renal or biliary excretion. Generally, drug metabolites have less or no therapeutic activity, although some metabolites may still have a strong cytotoxic effect. In some cases prodrugs are administered to patients, which require metabolism to their active forms, as is the case for cyclophosphamide. Many enzymes are implicated in the biotransformation of drugs, of which the cytochrome P450 isoenzymes, the glucuronidation pathways, and detoxifying enzymes implicated in glutathione metabolism are most relevant. The activity of these enzymes influences drug plasma concentrations and thus concentrations in tumour tissue.

It is useful to know the metabolic pathways of drugs in order to identify potential drug interactions. Hepatic mechanisms, such as CYP450 enzyme induction or inhibition, may dramatically alter the metabolism and hence the efficacy of a cytotoxic drug. Antiepileptics are well known to induce the activity of the CYP3A4 and CYP2C9 isoenzymes, and thus increase the biotransformation and clearance of many cytotoxic drugs. On the other hand, drugs such as azoles may inhibit the activity of several CYP isoenzymes, resulting in higher plasma concentrations and increasing toxicity of cytotoxic drugs, such as vincristine. Drug interactions should be taken into account when prescribing both chemotherapeutic and other drugs used for supportive care.

As the influence of these pharmacokinetic modifying enzymes has emerged, population-based studies of pharmacogenetics have been undertaken. Genetic polymorphisms of these or other enzymes may cause variable phenotypes, resulting in different enzyme activities from patient to patient and, thus, differences in drug clearance. An example of pharmacogenetic variability is encountered in the metabolism of 6-mercaptopurine (6-MP). This drug is inactivated by the enzyme thiopurine methyltransferase (TPMT) and patients with TPMT mutations require treatment with lower dosages of 6-MP to avoid excessive haematological toxicity. Another example consists of polymorphisms in the gene *UGT1A1* that lead to large differences in the glucuronidation of irinotecan metabolites and, thus, differences in systemic exposure of the active metabolite SN38. Future insights into genetic polymorphisms implicated in the metabolism of chemotherapeutics may facilitate individualization of treatment.

Therapeutic drug monitoring

An important approach to the treatment of children with cancer is the utility of therapeutic drug monitoring (TDM). This relates to the real-time quantification of drug levels in an individual patient, with a view to adapting the dose of drug administered to improve the likelihood of clinical response, whilst minimizing the incidence of toxicity. Many well-established cytotoxic drugs exhibit significant inter-patient pharmacokinetic variability and have steep dose–response relationships and narrow therapeutic windows—characteristics which very much lend themselves to TDM approaches. TDM approaches have been shown to be beneficial for several chemotherapeutics, including methotrexate, busulfan, and carboplatin, alongside some of the newer targeted anti-cancer drugs. For these drugs and others, the use of TDM approaches should be encouraged, particularly in relation to the treatment of patient subpopulations such as neonates and infants, anephric patients requiring dialysis, and patients receiving high-dose chemotherapy.

Drug development in paediatric oncology

Overview

There are several factors that influence the development of novel compounds, analogues, or formulations for children with cancer:

1. The need for appropriate safety and activity/efficacy studies in a paediatric population with biologically different subtypes of cancer compared to adults.
2. Reduction of side effects and studying the effect on growth and development or other long-term safety concerns.
3. Development of age-adapted paediatric formulations, and the ability to deliver oral compounds by nasogastric tube and/or with food.
4. Pharmacokinetic aspects, especially in children below the age of two years.
5. Market authorization/regulatory factors.

Potential pharmacokinetic differences between children and adults need to be evaluated to ensure paediatric dosing schedules are safe and effective. The use of population pharmacokinetic models has enabled the feasibility of such studies with limited sampling, and is being applied in paediatric oncology. However, in most studies the differences in pharmacokinetic properties between adults and older children are limited, and there is a relatively high correlation between the adult and paediatric MTD. This may be different in very young patients.

Until approximately a decade ago, there was limited interest from the pharmaceutical industry to perform clinical trials in children. By 2003, of more than a hundred drugs that had been approved by the Federal Drug Agency (FDA) for the treatment of cancer, information about paediatric use was available for less than 50% of those. In 2007, following an earlier similar initiative in the USA, new legislation governing the development of medicines for use in children was introduced in the European Union. Regulation EC no. 1901/2006 obliges pharmaceutical companies to explore paediatric indications when they want to have a new medicinal product authorized for an adult indication. Evidence shows that the regulation is positively influencing industry interest in paediatric drug development. Since the introduction of this legislation in Europe, more than eight hundred paediatric investigational plans (PIPs) have been submitted, of which 83 are in oncology (as of December 2015). This has resulted in four new drug approvals for cancer in children: everolimus, recombinant asparaginase, imatinib, and dintuximab. This has been supported in Europe through establishment of the European Network of Paediatric Research at the European Medicines Agency (Enpr-EMA) group—a consortium of research networks, investigators, and centres with recognized expertise in performing clinical studies in children. For paediatric oncology, this is the result of the achievements of major academic collaborative groups such as the European Innovative Therapies for Children with Cancer (ITCC) consortium, and the Phase I consortium of the Children's Oncology Group (COG) in North America.

A revised drug development model

A revised drug development model for paediatric cancers was created by the ITCC and others, in the era of molecularly targeted drugs, and includes the following steps:

1. Coordination of molecular profiling studies to identify new targets and potential predictive (selection) biomarkers, and to identify paediatric clinical patterns of drug targets matching with new (adult) compounds.
2. Biological and preclinical research to select the most promising drugs and combinations, and identification of the patient subgroups that could most benefit by matching the mechanism of action of the targeted agent with the biology of paediatric cancers.
3. First-in-child early phase I/II combination clinical studies with strong biological rationale, incorporating pharmacokinetic, pharmacodynamic, and predictive biomarker studies where possible. Studies designed to maximize efficiency, using the least number of patients to identify the recommended phase II dose, incorporating expansion cohorts for preliminary efficacy evaluation to gain further knowledge on the tumour types or biological entities of interest.
4. Drugs that are successful in first-in-child trials should be taken forward into randomized multi-arm trials in the relapse setting.
5. Drugs that have promising activity are then taken into the frontline setting in larger randomized clinical trials conducted by tumour-specific cooperative groups.

Novel drugs can be broadly categorized as follows, although significant overlap can exist:

1. Recently developed cytotoxic drugs.
2. Agents targeting specific molecular aberrations that are oncogenic drivers.
3. Agents targeting signalling pathways relevant to paediatric cancers.
4. Epigenetic agents.
5. Agents against tumour microenvironment and angiogenesis.
6. Targeted inhibitors of cell cycle and DNA repair.
7. Immunotherapy and monoclonal antibodies.

Over the following section, some examples are provided. A detailed description of agents and targets can be found in the 'Further reading' section.

Recently developed cytotoxic drugs

Several new cytotoxics and improved analogues have been relatively recently developed. Most new compounds have a slightly different cytotoxic mechanism of action and/or better pharmacological properties as compared to the conventional chemotherapies of the class to which they belong.

The alkylating agent temozolomide now has an established therapeutic role in the treatment of high-grade glioma with concurrent radiotherapy, although its single-agent activity against high-grade glioma and brainstem glioma is limited (response rates of 5–20%). It is possible that new metronomic dosing schedules may improve efficacy and/or may be more compatible with concurrent radiotherapy. Temozolomide also seems to be active against medulloblastoma and NBL, although it has not yet been integrated into first-line chemotherapeutic regimens and is mostly used as salvage regimen.

Taxanes and gemcitabine have also been explored in children but, so far, have not shown sufficiently promising results to be evaluated in frontline trials. Clofarabine is a novel deoxyadenosine analogue which has been registered in Europe for use in children with relapsed/refractory ALL. Interestingly, clofarabine is one of the few drugs where a label was first obtained in paediatrics. Clofarabine can either be used as a single agent or in combination with cyclophosphamide and etoposide. In AML, it is used in combination with cytarabine, replacing fludarabine in the FLA (fludarabine and high-dose cytarabine) regimen. Nelarabine is a purine nucleoside analogue (ARA-G) and is registered for use in paediatric relapsed/refractory T-cell ALL and NHL. In COG, the use of nelarabine in up-front protocols for T-cell disease is currently being evaluated.

Agents targeting specific molecular aberrations that are oncogenic drivers

Tyrosine kinase inhibitors inhibiting the *ABL* gene

Imatinib mesylate is a small molecule drug and the prime example of successful inhibition of the tyrosine kinase ABL, which is constitutively active as a result of a translocation between the *BCR* gene on chromosome 22 and the *ABL* gene on chromosome 9 (the Philadelphia chromosome) in chronic myelogenous leukaemia (CML) or Philadelphia-chromosome positive (Ph+) ALL. Only limited phase I and II studies have been performed in paediatrics and approval for use in children was mainly granted on extrapolating adult data. In CML, imatinib has changed the existing paradigms of treatment with cytarabine/interferon followed by stem-cell transplantation and is now a first-line treatment for this disease, achieving high rates of remissions. Given the relatively recent introduction of BCR-ABL tyrosine kinase inhibitors (TKIs) and the durable exposure to these agents, long-term toxicities need to be carefully monitored. In Ph+ ALL, a recent COG study combining imatinib with chemotherapy showed a clear improvement in outcome for children treated with the combination compared to historical data. Current studies in Ph+ ALL aim to decrease chemotherapy while maintaining cure rates.

Imatinib also inhibits the targets c-Kit, and PDGFR-α and β—a finding which led to its successful introduction in specific solid tumours, notably gastrointestinal stromal tumours and dermatofibrosarcoma protuberans, especially when radical surgery fails. Other disease indications are the Philadelphia-like cases of ALL with fusions of ABL-class kinase genes, including *ABL1, ABL2, CSF1R,* and *PDGFRB* gene fusions. Imatinib is also registered for hypereosinophilic syndrome.

Despite the success story of imatinib in CML, it was quickly apparent that new drugs might also give rise to old problems, in terms of development of resistance, in this case through mutations in *ABL*. These mutations prohibit effective binding of imatinib to the kinase pocket and hence cause resistance. Several second-generation kinase inhibitors are now available, which can still bind despite the presence of a mutation. The best-studied second-generation inhibitor in children is dasatinib. In general, the drug was better tolerated than in adults and appeared effective as salvage treatment in CML and Ph+ ALL, although responses were of short duration in the latter group. Studies with nilotinib and bosutinib are in progress.

Tyrosine kinase inhibitors inhibiting anaplastic lymphoma kinase (ALK)

Anaplastic lymphoma kinase (*ALK*) translocations were initially identified in anaplastic large-cell lymphoma (ALCL), but, more recently, point mutations and amplifications have been discovered in NBL, and translocations in patients with inflammatory myofibroblastic tumours (IMT) (a rare type of sarcoma). Crizotinib is a first-in-class ALK inhibitor, which also inhibits MET and ROS, and was developed in adults with *ALK*-translocated non-small-cell lung cancer (NSCLC). In a paediatric study, the recommended phase II dose was 280 mg/m^2 twice daily—much higher than the approved dose for lung cancer in adults. Anti-tumour activity was outstanding for tumours with *ALK* translocations such as ALCL, NSCLC, and IMT, but disappointingly low for tumours with *ALK* mutations such as NBL. Preclinical evidence suggests that the resistance to *ALK*-mutated NBL can be overcome by more potent inhibitors such as lorlatinib, or combination strategies with other targeted agents or chemotherapy. Further studies of crizotinib and ceritinib (LDK378) have confirmed the positive results for *ALK*-translocated cancers. Important questions relating to long-term safety, CNS penetrance, and secondary resistance mutation development still need to be answered.

Tyrosine kinase inhibitors inhibiting BRAF and MEK

BRAF (serine/threonine-protein kinase B-raf) inhibitors have been successfully developed to treat adults with melanoma harbouring the *BRAF V600E* mutation. While melanomas are very rare in paediatrics, other tumour types harbour the same mutation, which is an oncogenic driver, and these patients have experienced significant benefit from treatment with BRAF inhibitors. Approximately 10% of cases of low- and high-grade glioma have these mutations, as well as a significant proportion of children with Langerhans cell histiocytosis (LCH). Response rates above 60% in patients with heavily pretreated relapsed or refractory *V600E* positive tumours have been shown for dabrafenib, with an acceptable toxicity profile mainly consisting of rash, fever, and arthralgia.

MEK (mitogen-activated protein kinase kinase) is an intracellular kinase downstream of BRAF, with MEK inhibitors developed to overcome resistance to BRAF inhibition in adult patients with melanoma. In addition to paediatric patients with *V600E* mutant cancers, MEK inhibitors have also proven promising in other RAS-driven cancers such as plexiform neurofibroma related to NF1, and might have a role in other tumour types such as gliomas harbouring *BRAF* fusions, NBL, or other tumour types that acquire pathway mutations at relapse. Various leukaemias also carry mutations in the RAS pathway, most typically juvenile myelomonocytic leukaemia (JMML), and need to be studied. So far, three MEK inhibitors have been tested in paediatrics in early clinical trials: selumetinib, trametinib, and cobimetinib. For selumetinib (the first with phase I completed), most common toxic effects included acneiform rash, gastrointestinal effects, and asymptomatic creatine kinase elevation.

Agents targeting signalling pathways relevant to paediatric cancers

Sorafenib

Sorafenib was initially developed as a targeted compound against melanoma given its selectivity against BRAF, especially its mutant variant *V600E*. However, the compound proved to be a multi-target TKI, with broad selectivity against the receptor tyrosine kinases VEGFR-1 and -2, PDGFR, c-KIT, and RET. Sorafenib is active against renal cell carcinoma and hepatocellular carcinoma. In paediatrics, the recommended phase II dose of sorafenib administered every 12 hours continuously for children with solid tumours is 200 mg/m^2/dose and 150 mg/m^2/dose for children with leukaemias. Sorafenib is currently used off-label as a FLT3-inhibitor in combination with chemotherapy in various collaborative group paediatric AML studies, with comparable toxicities observed in children and adults.

Agents targeting epidermal growth factor receptors

Several compounds targeting the epidermal growth factor receptors (EGFRs)—a member of the ErbB family of receptors (EGFR (ErbB-1), HER2/c-neu (ErbB-2), Her 3 (ErbB-3), and Her 4 (ErbB-4))—have been developed in adult oncology, and include monoclonal antibodies and small molecules. FDA approval was obtained for the treatment of patients with NSCLC (gefitinib, afatinib, and erlotinib), colorectal cancer (cetuximab and panitumumab), head and neck cancer (cetuximab), pancreatic cancer (erlotinib), and breast cancer (lapatinib).

The potential role of these compounds in paediatric oncology seems limited to high-grade glioma (HGG) in which *EGFR* overexpression, amplification, or mutation can be found. Erlotinib has been evaluated in a phase I study in children with brain tumours, either as a single agent or with radiotherapy. However, a phase II study in patients with HGG failed to show clear benefit. In a phase I paediatric study, a recommended phase II dose of 900 mg/m^2 twice daily was established for lapatinib. High-level expression of phosphorylated EGFR and ERBB2 receptors was observed particularly in ependymomas, which showed prolonged stable disease on lapatinib. In a phase II study however, activity in medulloblastomas and ependymomas was limited. The failure of the anti-EGFR agents to improve outcome in brain tumours is probably related to limited drug penetration, a low frequency of mutations, and the failure to significantly affect downstream signalling with activation of parallel signalling pathways. Currently, paediatric studies are initiated with afatinib, which aims, in the expansion phase, to limit treatment to a biomarker-selected group of patients and the antibody drug conjugate ABT-414, which is an anti-EGFR antibody linked to an anti-microtubule agent.

Agents targeting insulin growth factor receptors

Various compounds targeting the insulin growth factor receptor IGF1R have been investigated in phase I/II trials in paediatrics, since there is significant preclinical evidence that IGF1R signalling seems to contribute to the malignant behaviour of various sarcomas. At least five different antibodies targeting IGF1R have recently been tested. However, most of these compounds have since been taken off the market as results in adults were not sufficiently convincing. In patients with Ewing sarcoma family of tumours, the objective response rate was around 10% across phase I/II studies, although these patients derived significant benefit since the responses were maintained for several years. In rhabdomyosarcoma, osteosarcoma, synovial sarcoma, and other sarcomas, the response rate was only 2.5%.

Mammalian target of rapamycin (mTOR) inhibitors

Mammalian target of rapamycin (mTOR) inhibitors that are analogues of rapamycin—so-called rapalogues such as sirolimus, everolimus, ridaforolimus, and temsirolimus—are being developed in paediatric oncology in several phase II combination studies. Everolimus was recently approved for use in children with unresectable subependymal giant-cell astrocytoma.

Epigenetic agents

An area of active clinical research is the inhibition of histone deacetylases (HDACs), which is thought to re-activate silenced tumour suppressor pathways. HDAC inhibitors have been widely investigated preclinically *in vitro* and *in vivo*, and showed positive results for leukaemia, CNS tumours, and NBL. Both vorinostat and panobinostat have entered paediatric phase I studies. Another strategy comprises hypomethylating agents such as decitabine and azacitidine, which are being tested in paediatric trials for myelodysplastic syndromes, AML, and some solid tumours. The inhibition of BET (Bromodomain and extra-terminal) proteins to target *MYC*-amplified tumours is another strategy. BET is an important transcription factor of the MYC family of proteins. However, BET inhibitors have still not entered paediatric clinical trials.

Agents against tumour microenvironment and angiogenesis

Several strategies have been developed to interfere with the process of tumour angiogenesis. Such compounds may decrease signalling through VEGF/VEGFR by inhibiting either the ligand VEGF or one of the receptors of VEGF (flt-1, KDR, flt-4), or inhibit the signalling pathways through PDGF and its receptors (PDGFRα and β).

The antibody bevacizumab (Avastin®) was the first to demonstrate clinical proof of principle, and has been approved for use in adults. A paediatric phase I trial was conducted by the COG, with bevacizumab administered intravenously every two weeks in 28-day courses in children with solid tumours. No dose-limiting toxicities were observed; adverse events included infusion reaction, rash, mucositis, proteinuria, and lymphocytopenia. Randomized trials have shown that the addition of bevacizumab in combination with standard chemotherapy did not improve survival in metastatic soft tissue sarcoma and HGG. A randomized phase II trial in NBL continues recruiting and results will soon be available. Other more potent inhibitors—VEGFR tyrosine kinase inhibitors such as axitinib, pazopanib, and lenvatinib (as opposed to bevacizumab which is a monoclonal antibody against VEGF)—are being evaluated in paediatrics.

Monoclonal antibodies and immunotherapy

Monoclonal antibodies in haematological malignancies

Several antibodies are being tested in various stages of development. Rituximab, a chimeric naked anti-CD20 monoclonal antibody, has been used in salvage treatment for CD20-positive NHL, in combination with ICE (ifosfamide, carboplatin, etoposide). In a phase II window study in 136 children with newly diagnosed Burkitt lymphoma or diffuse large B-cell NHL, rituximab was well tolerated, with a response rate of 41.4%. Recently, results of a phase III trial with rituximab added to chemotherapy in frontline high-risk B-NHL became available, and randomization was stopped as the experimental arm with rituximab showed a clinically meaningful improvement for EFS of 84% in the standard chemotherapy arm versus 95% in the rituximab plus chemotherapy arm.

Gemtuzumab ozogamicin (GO), an anti-CD33 antibody linked to the cytotoxic compound calicheamicin, has been tested as a single agent or in combination with standard chemotherapy in relapsed/refractory and upfront paediatric AML. Despite clear efficacy in early clinical studies, GO was recently taken off the market outside Japan, but regained approval, given that studies in upfront adult AML have shown evidence of benefit using a fractionated schedule of GO in combination with chemotherapy. Of interest is the development of a combination of an anti-CD22 antibody linked to calicheamicin (inotuzumab ozogamicin), which will be evaluated in paediatric ALL, following studies in adult ALL showing improved remission induction and survival rates compared to standard-of-care chemotherapy.

Epratuzumab is a naked antibody directed against CD22, which is being tested in a randomized fashion in standard-risk relapsed ALL in the IntReALL study. This follows an initial single-arm phase I/II study in North America in which it was combined with reinduction chemotherapy in relapsed ALL, which showed tolerance and suggested an improved MRD response.

Blinatumomab is an example of a BITE (bispecific T-cell engaging) antibody, linking CD19 expressed on B-cell precursor ALL cells to CD3 expressed on T-cells. Results of a phase I/II study have recently been reported: among the 70 patients who received the recommended dosage, 39% achieved complete remission within the first two cycles, 52% of whom were MRD-negative. The most frequent grade 3 or higher adverse events were anaemia (36%), thrombocytopenia (21%), and hypokalaemia (17%). Four patients had a grade 3 or higher cytokine-release syndrome. Two patients interrupted treatment after grade 2 seizures. Blinatumomab is now being studied in relapsed and upfront ALL trials.

Brentuximab vedotin is a conjugated antibody linking a chimeric anti-CD30 antibody to the antimitotic agent monomethyl auristatin E (MMAE), and has been studied in paediatric Hodgkin lymphoma (HL) and ALCL, diseases in which CD30 is expressed. The first results in paediatric HL show that Brentuximab vedotin 1.8 mg/kg every three weeks (RP2D) was generally well tolerated and demonstrated preliminary evidence of activity, with an objective response rate of 64%. Based on these data, brentuximab vedotin is now being studied in newly diagnosed HL in a COG study, and brentuximab vedotin and crizotinib in combination with standard chemotherapy, in upfront ALCL.

Anti-GD2 monoclonal antibodies in neuroblastoma

The first monoclonal antibodies that specifically targeted the disialoganglioside GD2 on tumour cells of neuroectodermal origin entered clinical trials in 1992. In addition to being identified in virtually all NBL, GD2 expression has also been identified in other tumour types such as soft-tissue sarcomas, Ewing sarcoma, osteosarcomas, small-cell lung cancers, and melanoma. The chimeric anti-GD2 monoclonal antibody dinutuximab entered paediatric phase I trials both in Europe and USA shortly after development. The COG phase III study (ANBL0032) demonstrated significant improvement of overall survival with immunotherapy using dinutuximab in combination with IL2 and GM-CSF compared with standard therapy. The SIOPEN group has developed another antibody called dinutuximab-beta that is given in a long-term infusion and appears to have more tolerable side effects. The role of other cytokines such as IL2 or GM-CSF has still not been established and efforts continue to identify more tolerable regimens to administer immunotherapy with anti-GD2 monoclonal antibodies.

Immunotherapy

The CTLA4 inhibitor ipilimumab and the checkpoint inhibitors (anti-PD1 and anti-PD-L1) are discussed elsewhere in this book (Chapter xx).

Miscellaneous

Differentiation induction, resulting in a maturation of tumour cells, has been utilized as a strategy both in acute promyelocytic leukaemia (APL) and in NBL. In APL, the value of all-*trans* retinoic acid (ATRA) is mainly in reducing early death by quickly diminishing the bleeding tendency that is characteristic of this disease. Current studies in APL are focusing on the combination of ATRA with arsenic trioxide, which showed improved results compared to combined ATRA and chemotherapy regimens. Moreover, data from the use of 13-*cis*-retinoic acid in NBL, given in a MRD setting, now shows clear evidence of survival benefit.

Another interesting compound is the recombinant human arginase BCT-100, designed to interfere with the arginine addiction of tumour cells, which will be studied in paediatric malignancies in the near future.

Finally, compounds inhibiting proteins involved in apoptosis regulation (BCL-2, survivin) are also being explored in preclinical paediatric tumour models. There is so far no firm paediatric clinical experience with these compounds, but a paediatric phase I/II basket trial with the BCL-2 inhibitor venetoclax is imminent.

FURTHER READING

Adamson PC, et al. (2014) Drug discovery in paediatric oncology: roadblocks to progress. *Nat Rev Clin Oncol* **11**(12), 732–9.

Cheymol G (2000) Effects of obesity on pharmacokinetics: implications for drug therapy. *Clin Pharmacokinet* **39**, 215–31.

European Medicines Agency (2018) *Annual Report 2017*. Available at: www.ema.europa.eu.

Gore L, et al. (2013) Targeting developmental pathways in children with cancer: what price success? *Lancet Oncol* **14**, e70–8.

Haidar C, Jeha S (2011) Drug interactions in childhood cancer. *Lancet Oncol* **12**, 92–9.

Hanahan D, Weinberg RA (2011) Hallmarks of cancer: the next generation. *Cell* **144**, 646–74.

Hirsch S, et al. (2015) Targeted approaches to childhood cancer: progress in drug discovery and development. *Expert Opin Drug Discov* **10**, 483–95.

Kearns GL, et al. (2003) Developmental pharmacology—drug disposition, action, and therapy in infants and children. *N Engl J Med* **349**, 1157–67.

Lee DP, et al. (2005) Pediatric phase I trials in oncology: an analysis of study conduct efficiency. *J Clin Oncol* **23**, 8431–41.

Mossé YP, et al. (2013) Safety and activity of crizotinib for paediatric patients with refractory solid tumours or anaplastic large-cell lymphoma: a COG phase 1 consortium study. *Lancet Oncol* **14**, 472–80.

Norris RE, Adamson PC (2012) Challenges and opportunities in childhood cancer drug development. *Nat Rev Cancer* **12**, 776–82.

Panetta JC, et al. (2003) The importance of pharmacokinetic limited sampling models for childhood cancer drug development. *Clin Cancer Res* **9**, 5068–77.

Pearson AD, et al. (2016) Implementation of mechanism of action biology-driven early drug development for children with cancer. *Eur J Cancer* **62**, 124–31.

Schultz KR, et al. (2009) Improved early event-free survival with imatinib in Philadelphia chromosome-positive acute lymphoblastic leukemia: a COG study. *J Clin Oncol* **27**, 5175–81.

Van den Berg H, et al. (2012) Cytostatic drugs in infants: a review on pharmacokinetic data in infants. *Cancer Treat Rev* **38**, 3–26.

Vassal G, et al. (2013) New drugs for children and adolescents with cancer: the need for novel development pathways. *Lancet Oncol* **14**, e117–24.

Vassal G, et al. (2013) Is the European pediatric medicine regulation working for children and adolescents with cancer? *Clin Cancer Res* **19**, 1315–25.

Von Stackelberg A, et al. (2016) Phase I/phase II study of blinatumomab in pediatric patients with relapsed/refractory acute lymphoblastic leukemia. *J Clin Oncol* **34**, 4381–9.

Yu AL, et al. (2010) Anti-GD2 antibody with GM-CSF, interleukin-2, and isotretinoin for neuroblastoma. *N Engl J Med* **363**, 1324–34.

Zwaan CM, et al. (2013) Dasatinib in children and adolescents with relapsed or refractory leukemia: results of the CA180-018 phase I dose-escalation study of the Innovative Therapies for Children With Cancer Consortium. *J Clin Oncol* **31**, 2460–8.

4

Radiotherapy in Paediatric Oncology

Mark Gaze and Tom Boterberg

Introduction

Radiotherapy is a key component of treatment for many childhood cancers. The role is usually to improve local control, which may often enhance the probability of survival, but in some cases additionally it is part of a curative strategy for metastatic disease. Radiotherapy may also be used in the salvage of relapsed patients and for palliation.

The patient's pathway through radiotherapy

Treatment centres

Children should only receive radiotherapy in centres suitably equipped, staffed, and experienced in paediatric radiotherapy, supported by the necessary paediatric backup facilities. This includes radiation oncologists with training and experience in paediatric radiotherapy fully integrated into the core paediatric oncology multidisciplinary team, the availability of play specialists and paediatric anaesthetic facilities, and sufficient on-site paediatric support to deal with emergencies. This may mean that some children cannot receive treatment in the radiotherapy centre closest to their homes. It will need to be explained to families that this inconvenience is offset by improved safety and quality.

Decision making

It is essential that radiation oncologists meet regularly with paediatric haematology and oncology colleagues, radiologists, pathologists, and surgeons to discuss the management of all patients in the light of full diagnostic and prognostic information.

While the decision to treat with radiotherapy is often straightforward, in many cases it is not simple, and discussion is vital. Children with cancer should be treated where possible in appropriate clinical trials, and outside trials, radiotherapy should be given according to approved guidelines.

Assessment

The initial consultation will help to make it clear that radiotherapy is an important part of treatment, and confirm that the radiotherapy team is part of the overall team caring for the child. An early introduction to the radiotherapy team is important as it may prevent the family from feeling that radiotherapy is an afterthought, or has been suggested because things have not gone according to plan. A frank discussion should help to allay any misunderstandings about radiotherapy. Early familiarity with the team will reduce subsequent anxieties, and will help to prevent the problems which can arise after delayed referral.

An important part of the initial assessment is to decide whether it is likely that the child will be able to cooperate with the radiotherapy team, be able to tolerate the requirements of immobilization while awake, and feel comfortable being left alone in the treatment room. Some time spent with a radiotherapy play specialist can transform an initially scared and uncooperative child into one who happily complies with treatment. If not, arrangements will have to be made for preparations and treatment under general anaesthesia.

Informed consent

It is important that families receive accurate and complete information about the indications for, practicalities of, and likely early and late side effects of the radiotherapy required. This should be given verbally by members of the radiotherapy team, and be supplemented by written information. Children should be given relevant information in a sensitive and age-appropriate manner, which may include comics or videos. Families speaking other languages should have the services of an interpreter available at every interaction with the radiotherapy team. Children and their families should have an opportunity for their questions to be answered in full and in an unhurried manner. Often, if there are anxieties about radiotherapy, it is recommended that families have more than one opportunity to discuss the information and ask questions. Finally, the receipt of informed consent for radiotherapy treatment should be documented according to local practice.

Positioning and immobilization

It is essential for the accurate and safe delivery of radiotherapy that the patient does not move during imaging for planning, or during treatment. As indicated above, this may require the use of daily general anaesthesia. For young children who are to be treated awake, the input of an experienced play specialist in the preparation can be indispensable. To minimize movement, an immobilization device may be necessary, for example a head and neck shell fixed to a base board. This will ensure accurate reproducibility of set-up on a daily basis.

Imaging and target volume definition

The art of radiotherapy is to ensure that all areas involved by tumour get an adequate radiation dose, while uninvolved normal tissues receive as little radiation as possible, in order to minimize the risk of adverse effects. To achieve this, a series of targets is defined on the basis of imaging which is interpreted in the light of the known pathology and likely patterns of spread, and natural barriers. Usually, prior to radiotherapy, a CT scan is performed in the radiotherapy department with the patient immobilized in the treatment position. Intravenous contrast may be required. The images obtained can be fused with other imaging, for example MRI or PET scans, which define the extent of tumour at critical times such as at diagnosis, following induction chemotherapy, or following surgery. Sometimes, if the tumour or normal organs may move with the respiratory cycle, a movie loop with four dimensional CT (4DCT) is performed to allow the variable position to be demonstrated and taken into account accurately.

The first step in target volume definition is usually to define the gross tumour volume (GTV) by contouring it, slice by slice, on the planning CT scan. Even if the tumour has shrunk as a result of chemotherapy, it may still be helpful to outline the original GTV on earlier scans. When this volume is then transferred to the radiotherapy planning CT scan, it indicates the area at risk of recurrence. The GTV will then be expanded into a clinical target volume (CTV). The CTV includes the original tumour volume plus a margin to encompass any subclinical extension of disease. The CTV margin may be cut back to natural barriers of spread, such as the skull in the case of brain tumours, or if previously displaced uninvolved normal organs like the liver have returned to their normal position following treatment of the tumour with chemotherapy and surgery. The CTV is then expanded by another margin to create the planning target volume (PTV), which takes into account errors and uncertainties in planning and set-up, and internal and external motion. The margin between CTV and PTV will depend on the anatomical site and accuracy of immobilization as determined by departmental audit.

It is also necessary to outline organs at risk so that dosimetrists and planning systems can limit the dose received by healthy normal tissues, especially those that are most sensitive to adverse effects from radiation.

It is good practice, if possible, for volumes to be checked and approved by another experienced clinician. This may be done within one centre, or remotely as part of a clinical trial quality assurance programme.

Planning and dosimetry

Dosimetrists, working under the guidance of the responsible doctors, will prepare treatment plans, which indicate how the treatment will be delivered, and the doses received by the tumour and normal tissues. Plans should take into account the need to give homogenous irradiation to the PTV while minimizing exposure to organs at risk.

Dose volume histograms (DVHs) that show the planned dose to the target volumes and relevant organs at risk should be produced. These allow the doctor to check that the target is receiving full irradiation, and that doses to organs at risk are acceptable. Sometimes achievement of these two things is not practicable. A compromise is then needed with part or all of the PTV receiving less than the ideal radiotherapy dose and/or organs at risk receiving more than is usually recommended. The doctor then approves the best plan, and the DVHs document the doses received as a guide to follow-up.

Prospective radiotherapy quality assurance, with review of treatment plans by other clinicians, is increasingly being introduced in clinical trials.

Dose prescription and fractionation

The clinician will specify the total dose to the tumour and the number of fractions in the course (hence the dose per fraction), the course duration, and the type of radiation and its energy. Typically in paediatric radiotherapy, a dose per fraction of 1.5 to 1.8 Gy is used, smaller than the 2 to 2.67 Gy fraction sizes often used in adult practice. This is because smaller fraction sizes allow better sparing of vulnerable normal tissue from late effects. Normally, treatments are given once each day, five days per week.

There is evidence that prolongation of the overall treatment time may compromise outcome. Compensation should therefore be made for any gap so that the overall treatment time does not exceed that intended. The simplest and best ways of doing this are to treat on days which are normally days off (for example, treat on Saturdays around public holidays) or to give two treatments per day, with a minimum inter-fraction interval of six hours.

In some cases, hyperfractionated (a larger number of smaller fractions than standard) and accelerated (given in a shorter than standard overall time) schedules are used to reduce late effects and overcome repopulation in highly proliferative tumours. This requires more than one treatment a day, and the inter-fraction interval should be at least six hours, preferably eight hours for radical brain treatments. In other cases, hypofractionation (a smaller number of larger than standard fractions) is used for stereotactically guided treatment of small volumes or in palliation.

Verification of treatment accuracy

It is important that radiotherapy is delivered to the highest possible standards. Quality assurance procedures for radiotherapy delivery, particularly geometric variation for set-up errors, are essential. This is usually done with electronic portal imaging or integrated (cone beam) CT scanning. Dose verification may be done with *in vivo* dosimetry, and is recommended as an additional quality assurance measure.

Supportive care

The blood count should be checked before treatment. Irradiation of anaemic children should be avoided, as anaemia is known to compromise the outcome of radiotherapy. If necessary, a blood transfusion should be given to bring the haemoglobin up to 120 g/l. Nausea and vomiting can usually be prevented by the use of antiemetics. Radiotherapy may cause loss of appetite, and nutrition is important, especially in children receiving daily general anaesthesia. The advice of a paediatric dietician and nutritional supplements, nasogastric or gastrostomy feeding, or even total parenteral nutrition may be needed.

Radiotherapy can be stressful for children, their parents, and other family members. This can have both a psychological and practical basis. Psychological supportive care for the family can be very beneficial. Travelling for radiotherapy, or staying away from home, can be expensive. Availability of (free) family accommodation in a nearby hotel or dedicated hostel for children and young people with cancer is ideal. Families should have access to support from social workers or other appropriate healthcare professionals who can advise on benefits and other practical issues.

Documentation

It is important that there is a summary of radiotherapy treatment, which is accessible to treating paediatric oncologists and is also available in long-term follow-up. This should include adequate patient identifiers and sufficient details of the diagnosis and other principal treatments (i.e. chemotherapy and surgery) to allow it to be read in context.

Follow-up

It is important that the patient is followed up in the long term with regard to late effects as well as for local tumour control and survival. Periodic assessments of relevant normal organ function should be systematically documented. Appropriate psychosocial support should be available as the child grows up and reaches maturity, to answer questions that might arise and to address proactively other survivorship issues.

Types of radiotherapy

Conventional external beam radiotherapy

The technical aspects of radiotherapy are evolving continuously, so it is difficult to define what might be considered 'conventional' or standard therapy compared with what is historic and what is innovative. Advances in diagnostic imaging and computer science have largely led this progress.

Nowadays, conventional radiotherapy usually implies the use of:

- megavoltage photons (or sometimes electrons for superficial lesions) from a linear accelerator;
- target volume definition based on images acquired on a CT simulator;
- three-dimensional planning with two or more shaped beams in the same plane or in several planes to allow conformal treatment of an irregular volume.

Intensity-modulated radiotherapy

Intensity-modulated radiotherapy (IMRT) is a way of changing the dose distribution of radiation in tissue by using beams where the amount of energy varies in different parts of the beam. The aim is to achieve the best possible dose distribution, especially where the target has a complex shape and there are adjacent critical structures. This can be achieved in a number of ways of increasing complexity.

The use of additional smaller segment fields to supplement a principal field, or field-in-field boost, is a relatively straightforward method for forward-planned IMRT to reduce non-homogeneity of the delivered dose within a target volume. Inverse-planned IMRT requires the clinical oncologist to define target volumes and organs at risk, as with conventional conformal radiotherapy, and to specify the desired target dose and constraints on the dose which an organ at risk may be allowed to receive. The planning computer used by the dosimetrist then calculates the best field arrangement to deliver this. This usually uses a larger than conventional number, often five or seven, of beam alignments which may be non-co-planar. A step-and-shoot approach entails movements of the linear accelerator gantry and multi-leaf collimator between the delivery of each treatment field. Alternatively, a sliding-window technique is used, where the leaves move during delivery of one beam, instead of being placed at several fixed positions before irradiation starts, as in step-and-shoot mode. A more sophisticated delivery, intensity-modulated arc therapy, involves dynamic gantry and multi-leaf collimator movements with the beam on, and is becoming more widely available.

Whatever form of IMRT is used, the result is to better conform the shape of the high-dose volume to the shape of the target, and to diminish the volume of healthy normal tissue that is incidentally included in the high-dose volume. The price of this is usually low-dose irradiation of a much larger volume of normal tissue than is the case with conventional radiotherapy.

There have been concerns that the low-dose bath effect seen with IMRT may result in a greater number of second cancers than has been the case with conventional radiotherapy. These anxieties have sometimes limited the use of IMRT in children. However, IMRT does allow full irradiation of the tumour in some circumstances where, with conventional radiotherapy, it has been necessary to compromise the dose to the tumour in order to respect normal tissue tolerance. Also, it has been recognized that most second cancers occur in or adjacent to the high-dose volume (which is usually significantly smaller with IMRT compared with conventional radiotherapy) rather than in the low-dose area, so the hazards of using IMRT in children may have been overstated. Furthermore, emerging long-term follow-up data have been reassuring. As always in paediatric radiotherapy, it is important to weigh up the likely benefits and potential risks of any proposed treatment very carefully, and make a balanced judgement of what is in the child's best interests.

Stereotactic radiotherapy

Stereotactic radiotherapy has been used for quite some time to treat small intracranial lesions. Accuracy of treatment of small volumes with narrow margins is achieved with the use of a fixed headframe (for a single treatment or radiosurgery) or relocatable headframe (for fractionated courses of treatment).

More recently, interest has developed in stereotactic body radiotherapy for small lesions in, for example, the lungs or liver. As external frames would not be helpful, image guidance is used to ensure accuracy of treatment delivery. Hypofractionated or single treatments are used, rather than fully fractionated courses of treatment. So far there has been only limited use of stereotactic body radiotherapy in children.

Image-guided and adaptive radiotherapy

The term image-guided radiotherapy (IGRT) is potentially misleading, as target volume definition has been based on imaging for years. IGRT refers instead to the use of imaging equipment integrated into treatment units to ensure accurate delivery of treatment. The position of the target may be indicated by implanted fiducial markers or by normal anatomy. Imaging, which may simply be orthogonal radiographs or more sophisticated cone beam CT images, is used with each fraction of treatment to ensure that the irradiated volume covers the target volume, which may move during (as with respiration) or between treatments.

Adaptive radiotherapy implies the ability to change the irradiated volume during a course of treatment in response to a change in the target volume. It is dependent on image guidance, and is so far little used in paediatric radiotherapy. Linear accelerators with integrated MRI are being developed, which may in due course bring greater accuracy to IGRT and adaptive radiotherapy.

Proton beam radiotherapy

This is a form of particle radiotherapy using high-energy protons produced by a cyclotron or synchro-cyclotron. The advantage lies in the dose distribution that can be achieved with protons. Unlike photons which are exponentially attenuated as they pass through tissue, protons travel for a finite distance, and deposit most of their energy towards the end of their path, the Bragg peak. This means that it is possible to spare, theoretically completely, normal tissues beyond the target.

In the treatment of relatively radio-resistant well-defined skull base tumours, cure rates may be increased as higher doses can be delivered to the target with effective sparing of adjacent critical structures like the brainstem. In other circumstances, the dose distributions that can be achieved with protons are advantageous because the dose to normal tissues for a given target dose can be reduced, thereby limiting normal tissue toxicity.

Although proton beam therapy has a long history, there is very little level-one evidence of benefit in the patient's outcome in comparison with photon radiotherapy. Most of the case for the use of proton beam therapy has been made from theoretical predictions. However, with the increasing use of proton radiotherapy in selected patients, more outcome data (in relation to both disease control and late effects) are emerging, and support its use, although also some unexpected toxicity has been described (e.g. brainstem necrosis in patients treated for CNS tumours). Although the availability of proton beam therapy has been limited, an increasing number of centres are being opened, and soon it should be available in most large developed nations. As with photon-based radiotherapy, technical advances in proton beam therapy equipment, including spot scanning (as opposed to passive scattering) and improved image guidance, have allowed the development of intensity-modulated proton therapy, which should be more advantageous.

Brachytherapy

Brachytherapy, with direct implantation of radioactive sources, was a valuable form of treatment decades ago. Interest waned with the introduction of the linear accelerator, which made treatment of deeply seated tumours much easier, with the increasing awareness of radiation protection hazards, and the difficulties of achieving a perfect geometrical implant. With the development of machines for remote afterloading of implanted catheters, the radiation protection risks have largely been overcome. The ability to use CT- and MRI-based planning with varying position and dwell times for the source has reduced the need for perfect geometry. These technical advances have led to a resurgence of interest in brachytherapy in paediatric oncology. In some childhood cancers, brachytherapy allows conformal irradiation of small target volumes with greater sparing of normal tissues than is possible with external beam radiotherapy.

Molecular radiotherapy

This is essentially the use of radiotherapy as a drug. It is possible where a metabolic pathway can be used to allow accumulation of a radionuclide within tumour cells. For example, in patients with well-differentiated thyroid cancer of follicular cell origin, radioactive iodine (^{131}I) can be biologically targeted into residual normal thyroid tissue and metastases. In children, lymph node and distant metastases are more common than in adults with thyroid cancer, yet thanks to the use of radioactive iodine this is a highly curable disease.

In neuroblastoma, the catecholamine analogue meta-iodobenzylguanidine (mIBG) can be used for diagnostic scintigraphy (^{123}I-mIBG) and for therapy (^{131}I-mIBG). Therapeutic mIBG is recognized as an established palliative treatment, and it may also have value if used intensively in patients with refractory disease as part of a multi-modality strategy for cure.

Additional types of molecular radiotherapy are being evaluated in clinical trials.

Side effects of treatment

Factors affecting radiation injury to normal tissues

The incidence and severity of adverse reactions to radiotherapy among children treated for cancer are related to several factors, knowledge of which allows new strategies to be devised that may reduce adverse effects without compromising the chances of cure. These factors include whether or not radiotherapy is used at all, the total dose used, the dose per fraction, the volume and type of tissue irradiated, the type of radiation used, the use of concomitant chemotherapy, and, not least, the age of the patient at the time of treatment.

Early side effects

Early or acute side effects occur during, or in the first weeks after, radiotherapy. They are usually the result of the depletion of stem cells in the healthy tissue surrounding the tumour area to be irradiated. In most cases they subside with time or supportive therapy only, although some of them may be life-threatening and require early interruption of therapy.

The most common early side effects are skin reactions (like erythema and alopecia) and mucositis (like stomatitis, oesophagitis, cystitis, and diarrhoea), all depending of the site of the body being treated. Nausea and vomiting may occur in case of abdominal irradiation. Fatigue is a general and frequently encountered early effect which may take several months to resolve. Many of these side effects can also be aggravated by the concurrent use of chemotherapy, especially actinomycin and anthracyclines. Subsequent chemotherapy may even mimic the cutaneous side effects of radiotherapy at sites where radiation previously entered the body, the so-called 'radiation recall' reaction, requiring appropriate care and explanation to the parents.

Late side effects

Late side effects are defined as toxicity occurring or persisting from three months onwards after radiotherapy. They are usually irreversible and sometimes worsen with time. Therefore, all care should be given to prevent this type of side effect. On the other hand, some of these side effects are very difficult to prevent and should be considered as 'the price to be paid' for cure. Finding the right balance is a huge challenge for doctors, patients, and their parents.

Late central nervous system side effects

Although the number of neurons usually does not increase after birth, the brain matures by the development and branching of axons and the formation of new synapses. This process mostly takes place within the first three years of life and is almost complete by the age of six, although it continues at a much lower rate till the end of puberty. Radiotherapy may affect this process by killing astrocytes and oligodendrocytes, thus causing demyelinization. Radiotherapy also affects vascular endothelial cells. Mostly these effects are irreversible, although sometimes a transient somnolence syndrome is seen. This is characterized by drowsiness, apathy, and irritability, and usually occurs one to two months after the end of treatment. It is self-limiting within 12 weeks of its onset.

Even at rather low doses, whole brain irradiation may lead to functional disturbances in the brain, although no obvious structural changes can be observed. The most common side effects are neurocognitive deficits: lower IQ, worse short-term memory, lower speed of processing new information, and concentration difficulties. In medulloblastoma, safe replacement of craniospinal irradiation by chemotherapy has proved challenging. Despite its risk for late central nervous systems (CNS) side effects, craniospinal irradiation is still standard treatment for older children, and parents should be well informed about this. Chemotherapy can be used to allow postponing radiotherapy until the child is of a more suitable age to receive radiotherapy to the brain. Proton beam therapy is of particular value in treating small localized brain tumours, with less irradiation of non-target healthy brain tissue than is possible with photon techniques. However, it should be noted that the neurocognitive deficits are usually limited if small volumes are treated, even at high doses and in small children.

High doses or re-irradiation may lead to brain necrosis. This may develop years after treatment and may even mimic tumour recurrence. Steroids are commonly used for treatment, and in some cases resection may be necessary to stop the process. Concurrent radiosensitizing chemotherapy increases the risk of developing brain necrosis. Necrosis of the spinal cord is a very serious complication leading to irreversible paralysis. Fortunately it is only very rarely encountered as great care is taken to keep the dose to the spinal cord within safe limits.

Radiotherapy may damage blood vessels, and this in turn can lead to neurotoxicity. Patients with neurofibromatosis type 1 are at increased risk. Moya moya may lead to strokes. Cavernous haemangiomas or cavernomas are being recognized increasingly commonly after brain radiotherapy. Usually these are incidental findings on surveillance MRI scans. Sometimes a cavernoma may bleed into the brain. This may be either a minor bleed without overt brain damage or, rarely, a catastrophic haemorrhage with resulting neurodisability or death.

Late renal side effects

Acute renal side effects are usually rare, but long-term effects may be important and include chronic renal failure, hypertension, and anaemia. The development of these conditions is insidious and takes several years after treatment. Careful follow-up of patients who received abdominal radiotherapy is therefore very important. Concurrent chemotherapy like cisplatin or previous surgery to the kidney may necessitate lowering the dose, at least to part of the kidney. In patients who have undergone nephrectomy, special attention is needed to spare the contralateral kidney as much as possible, not only to preserve its function per se, but also not to hinder the compensatory hypertrophy.

Late musculoskeletal and soft-tissue side effects

In adults, muscles and bones are very radio-resistant. In children, muscles and bones are in full development and these dividing tissues are therefore very sensitive to radiation, especially the epiphyseal growth plates. A dose around 12–15 Gy will impair the chondroblast function and have an adverse effect on bone growth. It is clear that there is not a threshold dose, and the degree of growth impairment is related to the age of the child, the volume of bone irradiated, and the dose given. Avascular necrosis is also possible, and the risk is higher if concurrent steroids are to be given. The effect on growth is usually greatest following the onset of puberty, when the growth spurt starts. Disproportion between body parts may not only have functional implications but also leads to psychological and social problems.

Spinal irradiation will result in shorter height, but may also be accompanied by deformities. Even if all care has been taken to uniformly irradiate the involved vertebrae, flank surgery and radiation-induced hypoplasia of the unilateral paraspinal and abdominal muscles may contribute to the development of scoliosis. Partial irradiation of the head and neck region can lead to facial bone hypoplasia and consequent asymmetry of the face. When growth is complete, plastic surgery may sometimes be used to improve cosmetic appearances. Radiation-induced impaired dental development may be aggravated by an increased risk of dental caries if xerostomia develops after irradiation of the salivary glands higher than 25–30 Gy.

Thoracic irradiation including the breast bud, or the developing breast in pubertal girls, may lead to hypoplasia. Plastic surgery for breast augmentation to restore symmetry may be considered once growth is complete. Irradiation of the developing breast raises the risk of breast cancer developing subsequently. Patients at risk should have screening performed as part of their long-term follow-up from an earlier age than is standard for breast cancer screening.

Late pulmonary side effects

Radiation pneumonitis usually develops between three and six months after radiotherapy. Cough and dyspnoea are the most common symptoms, and diffuse infiltrates can be seen on imaging. If no spontaneous remission occurs, steroid treatment may be needed. In some cases, pneumonitis will lead to lung fibrosis, although fibrosis can also be seen without preceding pneumonitis. Whole-lung irradiation to doses of 15 Gy is considered safe and without clinically important consequences, although lung function tests usually reveal some degree of restrictive disease at adult age. Bleomycin, actinomycin, and busulfan are radiosensitizing chemotherapeutic agents and should be avoided or only used with great care in combination with radiotherapy on the lungs. Anaesthetists should be aware of oxygen toxicity in patients treated with bleomycin and radiotherapy. Obviously, smoking should be firmly discouraged, but especially following lung radiotherapy.

Late cardiac side effects

Severe cardiac damage, including cardiomyopathy, valvular disease, and myocardial infarction, has been seen in the past, especially in patients treated for Hodgkin lymphoma. However, it should be noted that these patients had large volumes (often nearly the whole heart) treated with high doses, up to 45 Gy or higher. Currently, the use of radiotherapy has been reduced, as have volume and dose. Nowadays, the main reason for cardiac toxicity is probably not the dose to the ventricles (which may, in part, tolerate doses of 50 Gy or more) but to the valves and coronary arteries. Even much lower doses may still affect subsequent cardiac function, and the mean heart dose should be kept as low as reasonably achieveable. Following incidental cardiac irradiation, patients should be encouraged to have a healthy life style with enough physical exercise, regular blood pressure checks, and without smoking or excessive intake of fatty food. Finally, the use of anthracyclines also plays a role in the development of cardiomyopathy.

Late endocrine side effects

Most endocrine deficiencies result from irradiation of the hypothalamic–hypophyseal axis. They may develop very insidiously and years after radiotherapy, so close follow-up is necessary. Doses as low as 18 Gy can be sufficient to impair growth hormone secretion after a period of 18 months or two years. Above 36 Gy, growth hormone secretion may be totally stopped; and at doses above 40 Gy, other hormones like adrenocorticotropic hormone (ACTH), thyrotropin-releasing hormone (TRH), and the gonadotrophins may be affected. Hyperprolactinaemia and early puberty may also develop. Hormone replacement therapy should be started as soon as it is judged safe.

Radiotherapy above about 20 Gy to the thyroid gland increases the risk of primary hypothyroidism. In patients treated with doses around 40 Gy, the risk of developing hypothyroidism is as high as 50%. Even compensated hypothyroidism, where the thyroid-stimulating hormone (TSH) is elevated but the T3 and T4 are within the normal range, should be treated with thyroid hormone replacement therapy to reduce the risk of a raised TSH level over a prolonged period, stimulating the development of thyroid cancer.

Late side effects on fertility

Spermatogenesis is especially radiosensitive. A dose as low as 15 cGy (0.15 Gy) is enough to result in a reversible reduction of the sperm count, and permanent sterilization has been observed at cumulative doses of 1–2 Gy. Small fractionated doses seem to be more toxic than a single fraction dose. Therefore adequate shielding of the testicles from radiation, for example during pelvic radiotherapy, should be undertaken if possible. A dose above 10 Gy usually results in permanent azoospermia. If possible and indicated, semen cryopreservation or testicle biopsy cryopreservation should be organized in (post-) pubertal boys before any radiotherapy starts. Testosterone production by the Leydig cells is usually not affected by doses below 20 Gy.

In girls, permanent sterility can be seen at an ovarian dose of 8 Gy or higher. Hormonal deficit develops from 12 Gy onwards and is usually permanent above 20 Gy. Until some years ago, avoiding irradiation of the ovaries or oophoropexy (surgical relocation of the ovary outside the irradiated volume) were the only possibilities to protect the ovarian function in prepubertal girls who needed radiotherapy to the pelvic region. Partial ovarian cryopreservation and follicle cryopreservation are new techniques that may allow preservation of fertility. However, even partial irradiation of the uterus results in a higher risk of intra-uterine death, stillbirth, or a child with a low birthweight, due to the uterus or cervix being partially less well developed. Sometimes treatment does not lead to complete infertility, but female survivors of childhood cancer may have their reproductive period reduced by premature ovarian failure and an early menopause. This should be discussed with young women attending long-term follow-up clinics.

Late ocular side effects

The radiosensitivity of the eye depends on which part is irradiated. The retina and optic pathways are relatively resistant and may tolerate doses of 45 to 54 Gy without major toxicity. Dose constraints of 45 Gy for the retina, 50 Gy for the optic nerves, and 54 Gy for the optic chiasm, are often specified. Above 54 Gy, optic neuritis and permanent blindness may develop. By contrast, the lens is very radiosensitive and cataract formation may occur after doses as low as 2–6 Gy. However, lens replacement is an effective and safe treatment for these patients. Irradiation of the lacrimal gland may result in dry eye syndrome, a very painful condition that may require enucleation. The dose constraints are not very clear: 40 Gy is considered as acceptable, although less than 26 Gy to 50% of the volume is probably safer.

Late hepatic side effects

The tolerance of the liver for hepatitis and liver failure due to atrophy and the development of fibrosis depends on the total dose, the volume, concurrent chemotherapy, and previous surgery. A mean dose of 30 Gy to the entire liver can be safe if part of it (at least 25%) receives a dose of 10 Gy or less and no previous surgery was performed or concurrent chemotherapy is needed. After partial hepatectomy, irradiation of the regenerating liver should be performed with great care, excluding as much liver as possible. Combined with actinomycin, the upper dose limit may need reduction to 15 Gy. Total body irradiation (TBI), or other hepatic radiotherapy combined with chemotherapy, may result in veno-occlusive disease (VOD), currently usually called hepatic sinusoidal obstructive syndrome (SOS). Caution should be exercised in irradiating the liver if there is pre-existing hepatic dysfunction.

Metabolic syndrome

A more recently recognized long-term side effect of especially abdominal radiotherapy is the metabolic syndrome. It is characterized by higher blood pressure, increased levels of triglycerides, cholesterol, and free fatty acids, and increased adiposity. Prevention being difficult, adequate follow-up for early detection and treatment are important countermeasures.

Second cancers

All patients who have survived cancer are at risk of developing a second cancer. This may be due to their genetic background, epigenetic risk factors, and, last but not least, previous treatment with chemotherapy and radiotherapy. All of these factors may influence each other, making it even more complicated to assess that risk and to counsel patients with regard to secondary prevention. Patients with DNA repair deficiencies like xeroderma pigmentosum are particularly sensitive to radiotherapy and the development of second tumours after radiotherapy. Girls treated at or just before puberty for mediastinal Hodgkin lymphoma are at higher risk to develop breast cancer and should therefore be screened earlier than the general population. Basal cell carcinomas are often seen on irradiated skin.

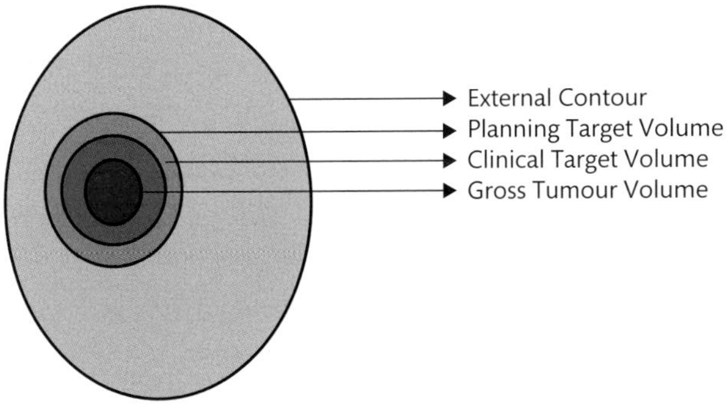

Figure 4.1 Stylised axial CT slice of body to show the position of the gross tumour volume (GTV), expanded to cover areas of subclinical potential spread forming the clinical target volume (CTV), and expanded again to form the planning target volume, allowing for inaccuracies and uncertainties in set-up.

Radiotherapy to the thyroid may not only result in hypothyroidism but also in the development of thyroid cancer.

Compromising the chance of survival by omitting radiotherapy in the hope of minimizing late effects, including second malignant neoplasms, is not an attractive option. Therefore, patients should receive radiotherapy where indicated. The knowledge that they are at risk of developing a second tumour or other late effects justifies their life-long follow-up by a multidisciplinary team.

FURTHER READING

Alvarez JA, et al. (2007) Long-term effects of treatments for childhood cancers. *Curr Opin Pediatr* **19**, 23–31.

Bhandare N, et al. (2008) Hypopituitarism after radiotherapy for extracranial head and neck cancers in pediatric patients. *Am J Clin Oncol* **31**, 567–72.

Bölling T, et al. (2008) Late effects of thoracic irradiation in children. *Strahlenther Onkol* **184**, 289–95.

Bölling T, et al. (2010) Dose-volume analysis of radiation nephropathy in children: preliminary report of the RiSK Consortium. *Int J Radiat Oncol Biol Phys* **80**, 840–4.

Boterberg et al. (Eds). (2020) Radiotherapy and cancers of children teenagers and young adults. Oxford: Oxford University Press.

Carver JR, et al. (2007) ASCO Cancer Survivorship Expert Panel. American Society of Clinical Oncology clinical evidence review on the ongoing care of adult cancer survivors: cardiac and pulmonary late effects. *J Clin Oncol* **25**, 3991–4008.

Castellino S, et al. (2010) Hepato-biliary late effects in survivors of childhood and adolescent cancer: a report from the Children's Oncology Group. *Pediatr Blood Cancer* **54**, 663–9.

Fossati P, et al. (2009) Pediatric medulloblastoma: toxicity of current treatment and potential role of protontherapy. *Cancer Treat Rev* **35**, 79–96.

Gains JE, et al. (2013) Intensity-modulated arc therapy to improve radiation dose delivery in the treatment of abdominal neuroblastoma. *Future Oncol* **9**, 439–49.

Gan HW, et al. (2015) Neuroendocrine morbidity after pediatric optic gliomas: a longitudinal analysis of 166 children over 30 years. *J Clin Endocrinol Metab* **100**, 3787–99.

Haas-Kogan D, et al. (2018) National Cancer Institute Workshop on Proton Therapy for Children: considerations regarding brainstem injury. *Int J Radiat Oncol Biol Phys* 101(1), 152–68.

Hodgson DC, et al. (2007) Pediatric Hodgkin lymphoma: maximizing efficacy and minimizing toxicity. *Semin Radiat Oncol* **17**, 230–42.

Indelicato DJ, et al. (2008) Definitive radiotherapy for Ewing tumors of extremities and pelvis: long-term disease control, limb function, and treatment toxicity. *Int J Radiat Oncol Biol Phys* **72**, 871–7.

Ness KK, et al. (2010) Physical performance limitations among adult survivors of childhood brain tumors. *Cancer* **116**, 3034–44.

Puri DR, et al. (2006) The challenging role of radiation therapy for very young children with rhabdomyosarcoma. *Int J Radiat Oncol Biol Phys* **65**, 1177–84.

Schoot RA, et al. (2015). Adverse events of local treatment in long-term head and neck rhabdomyosarcoma survivors after external beam radiotherapy or AMORE treatment. *Eur J Cancer* **51**, 1424–34.

Selo N, et al. (2010) Acute toxicity profile of radiotherapy in 690 children and adolescents: RiSK data. *Radiother Oncol* **97**, 119–26.

The Royal College of Radiologists (2018) *Good Practice Guide for Paediatric Radiotherapy, second edition.* London: The Royal College of Radiologists.

Timmermann B, et al. (2007) Spot-scanning proton therapy for malignant soft tissue tumors in childhood: first experiences at the Paul Scherrer Institute. *Int J Radiat Oncol Biol Phys* **67**, 497–504.

van Waas M, et al (2012) Abdominal radiotherapy: a major determinant of metabolic syndrome in nephroblastoma and neuroblastoma survivors. *PLoS ONE* **7**(12), e52237.

Vivekanandan S, et al. (2015) The UK experience of a treatment strategy for pediatric metastatic medulloblastoma comprising intensive induction chemotherapy, hyperfractionated accelerated radiotherapy and response directed high dose myeloablative chemotherapy or maintenance chemotherapy (Milan strategy). *Pediatr Blood Cancer* **62**, 2132–9.

Waber DP, et al. (2007) Neuropsychological outcomes from a randomized trial of triple intrathecal chemotherapy compared with 18 Gy cranial radiation as CNS treatment in acute lymphoblastic leukemia: findings from Dana-Farber Cancer Institute ALL Consortium Protocol 95-01. *J Clin Oncol* **25**, 4914–21.

Wright KD, et al. (2009) Late effects of treatment for Wilms tumor. *Pediatr Hematol Oncol* **26**, 407–13.

5
Clinical Trials in Childhood Cancer

Maria Grazia Valsecchi, Stefania Galimberti, and Pamela Kearns

Introduction

Childhood cancer was regarded as almost universally fatal until the first clinical trials performed by Sidney Farber in the late 1940s showed that it was possible to induce temporary remissions in childhood leukaemia. Over the ensuing decades, clinicians have organized themselves into national and then international co-operative groups, with the aim of conducting clinical trials to improve outcomes in these rare diseases. Such collaborative efforts have optimized the dose intensity and combinations of multi-agent conventional chemotherapy, and have helped define the role of surgery and radiotherapy to achieve maximum overall survival. This means that in the early twenty-first century, approximately 80% of children newly diagnosed with cancer, who are treated in countries where participation in clinical trials is widely available, can expect to be long-term survivors. However, these high overall survival rates present challenges for future trial design, to secure further incremental improvements in survival or to demonstrate survival equivalence from the promising new agents that may have reduced side effects.

Recent advances in understanding cancer biology have defined even smaller subgroups of childhood cancers according to molecular signatures. This means that international recruitment is essential to conduct trials within a reasonable time frame. Such collaboration across linguistic and cultural boundaries presents not only legal and regulatory hurdles but also challenges the childhood cancer research community to reappraise their individual therapeutic preferences. Paediatric regulations in North America and Europe should encourage manufacturers of new anti-cancer drugs to support the whole process, possibly with an adequate structure of incentives. In the last decade, since the introduction of the EU Paediatric Regulation (EC) 1901/2006 and Amendment Regulation (EC) 1902/2006, very few new compounds among those available for adult cancers have completed a paediatric investigation plan (PIP) or have reached marketing authorization for children. It should be ensured, in particular, that a PIP is based on how a drug works and its capacity to address unmet medical needs in children and adolescents, rather than on the type of disease in adults for which it was introduced. Mechanisms to prioritize drug development in relation to real needs of children and to make a more efficient use of trial methodology are required.

This chapter will review how the conventional approaches to reliably defining the benefit of a new drug or a new treatment strategy must be adapted.

Design and implementation of clinical trials

For a clinical trial to have the best chance of success, it must ask a clear question that is seen as important both to the clinicians who will implement the trial and the patients who will participate. For these reasons, early engagement with families affected by childhood cancer is key: if a trial question cannot be explained easily to those who represent the patient group, then it will be even more difficult to be understood by parents, especially at the distressing time of initial diagnosis of cancer in their child. The issue of study design is equally crucial and, quoting Sir David R. Cox (2007): 'A seriously defective design may be incapable of rescue even by the most ingenious of analyses; a good design may lead to conclusions so clear that simple analyses are enough.' The design of a study basically aims at answering, reliably, the research question by both minimizing biases (i.e. systematic errors that may deviate the estimate of interest from its 'true' unknown value) and by maximizing precision (i.e. minimizing variability of estimates, through control of random errors with appropriate sample size).

Background definitions

Clinical trials are traditionally classified into four phases, from Phase I to Phase IV, following the stages of pharmacological development of new drugs for human use. **Phase I** is the earliest stage, carried out to investigate pharmacokinetics and safety of the new product, so as to establish the most tolerable dose. **Phase II** trials study the safety and the activity profiles on a larger scale. They may define disease types or subgroups with better response rates and, hence, lead to **Phase III** trials, in which the new treatment is compared to an alternative (an established 'standard of care' or placebo). Here, the aim is to demonstrate improved efficacy or increased safety with equal efficacy. **Phase IV** trials are performed, usually on an observational basis, after the new intervention has received regulatory approval, and aim at obtaining additional information about risks (e.g. rare but serious side effects, long-term side effects), benefits (long-term outcomes), and optimal use. Of note, in these definitions, the new product's beneficial property is either referred to as **activity** or **efficacy**, with two different meanings. Activity relates to the biological activity and to disease control, while efficacy relates to an outcome measure that unequivocally reflects tangible benefits to patients. Examples are the impact of a drug/therapeutic strategy on response, either morphological or molecular (activity), as compared to the impact on event-free survival or survival (efficacy).

This classification into Phase I–IV trials has recently been criticized because it does not provide a general terminology able to accommodate the development of medical products that do not necessarily fit that of traditional pharmaceuticals (e.g. biologically targeted agents). A more flexible and general approach, that classifies studies on the basis of their principal aim, is as follows: (a) early-development studies (translational or treatment-mechanism testing studies), (b) middle-development studies (assessing treatment tolerability), and (c) late-development studies (including comparative studies as well as expanded safety or post-marketing studies). The traditional classification is easily recognized within this new 'descriptive' one.

Early-development studies include translational trials and the name reflects their purpose—connecting laboratory findings to clinic and vice versa. A more traditional early-phase study is the one focused on understanding the treatment mechanism and the dose–safety profile, in a context guided by a biological model. At this stage, biomarkers that are associated with the desired effect on the biological target should be developed (pharmacodynamic studies).

Assessment of the clinical outcome of the new treatment is formally introduced in **middle-development studies**, where its relationship to safety and activity is studied. This stage is particularly important when various new compounds/interventions are available and it is necessary to select out the more promising ones. Phase II trials are a typical example. Given the developmental purpose, they usually involve a broader definition of activity, for instance utilizing biomarkers (e.g. tumour or host genotype or marker in peripheral blood lymphocytes associated with target inhibition) or an early response (e.g. complete remission rate in leukaemia) to better identify the patient population who may benefit. In specific circumstances, middle-development studies can comprise a randomized question, when there are two or more new promising treatments and the primary objective is to select the one to be considered for a successive comparative trial.

Comparative trials are the most important among **late-development studies** and are focused on questions of comparison of treatment efficacy (and as such they correspond to classical Phase III trials). These represent the gold standard for gathering evidence in medical research as they are designed to minimize bias through control over treatment assignment, systematic errors, and ascertainment of endpoints, and are completed by predefined analysis. Replication of trials and consolidation of their results with meta-analyses further increase the credibility of conclusions. A key feature in comparative trials is equipoise, defined as the state in which any rational, informed person (patient, clinician, or researcher) does not favour a treatment over the other(s) being studied. This condition of genuine uncertainty is fundamental in clinical research comprising a randomization procedure.

Overview of clinical studies in childhood cancer

Phase I trials

Phase I trials are nearly always 'first in child' studies rather than 'first in man'. In other words, a new anti-cancer drug is only offered to children with cancer when there is already some knowledge of the dose tolerated by adults and the expected side effects. This reduces the number of children who may otherwise be exposed to a potentially subtherapeutic dose, and gives clinicians and families some reassurance about what toxicities to expect. However, there may be unpredictable side effects in children, especially because the side effects may be related to growth, and there is also a need for caution in very young infants/neonates, whose physiology is more immature and therefore may handle drugs differently in terms of pharmacokinetics. The second point that motivates studies in children is that with the evolution of more targeted therapies, there are now examples where the target is unique to paediatric cancers (such as GD2 in neuroblastoma).

A conventional phase I trial determines the maximum tolerated dose (MTD) of a drug in the patient group under investigation, and gives a preliminary indication of the toxicity profile and whether the acute phase is reversible. In adults, blood sampling for pharmacokinetic analysis is mandatory, in order to determine if the dose and schedule achieves sustained blood levels of the active agent equivalent to those required for activity in preclinical models. A phase I study defines a starting dose and a modality of dose escalation based on the assumption that the greater the dose, the greater the likely anti-tumour activity. The MTD is obtained as the maximum dose at which the target toxicity level (TTL) defined as acceptable is not exceeded.

Phase I designs can be broadly classified as 'rule-based' or 'model-based'. Among the 'rule-based', the conventional '3 + 3' design is still most commonly used: three patients are entered at each dose level and if none of the patients experience the type of toxicity defined to be relevant (the so-called dose-limiting toxicity, DLT) (i.e. grade 3 or 4 toxicity of given type), the dose is escalated to the next predetermined level. If one patient experiences a DLT (corresponding to a fixed 33% TTL), then the cohort is expanded to six patients. This cycle continues until two patients (out of three or six) experience DLT; the MTD is then specified as the previously tested dose level. Sometimes, a predetermined maximum feasible dose is specified, based on the pharmaceutical properties of the agent.

Variations to the '3 + 3' design have been proposed to accelerate patient recruitment and reduce the time periods for which a trial is suspended for observation for potential toxicity. The 'rolling 6' design permits continued enrolment of up to six patients at each dose level, pending toxicity evaluation of the first three patients enrolled.

Among the 'model-based' designs, the continual reassessment method (first introduced in 1990) adopts a Bayesian approach (see the section 'Novel strategies for clinical trial design') with a parametric dose–response curve (e.g. logistic) which is updated after each patient (or cohort) is enrolled at the current best estimate of the MTD using all information available after the first DLT is observed and avoiding waiting between subsequent cohorts. This design may be useful in shortening the dose determination phase but tends to expose more patients at MTD and higher doses. To reduce this risk, a methodological adaptation (escalation with overdose control) has been proposed. Other methodological adaptations have been developed to include 'time to event' continual reassessment method (CRM) in modelling the dose–toxicity relationship and summary toxicity scores that can take account of a multiplicity of organ toxicities and moderate-grade events, all of which may be important considerations in testing new drugs in young children.

Interval-based designs have been recently proposed as a new option. The modified toxicity probability interval (mTPI) and the Bayesian optimal interval (BOIN) define an interval of acceptable toxicity around the target DLT probability and two additional subintervals of low and high toxicity rates. Dose adaptation is made on the posterior probabilities for the three subintervals using a Bayesian model and observed data at each dose level in the mTPI design and on the observed toxicity rate in the BOIN design. This latter is a Bayesian design in that it selects optimal interval boundaries minimizing the decision errors of dose assignment under a Bayesian framework. Interval-based designs, that are a mixture of rule-based and model-based designs, are attractive as they are flexible, well-performing (they show operative characteristics that compete with CRM), and represent a good compromise between 3+3 and CRM.

Phase II trials

A phase II trial is designed to obtain an initial estimate of the anti-tumour activity of an agent. The purpose is to determine, with a reasonable degree of confidence, whether the new anti-cancer agent has sufficient activity against a specified tumour type as to warrant its further development or evaluation in that tumour type. A further consideration is to minimize the number of patients treated with a drug of low activity.

The classical study design (phase IIA) comprises a single-arm, multi-stage recruitment plan with the endpoint of anti-tumour activity generally based on categorical response criteria (complete and partial response). The presence of multiple stages, usually two, ensures that the study continues to the second stage of recruitment only if in the first stage, on fewer patients, a minimal response rate is reached according to a predefined statistical design. Such a design presents practical problems in childhood cancer studies. First, the endpoint of response may take several weeks to manifest, leading to periods of suspension of recruitment between the first and second stage, which can present difficulties for clinicians and patients waiting to be enrolled. Second, the fortunate reality is that there are very few available patients who are eligible for early phase trials in childhood cancer, due to the effectiveness of current therapies for most newly diagnosed patients. Third, many of the patients with relapsed or progressive disease do not have 'measurable' disease according to response evaluation criteria in solid tumours (RECIST) (see Chapter 2 'Imaging in Paediatric Oncology'), which require a soft-tissue lesion visible on cross-sectional imaging. Instead, children with relapsed neuroblastoma and sarcomas may have only bone or bone marrow disease, reducing the number of eligible patients. Hence, a classical phase II trial testing efficacy in a single or restricted range of childhood cancers inevitably requires international collaboration in order to recruit in a reasonable time frame of 18–24 months. This presents practical and financial challenges for implementation. Fourth, the response criteria need to be reassessed in the light of new biological findings and, for instance, considered as continuous variables rather than categorical variables. This could be the case in using the level of minimal residual disease as a measure of response in acute lymphoblastic leukaemia (ALL). Also, for some targeted treatments in paediatric tumours, especially tumours of the central nervous system (CNS), prolonged stable disease could be a valuable endpoint yet requiring a longer time of observation.

Early drug development studies of targeted therapies in childhood cancer present new challenges. For example, only rare subpopulations of childhood leukaemias would theoretically benefit from tyrosine kinase inhibitors for BCR-ABL + ALL or FLT3 inhibitors in acute myeloid leukaemia (AML) (or infants with ALL) whose leukaemic cells have FLT3 internal tandem duplications. These therapies open a different scenario as the DLT approach is generally not appropriate and because the clinical development may be aimed primarily at assessing the combination of the target agent with standard agents. When a phase II trial does not use the new drug as a single agent, activity data become difficult to interpret because there might be an unquantifiable response due to the underlying therapy. Even if historical data are available on the adopted underlying standard therapy, these may not be fully appropriate for the patient mix on which the phase II study is conducted. These considerations stimulated the development of randomized phase II designs such as the screening design.

Randomized phase II (or phase IIB) studies are smaller than phase III studies, as they look for large differences and relax the type I and II error rates, and they tend to be quicker, as they assess activity (or early intermediate endpoints) rather than efficacy. They may be of value in high-risk patient populations (i.e. patients whose disease behaves aggressively and there is a high event rate in terms of disease progression), but also in good-prognosis diseases where randomization is used to have an unbiased evaluation with an internal control. For these reasons they should not compromise the conduct of a definitive phase III study on the promising new drug combination on the most appropriate patient population, which may be newly diagnosed patients. The definition of the endpoint is here a key issue and, recently, a lot of attention has been stimulated on adopting early activity endpoints that could be regarded as surrogate biomarkers for the clinical outcome of efficacy that requires longer-term evaluation (event-free survival or survival). Surrogacy requires a proper validation; without that a dangerous claim could be made on the long-term advantage of a given treatment based on the early advantage seen on the biomarker. The debate is open on minimal residual disease (MRD) as a candidate, but evidence on its surrogate value is not available.

Seamless phase I/II trials can be designed which streamline the transition between the two phases, reducing patients' exposure to ineffective doses as well as saving time and money. An example is the so-called 'dose expansion-cohort' approach: after the MTD is detected, additional patients are treated at MTD and toxicity is recorded through the whole trial (pre and post expansion), while activity is evaluated on patients belonging to the cohort at MTD as a secondary endpoint.

Phase III trials

Phase III trials in childhood cancer are generally offered to newly diagnosed patients or, for some diseases with standard effective salvage therapies, to patients at first relapse. They are designed to be 'low risk' to participants in terms of not compromising their chance of cure. These trials usually compare the current best-known treatment (the standard arm) against a modification of that treatment (the experimental arm), and are designed to test whether there is either an improvement in efficacy or the same efficacy with reduced toxicity.

In designing a trial, the number of children who can potentially be recruited in order to ensure sufficient statistical power must be anticipated. For most childhood cancers, the numbers that need to

Table 5.1 Approximate number of newly diagnosed cases per year and expected number of deaths per year for the more common subgroups of childhood cancer diagnosed before age 15 years, expected in a European country, total population approximately 60 million.

Diagnostic subgroup	Expected no. of cases per yr*	Expected no. of deaths per yr*
Acute lymphoblastic leukaemia	372	71
Acute myeloid leukaemia	69	26
Hodgkin lymphoma	58	<2
Non-Hodgkin lymphoma	82	16
Medulloblastoma	70	31
Astrocytoma	155	33
Neuroblastoma	89	38
Retinoblastoma	43	2
Renal tumour	81	13
Hepatoblastoma	11	3
Osteosarcoma	31	10
Ewing sarcoma	22	6
Rhabdomyosarcoma	55	17
Malignant germ-cell tumour	31	2

*Estimated from population-based registration and mortality figures for Great Britain (Stiller, 2007) and Europe (Steliarova-Foucher et al., 2006).

Source: data from Stiller C (Ed), Childhood Cancer in Britain: Incidence, Survival, Mortality (2007), Oxford University Press, Oxford, UK; and Steliarova-Foucher E et al. (Eds), 'Cancer in Children and Adolescents in Europe', European Journal of Cancer Special Edition (2006), Volume 42, pp. 1913–2190.

be recruited into a randomized trial are large in comparison with the annual numbers of children diagnosed in an average-sized European country per year (Tables 5.1 and 5.2). Optimal sample size in clinical trials depends largely on the target difference the trial aims to detect: the smaller the difference, the greater the number of participants that needs to be enrolled. The required sample size can easily reach thousands of patients when the study is powered to detect less than a 10% absolute increase in event-free survival (EFS). Such relatively modest yet clinically important improvements are to be expected with more efficient definition of therapeutic strategies using existing chemotherapeutic agents. Even for the high-risk cancers, where patients have a dismal prognosis and new experimental therapeutic approaches offer hope of more marked improvements, required sample sizes are in the hundreds, yet these high-risk cancers generally represent small subgroups. Also in this context, it is important to make every effort not to revert to the use of single-arm studies and historical controls in order to have sound and unbiased estimates.

Since the 1970s, many countries have developed national childhood cancer study groups which have stimulated the development of tumour-specific committees to design and run clinical trials. High rates of participation in national clinical trials have been achieved through the active engagement of clinicians and patients in specialist treatment centres and through national consensus. However, even for the more common childhood cancers, achieving the numbers required for a robustly powered trial within a reasonable time-span (normally five years of recruitment) ideally requires participation from several countries. This adds to the expense and the time required to design and implement such trials and can mean national compromise in terms of accepting what is defined as the 'standard' arm. Nonetheless, expansion of recruitment from national to international communities has been largely successful, although it has sometimes required an innovative approach. For example, a study design that prospectively used the principles of meta-analysis was adopted in an international trial on intensification of maintenance treatment in ALL.

In the rarer paediatric cancers or in specific subgroups, international cooperation is often the only way to produce solid evidence and to improve clinical practice. Thus, when the SIOPEL group of the International Society of Paediatric Oncology (SIOP) commenced clinical trials in the very rare tumour group, hepatoblastoma, this led to considerable improvements in survival in participating countries (Figure 5.1).

Very large numbers are also needed for non-inferiority trials. These are typically used when the aim is to reduce treatment burden, toxicity, and long-term side effects for patients who have a good

Table 5.2 Number of subjects needed in different scenarios of superiority and non-inferiority trials with two parallel groups of equal allocation and comparison of event-free survival (EFS) based on log-rank test (one-sided test, type I error 0.025 and 0.80 power).

Standard treatment 5-year EFS	Standard treatment Δ in 5-year EFS*	Total number of subjects (events)
25%	+20%	167 (109)
25%	+15%	280 (189)
60%	+10%	711 (249)
60%	+5%	2,897 (1,086)
90%	-4%	2,077 (249)
90%	-3%	3,554 (409)

*A positive Δ indicates the target improvement and a negative Δ indicates the target non-inferiority margin that the trial aims to detect. The number of subjects to be enrolled in each treatment group is half the total number reported in the last column (software PASS 11. NCSS, LLC. Kaysville, Utah, USA).

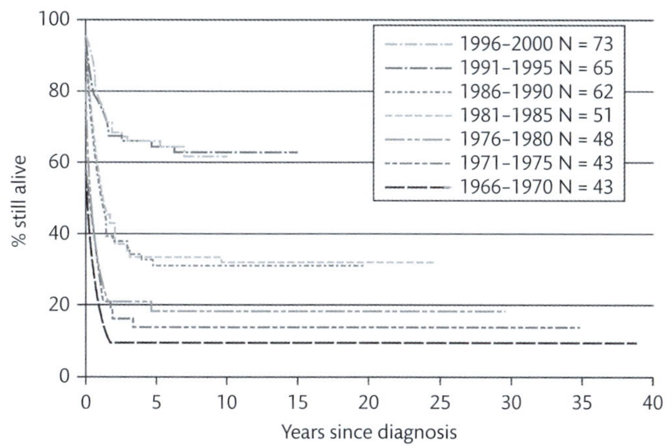

Figure 5.1 Rapid improvement in survival of children with hepatoblastoma (average 11 cases per year) in Great Britain following the introduction of participation in the SIOPEL clinical trials in 1991. The number of cases diagnosed per quinquennium is indicated.

Reproduced with permission from Stiller C (Ed), *Childhood Cancer in Britain: Incidence, Survival, Mortality*, Table 5.26, p. 204, Oxford University Press, Oxford, UK, Copyright © 2007.

risk profile, without compromising overall survival rates. For instance, in ALL, they are useful in patients with very good clinical outcome (at least 90–95% five-year EFS), for whom the aim is to optimize therapy under controlled conditions, de-intensifying certain therapy elements with known short- or long-term side effects, without compromising the EFS outcome. Up to 30% of children with ALL treated in current protocols in North America and Western Europe may be candidates for this type of trial. In general, however, non-inferiority 'head-to-head' trials, where a novel drug replaces an existing one, are often viewed with suspicion, as they may be used to promote drugs of less therapeutic value. Switching the objective of a trial from superiority to non-inferiority can be much more seriously misleading than vice versa as, for instance, a poorly conducted or an underpowered superiority trial may easily lead to a non-significant result, because treatment effect is diluted or it has wide confidence intervals. Whenever appropriate, based on the objective and trial recruitment, the design can include a preplanned schedule of interim analyses on the primary endpoint and guidelines for stopping rules on selected aspects (e.g. toxicities).

As a final consideration, trial design requires that experts in various fields (clinical, biological, pharmacological, biostatistical) cooperate to formulate in advance, as clearly and precisely as possible, based on up-to-date knowledge, the objectives and hypothesis of the trial. Data from a trial where the results support a sound, prespecified hypothesis is more persuasive than one where the results are 'surprising', and unplanned testing for non-inferiority in trials designed for superiority should be discouraged. Study designs that incorporate both non-inferiority and superiority testing are possible, and may be useful and applicable in selected contexts.

Novel strategies for clinical trial design

The issues raised by the more precise characterization of subgroups in paediatric oncology continue to grow in importance. Advances in understanding the molecular basis of many childhood cancers and the development of more sensitive methods for assessing response mean that even the common childhood cancers such as ALL are now being subdivided into ever smaller subgroups (e.g. infants, Philadelphia-positive patients), each with their own different survival profiles and therapeutic questions. New statistical approaches to design are therefore needed to address important therapeutic questions. These include increased efficacy for those subgroups where survival is still very poor. They also include optimizing the design of phase I and II studies, given the limited number of patients available and the growing number of new drugs that must be evaluated for toxicity and activity. These kinds of questions have stimulated the development of adaptive designs. Such designs may be most useful when drug activity is evaluated in terms of early response to treatment, rather than in phase III studies, where efficacy is measured by long-term evaluation of event-free and overall survival.

A broad range of design modifications—for instance, sample size re-estimation, discontinuation of treatment arms, changes in the primary measure of treatment response—is allowed for adaptive designs. Adaptive designs make use of known interim findings to modify the sampling plan and are therefore data-driven. For this reason, they raise concern about the unintended consequence of introducing bias and imprecision in the estimates. In addition, the adoption of an adaptive design for a phase III trial could be seen as a main contradiction to the confirmatory nature of such late-development studies, especially if these are pivotal trials aiming at approval of a new product.

Adaptive approaches are justified by the need to cope with difficult experimental situations, where the paucity of available knowledge determines uncertainty about crucial aspects of the study. These difficulties must be acknowledged in advance, so that any modification of the trial design (e.g. sample size re-estimation) is anticipated and justified in the study protocol. Adaptive designs cannot in fact be used as a remedy for poor trial planning, but actually require more upfront planning, both statistically and in managing logistics and implementation. In short, a proper adaptive design must control potential sources of bias, first of all by ensuring that type-I error is fully preserved and valid estimates and confidence intervals for the treatment effect will be available as a summary of the totality of evidence. Additional measures to be taken operationally, in order to maintain the integrity of the trial, include the careful disclosure of interim analyses. In practice, access to the available data and related results must be limited (it is recommended that the trial's clinical team be isolated from both) and communication of interim analysis decisions is to be preferred over communication of interim results.

A general concern about monitoring designs is heterogeneity in treatment effects estimated from the different stages of the trial. This may be due to random variation, but in practice it cannot be excluded that a calendar time effect might be present, for instance because of a learning process or a change in important prognostic factors occurring over time. Heterogeneity in stage results can be detected by applying a heterogeneity test, although its statistical power is generally limited. Should it indicate that a discrepancy exists, further investigation into possible causes is recommended.

An interesting example of adaptive design is the so-called adaptive 'seamless' design, in which two separate phases of drug development, that could be conducted as separate trials, are in fact combined into a single one, both operationally and inferentially. Data gathered from the first, **learning** stage (e.g. dose selection) are used to adapt the trial plan of the second, **confirming** stage, and data from both are used to run the final analysis and answer study questions. This adaptive 'seamless' design does not simply select out the most promising treatment option, but actually allows continuation of the preferred arm without the need to start a new trial (see Figure 5.2). Application of this type of study requires that the endpoint for the learning phase be immediately available for continuation with the confirming stage and that it also be adopted as a primary endpoint, to answer the study question. A multi-arm, multi-stage trial design was recently proposed to compare many new therapies simultaneously against a control treatment and reject insufficiently active therapies in a randomized pairwise comparison with the control, performed at different stages, with a seamless move from one stage to the next.

Bayesian designs

Bayesian statistics is a methodology, used both in the design and in the analysis stage of a trial, that provides a coherent method for learning from evidence as it accumulates. This is performed by combining prior information with accumulating evidence through a mathematical model, and leads to the so-called 'posterior distribution' of the clinical endpoint of interest.

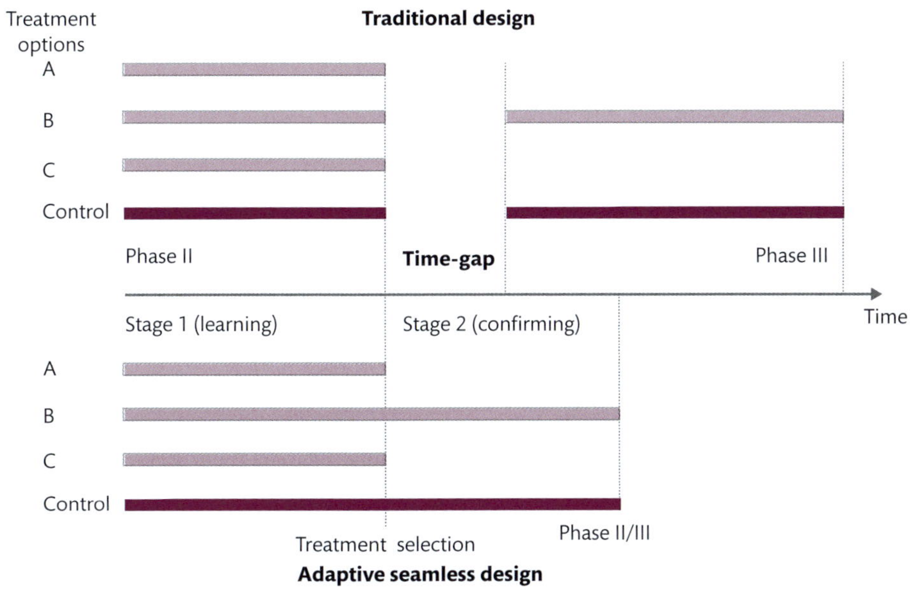

Figure 5.2 Comparison of adaptive seamless and traditional design.

The Bayesian approach may be useful especially when good prior information on clinical use of a device or treatment exists, so that incorporating it in the design and analysis of the future trial may result in a smaller-sized or shorter-duration study. It can also be used when prior information is only partially (or not) informative, because it can provide flexible methods for interim analyses and modifications of on-going trials (e.g. changes to sample size, changes in the randomization scheme).

Usually, the Bayesian approach for trial design does not determine sample size in advance; instead, it may specify a particular criterion to stop the trial. Appropriate stopping criteria may be based on a specific amount of information about the clinical measure of interest (e.g. a sufficiently narrow credible interval, as defined below) or an appropriately high probability for a prespecified hypothesis.

At any point during a Bayesian clinical trial, it is possible to update the computation of the expected additional number of observations needed to meet the stopping criterion. Because the sample size is not explicitly part of the stopping criterion, the trial can be terminated whenever enough information has been collected to answer the trial questions. When sizing a Bayesian trial, it is recommended that the minimum sample size is prespecified according to safety and effectiveness endpoints. It is also wise to anticipate a minimum level of information from the current trial needed to verify model assumptions and appropriateness of prior information used.

Prespecified interim analyses can be part of a Bayesian trial, and various methods are available. The final analyses within the Bayesian approach include hypothesis testing and interval estimates. For Bayesian hypothesis testing, the posterior distribution can be used to calculate the probability that a particular hypothesis regarding the endpoint is true, given the observed data. Interval estimates in the Bayesian context are called **credible intervals**: a 95% credible interval is the interval with 95% posterior probability of including the 'true' unknown treatment effect. Of note, Bayesian methods for interim monitoring of futility or efficacy can also be applied in the setting of a traditional trial. For example, guidelines based on predictive probability can be used to calculate how likely it is to reach the study aim, should the current observed trend continue and the trial be continued to the end of planned recruitment.

A Bayesian approach can be used in phase I studies (as shown in the section 'Design and implementation of clinical trials'). It can also be used to design phase II trials more efficiently by thinking of them as randomized selection trials comparing several therapies. Thus, in rare subgroups, it has been proposed to formally combine, at the design stage, the expected outcome of the new small trial being planned with the prior information on treatment effect generated by earlier studies. A Bayesian approach of this kind provides an estimate of the potential contribution to the demonstration of treatment effect of the new trial which, if seen in isolation, would be underpowered.

Regulatory agencies have recently issued guidelines on clinical trials in small populations that indicate the possibility of using non-standard designs. These guidelines propose that there are no special methods for designing, carrying out, or analysing clinical trials in small populations. They note though that the need for statistical efficiency should be weighed against the need for clinically relevant/interpretable results, the latter being more important. While frequentist formulations of analysis are typically best suited for careful assessment of the strength of evidence, Bayesian formulations may allow the insertion of additional information which may open the route to bolder speculations, sometimes providing an alternative to sensitivity analysis.

Practical considerations in conducting clinical trials

The conduct of clinical trials is a highly regulated process, designed to give maximum safety to patients whilst allowing them access to innovation in a well-designed, controlled scientific study that has a high chance of achieving its aims. Each country has its own legal framework for ethical review procedures and regulatory approval processes. Ensuring consistent data quality when working across national, cultural, legal. and linguistic boundaries adds further to the challenges. Hence, multinational trials require additional time to design and implement.

The implementation of the Clinical Trial Directive 2001/20/EC (EUCTD) and its translation into law throughout the European Union in 2004 aimed to provide a common set of regulations and defined standards of quality of clinical studies across member states. Although the overall aim of the EUCTD is to protect the safety and rights of patients and the integrity of trial data, the implementation of the legislation has proved difficult, and it is well recognized that it significantly delayed academic-driven clinical research and has significantly increased the cost and bureaucracy for non-commercial trials conducted by universities and public research institutions.

A key problem is the Directive's requirement for equal application of a high level of regulation and governance to all clinical trials that investigate the effects of drugs, regardless of the existing knowledge and experience in using that drug. The EUCTD does not differentiate between trials investigating unlicensed medicinal products, licensed products used within their marketing authorization, or those used 'off-label', as in many cancer indications. For the majority of late-development clinical trials in childhood cancer, the drugs in the treatment regimens being investigated have marketing authorization, although are not necessarily being used according to their licensed indication (i.e. off-label use). This off-label use is supported by considerable published experience and safety data relating to the use of these regimes in the paediatric cancer population.

The need for a more proportionate, risk-adapted approach to regulation of clinical trials was recognized by the European Commission and was a major factor that led to a revision of the EU's clinical trial legislation. The new law, the Clinical Trial Regulation (CTR), is anticipated to be implemented in early 2020. The basic requirement that each trial should have an overall sponsor—taking the legal responsibility for the conduct of the trial including obtaining a clinical trial authorization from the competent authorities, ensuring the suitability of each participating institution and of investigators, overseeing pharmacovigilance, and ensuring the integrity of clinical trial data—will continue. Nevertheless, the CTR introduces the concept of proportionate regulation and oversight of clinical trials according to risk. For example, it incorporates a category of 'low-intervention trial'. This category will apply to clinical trials in which licensed drugs are used, either in their licensed indication or according to standard clinical practice, and in which the trial interventions pose no more than minimum additional risk or burden to the safety of the participants. For a trial that complies with the definition of low intervention, the regulatory requirements will be proportionately reduced, acknowledging that investigational medicinal products in such trials are licensed products that are prescribed routinely outside the context of clinical trials and for which extensively documented safety profiles exist. This, amongst other pragmatic changes in the CTR, will have an important effect in reducing the unnecessary administrative and financial burdens for many late-development clinical trials in paediatric oncology, where the principal aim is to optimize the use of currently available, licensed drugs to guide best clinical practice.

Although there are many ethical considerations in undertaking clinical research on children, a 'therapeutic alliance' begins between doctors and families when a child is first diagnosed with cancer. All parents want their child to access the best treatment available, and entry into a phase III trial is generally considered 'best practice' in paediatric oncology. More research is needed, however, to understand how best to present the alien concept of a randomized clinical trial at this stressful time and to understand why there are differences in randomization rates between countries participating within the same clinical trial. Also, given the success in treating various childhood cancers, attention must be paid to long-term quality of life and health challenges, with strategies in place to capture all relevant late effects.

Engaging families as informed partners in clinical trials is a key goal of sound practice, but is far from straightforward in its achievement. One key issue concerns whether to involve a child with cancer in the decision about participating in a trial. The principle that children should be consulted, informed, and involved in decisions affecting them, but not have the final authority over decisions, is enshrined in the UN Convention of the Rights of the Child (UNCRC). The guiding principle of the UNCRC is that the 'best interests' of the child must be promoted, but differences of opinion between parents, children, and professionals about the 'best interests' of the child will sometimes need to be resolved. Involving a child in a decision about participation in a cancer trial may be especially complex in those situations where parents, struggling to come to terms with the diagnosis themselves, prefer to defer telling the child the full diagnosis and its implications, perhaps until treatment is established and the parents are better able to cope with their own emotions. Some parents may see a demand to involve the child in the decision—and, by definition, disclose the diagnosis—as interfering with their autonomy as parents. Further complexity arises because of varying definitions of minors and of the legal age of consent between different countries. Additionally, some jurisdictions rely on the assessment of 'competence' rather than specifying a particular age of consent.

Patient 'misunderstandings' of concepts such as randomization are often assumed to arise from incomplete, badly written, or misleading information. Much attention, particularly from research ethics committees, tends to focus on the detail of patient information sheets (PIS). However, the role of written information in this context remains poorly understood, and parents may find discussion with staff more helpful than the consent document·

Summary

Despite the progress made in curing children with cancer, there is little room for complacency and, if progress is to be sustained, formidable challenges must be faced. These include the scientific challenge of studies in small populations, the complexities of the regulatory environment, ethical and organizational constraints, the emotional context, and the attitudes of individual families and physicians. All efforts should be made to ensure that clinical efficacy of a treatment is scientifically established for future generations of children and adolescents. Some of these issues may be addressed by innovative trial design and implementation, but all will require engagement with the communities of families and physicians on whom trials depend. Clinical research must include a well-designed social science and ethical evaluation of how best to inform and engage the patient community who need clinical trials to continue in order for progress to be made.

FURTHER READING

Cox, DR (2007) Applied statistics: a review. *Ann Appl Stat* **1**, 1–16.

Dupont JC, et al. (2016). Ethical issues of clinical trials in paediatric oncology from 2003 to 2013: a systematic review. *Lancet Oncol* **17**(5), e187–97.

Galimberti S, Devidas M, Lucenti A, Cazzaniga G, Möricke A, Bartram CR, Mann G, Carroll W, Winick N, Borowitz M, Wood B, Basso G, Conter V, Zimmermann M, Suciu S, Biondi A, Schrappe M, Hunger S, Valsecchi MG (2018) Evaluation of minimal residual disease as a potential surrogate endpoint for event free survival in randomized childhood B-lineage acute lymphoblastic leukemia clinical trials. *Journal of the National Cancer Institute Cancer Spectrum*, 2(4).

European Medicines Agency: Committee for Medicinal Products for Human Use (CHMP) (2006) Guideline on clinical trials in small populations. CHMP/EWP/83561/2005, July 2006. Available at: http://www.ema.europa.eu/docs/en_GB/document_library/Scientific_guideline/2009/09/WC500003615.pdf (accessed May 2017).

European Medicines Agency: Committee for Proprietary Medicinal Products (CPMP) (2000) Points to consider on switching between superiority and non-inferiority. CPMP/EWP/482/99, July 2000. Available at: http://www.ema.europa.eu/docs/en_GB/document_library/Scientific_guideline/2009/09/WC500003658.pdf (accessed May 2017).

Freedman, B (1987) Equipoise and the ethics of clinical research. *New Engl J Med* **317**, 141–5.

Garattini S, Bertelè V (2007) Non-inferiority trials are unethical because they disregard patients' interests. *Lancet* **370**, 1875–7.

Hearn J, Sullivan R (2007) The impact of the 'Clinical Trials' directive on the cost and conduct of non-commercial cancer trials in the UK. *Eur J Cancer* **43**, 8–13.

Kumar A, et al. (2005) Are experimental treatments for cancer in children superior to established treatments? Observational study of randomised controlled trials by the Children's Oncology Group. *BMJ* **331**, 1295.

Lee DP, et al. (2005) Pediatric phase I trials in oncology: an analysis of study conduct efficiency. *J Clin Oncol* **23**(33), 8431–41.

Machin D, et al. (1997) *Sample Size Tables for Clinical Studies* (2nd edn). Malden, MA: Blackwell Science.

Moroz V, et al. (2014) Comparison of anticipated and actual control group outcomes in randomised trials in paediatric oncology provides evidence that historically controlled studies are biased in favour of the novel treatment. *Trials* **10**(15), 481.

Parmar MKB, et al. (2008) Speeding up the evaluation of new agents in cancer. *J Nat Can Inst* **100**(17), 1204–14.

Piantadosi S (2005) Clinical Trials: A Methodologic Perspective (2nd edn). New York: Wiley.

Pritchard-Jones K, et al. (2008) Improving recruitment to clinical trials for cancer in childhood. *Lancet Oncol* **9**(4), 392–9.

Rubinstein LV, et al. (2005) Design issues of randomized phase II trials and a proposal for phase II screening trials. *J Clin Oncol* 23(28), 7199–206.

Scott M, et al. (2010) *Bayesian Adaptive Methods for Clinical Trials*. Florida: CRC Press.

Simon CM, et al. (2004) Comparison of the informed consent process for randomized clinical trials in pediatric and adult oncology. *J Clin Oncol* **22**(13), 2708–17.

Simon R (1989) Optimal two-stage designs for phase II clinical trials. *Control Clin Trials* **10**, 1–10.

Steliarova-Foucher E, et al. (eds) (2006) Cancer in children and adolescents in Europe. *Eur J Cancer Special Edn* **42**, 1913–2190.

Stiller C (ed.) (2007). *Childhood Cancer in Britain*. London: Oxford University Press.

Sullivan R, et al. (2013) New policies to address the global burden of childhood cancers. *Lancet Oncol* **14**(3), e125–35.

Valsecchi MG, Masera G (1996) A new challenge in clinical research in childhood ALL: the prospective meta-analysis strategy for intergroup collaboration. *Ann Oncol* **7**, 1005–8.

Valsecchi MG, et al. (2008) Web-based international studies in limited populations of pediatric leukemia. *Pediatr Blood Cancer* **50**, 270–3.

Vassal G, et al. (2013) New drugs for children and adolescents with cancer: the need for novel development pathways. *Lancet Oncol* **14**(3), e117–24.

6

Evidence-Based Paediatric Oncology

Leontien C.M. Kremer, Erik A.H. Loeffen, and Robert S. Phillips

History

The term evidence-based medicine was introduced by a research group led by David Sackett and Gordon Guyatt from the McMaster Medical School in Canada, in 1992, with one of the first publications about evidence-based medicine appearing in the *Journal of the American Medical Association*. The work built on strong foundations, particularly a book published in 1972 by a Scottish epidemiologist called Archie Cochrane—*Effectiveness and Efficiency: Random Reflections on Health Services*—which outlined the concepts of evidence-based practice. The Cochrane Collaboration (based on these ideas) was founded in 1993 and continues to grow. It is dedicated to making up-to-date, accurate information about the effects of healthcare readily available worldwide. The practice of evidence-based medicine is very important in delivering optimal patient care, and the terms evidence-based medicine, or evidence-based practice, are used all around the world. The *British Medical Journal* listed evidence-based medicine as one of the 15 most important medical advances since 1840.

What is evidence-based medicine?

Evidence-based medicine (EBM) is the practice of identifying the best available research evidence, utilizing a process of systematically finding, appraising, and interpreting research findings, and integrating these with clinical expertise and patient values to come to a clinical decision (see Figure 6.1). It has been strikingly defined by Sackett et al. as 'the conscientious, explicit, and judicious use of current best evidence in making decisions about the care of individual patients'. It describes a philosophy of care which integrates the highest quality scientific research, the treating clinician's expertise, and the child's (and his/her family's) specific medical, psychological, and social condition. It is a heuristic way of thinking—not a recipe or fixed set of instructions.

The different roles for evidence-based medicine in paediatric oncology

There is a daily need for valid information about therapy, diagnosis, prognosis, aetiology, and prevention for children with cancer. There is an overwhelming amount of information available; however, this information is rarely summarized and the conclusions may be conflicting. Even in 1995, the scale of this problem was already estimated as requiring that a physician would need to read 17 journal articles a day, all year round, in order to keep up to date with all research relevant to a particular area of clinical practice. With the number of studies published annually having more than doubled since then, one can imagine that this is an unattainable effort.

In this chapter, we will give an overview how EBM can be used in a non-exhaustive but still comprehensive way in daily practice of care for children with cancer, and which tools are available for paediatric oncologists.

Three different roles for practice of EBM have been proposed: replicator, user, and doer. The **replicator** describes the doctor who copies, knowingly or unconsciously, the actions and practices of a trusted colleague. This is hopefully a mentor whose work is centred on the delivery of EBM. The **user** is the commonest practice of taking evidence-based resources such as randomized controlled clinical trials (RCTs), systematic reviews, or evidence-based guidelines, and using them to guide clinical problem solving. When the resources that the doctor is using are solidly based on the best-quality evidence that exists, this is an extremely efficient way of practicing EBM. This is the most practical and widely used way of putting evidence-based paediatric oncology into action, and the majority of this chapter will focus on how to learn to become a skilled user of EBM.

The **doer** refers to performing EBM in detail; full expression of the structured question, broad search and detailed appraisal of the evidence identified, summarizing the evidence, followed by a careful decision and implementation plan. This is infrequently undertaken by a paediatric oncologist in daily clinical practice, but more common in the development of local policies, systematic reviews, or guidelines. It is the most thorough but also the most time-consuming and technically demanding of the three roles, and learning this one requires a level of detail well beyond this chapter. We will only give some insight into the Grading of Recommendations, Assessment, Development, and Evaluation (GRADE) methodology for guideline development.

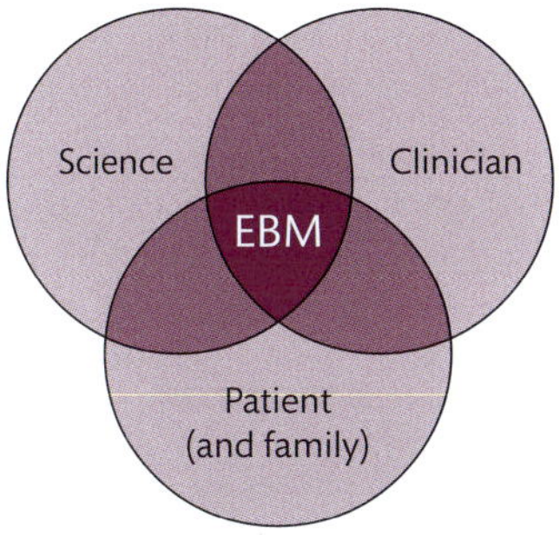

Figure 6.1 The integration of the triad of patients, physicians, and publications.

Steps in evidence-based paediatric oncology for a user of evidence-based medicine

The practical output of EBM in daily practice, as a user of EBM, can be viewed as a four-step process:

1. Ask a structured clinical question.
2. Acquire relevant research.
3. Appraise the identified evidence for its validity, importance, and applicability.
4. Apply the results in practice.

First step: ask . . . and it might be given unto you

Asking an answerable question can prove terribly difficult, but when good questions are dissected, the physiology becomes clear. The first step in deconstructing the anatomy of inquiry is to ask 'What sort of question is being asked?' Clinical questions can be grossly categorized as 'foreground' and 'background'. Background questions are generally broad, and can be caricatured as those asked by a medical student. They are often of the 'what is' or 'what causes' type: for example, 'What is a pilomyxoid astrocytoma?', 'What causes leukaemia in childhood?' Foreground questions are specific, have intent, and can be asked in the domains of therapy (efficacy or harm), diagnosis, prognosis, aetiology, or prevention. They frequently have three or four components, summarized in the acronym 'PICO':

Patient, **p**roblem, or **p**opulation (the group to which the question applies)
Intervention (or diagnostic test, or exposure, or prognostic marker)
Comparison (not always necessary)
Outcome(s) of interest (which should include patient-relevant, adverse, and beneficial measures)

An example might be 'In children with metastatic rhabdomyosarcoma [population], does high-dose therapy with stem-cell rescue [intervention] compared with intensive conventional chemotherapy [comparison] increase five-year overall survival [outcome]?' Questions of therapy can usually fit quite easily into this PICO frame.

As a final aside in the description of structured clinical questions, it is worth reflecting on how to choose which outcomes to look at. Do doctors really know what outcome their patients and families most value, or do physicians presume? If the question is highly particular to one patient and their family, it may be pertinent to ask the patients and their families directly, to frame the PICO to actually answer their question. In this effort, it might also be worthwhile to a priori decide which outcomes are most important for decision making, as there is a chance the identified evidence is incomplete or conflicting on various outcomes (i.e. improvement on one outcome, worsening on another outcome).

Second step: acquisition is not a vice

Timely supply of useful evidence from the scientific medical literature is essential for the optimal care of children with cancer, and professionals have a responsibility to keep up to date with research findings to ensure that their practice remains effective. These needs can be characterized by those of keeping up to date ('just in case' information) and answering day-to-day clinical questions ('just in time' information).

Summary or alerting systems can be useful for keeping abreast of new information. 'EvidenceAlerts', a service from DynaMed Plus and McMaster University, alerts subscribers by email to new studies (https://plus.mcmaster.ca/EvidenceAlerts/). EvidenceAlerts uses highly trained research staff to select papers based on methodological quality from over 110 premier clinical journals. At least three members of a worldwide panel of practicing physicians then rate the papers for clinical relevance and interest, and often leave contextual comments which can be really useful to practicing clinicians. In addition, in most electronic databases, such as PubMed, it is also possible to create a periodical alert for new results of a user-specified search.

A widely described hierarchy of information resources to address the day-to-day clinical questions is that of the '5S' pyramid (Figure 6.2). In the ideal situation, evidence from applicable research is integrated into computerized systems that aid in decision making, such as electronic care pathways. If this is not available, then summaries in a guideline or protocol could deliver the right answers in an evidence-based fashion. If these cannot be found, then specific questions can be effectively answered if others provide a resource that finds, appraises, and summarizes the key evidence related to a specific topic. These synopses can be incredibly useful to both answer specific questions and to try to keep up to date with the new knowledge that is flooding out of medical research. Without these, then a systematic review can provide a synthesis of the breadth of the best evidence to answer specific questions. Lastly, and only rarely, should we need to rely on looking at single, individual studies to answer our common queries.

We highlight examples of the 5S pyramid in the rest of this section and in Table 6.1. There are also various meta-search engines that search in multiple layers of the 5S pyramid: examples are TRIP (www.tripdatabase.com) and SUMsearch2 (www.sumsearch.org).

Systems: computerized decision-support and care pathways

There are few opportunities in paediatric oncology to use computerized decision-support systems where evidence-based guidelines are included in computer systems for daily practice. But the idea of having a 'pathway' of care, based on the best available evidence, is not new to paediatric oncologists. Every treatment protocol we use has, built into it, a plan of investigation, treatment, response assessment, and follow-up. The use of care pathways has been demonstrated to have good improvements in patient-related outcomes in a number of adult and paediatric specialty areas, although no direct evidence exists for children with malignancies. In the (near) future,

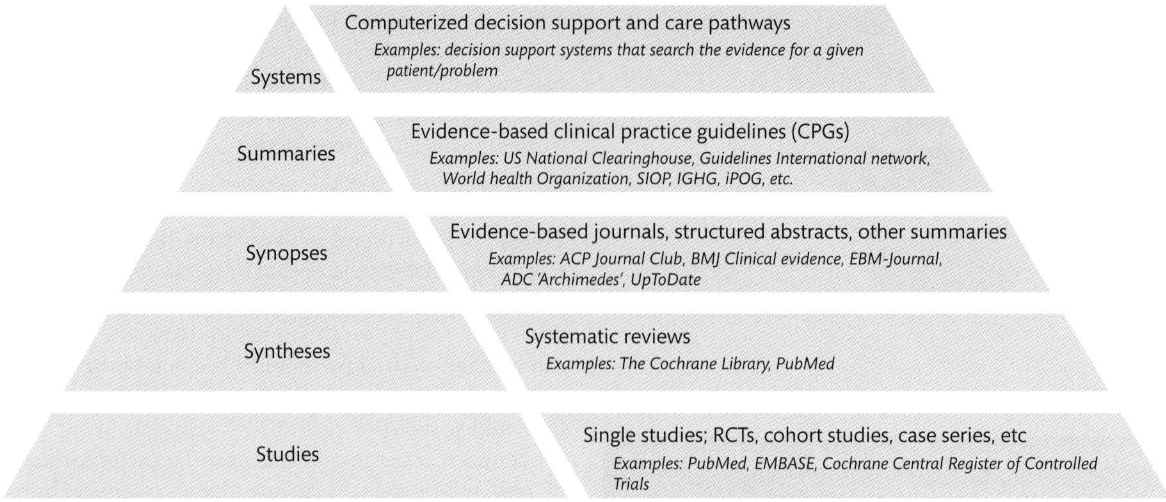

Figure 6.2 The '5S' pyramid.

we expect to see computerized decision-support software, based on the flow charts of clinical practice guidelines, being integrated more fully in electronic health record systems.

Summaries: evidence-based clinical practice guidelines

The Institute of Medicine defined clinical practice guidelines (CPGs) as 'statements that include recommendations, intended to optimize patient care, that are informed by a systematic review of evidence and an assessment of the benefits and harms of alternative care options'. Guidelines are frequently produced by multidisciplinary teams which include healthcare professionals of different types, guideline methodologists, health economists, and patient advocates.

The development of a CPG can be divided into five phases:

1. Preparation—selecting topic, identification of existing CPGs, formulating clinical questions
2. Search and selection—performing the systematic search, selecting citations based on predefined inclusion and exclusion criteria
3. Extraction and appraisal—extracting the data using standardized data extraction forms and appraising the methodological quality of the included evidence
4. Summarization and formulation of recommendations—the included evidence is summarized, whereafter the panel discusses the benefits, harms, patient values, and other important factors, and formulates recommendations
5. Writing, review, and publication—the CPG is written (with a specific description of the process, and the choices made in formulating recommendations) and sent out for external review, whereafter it is published.

Guidelines can have pitfalls, as can all forms of research. For example, the high number of topics to be covered by a guideline in a limited time may mean the evidence summaries are suboptimal, and guidelines may become 'stale' as it is difficult to refresh them frequently and keep the knowledge up to date. The term 'evidence-based' should be reserved for guidelines that followed the structured process of CPG development. It is important to realise that the term 'evidence-based' does not only apply to those recommendations where strong evidence supports the choice for a clinical decision but also, rather, refers to the process of generating the guidance.

Clinical guidelines might require adaptation before use in a local healthcare environment. The ADAPTE toolkit provides a helpful approach to doing so (www.g-i-n.net/working-groups/adaptation/history). Some useful sites to find guidelines related to paediatric oncology are in **Table 6.1**.

Synopses: evidence-based journals, structured abstracts, and other summaries

Several journals present evidence-based summaries of the knowledge in healthcare: examples are *ACP (American College of Physicians) Journal Club, BMJ (British Medical Journal) Clinical Evidence*, and *Evidence-Based Medicine* (*EBM Online*). These journals focus on a general medical audience, sometimes with paediatric issues being included. The 'Archimedes' section of *Archives of Diseases of Childhood* provides short evidence-based overviews of paediatric topics.

A further resource is UpToDate (www.uptodate.com). This is an internet-based electronic textbook that offers clinical decision-support information using current evidence to answer clinical questions. All topics are peer reviewed. However, all the steps of EBM are not clearly described which makes it difficult to judge the influence of bias. UpToDate covers around 8,000 topics but only a few topics important for the care of children with cancer are included.

Syntheses: systematic reviews in childhood cancer

The synthesized evidence in systematic reviews can help healthcare professionals to keep up to date. In a systematic review, the three first steps of EBM are included—formulating a clinical relevant question, performing an extensive search for literature, and assessing the methodological quality of the selected studies. Furthermore, a meta-analysis can be included. A systematic review aims to minimize the occurrence of bias through a systematic search, selection, and assessment of methodological quality and to reduce random error by using quantitative methods (i.e. meta-analysis) where appropriate. In paediatric oncology, 117 systematic reviews, including 18 Cochrane reviews, had been published between 1988 and November 2006. Unfortunately, the methodological quality of most of the systematic reviews in paediatric oncology seemed to have serious methodological flaws, leading to a high risk of bias.

Table 6.1 Examples for the '5S' evolution of information services for evidence-based healthcare decisions

5S	Examples	Websites
Systems	Decision-support systems that search the evidence for a given patient/ problem	
Summaries	**General (examples)**	
Clinical practice guidelines	US National Clearinghouse	www.guidelines.gov
	Guidelines International Network	www.g-i-n.net
	UK National Institute for Health and Clinical Excellence	www.nice.org.uk
	Scottish Intercollegiate Guidelines Network	www.sign.ac.uk
	Australian Clinical Practice Guidelines	www.clinicalguidelines.gov.au
	World Health Organization	www.who.int
	Evidence-based guidelines	www.ebm-guidelines.com
	Paediatric oncology (examples)	
	SIOP (Society of Paediatric Oncology)	www.siop.nl
	Children's Oncology Group	www.childrensoncologygroup.org
	International Late Effects of Childhood Cancer Guideline Harmonization Group (IGHG)	www.ighg.org
	International Paediatric Oncology Guidelines in Supportive Care Network (iPOG)	www.sickkids.ca/Research/iPOG
Synopsis	*ACP Journal Club*	annals.org/aim/journal-club
	BMJ Clinical Evidence	www.clinicalevidence.bmj.com
	Evidence-Based Medicine (EBM Online)	www.ebm.bmj.com
	'Archimedes'/'Picket' section of *Archives of Diseases of Childhood*	adc.bmj.com
	UpToDate	www.uptodate.com
Synthesis	The Cochrane Library (Cochrane database of systematic and Dare; non-Cochrane reviews)	www.cochranelibrary.com
	PubMed	www.pubmed.com
Single studies	PubMed	www.pubmed.com
	Embase	www.embase.com
	Cochrane Central Register of Controlled Trials (CENTRAL)	www.cochranelibrary.com/central

The largest single provider of systematic reviews for healthcare is the Cochrane Collaboration, with approximately 6,000 systematic reviews included in the Cochrane Library. The Cochrane Collaboration developed standardized methods to perform systematic reviews and, since 2006, Cochrane Childhood Cancer (CCC) has been registered within the Cochrane Collaboration (www.ccg.cochrane.org). The aim of CCC is to conduct and maintain systematic reviews on interventions and diagnosis for cancer in children and young adults with respect to prevention, treatment, supportive care, psychosocial care, palliative and terminal care, nursing care, and late effects of treatment. As of 2017, 75 author groups from all around the world have been preparing and updating Cochrane systematic reviews in collaboration with CCC. Those who prepare systematic reviews for CCC are mostly volunteers.

Studies

If no other sources are available, the only option to get scientific information is to identify as many single studies as are relevant to the question in PubMed or similar bibliographical databases. Each type of question (i.e. therapy (efficacy or harm), diagnosis, prognosis, aetiology, or prevention) is best answered by a different study design.

Third step: appraisals are more than criticism

The process of critical appraisal is to examine a study in detail, in order to determine if it provides a valid, important, and applicable answer to a specific clinical question. It is not the process of finding flaws and destroying research: it is evaluating strengths and weaknesses and coming to a conclusion in clear sight.

There are a wide range of structured checklists, which differ according to the study type that is being appraised. We favour the Cochrane risk of bias tool for randomized studies and the ROBINS-I tool for non-randomized studies. For other study types, guidance is provided in the *JAMA Users Guides* (www.jamaevidence.com). The methodological quality of synthesized evidence (like systematic reviews or guidelines) can be appraised in a systematic manner by using the AMSTAR tool or ROBIS tool for systematic reviews, and the AGREE instrument for guidelines.

Fourth step: apply the results in practice

After the first three steps of EBM, a decision should be made on how to apply the results to your patient(s) or how to formulate recommendations for (a group of) patients.

For only 20% of the interventions in clinical practice do we know that the treatment is beneficial or we know that there is a trade-off between benefits and harms. Even in these cases, a weighting of the evidence, clinical expertise, patient values, and sociocultural values will be essential. When the evidence is uncertain, making these decisions and trade-offs explicit and insightful becomes even more important. Furthermore, the costs and resources used or saved should be taken into account.

In the world of paediatric oncology, there are frequently times when the rarity of the condition makes 'gold standard' or high-quality, directly applicable evidence unobtainable. For these sorts of situations, Jeremy Howick, Paul Glazsiou, and Jeffrey Aronson have revisited the Revised Bradford-Hill Guidelines for Causation and developed the concept of categories of evidence: a trio of the main category (direct evidence) and two subsidiary categories (mechanistic and parallel evidence).

Direct evidence is the data we rely on most securely: the RCT gives results of a therapy being effective, or when an exceptionally effective intervention is considerably better than all others (like when insulin was first used in diabetic ketoacidosis).

Parallel evidence is used in paediatrics a great deal: similarities exist between the direct evidence in other populations and the ones we treat, and by replication of results across different areas.

Mechanistic evidence is the shakiest: coherence with other theories of how things work, and a plausible biological explanation.

Another reason why evidence could be difficult to translate directly to practice is when, for instance, the results of a systematic review are focused on concepts. For example, a systematic review of antiemetics to prevent nausea and vomiting after chemotherapy tells you 'antiemetics work'. However, you cannot just prescribe 'antiemetics', so how can you transfer the review result into clinical practice? A couple of suggestions have been offered, and both have clinical common sense:

1. Go for the strategy of the largest trial (it has the most weight in the review, so has the 'most' evidence).
2. Go for the most often-used dose/drug/approach (it was shown to be feasible the most often).

This clear conceptualization of the various guises in which evidence exists can help us decide what works, what works best, and what is likely to work for this patient.

Steps in guideline development as a doer of evidence-based medicine

A more rigorous approach to answering a question is to complete a GRADE evidence to decision (EtD) framework for the clinical question at hand. This framework helps to systematically and transparently assess things like benefits, harms, use of resources, acceptability, and feasibility of a treatment option, and thus aids in making a clinical decision. This approach comprises two major steps: summarizing the evidence and formulating one or more recommendations.

In the first step, the GRADE system is used to determine the so-called 'body of evidence' per outcome. For each outcome of interest, a different combination of studies can be included. Therefore, for each outcome the quality of evidence is determined separately on a four-level scale—high, moderate, low, or very low. The initial quality depends on the included type of studies: randomized controlled trials are regarded as high-quality, observational studies are regarded as low-quality. These levels of evidence can then be downgraded due to risk of bias (see step 3: appraisal), inconsistency, indirectness, imprecision, and/or publication bias. Upgrading the level of evidence is also possible due to the magnitude of effect, identified dose–response gradient, or identified plausible confounders that would have reduced the effect. There is an excellent series of articles in the *Journal of Clinical Epidemiology* teaching the reader how to use this system. (Details of the first of these articles, by Guyatt et al., can be found in 'Further reading'). The GRADE system is being increasingly adopted by organizations other than the GRADE working group: for instance, the Cochrane Collaboration recommends this approach in assessing the quality of evidence in their reviews.

In the second step, the GRADE EtD framework is completed, in which questions are answered regarding the priority of the problem, anticipated benefits and harms (using the evidence and its determined quality level), resource use, equity, acceptability, and feasibility. This leads to an overall balance of desirable and undesirable consequences, from which a recommendation is distilled. This recommendation to do or not do something can either be strong ('you should', 'we recommend') or weak ('you might', 'we suggest'). For each recommendation, the accompanying quality of evidence is provided, where it should be noted that high-quality evidence does not automatically lead to a strong recommendation or low-quality evidence to a weak recommendation. A strong recommendation based on very low-quality evidence (e.g. small, observational studies with large effect on pivotal outcome) or a weak recommendation based on high-quality evidence (e.g. large, randomized trials with a marginal beneficial effect) is also possible.

We would not advise to follow this EtD methodology strictly and extensively when in need of an answer for a specific patient question, as this is very time-consuming and more appropriate for true guideline development. However, it is beneficial to familiarize oneself with this way of thinking about/coming to a decision, as it might be extremely useful when weighing the options and the evidence for a specific patient question.

In conclusion, there are various methods for deriving a clinical decision from the available evidence, of which critical appraisal of the identified evidence is always a pivotal step. For each clinical decision the (quality of) available evidence, values of patients, cultural values, clinical expertise, and the resource use should be taken into account.

Common criticisms of evidence-based medicine

Since the introduction of EBM, criticisms of this paradigm shift have been described which can be divided into 'limitations universal to the practice of medicine', 'misperceptions of EBM', and 'genuine limitations of EBM'.

Within the group of 'limitations universal to the practice of medicine' fall criticisms such as 'There is a shortage of coherent, consistent scientific evidence' or 'There is no evidence available', along with complaints stating 'It is difficult to translate evidence to the care of an individual patient'. In instances like this, the methods of EBM can be used to assess these shortages and difficulties systematically, and thus identify research gaps for further study.

The second group of criticisms of EBM are based on misperceptions. For example, criticisms that EBM 'denigrates clinical expertise' or 'ignores patients' values' or 'promotes "cookbook" medicine' arise through a failure to include all the important steps of EBM. EBM is a guide in science and aids decision making; it is not a law, nor it is a system that will make a decision for you. A further example of misperception is that 'only randomized trials or systematic reviews' constitute the 'evidence' in EBM. This is not true, and several sources of best available evidence may inform clinical decision making. For instance, if RCTs to answer your clinical questions are lacking, you can choose to divert to RCTs in other populations, but in certain scenarios it might be more suitable to divert to other study designs, such as non-randomized comparison studies or cohort studies, in your own target population.

Finally, some of the criticisms of EBM are genuine limitations of the process: there is a need to develop new skills and apply the process during limited time and with limited resources. To overcome this barrier, we believe an increasing number of prepared evidence-based products and training programmes will be available in the future.

The way forward

To take paediatric oncology further forward, in developing its evidence base and the implementation of that evidence, we need to continue doing lots of what we are doing:

- We need to work as international collaborators, focused on the cure and support of children with malignancies by engaging in high-quality research, including our patients, their families, and our colleagues in other specialties.
- We need to continue to collaborate in developing high-quality trials in paediatric oncology. As previously stated by Caldwell and colleagues in the *Lancet*: 'Participation in protocol-driven clinical research is clearly better than the ad hoc patterns of non-protocol treatments, paediatric cancer trials offer a paradigm for paediatric clinical research'.
- We need to collaborate in summarizing the evidence. CCC offers a unique possibility to collaborate worldwide in preparing scientific summaries of evidence. We should strive towards making the evidence easily accessible and usable, for instance with the development of summaries of findings tables.
- We need to collaborate in producing evidence-based guidelines. For this purpose, various international initiatives have been undertaken, such as the International Late Effects of Childhood Cancer Guideline Harmonization Group (IGHG) and the International Paediatric Oncology Guidelines in Supportive Care Network (iPOG). International collaboration is of the utmost importance to reduce duplication of work and maximize results from the available time and effort.
- We need to develop new systems and strategies to implement up-to-date high-quality scientific knowledge in daily practice.
- We need to develop training for researchers and clinicians in clinical epidemiology and EBM methods.

In conclusion, we need interventions to bridge the gap between science and practice in paediatric oncology worldwide and make our daily practice as evidence-based as possible.

FURTHER READING

Alonso-Coello P, et al. (2016) GRADE evidence to decision (EtD) frameworks: a systematic and transparent approach to making well informed healthcare choices. 1: Introduction. *BMJ* **353**, i2016.

Caldwell PH, et al. (2004) Clinical trials in children. *Lancet* **364**, 803–11.

Davidoff F, et al. (1995) Evidence based medicine. *BMJ* **310**, 1085–6.

Evidence-Based Medicine Working Group (1992) Evidence-based medicine. A new approach to teaching the practice of medicine. *JAMA* **268**, 2420–5.

Godlee F (2007). Milestones on the long road to knowledge. *BMJ* **334**(Suppl 1), s2–3.

Graham R, et al. (2011) *Clinical Practice Guidelines We Can Trust.* Washington DC: The National Academies Press.

Guyatt G, et al. (2011) GRADE guidelines: 1. Introduction—GRADE evidence profiles and summary of findings tables. *J Clin Epidemiol* **64**, 383–94.

Haynes RB (2006) Of studies, syntheses, synopses, summaries, and systems: the '5S' evolution of information services for evidence-based healthcare decisions. *Evid Based Med* **11**, 162–4.

Higgins JPT, et al. (eds) (2019) *Cochrane Handbook for Systematic Reviews of Interventions, Version 6.0*. Available from: www.training.cochrane.org/handbook

Higgins JPT, et al. (eds) (2019) *Cochrane Handbook for Systematic Reviews of Interventions* (2nd edn). Chichester, UK: Wiley.

Howick J, et al. (2009) The evolution of evidence hierarchies: what can Bradford Hill's 'guidelines for causation' contribute? *J R Soc Med* **102**, 186–94.

Lundh A, et al. (2009) *Quality of systematic reviews in pediatric oncology—a systematic review. Cancer Treat Rev* **35**, 645–52.

Phillips R, Glasziou P (2008) Evidence based practice: the practicalities of keeping abreast of clinical evidence while in training. *Postgrad Med J* **84**, 450–3.

Rotter T, et al. (2010) Clinical pathways: effects on professional practice, patient outcomes, length of stay and hospital costs. *Cochrane Database Syst Rev* **17**, CD006632.

Sackett DL, et al. (1996) Evidence based medicine: what it is and what it isn't. *BMJ* **312**, 71.

Shea BJ, et al. (2009) AMSTAR is a reliable and valid measurement tool to assess the methodological quality of systematic reviews. *J Clin Epidemiol* **10**, 1013–20.

Sterne JAC, et al. (2016) ROBINS-I: a tool for assessing risk of bias in non-randomised studies of interventions. *BMJ* **355**, i4919.

Straus SE, McAlister FA (2000) Evidence-based medicine: a commentary on common criticisms. *CMAJ* **163**, 837–41.

Whiting P, et al. (2016) ROBIS: a new tool to assess risk of bias in systematic reviews was developed. *J Clin Epidemiol* **69**, 225–34.

7

Allogeneic Stem-Cell Transplantation in Children and Adolescents with Malignancies

Adriana Balduzzi, Giovanna Lucchini, Jean-Hugues Dalle, and Rupert Handgretinger

History of stem-cell transplantation

The incipit

The first allogeneic haematopoietic stem-cell transplantation (HSCT) was pioneered by E. Donnall Thomas and reported in the *New England Journal of Medicine* in 1957. Radiation and chemotherapy, followed by intravenous infusion of bone marrow (BM) from a normal donor, led to haematological reconstitution and leukaemia eradication. Despite the fact that no patients transplanted in the late 1950s and early 1960s survived—due to graft failure, rejection, graft-versus-host disease (GvHD), or opportunistic infections—three major principles of allogeneic HSCT were demonstrated:

1. the role of the preparative anti-leukaemic regimen,
2. the ability of the new engrafted immune system to prevent leukaemia relapse, and
3. the activity of the engrafted immune system against the recipient.

It was a proof of principle. The bone marrow transplantation era had begun.

After van Rood's recognition of anti-HLA antibodies in pregnant women in 1958, the discovery of the role of human leukocyte antigen (HLA) in tissue transplantation, and van Bekkum's animal models, three patients with congenital immunodeficiencies were transplanted from their HLA-identical siblings, in the United States and in the Netherlands, in 1968. Thomas then reported the first allografting experience in patients with severe aplastic anaemia in 1972, in 100 advanced acute leukaemia patients in 1977, after which 13 patients were alive without disease, and in acute myeloid leukaemia (AML) patients in first remission in 1979, achieving a cure rate of 50%. In 1990, E. Donnall Thomas won a Nobel Prize 'for his discoveries in cell transplantation in the treatment of human diseases'.

During the past 50 years, the role of HSCT has changed from a desperate therapeutic approach to a curative treatment modality for thousands of patients with haematological diseases.

Recent developments

The myeloablative effect of the conditioning regimen and the alloreactivity of donor cells, potentially eradicating residual malignant cells in the patient, play crucial role in transplantation.

Even though, in the current era, higher resolution of HLA typing—allowing strict donor–recipient matching—and better management of infection and graft-versus-host disease (GvHD) lessen—the incidence of complications, the risk of morbidity and, mainly, mortality (defined as transplant-related mortality, TRM) remain definitely higher than with chemotherapy alone. The use of peripheral blood stem cells (PBSC) or cord blood (CB), instead of BM, for HSCT, has become a routine part of transplantation.

In the mid 1990s, alongside myeloablative (MA) conditionings, non-MA or reduced-intensity (RI) conditionings were introduced. As expected, non-MA and RI conditionings broadened the eligibility for HSCT to include patients with comorbidities.

Donor type

The human leukocyte antigen barrier

After van Rood's pivotal discovery and the subsequent studies which unravelled the genetics of HLA, allowing better donor selection, a major concern in the 1970s was the limitation of allogeneic grafting only to those patients who had an HLA-identical sibling available. In 1979, Hansen performed the first successful marrow graft from an unrelated donor (URD) for a patient with leukaemia. Since then, the establishment of URD registries has facilitated HSCT worldwide and dramatically increased the odds for finding a match, which have risen from 25% to 75% for Caucasian patients.

Donor and patient registries

In 1972, the International Bone Marrow Transplant Registry (IBMTR) and, in 1974, the European Group for Blood and Marrow Transplantation (EBMT) were established for documenting HSCT outcome data and facilitating cooperative studies. Between 1989 and 1995, the use of volunteer URDs was extended and reported in children affected with congenital disorders or malignancies by many groups. TRM was a major obstacle; relapse remained the most frequent cause of treatment failure in malignancies.

Human leukocyte antigen typing

Nowadays, HLA compatibility with the donor, either related or unrelated, is defined by high-resolution typing (four digits) for HLA-A, -B, -C, -DR, -DQ HLA alleles. All the ten alleles are usually matched in paediatrics, but also matching for all but DQB1 alleles is commonly accepted.

According to the Paediatric Diseases Working Party of the European Bone Marrow Transplantation association (EBMT) and the HSCT Committee of the International BFM (Berlin–Frankfurt–Munster) Study Group (I-BFM SG), donors are defined as matched siblings (MSD) if they are HLA-identical to their recipients, as each donor and recipient inherited the same parental haplotypes. Regardless of their relationship, donor–recipient pairs are defined as HLA-matched donors (MD) if they are fully matched (10/10 or 8/8) or have a single allelic or antigenic disparity (9/10 or 7/8). Donors are defined as mismatched donors (MMD) if they have two (8/10 or 6/8) or more allelic or antigenic disparities, up to a different haplotype. Any donor who is not an HLA-identical sibling or a MD, as defined above, is to be considered a MMD. By definition, both an MD and MMD could be either related or unrelated to their recipient, regardless of cell source.

Cord-blood matching

As a matter of fact, the concept of 'compatibility' for CB donor–recipient pairs is still under debate. In the past, any CB unit which was 6/6 or 5/6 matched was labelled HLA compatible (MD), as defined by low-resolution typing at A and B loci and high-resolution at the DRB1 locus; more recently, high-resolution typing for at least A, B, C, DRB1 loci has been requested and, progressively, the same criteria used for volunteer donors has come to define CB HLA matching.

Donor selection

It is known that multiple factors have an impact on transplantation outcome; the most crucial ones are disease-related (e.g. disease refractoriness and phase, clonal abnormalities in malignancies; disease type and associated rejection risk in non-malignant diseases) or patient-related (e.g. age, comorbidities, infectious diseases/colonization), but many are donor-related.

Human leukocyte antigen compatibility

The outcome of HSCT depends on the matching between the donor and the recipient for the HLAs, encoded by a group of genes on chromosome 6; genes and products are labelled as major histocompatibility complex (MHC). The most relevant genes for transplantation belong to class I (HLA-A, -B, and -Cw) and class II (HLA-DR, -DQ, and -DP). Class I specificities are present on all nucleated cells of an individual, whereas class II genes are found primarily on cells of the immune system, such as B lymphocytes and macrophages. In contrast to previous serological methods, HLA specificities are nowadays mostly identified by DNA sequencing. A locus name is followed by a one- or two-digit number, indicating a serological-defined specificity (e.g. HLA-A2). A DNA sequence registered with the World Health Organization (WHO) is assigned a number with the first digits usually related to the closer serological equivalent, such as HLA-A*02:01, and the following digits representing the order of sequence registration for alleles of that group (e.g. HLA-A*02:01:01:01). The asterisk indicates that data are assessed by molecular typing.

Individuals inherit a set of HLA, called a haplotype, from each parent; therefore, the probability that a child shares both haplotypes with a full sibling is 25%, the chance of sharing one haplotype is 50% and the chance of sharing neither haplotype is 25%. An HLA-identical sibling is considered an optimal donor.

The HLA system has proven to be the most polymorphic genetic region known in the human genome; nevertheless, the HLA genes are closely linked and the recombination rate is therefore limited. Unfortunately, the likelihood of identifying a URD decreases with the requested degree of matching.

Donor-related issues

Besides HLA compatibility and stem-cell source, donor age, gender, female parity, weight, ABO blood group, and viral serological status should also be considered in the decision-making process for donor selection, whenever more than one donor is available (which may not often be the case). Most studies report that a young donor is better than an older one, and a male donor is better for a male recipient and better than a multiparous woman for any recipient, even though there is no consensus on this issue. Unfavourable weight disparity, with donors weighing less than their recipient, should be avoided, when possible. CMV (cytomegalovirus)-IgG-positive and EBV (Epstein-Barr virus)-positive patients should be grafted from CMV- and EBV-positive donors, respectively. ABO matching is usually preferred, especially instead of a major or even minor incompatibility. Donor location might also be considered, as overseas deliveries increase the time elapsing between collection and infusion, thus reducing cell viability and potentially jeopardizing engraftment. More recently, killer-cell immunoglobulin-like receptor (KIR) genotyping has allowed identification of alloreactive donors who may help to prevent relapse.

Hierarchy

Even though it is mainly clear which variant should be preferred within each feature, there is no consensus regarding the hierarchical order by which the aforementioned factors should be combined. In a recent survey within the Paediatric Diseases Working Party of the EBMT, the features were generally listed in the following order of importance, although evaluations widely differed among responders: HLA compatibility, CMV serological status in case of positive recipients, stem-cell source, donor age, donor gender, ABO major incompatibility, donor-centre location, ABO minor incompatibility (unpublished data).

Haploidentical transplant: history and recent development

Unmanipulated bone marrow

The first haploidentical transplantations, performed in the 1980s with unmanipulated BM, were complicated by severe and often lethal side effects, such as pulmonary oedema and multi-organ failure, most likely caused by severe GvHD. Attempts were then made to remove T-cells from BM grafts by means of soybean agglutinin and rosette formation with sheep red-blood cells in children with immunodeficiencies.

Ex vivo T-cell depletion

Subsequently, Henslee-Downey and colleagues introduced partial *in vitro* T-cell depletion of BM grafts by means of anti-CD3 antibodies (T10B9 or OKT-3) with a 1–1.5 log T-cell reduction and post-transplant pharmacological GvHD prophylaxis. Out of the 201 patients treated, 98% engrafted, and the five-year cumulative incidence of relapses was 31% and TRM was 51%.

CD34+ positive selection

The introduction of CD34+ cell positive selection methods from mobilized PBSCs allowed the transplantation of high numbers of CD34+ stem cells and the efficient depletion of T-cells. Haploidentical transplantation was performed in adults and children without, or with only minimal, pharmacological GvHD prophylaxis. However, the immune reconstitution was delayed, resulting in viral and bacterial infections.

With the CD34+ cell positive selection, no other cells are co-transplanted, whereas with negative depletion strategies, large numbers of other cells (e.g. NK cells, monocytes, dendritic cells) are infused together with high numbers of CD34+ stem cells. Therefore, innovative methods were developed to negatively deplete T-cells (and also B-cells) from PBSCs.

CD34+ negative selection

Depletion of CD3+ T-cells enabled a T-cell depletion of 3.5–4 log. Various clinical studies using this method were performed in children and in adults. The engraftment was rapid and an accelerated recovery of natural killer (NK) cells was observed. The rate of GvHD was acceptable and the risk of infectious complications was lower in children compared to adult patients.

Since the efficacy of the CD34+ negative selection (i.e. CD3+ depletion method was 1-log lower compared to the previous CD34+ positive selection methods), attempts were made to improve the negative depletion efficacy by the removal of TCRαβ+ T-lymphocytes. TCRαβ+ depletion yields a 4–4.5 log CD3+ depletion, comparable to the CD3 depletion which can be achieved with the CD34+ positive selection method. In addition, non-alloreactive γδ T-lymphocytes remain within the graft, which might induce anti-infectious and anti-leukaemic effects.

TCRαβ depletion

An improved immune recovery after TCRαβ-depleted stem cells from haploidentical donors in paediatric patients was reported by Lang and colleagues. In another study in children with acute leukaemias, the outcome of TCRαβ-depleted stem cell transplantation was similar to children who grafted from matched siblings or matched URDs. Promising results with the same approach were reported in children with non-malignant diseases and confirmed by a multicentre phase I/II study recently performed in children with various diseases.

In vivo T-cell depletion

An alternative approach to the *ex vivo* T-cell depletion is the use of unmanipulated BM (T-replete BM), with or without PBSCs with extensive GvHD prophylaxis. Huang and colleagues have pioneered the use of granulocyte colony-stimulating growth factor (G-CSF)-primed BM, together with PBSCs, in adult patients. Grade II–IV acute and chronic GvHD were observed in 78% and 73% of the patients, respectively. The use of (G-CSF)-mobilized PBSCs alone was inferior compared to the use of G-CSF-primed BM together with PBSCs. G-CSF-primed BM was also used in paediatric patients with haematological malignancies, with a two-year disease-free survival of 53%.

Post-transplant cyclophosphamide

A more recently developed approach of T-replete transplantation of either BM or peripheral blood (PB) is the use of post-transplant cyclophosphamide (PT-Cy) to induce tolerance of donor-derived T-lymphocytes. In an initial study in 68 adult patients with haematological malignancies, cyclophosphamide (50 mg/kg) was given on day three, or days three and four, after transplant. Graft failure was seen in 13% of the patients and cumulative incidence of grade II–IV, grade III–IV acute GvHD, and chronic GvHD was 34%, 6%, and 22%, respectively. The two-year event-free survival was 26%. Based on the feasibility of this approach, PT-Cy is increasingly used, mainly in adult patients. Less experience exists in paediatric patients, but reports are promising so far. Whether the risk of relapse in children with haematological malignancies will increase due to heavier immune suppression needs to be assessed in future prospective clinical studies.

Summary

Overall, haploidentical transplantation in children has evolved as a realistic alternative for patients in need of a transplant lacking a suitable donor. In children, haploidentical donors are mainly three-loci mismatched parental donors, but haploidentical relatives can also be included in the rare cases where parents are not medically fit to donate.

Currently, the choice between T-depleted versus T-repleted grafts depends on the experience of the transplant centre with each different method, while a prospective study comparing the two different approaches would be desirable.

Stem-cell source

As for adult patients, three different stem-cell (SC) sources may be used for paediatric HSCT: BM, PBSC obtained after donor mobilization with G-CSF, and CB—or a combination of the three.

Bone marrow

For many years and for historical reasons, BM was the most common source used in the allograft setting and still remains the 'gold standard' in paediatrics, as it offers the most consolidated results. The graft should contain at least 3×10^8 nucleated cells/kg recipient body weight and 3×10^6 CD34+ cells/kg body weight, in order to yield more than 95% neutrophil engraftment chances at a median of 21 days in the setting of haematological malignant diseases.

Peripheral blood

Mobilized PB as a SC source has become more and more common over the years (initially in adults, and eventually in children) mainly due to its higher cell content, especially CD34, allowing faster engraftment.

Haploidentical setting

PBSCs are also used in the setting of T-cell-depleted haploidentical transplantation, after the concept of mega-cell dose, in order to overcome HLA disparity and ensure engraftment.

Impact of stem-cell source on graft-versus-host disease and relapse

The possible increased risk of both acute and chronic GvHD after PBSC transplantation, as compared to BM transplantation, is still debated. In a recent European retrospective study, including 2,584 paediatric patients transplanted from 2003 to 2012 for acute lymphoblastic leukaemia, both TRM and chronic GvHD appeared significantly higher after PBSC, as compared with other SC sources, despite that overall survival (OS) was similar for both stem-cell sources. In the prospective ALL-SCT-BFM 2003 Study chaired by Peters, the same OS was reported, and no difference could be demonstrated in TRM, GvHD, and relapse, whichever the stem-cell source in the two cohorts of patients transplanted from HLA-identical siblings and other matched donors. Nevertheless, within patients transplanted from HLA-identical siblings, the cumulative incidence of chronic GvHD was higher in PB compared with BM recipients.

Nowadays, in the ongoing prospective ALL-I-BFM HSCT trial (FORUM), the algorithm for choosing stem-cell source recommends BM as the first choice. Reinforced GvHD prophylaxis may be recommended when PBSC are used, mainly when no serotherapy is included as for GvHD prophylaxis, as in most protocols in the HLA-identical sibling setting.

To date, there is no demonstration for a better graft-versus-leukaemia effect after either BM or PBSC in the paediatric population.

T-cell replete haploidentical graft

Recently, T-cell repleted haploidentical transplantation was developed. So far, there are no available data to advocate for using BM or PBSC as the preferred stem-cell source, particularly in the paediatric population transplanted for malignant diseases.

Cord blood

From the first CB transplantation performed for a Fanconi anaemia patient in 1987, CB has appeared as a useful and efficient stem-cell source, due to two major features: high proliferative capacity (allowing engraftment despite 1-log fewer cells) and immune plasticity (allowing a wider HLA disparity within each donor–recipient pair).

The possibility to adopt less stringent HLA matching criteria enlarged the availability of grafts to at least 90% of the paediatric patients in need of an allogeneic transplant. According to Eurocord Consortium recommendations, unrelated CB with two or less HLA disparities typed in low resolution (i.e. two-digit) for class I (A and B loci) and high resolution (i.e. four-digit) for class II (DRB1 locus), and with more than 2.5×10^7 nucleated cell dose/kg or 2×10^5 CD34+ cells/kg are suitable for engraftment. Recent studies from Eurocord, Netcord, EBMT, and the Center for International Blood and Marrow Transplant Research (CIBMTR) recommend high-resolution HLA typing for A, B, C, and DRB1, and a maximum of one or two mismatched loci with a cellularity of 3×10^7 TNC/kg or higher.

Two prospective studies could demonstrate no benefit of double CB in paediatric patients transplanted for malignant diseases.

Minor sibling donors

Paediatricians have to take into special consideration minor sibling donors. As for any transplantation from living donors, it is mandatory that the healthy donor's safety should remain the most important issue of the procedure. However, minor donors are particularly fragile, as they do not really feel free regarding donation acceptance. Physicians have to ensure donor autonomy and both physical and psychological integrity as much as possible.

The American Academy of Pediatrics Committee on Bioethics (AAPCOB) deems the use of a child BM donor ethically appropriate when five conditions are met: no available matched adult donor; reasonable expected benefit for recipient; strong relationship between donor and recipient; medical, emotional, and psychological risk to the child donor minimal and reasonable in comparison to the benefit gained by the recipient; and, finally, parent consent and patient assent. This last point is the most difficult ethical issue. In order to ensure it, some countries or institutions provide independent committees to interview and evaluate minor donors.

Conditioning regimens

The struggle to reduce the use of radiotherapy in children

Total body irradiation (TBI) has been at the heart of conditioning regimens for malignancies in both adults and children since the beginning of the HSCT era. Despite its efficacy, the burden of long-term side effects, specifically in the paediatric population, has been a concern for transplanters all along. While fractionating radiation doses and lung shielding has proven efficacious in reducing, from 50% to 4%, the incidence of pulmonary complications, recent data confirms that TBI exposure is implicated in the long-term post-HSCT burden of diseases. Indeed, TBI significantly increases the cardiovascular risk in long-term transplant survivors, by increasing the risk of metabolic syndrome, specifically of hypertriglyceridaemia, hypercholesterolaemia, and insulin resistance. A strong association is also known between cataracts and TBI, with 28–78% of exposed patients presenting with this complication. In terms of endocrine dysfunction, a clear role for TBI versus alkylating agents such as busulfan (Bu) could not be found to support long-term thyroid impairment as well as ovarian failure/azoospermia, but TBI is definitely implicated in growth failure. Indeed, not only is growth hormone (GH) production reduced post TBI but also the growth spurt is absent due to low GH in combination with low sex hormones, and growth plates in long bones undergoing premature closure after TBI exposure.

With regard to lung function, it is unclear whether fractionated TBI plays a worse role than BU in causing restrictive lung function. Moreover, the specific role of TBI in undermining the cognitive functions of transplanted patients has been confirmed by some, but not by other, studies. In this regard, it is important to underline that all studies conclude that socioeconomic status, as well as pre-HSCT IQ, are the most important predictive factors for long-term cognitive functions in patients undergoing HSCT for malignant disorders. Dramatically though, secondary malignancies appear to be the most serious long-term effect of HSCT, with cranio-spinal irradiation being a significant risk factor. With an incidence of second tumour of up to 11% at 15 years post-HSCT and an age-dependent factor (patients receiving HSCT aged 10 years or younger are at a significantly higher risk of second tumour than older patients), this alone represents a significant reason to try and avoid TBI as much as possible in the preparation regimen of children.

Acute myeloid leukaemia

Thomas and colleagues were the first to describe the use of TBI for AML and reported a reduced toxicity by using a fractionated TBI schedule. Santos firstly described the use of Bu-based regimens associated with Cy 200 mg/kg. This regimen showed low cumulative incidence of relapse (CIR) but increased TRM, which could be corrected by reducing the Cy dose to 120 mg/kg as described by Tutschka and colleagues. Blaise and Ringden published two randomized trials, which compared TBI-Cy120 versus Bu-Cy120, and showed higher non-relapse mortality (NRM) and higher CIR in the Bu arm. Nevertheless, further updates on these studies provided longer follow-up and failed to document a worse outcome in Bu-treated patients. De Berranger and colleagues also concluded that there was no advantage of one regimen over the other when considering only a paediatric population with AML in CR1 at HSCT. A more recent prospective study from Ishida and colleagues confirmed no significant differences in outcome in children with AML in CR1/CR2 receiving TBI-Cy or IV Bu-Cy. Copelan and colleagues documented lower TRM and lower CIR in patients with AML in CR1 treated with IV Bu-Cy as compared to those treated with TBI-Cy, and lower CIR as compared to both TBI-Cy and oral Bu-Cy treatment. Overall, these data have resulted in a markedly reduced use of TBI-based conditioning regimens in the AML paediatric population.

Acute lymphoblastic leukaemia

In the context of ALL, it has been less easy to outplay TBI. Standard use of TBI combined with VP16 or Cy has been challenged by prospective and randomized studies comparing Bu-containing regimens with no benefit in terms of relapse rate and increased transplant-related toxicities in the non-TBI arm. Moreover, some cooperative groups showed a correlation between increasing the TBI dose and reducing relapse rate in paediatric and adult patients.

Given the small proportion of ALL-affected patients that need HSCT as a standard treatment, the implementation of an international randomized study was deemed necessary to finally answer the question of whether a TBI-containing regimen is superior to chemotherapy-alone regimens in the treatment of ALL in children. Such a study is currently open for recruitment in 20 countries worldwide, and aims at comparing the standard VP16 TBI 12-Gy conditioning regimen with Fludarabine/Thiotepa/IV Bu or Fludarabine/Thiotepa/Treosulfan regimens. While results of this study will be crucial to shape further HSCT ALL treatment, it has to be remembered that the role of TBI in the context of mismatched or haploidentical transplants is even more difficult to understand, with low patient numbers and numerous differences in conditioning regimen and HSCT approach jeopardizing the possibility of meaningful comparisons.

Reduced-intensity conditioning to reduce toxicity post stem-cell transplantation

The traditional aim of conditioning regimens in the malignancy setting had been that of eradicating residual disease and guaranteeing complete marrow ablation to allow donor cell engraftment. Data showing the role of donor T-cells in mediating graft-versus-tumour effect, and preclinical experiments documenting the possibility of engraftment despite reduced myeloablation, paved the way for the development of so-called 'reduced-intensity conditioning' (RIC). This definition underpins numerous conditioning regimens, the intensity of which varies considerably from minimal to little less than myeloablative. Overall, a consensus had been reached in 2009 with regard to the definition of RIC, which is still valid, despite novel agents entering the chemotherapy field.

Since the 1990s, the use of RIC regimens has been increasingly popular for older recipients with comorbidities which prevent the safe use of conventional myeloablative regimens. The intrinsic nature of RIC regimens has seen them being allocated to more vulnerable patients, making direct comparisons between RIC and myeloablative conditioning (MAC) regimens difficult. As children conventionally tolerate higher treatment exposures, the use of RIC in the paediatric population has remained quite limited so far. The possibility of expanding its use with the aim of limiting long-term post-HSCT sequelae is nevertheless appealing. Early data which still need to be confirmed and have been gathered in the context of non-malignant disorders, showed better gonadal function following RIC regimens, with hope for fertility preservation. It appears that thyroid dysfunction, as well as growth impairment, might remain significant, despite avoiding myeloablation, but the substantial question will be whether secondary malignancies could be significantly reduced after RIC.

Data obtained so far explore children mainly transplanted for non-malignant diseases, which may be influenced by genetic factors as well. Data on the use of RIC regimens for malignancies are rare in paediatric patients.

Reduced-intensity versus myeloablative conditioning in paediatric acute myeloid leukaemia

CIBMTR ran a case-control study on the use of RIC versus MA protocols for children receiving their first HSCT for AML. Case and controls were matched for age, disease status, cytogenetics, graft type, and year of HSCT. Thirty-nine patients receiving RIC were matched with 141 receiving MAC protocols. Not surprisingly, patients receiving RIC displayed a lower performance score. Overall, the two groups showed no statistically significant differences in terms of count recovery (RIC 87% versus MAC 84%), GvHD incidence (28% versus 39%), TRM (16% in both cohorts), relapse rate (39% in both cohorts), leukaemia-free survival (LFS) (46% in both cohorts), and OS (45% versus 48%). After adjusting for disease status at HSCT, cytogenetic risk group, graft type, and HSCT year, the only characteristic associated with higher LFS and OS was the patient performance score. It has to be underlined that these are retrospective, registry data, not accounting for MRD status. It has also to be noted that these results are different from the ones repeatedly reported in adult cohorts, in which the use of RIC for AML has often resulted in increased relapse rate but reduced TRM, thus achieving a similar OS to MAC-based HSCT, where toxicity was higher but relapse rate lower.

A recent meta-analysis of available data in this setting correctly underlined that in all previous studies, apart from a single randomized one, patients undergoing RIC regimens were older, and had a more advanced stage of disease and potentially lower performance scores than those allocated to MAC conditionings, thus leaving open the question of RIC versus MAC in a young cohort of patients.

There are currently two ongoing prospective trials in children assessing the use of RIC in AML (NCI NCT02724163 and NCT02626715), and one of those is a randomized trial which aims at comparing standard busulfan-cyclophosphamide association to busulfan-fludarabine association in AML CR1 high risk for MRD and/or cytogenetics.

Reduced-intensity versus myeloablative conditioning regimen in acute lymphoblastic leukaemia

Given the reduced evidence of a graft-versus-leukaemia effect in rapid-evolving diseases like ALL, less experience has been gathered on the use of RIC in this setting. Specifically, for paediatric patients receiving their first HSCT, two retrospective studies are available to describe the use of RIC conditioning. Verneris and colleagues collected data on 38 patients transplanted between 1995 and 2005 in several American centres. Median age at HSCT was 12 years; 22% of the patients had active disease at HSCT and different RIC regimens were used. This study observed three-year disease-free survival (DFS), in line with other paediatric studies using MAC, but significant three-year TRM of 32%, which is higher than the TRM reported in the only prospective study assessing the use of RIC in malignancies for children not eligible to MAC transplant. The increased TRM in this study has been attributed to the possible non-homogeneity of RIC used and to transplants performed in an earlier era than the Pulsipher study. Moreover, no clear identification of the reasons for allocating patients to RIC regimens is described in this study, though no patient was reported to have significant comorbidities at the time of HSCT.

The Japanese Society for HSCT reported recently on their retrospective experience on the use of RIC in paediatric ALL and its comparison with MAC: 1,201 patients undergoing MAC were compared with 133 patients receiving RIC between the year 2000 and 2010, with a median follow-up of five years post-HSCT. Most patients were in CR1 at the time of transplant, with disease phases being equally represented in RIC and MAC cohorts. In the RIC setting, a higher percentage of patients received HSCT from a MMD. In this context, relapse rate was found to be higher in patients receiving RIC (43% versus 33%; $p = 0.02$), while TRM rate was superimposable in both cohorts at 15%, and OS was 52% for RIC patients and 56% for MAC patients (p = ns). In the multivariate analysis—adjusted for age, gender, disease status, stem-cell source, conditioning regimen, and HLA matching—the conditioning regimen was no longer a significant prognostic factor for relapse.

Overall, while ALL-affected paediatric patients can be allocated to RIC regimens in case of unsuitability for MAC, there are currently no active studies investigating the use of RIC as primary conditioning for ALL in children.

Indications for stem-cell transplantation

The definition of the indications for HSCT in childhood is a dynamic process, requiring constant assessment of the likelihood of cure with chemotherapy only, in order to identify the subsets of children who would benefit from transplantation. Eligibility criteria have evolved over time, due to improvements in treatment outcome obtained with chemotherapeutic protocols and changes in transplantation outcome.

Randomized controlled clinical trials represent the gold standard by which treatment choices are made in modern medicine. Paediatric oncology has, par excellence, been one of the specialties that have adopted the approach of randomized controlled trials. Nevertheless, to date, the evidence upon which a decision is made to transplant a child or not has rarely been based on randomized trials. Reliance on data collected by retrospective studies, observational databases (e.g. EBMT), or prospective non-randomized studies mainly identifies the current role of HSCT in paediatrics.

The most frequent indication for HSCT in paediatrics is acute leukaemia. Other haematological malignancies, including myelodysplastic syndrome, non-Hodgkin lymphoma, chronic myeloid leukaemia, and other myeloproliferative neoplasms, may be treated with HSCT when they are refractory to conventional therapy.

Acute lymphoblastic leukaemia

ALL is the most common neoplastic disease in childhood, with an incidence of four new diagnoses per year out of 100,000 children below 18 years of age.

Almost 50 years have passed since the first reports that childhood ALL was no longer incurable. The improved outcome of paediatric ALL is one of the greatest successes in modern medicine, with a cure rate which has risen from 3% in the 1960s to the current 85%, at least in developed countries. These advances are the result of basic research, biological investigations, large clinical trials, and intensive collaboration of cooperative groups. Unfortunately, the remaining 15% of children relapse despite appropriate treatment.

In 2005, a cooperative prospective study, including 357 patients, demonstrated the benefit of HCT from HLA-identical siblings as compared to further intensified chemotherapy in improving the outcome of the commonly defined 'very high risk' (VHR) childhood ALL patients in first complete remission (CR1). At the time, VHR features were defined by the presence of at least one of the following criteria:

1. failure to achieve CR after the first four-drug induction phase;
2. t(9;22) or t(4;11) clonal abnormalities;
3. prednisone poor response (PPR) if associated with T immunophenotype and/or white blood-cell count equal to or greater than 100×10^9/L.

Patients were randomized by 'genetic chance', according to the availability of a compatible related donor or not. According to intention to treat, the five-year DFS was 40.6% (SE 3.1) and 56.7% (SE 5.7), (hazard ratio 0.67, $p = 0.02$), and the five-year survival was 50.1% (SE 3.1) and 56.4% (SE 5.9) ($p = 0.12$) in the 'No donor' and 'Donor' arms, respectively. The availability of a compatible related donor was associated with a better outcome, particularly for patients with the worst prognostic criteria (as the subset with 'induction failure'), and less evident for PPR-only patients.

In the last decade, the detection of minimal residual disease (MRD) in childhood ALL turned out to be the most sensitive method to evaluate treatment response and one of the strongest predictors of outcome. The inclusion of MRD into survival models decreased the predictive value of any other prognostic feature, to the extent that it overtook most 'biological' high-risk features.

Haematopoietic stem-cell transplantation in first complete remission

Nowadays, transplantation is recommended for less than 10% of paediatric patients with ALL at presentation. Within the AIEOP-BFM ALL 2009 Protocol, mainly patients having MRD levels greater than or equal to 5×10^{-4} after the second induction element are considered VHR and are therefore eligible for HSCT. Patients who fail to achieve CR after the first induction phase, carry the t(4;11) clonal abnormality, or experience PPR in T immunophenotype ALL are currently considered VHR only if their MRD level is greater than or equal to 5×10^{-4} after the first induction element or whenever their MRD is not available.

The t(9;22) translocation

Patients carrying the t(9;22) translocation are treated with chemotherapy associated with tyrosine-kinase inhibitors. Within the updated ESPHALL trial, 'Ph-positive' patients are considered at VHR when the MRD level is greater than or equal to 5×10^{-4} after the second element of induction or is positive at any level after the three high-dose blocks.

Infants

Infant patients are defined as VHR if they present with two or more of the following features: six months old or younger at diagnosis; carry mixed leukaemia lineage (MLL) gene rearrangement; present with a white blood-cell count greater than 300×10^{9}/L and/or PPR; MRD levels greater than or equal to 10^{-4} at the start of consolidation.

Haematopoietic stem-cell transplantation in second complete remission

HSCT is recommended for all patients relapsing in the BM early (less than 30 months) after diagnosis and generally for the majority of the patients who experience relapse, depending on early MRD response after initial relapse treatment.

Within the ongoing IntReALL Protocol, patients randomly allocated to arm A (previous ALL-REZ BFM 2002) are eligible for HSCT if MRD after induction (day one of week five) is greater than or equal to 10^{-3}, while those allocated to arm B (previous UK ALLR3) are eligible for HSCT if MRD after induction (day 1 of week 6) is greater than or equal to 10^{-4}.

Donor type according to patient risk profile

In the last decade, results of allogeneic HSCT from unrelated donors has improved to the extent that there is an increasing agreement that outcomes of transplantation from HLA-identical sibling and matched URD are comparable in paediatric ALL, even though there are no randomized trials nor studies on the 'intention-to-treat' concept in this regards.

According to the prospective multicentre BFM ALL SCT 2003 Study, held in Austria, Germany, and Switzerland, the outcome of transplantation from MD was not inferior to the outcome of transplantation from MSD in terms of EFS (67% versus 71%, $p = 0.05$) and CIR (22% versus 24%, $p = 0.4$), with NRM (10% versus 3%, $p = 0.017$) being higher for the former, as compared with the latter.

The role of donor type and compatibility in a broader network of countries has been evaluated within the International BFM Study Group (I-BFM-SG) ALL SCT 2007 Protocol, run in ten countries, which confirms the non-inferiority of MD versus MSD HSCT, in terms of EFS, OS, CIR, and NRM. Therefore, URD search activation and transplantation might be recommended in the future for virtually every child for whom an allogeneic transplantation is indicated.

Depending on the experience of each transplant centre, MMD might be preferred, carrying the advantage of prompt donor availability and flexible schedules, and bringing a higher degree of alloreactivity, potentially associated with lower relapse risk. HSCT from MMD is widely recommended in advanced diseases and relapses after transplant, when timing adjustment is crucial.

Disparities within donor and recipient pairs are progressively accepted as the risk profile of the patient worsens.

Outcome according to minimal residual disease at haematopoietic stem-cell transplantation

MRD status before and after HSCT is strongly associated with the outcome of paediatric patients undergoing allogeneic transplantation for ALL. HSCT in MRD-positive patients is significantly inferior in terms of both EFS (around 25%) and cumulative incidence of relapse (between 40% and 60%) compared with patients with MRD that is negative or less than 1×10^{-4}, for whom an EFS of more than 70% and a CIR of less then 20% are reported.

Whether additional intensified treatment with either chemotherapy (i.e. fludarabine-cytarabin +/− daunorubicin association) or innovative strategies (i.e. blinatumomab) given to patients with a pre-transplant MRD greater than or equal to 1×10^{-4} might be effective in improving outcome is still controversial. Early tapering of immunosuppression when HSCT is performed in MRD-positive patients may reduce the risk of relapse, and the timing of +55 to +200 days after transplant has been identified as the optimal window to initiate intervention to prevent relapse. In a 2012 study, Pulsipher demonstrated the combined effect of GvHD and MRD status in a cohort of 144 patients, suggesting a role for the graft-versus-leukaemia effect.

MRD positivity after transplantation does not necessarily imply relapse, but it is well demonstrated that ALL patients experiencing any MRD positivity after transplant have a worse outcome compared with patients for whom no MRD could be detected in the post-transplant course. Whether the dismal prognosis of MRD-positive patients could be reset by immunomodulatory strategies to enhance a graft-versus-leukaemia effect, such as early tapering/sudden discontinuation of immunosuppression and donor lymphocyte infusion (DLI) or other cell therapies, is still to be assessed.

MRD measurement by flow cytometry or molecular techniques yields consistent impact on outcome. Ideally, a more sensitive and specific method for identification of patients with impending relapse is desirable; next-generation sequencing might unravel the conundrum in the near future.

Relapse after transplant

The prognosis of patients who relapse after transplant is dismal. Nowadays, innovative tools such as chimeric antigen receptor T-cells, bispecific T-cell engagers, and advanced conjugated immunotoxins offer further chances of cure. Hopefully, tools to foresee impending relapse will gain better sensitivity and specificity, so that identified patients will be suitable candidates for MRD-driven targeted therapy.

Acute myeloid leukaemia

HSCT has been the cornerstone of consolidation treatment for AML in children according to many collaborative groups. The 1990s were dominated by allocation to allogeneic HSCT versus autologous HSCT or further consolidation chemotherapy, depending on the availability of a matched sibling donor and/or the cytogenetic risk group of the patient. More recently, the detection of molecular abnormalities in AML blasts allowed further refinement in the risk-group definition.

With this approach, data progressively showed no benefit of autologous HSCT over chemotherapy, thus causing the progressive abandonment of autologous HSCT as a consolidation strategy. On the contrary, indications for allogeneic HSCT in CR1 remained controversial. Multiple studies suggested a reduction in the CIR for the HSCT recipient, but this did not translate into better OS, given the high TRM. Moreover, the distinction between intermediate-risk and high-risk groups, as per cytogenetics/molecular abnormalities, remained non-homogeneous among groups, hampering the possibility of comparisons across studies.

Kasper, in 2007, showed that by using cytogenetic-based classification, different study groups would allocate 15–80% of their patients to HSCT in CR1. When disease stratification according to cytogenetics was taken into account, few retrospective studies were able to document a real benefit of HSCT over chemotherapy, although not all the risk groups were equally well represented in those studies.

While HSCT techniques, as well as supportive therapy, has progressively improved over time, allowing a reduction in TRM and improvement of OS for HSCT recipients, the need of exposing children affected with AML to the long-term toxicities of allogeneic HSCT is still debated. Moreover, a significant number of patients relapsing post the first AML diagnosis can achieve a second remission and proceed to HSCT in CR2, while disease relapse post HSCT in AML remains very hard to address. The introduction of MRD monitoring, either with flow cytometry or molecular polymerase chain reaction (PCR), might represent a key factor in harmonizing the use of allogeneic HSCT for patients in CR1.

So far, two prospective studies have shown MRD to be the single more significant prognostic factor to predict children at high risk of relapse. Both in the St Jude AML02 Study and in the NOPHO AML 2004 Study, MRD positivity at the end of induction identified a group of patients at high risk of disease recurrence. Significantly, in the AML02 Study, HSCT offered an advantage over chemotherapy when high risk was defined by MRD rather than by cytogenetics.

Nowadays, the current general approach to HSCT for AML in CR1 is based on a stratification that accounts for cytogenetics, molecular characteristics of the disease, and post-induction MRD. A classification combining all these features was proposed by Rubnitz in 2017.

Relapsed AML remains the most common indication for allogeneic HSCT. After relapsing, approximately 65% of paediatric AML patients will achieve a CR2 and their outcome, post HSCT, will yield a survival ranging between 10% and 50% depending on the patient risk factors. Key prognostic features in relapsed AML remain the time from diagnosis to relapse, cytogenetics risk group, disease response to re-induction treatment, and previous HSCT.

For HSCT in CR2, MDs (both family and unrelated) have been used with superimposable results, and even HSCT from MMDs has given good results in the absence of adequate MDs. Noticeably, recent developments in the haploidentical transplant setting have provided extremely positive outcomes when compared to matched URD transplants, in prospective single-centre trials. Further studies are required to confirm those promising reports.

The role of MRD pre HSCT in CR1 and CR2 has been investigated by few studies. In the St Jude AML02 trial, MRD pre HSCT showed a limited impact on the post-HSCT prognosis, not reaching statistical significance. The contrary has been proven in adult studies, where MRD risk could stratify patients pre HSCT and define long-term prognosis. Further paediatric data are warranted to understand the impact of pre HSCT MRD.

Patients with primary induction failure have been documented to benefit from HSCT as opposed to chemotherapy in prospective collaborative studies, with a potential EFS around 30%, depending on associated risk factors. HSCT in patients with active disease, either primary refractory or relapsed refractory disease, has been investigated by few studies. Blast counts and age at HSCT in these groups of patients have proven to be helpful in selecting a subgroup of children with extremely dismal prognosis who might therefore be allocated to experimental treatments in the attempt to reduce the blast burden pre HSCT.

With regard to the type of conditioning regimen recommended for AML in CR1, the use of TBI has shown no benefit over chemotherapy in multiple studies and should be abandoned given the well-known, long-term consequences of irradiation in children. Busulfan remains the most commonly used agent in conditioning, and its association with cyclophosphamide has been documented as efficacious by many studies. A further increase in the conditioning intensity by adding a third alkylating agent has been proven efficacious in reducing CIR, but often at the cost of increased TRM (specifically if used in older patients or in CR2). The use of clofarabine and fludarabine as alternative agents in AML conditioning is becoming more frequent and deserves attention.

Solid tumours

Currently, there are no standard indications for allogeneic transplantation in children with solid tumours. However, there are some hints that allogeneic transplantation might play a future role in the treatment of refractory/relapsed paediatric solid tumours.

Allogeneic HSCT led to the cure of an incurable patient after a non-myeloablative preparative regimen and tumour regression was associated with acute and chronic GvHD. A similar observation was made in a patient with relapsed disseminated Ewing sarcoma, who received an haploidentical transplantation and experienced impressive tumour regression, even of a cerebral metastasis in association with the development of chronic GvHD. Interestingly, this patient is still alive and tumour-free 18 years after transplantation.

In a retrospective analysis of allogeneic HSCT in paediatric patients with advanced rhabdomyosarcoma, the outcome of 30 patients who received llogeneic HSCT from a donor who was matched sibling (n = 17), matched unrelated (n = 6), or one or more allele mismatch (n = 7) was analysed. Ten patients received MAC, whereas 20 patients were conditioned with a RIC regimen. Three-year OS was 20% with a median survival time of 12 months. The cumulative risk of progression and TRM was 67% and 11%, respectively. A RIC regimen was also given to paediatric and young adults with solid tumours (n = 20), who received haploidentical BM transplantation followed by post-transplant cyclophosphamide. OS was 88%, 56%, and 21% at 6, 12, and 24 months, respectively. Paillard and colleagues also transplanted 20 patients with solid tumours with a RIC regimen. Three-year EFS was 28% for neuroblastoma and 22% for sarcoma patients. Earlier studies of allogeneic HSCT in neuroblastoma did not show an advantage of allogeneic HSCT versus autologous HSCT.

With current conventional transplant approaches, the outcome in disseminated sarcoma is still poor, and more research and prospective clinical trials are necessary to fully exploit the graft-versus-tumour (GvT) effect of allogeneic transplantation.

Strategies to exploit the graft-versus-tumour effect in solid tumours

Currently, no clear strategies are available to separate GvHD from GvTD. However, allogeneic HSCT could be a platform for further post-transplant immunotherapeutic approaches, as the use of cellular therapy and/or the application of antibodies against suitable target antigens. Haploidentical transplantation with *ex vivo* T-cell depleted grafts without post-transplant pharmacological GvHD prophylaxis and the adoptive transfer of donor-derived NK cells has been performed in children with refractory solid tumours. In this preliminary study, donor NK cells were stimulated *in vitro* with Interleukin 15 (IL-15) and adoptively transferred to the patient. Four patients died with progressive disease and two of TRM. It remains to be shown in future clinical trials whether the *in vivo* application of IL-15, such as the more recently described IL-15 superagonist complex, comprised of an IL-15N72D mutation and IL-15RαSu/Fc fusion (ALT 803), might induce GvTD without GvHD in humans, as it has been reported in mice.

These strategies aim at the activation of a newly established donor-derived NK-cell system, and favourable NK-cell activity has been reported after haploidentical transplantation in patients with relapses of disseminated Ewing sarcoma. The rapid recovery of NK cells after T-cell-depleted haploidentical transplantation and the omission of a long and intensive pharmacological GvHD prophylaxis is also the rationale for an ongoing trial (NCT02258815) of haploidentical transplantation followed by the post-transplant application of the monoclonal anti-GD2 antibody ch14.18 in patients with refractory/relapsed high-risk neuroblastoma. In this clinical study, ch14.18 is applied to induce antibody-dependent cellular cytotoxicity (ADCC) of the reconstituting donor-derived NK cells. This approach is feasible with low TRM (less than 5%) and shows promising clinical efficacy. However, longer follow-up is needed to draw final conclusions.

Another interesting approach could be the exploitation of the anti-tumour effect of γδ T-lymphocytes in the setting of allogeneic HSCT. These lymphocytes are non-alloreactive and their spontaneous cytotoxicity and their ADCC against solid tumours can be activated *in vitro* with bisphosphonates and Interleukin 2 (IL-2). It has been reported that those children with haematological malignancies who received an haploidentical graft depleted of TCRαβ+ T-cells and three or more infusions post-transplant of the bisphosphonate zoledronate had better survival compared to those who received only one or two infusions, suggesting that the *in vivo* activation of the γδ T-lymphocytes improved survival. Whether similar results could be obtained in patients with solid tumours should be the focus of future clinical trials.

Prompt donor availability in haploidentical transplantation would, especially, allow the post-transplant adoptive transfer of donor-derived NK cells, cytokine-induced killer (CIK) cells, γδ T-lymphocytes, and also of tumour-specific TCRαβ+ T-lymphocytes. Tumour-associated antigens, such as NY-ESO-1 which is widely expressed on solid tumours, could be a suitable target for T-cells, and large-scale clinical methods have been established to isolate NY-ESO-1-specific T-cells from healthy donors. In the autologous setting, objective clinical responses were observed in four out of six patients with metastatic synovial cell sarcomas after adoptive transfer of autologous T-cells transduced with a T-cell receptor against NY-ESO-1. Since NY-ESO-1-specific T-cells can be found in healthy persons, adoptive transfer of donor-derived NY-ESO-1-specific T-cells is possible, and future clinical trials are warranted using such an approach.

It is currently not known whether checkpoint inhibitors (PD-1/PD-L1 blockade) would have an additional impact on such T-cell-based approaches or whether they would, rather, increase the risk of GvHD as it has been observed in patients with relapsed lymphoma in whom PD-1 blockade post-allogeneic HSCT resulted in a high response rate but also in rapid onset of severe and treatment-refractory GvHD. Prospective clinical trials are necessary to investigate the role of checkpoint inhibitors post transplant in patients with solid tumours.

In summary, allogeneic HSCT and the establishment of a donor-derived immune system can provide a platform for various post-transplant immunotherapeutic strategies for patients with otherwise non-curable solid tumours, and prospective clinical trials are warranted.

Post-transplant immunotherapy

Chimerism monitoring post HSCT has been established as a useful tool to identify recurrence of recipient haematopoiesis. Post-myeloablative HSCT for malignant disorders, the detection of early mixed chimerism has been associated with impending relapse, while its role following RIC must be taken cautiously depending on regimen intensity. Post-HSCT chimerism assessment represents a standard monitoring to assess engraftment in most centres, and the availability of reliable techniques on PB, as well as on BM, makes its use practical. If assessed by means of short tandem repeat PCR, a sensitivity of 10–3 can be marginally increased if subsets of cells are sorted (typically CD3+ and CD34+ cells). The use of quantitative PCR to detect donor/recipient polymorphisms allows 2-log increased sensitivity. According to international recommendations, chimerism should always be assessed together with other more specific disease monitoring strategies (flow or quantitative/molecular PCR) to confirm the diagnosis of disease recurrence.

In the paediatric setting, data from both European and American centres are available with regard to the use of immunotherapy for halting immunosuppression and/or DLI to treat mixed chimerism and efficaciously prevent relapse both in AML and ALL. These data have been encouraging in showing limited GvHD post DLI, but the dosage and schedule of DLI administration differed significantly between the three studies, thus preventing strong recommendations in this regard. Crucial to all of these studies has been the intensity of chimerism monitoring in the post-transplant setting, with weekly assessments until day +100 in the American study and +200 in the German studies. It can be speculated that this represents a key component in the use of pre-emptive DLI, as it has been described that the quick kinetic of disease relapse often escapes the possibility of DLI treatment.

This argument has prompted multiple studies in which DLI has been administered prophylactically post HSCT, specifically after T-cell-depleted or RIC-conditioned HSCT. While the rationale of prophylactic DLI proved correct in increasing the survival probability of patients with high-risk diseases in multiple studies, this came at the high price of acute and chronic GvHD, specifically when DLI was administered in the first 100 days post HSCT. More recent experience with cautious DLI timing and dosing and/or modified DLI has proven better results. Nevertheless, the choice of prophylactic DLI specifically in paediatric patients must be heavily considered against the high risk of severe and potentially life-limiting GvHD.

Importance of long-term follow-up

As other paediatricians taking care of patients with severe diseases requiring intensive or prolonged therapy, paediatric transplanters are very concerned about the long-term side effects on their patients. Thanks to the improvements achieved in the HSCT setting, approximately 70% of the children transplanted for malignant diseases survive after transplantation and are virtually cured from their primary disease. Then, besides the goal to improve OS, the most important challenge for the transplant community is to improve patient quality of life by reducing sequelae without losing disease control.

Multiple national or international consortiums were developed in previous decades in order to better describe, understand, and treat the mid- and long-term complications of patients surviving after childhood cancer. The first long-term follow-up structured programme was the Childhood Cancer Survivor Study in the USA and Canada, reporting on more than 5,000 patients treated for acute leukaemia between 1970 and 1986. Unfortunately, there were no specific data regarding transplantation in this cohort. A European consortium created the Pancare programme dedicated to the same population and, finally, a French group built the Leucémie Enfants et Adolescents (LEA, i.e. leukaemia children and adolescents) cohort from 2004, including patients specifically treated for acute leukaemia with or without transplantation. Specific cohorts allowed for the description of both physical and psychological side effects experienced by survivors after childhood cancer and/or HSCT.

The amount of produced data is extremely impressive and somehow difficult to summarize due to confounding factors like recruitment bias, loss to follow-up growing with time, time-dependent evolution of both first and subsequent lines of therapy for primary malignancies as well as HSCT procedures, and, finally, methodology for data collection (e.g. questionnaires only, register studies, studies with or without clinical examination). However, it is now clearly demonstrated that transplanted patients experience more severe and more frequent sequelae than non-transplanted children and more often report worse quality of life.

The most frequent physical sequelae are metabolic syndrome (defined by dyslipidaemia, hypertension, glucose intolerance, and abdominal obesity), thyroid dysfunction, growth retardation (with low adult final height), hypofertility or sterility, cataract, heart injury, kidney-function injury, lung-function alteration, and second cancer. Moreover, transplanted patients describe less success in professional, social, and family life, with lower global well-being and quality of life as compared to the general population or even to patients treated for cancer during childhood in the same years but without HSCT. Overall, it appeared that myeloablative conditioning regimens, especially TBI-based ones, yielded the most severe and frequent sequelae.

In 2002, the International BFM Study Group initiated a prospective randomized study comparing a TBI-based versus a chemotherapy-based conditioning regimen for paediatric patients transplanted for acute lymphoblastic leukaemia, with long-term follow-up being one of the secondary endpoints of this study. An important achievement was the publication of guidelines for the population of patients transplanted during childhood and the development of specific long-term follow-up clinics in many centres. Specifically trained, multiple professional caregivers should offer comprehensive and global care and deal with issues in endocrinology, dermatology, cardiology, pulmonology, gynaecology, andrology, neurology, nephrology, internal medicine, ophthalmology, orthopaedics, physiotherapy, and psychology.

Recommendations may differ among countries and may depend on the type of conditioning regimen, patient age at the time of HSCT, and early and late complications occurring after HSCT. However, a minimal corpus of tests should include at least blood tests (haematology, immunology, metabolic tests, endocrinological functions, vitamin D level, ferritin); physical examination, with a special emphasis on skin (especially for patients who received TBI and/or experienced chronic GvHD) and growth (before, during, and after puberty); as well as imaging and diagnostics, with ultrasound echocardiography, lung-function tests, dual X-ray absorptiometry (DEXA) for bone metabolism, eye examination, and limb MRI in case of avascular necrosis symptoms. This test set has to be performed regularly after HSCT, within one year after transplant, and then repeated on a yearly basis up to adulthood.

As for any other chronic paediatric disease, transition from the paediatric to the adult medical environment represents a very critical period and challenge, and has to be anticipated, well organized, and accompanied. Patients surviving after childhood HSCT have to be well informed about the treatment they received and their potential late sequelae in order to play as primary actors in their subsequent medical life.

Nowadays, it is mandatory that prevention, early diagnosis, and treatment of long-term side effects are integrated in the care of transplanted paediatric patients, without which the whole work of any transplanting physician would be valueless.

FURTHER READING

Abdul Wahid SF, et al. (2014) Comparison of reduced-intensity and myeloablative conditioning regimens for allogeneic hematopoietic stem cell transplantation in patients with acute myeloid leukemia and acute lymphoblastic leukemia: a meta-analysis. *Stem Cells Dev* **23**(21), 2535–52.

Ash RC, et al. (1990) Successful allogeneic transplantation of T-cell-depleted bone marrow from closely HLA-matched unrelated donors. *N Engl J Med* **322**(8), 485–94.

Baker KS, et al. (2010) The burden of cure: long-term side effects following hematopoietic stem cell transplantation (HSCT) in children. Pediatr Clin North Am **57**(1), 323–42.

Balduzzi A, et al. (1995) Unrelated donor marrow transplantation in children. Blood **86**(8), 3247–56.

Bashey A, Solomon SR (2014) T-cell replete haploidentical donor transplantation using post-transplant CY: an emerging standard-of-care option for patients who lack an HLA-identical sibling donor. *Bone Marrow Transplant* **49**(8), 999–1008.

Beck F et al. (2015) Survivorship after childhood cancer. PanCare: a European Network to promote optimal long-term care. *Eur J Cancer* **51**(10), 1203–11.

Biondi A, et al. (2012) Imatinib after induction for treatment of children and adolescents with Philadelphia-chromosome-positive acute lymphoblastic leukaemia (EsPhALL): a randomised, open-label, intergroup study. *Lancet Oncol* **13**(9), 936–45.

Blaise D, et al. (1992) Allogeneic bone marrow transplantation for acute myeloid leukemia in first remission: a randomized trial of a Busulfan-Cytoxan versus Cytoxan-total body irradiation as preparative regimen: a report from the Group d'Etudes de la Greffe de Moelle Osseuse. *Blood* **79**(10), 2578–82.

Bonneville M, et al. (2010) Gammadelta T cell effector functions: a blend of innate programming and acquired plasticity. *Nat Rev Immunol* **10**(7), 467–78.

Conter V, et al. (2010) Molecular response to treatment redefines all prognostic factors in children and adolescents with B-cell precursor acute lymphoblastic leukemia: results in 3184 patients of the AIEOP-BFM ALL 2000 study. *Blood* **115**, 3206–14.

Copelan EA, et al. (2013) Better leukemia-free and overall survival in AML in first remission following cyclophosphamide in combination with busulfan compared with TBI. *Blood* **122**(24), 3863–70.

de Berranger E, et al. (2014) Impact on long-term OS of conditioning regimen in allogeneic BMT for children with AML in first CR: TBI+CY versus BU+CY: a report from the Societe Francaise de Greffe de Moelle et de Therapie Cellulaire. *Bone Marrow Transplant* **49**(3), 382–8.

Eapen M, et al. (2017) Allele-level HLA matching for umbilical cord blood transplantation for non-malignant diseases in children: a retrospective analysis. *Lancet Haematol* **4**(7), e325–33.

Gluckman E, et al. (1989) Hematopoietic reconstitution in a patient with Fanconi's anemia by means of umbilical-cord blood from an HLA-identical sibling. *N Engl J Med* **321**(17), 1174–8.

Hasle H (2014) A critical review of which children with acute myeloid leukaemia need stem cell procedures. *Br J Haematol* **166**(1), 23–33.

Hjorth L, et al. (2015) Survivorship after childhood cancer. PanCare: a European Network to promote optimal long-term care. *Eur J Cancer* **51**(10),1203–11.

Horan JT, et al. (2008) Impact of disease risk on efficacy of matched related bone marrow transplantation for pediatric acute myeloid leukemia: the Children's Oncology Group. *J Clin Oncol* **26**(35), 5797–801.

Hunger SP, Mullighan CG (2015) Acute lymphoblastic leukemia in children. *N Engl J Med* **373**(16), 1541–52.

Kato K, et al. (2015) Comparison of transplantation with reduced and myeloablative conditioning for children with acute lymphoblastic leukemia. *Blood* **125**(8), 1352–4.

Kuhlen M, et al. (2018) Outcome of relapse after allogeneic HSCT in children with ALL enrolled in the ALL-SCT 2003/2007 trial. *Br J Haematol* **180**(1), 82–9.

Kupst MJ, et al. (2002) Cognitive and psychosocial functioning of pediatric hematopoietic stem cell transplant patients: a prospective longitudinal study. *Bone Marrow Transplant* **30**(9), 609–17.

Lang P, et al. (2015) Improved immune recovery after transplantation of TCRalphabeta/CD19-depleted allografts from haploidentical donors in pediatric patients. *Bone Marrow Transplant* **50**(Suppl 2), S6–10.

Llosa NJ, et al. (2017) Reduced-intensity haploidentical bone marrow transplantation with post-transplant cyclophosphamide for solid tumors in pediatric and young adult patients. *Biol Blood Marrow Transplant* **23**(12), 2127–36.

Locatelli F, et al. (2017) Outcome of children with acute leukemia given HLA-haploidentical HSCT after alphabeta T-cell and B-cell depletion. *Blood* **130**(5), 677–85.

Mertens AC, et al. (2015) Conditional survival in pediatric malignancies: analysis of data from the Childhood Cancer Survivor Study and the Surveillance, Epidemiology, and End Results Program. *Cancer* **121**(7), 1108–17.

Panasiuk A, et al. (2015) Gonadal function and fertility after stem cell transplantation in childhood: comparison of a reduced intensity conditioning regimen containing melphalan with a myeloablative regimen containing busulfan. *Br J Haematol* **170**(5), 719–26.

Pérez-Martínez A, et al. (2015) A phase I/II trial of Interleukin-15—stimulated natural killer cell infusion after haploidentical stem cell transplantation for pediatric refractory solid tumors. *Cytotherapy* **17**(11), 1594–603.

Peter J, et al. (2017) Safety and efficacy of Tcralpha/beta and CD19 depleted haploidentical stem cell transplantation following reduced intensity conditioning in children: results of a prospective multicenter phase I/II clinical trial. *Blood* **130**, 214.

Peters C, et al. (2015) Stem-cell transplantation in children with acute lymphoblastic leukemia: a prospective international multicenter trial comparing sibling donors with matched unrelated donors—The ALL-SCT-BFM-2003 trial. *J Clin Oncol* **33**(11), 1265–74.

Powles RL, et al. (1983) Mismatched family donors for bone-marrow transplantation as treatment for acute leukaemia. *Lancet* **1**(8325), 612–15.

Rettinger E, et al. (2011) Preemptive immunotherapy in childhood acute myeloid leukemia for patients showing evidence of mixed chimerism after allogeneic stem cell transplantation. *Blood* **118**(20), 5681–88.

Robinson TM, et al. (2016) Haploidentical bone marrow and stem cell transplantation: experience with post-transplantation cyclophosphamide. *Semin Hematol* **53**(2), 90–7.

Rubnitz JE, et al. (2010) Minimal residual disease-directed therapy for childhood acute myeloid leukaemia: results of the AML02 multicentre trial. *Lancet Oncol* **11**(6), 543–52.

Schlegel P, et al. (2015) Favorable NK cell activity after haploidentical hematopoietic stem cell transplantation in stage IV relapsed Ewing's sarcoma patients. *Bone Marrow Transplant* 50(Suppl 2), S72–6.

Socie G, et al. (2000) New malignant diseases after allogeneic marrow transplantation for childhood acute leukemia. *J Clin Oncol* **18**(2), 348–57.

Thiel U, et al. (2013) Allogeneic stem cell transplantation for patients with advanced rhabdomyosarcoma: a retrospective assessment. *Br J Cancer* **109**(10), 2523–32.

Thomas ED, et al. (1957) Intravenous infusion of bone marrow in patients receiving radiation and chemotherapy. *N Engl J Med* **257**, 491–6.

Verneris MR, et al. (2015) HLA mismatch is associated with worse outcomes after unrelated donor reduced-intensity conditioning hematopoietic cell transplantation: an analysis from the Center for International Blood and Marrow Transplant Research. *Biol Blood Marrow Transplant* **21**(10), 1783–9.

8

Cancer Immunotherapy in Children

Koichi Hirabayashi, Gianpietro Dotti, and Barbara Savoldo

Introduction

Chemotherapy and radiotherapy play a critical role in promoting a high cure rate in several paediatric malignancies. However, the long-term toxicities associated with these treatments remain significant. Furthermore, patients with tumours relapsing after chemotherapy and/or radiotherapy, or resistant to these treatments, do not have effective alternative therapeutic options.

In addition to toxic agents, tumour cells can be eliminated through other mechanisms including the cytolytic effects mediated by cellular components of the immune system, or by antibodies targeting surface antigens expressed by tumour cells and activating either the complement or immune cells, or by delivering conjugated toxins. Cellular and humoral immunotherapy approaches are thus explored in cancer patients with the goal to offer less toxic therapies, overcome tumour chemo/radio resistance and prevent relapse, or treat minimal diseases.

In this chapter, we will discuss the principle of cancer immunotherapy in paediatric patients starting with the most common form of cellular immunotherapy: allogeneic haematopoietic stem-cell transplantation (HSCT). We will then discuss specific immunotherapy strategies based on the administration of classic monoclonal antibodies (mAbs) targeting tumour-associated antigens, novel bispecific antibodies that simultaneously target tumour-associated antigens and activate CD3+ T lymphocytes, and mAbs that block key inhibitory molecules of the immune system (checkpoint blockade). Finally, we will describe specific cellular immunotherapy approaches, such as tumour vaccine and adoptive transfer of immune cells. Although only a few immunotherapies have so far been incorporated into standard practice for paediatric cancers, their role is enjoying a new revival, after the promising results obtained in recent clinical trials. The great majority of clinical studies are conducted in patients with relapsed cancer, and consist of Phase I trials. Here, we only outline the most innovative ones and/or those that have reached Phase II/III (Table 8.1).

Allogeneic haematopoietic stem-cell transplantation

Allogeneic haematopoietic stem-cell transplantation (HSCT) is currently considered the standard of care for paediatric patients with haematological malignancies such as high-risk acute lymphoblastic leukaemia (ALL) and acute myeloid leukaemia (AML), relapsed/refractory lymphoma, juvenile myelomonocytic leukaemia, and myelodysplastic syndrome. The inclusion of HSCT as a form of cellular immunotherapy, called graft-versus-leukaemia (GvL), or more generally graft-versus-tumour (GvT), stems from the observation that tumour relapse rate is reduced in patients developing graft-versus-host disease (GvHD). Furthermore, lower relapse rates are observed in patients receiving non-T-cell-depleted allografts and experiencing GvHD, as compared to those receiving T-cell-depleted allografts without occurrence of GvHD. The critical role of GvT effects were further supported by the re-induction of remission upon donor lymphocyte infusion (DLI) in patients who relapsed after HSCT. Currently, HSCTs are safely, widely, and more effectively performed by virtue of the diversification of donor sources, reduced toxicity associated with conditioning regimens, and better supportive therapies. As a result, prognoses of paediatric patients with haematological malignancies have significantly improved upon HSCT.

Separating graft-versus-tumour versus graft-versus-host disease effects

GvHD is mediated by both donor T-cell responses to host alloantigens and the concomitant dysregulation of inflammatory cytokines cascade that follows the HSCT procedure. The most critical trigger for acute GvHD is found in disparities in major histocompatibility complex (MHC) molecules. Minor histocompatibility antigens and donor/recipient differences in the killer immunoglobulin-like receptor (KIR) and KIR-ligand (KIRL) interactions also affect the risk of acute GvHD. Natural killer (NK) cells participate in the GvT effects through KIRL mismatches. NK cells exert their alloreactivity by sensing missing-self on leukaemia cells, especially in adult patients with AML and paediatric patients with B-cell precursor ALL.

A major goal in the setting of HSCT is to suppress GvHD while maintaining or promoting GvT. In animal models, controlling the proliferation of alloreactive T cells is an effective strategy to uncouple GvT from GvHD. The clinical translation of these observations has been pursued for the past three decades by administering immunosuppressive agents or by T-cell depletion of the graft. In recent years, the most innovative approaches to control GvHD, especially in the setting of haploidentical transplant, consist of the administration of cyclophosphamide in the post-transplant setting and/or in selective

Table 8.1 Summary of the clinical studies in paediatric patients with anti-tumour antibody agents

Trial	Phase	Agents	Disease	Number of patients	Age in years (range)	Outcome	Reference
Goldman et al.	III	Rituximab	Burkitt lymphoma / leukaemia	40	11(3–23)	90% (3-year OS and EFS; 95% CI, 76–96%)	*Br J Haematol* (2014), 167, 394–401.
Meinhardt et al.	II	Rituximab	Mature B-cell NHL and Burkitt leukaemia	87	10.4(1.5–17.5)	41.4% (RR) (95% CI, 31–52%)	*J Clin Oncol* (2015), 28, 3115–21.
Raetz et al.	II	Epratuzumab (weekly)	ALL	54	8.4	49.3% ± 8.1% (2-year OS), 39.9 ± 8.0% (2-year EFS), 66% (CR)	*Pediatr Blood Cancer* (2015), 62, 1171–5.
		Epratuzumab (twice-weekly)		60	(4–15)	60% (RR), 40% (CR)	
Rytting et al.	II	Inotuzumab ozogamicin	B-cell ALL	5	(4–15)	60% (RR), 40% (CR)	*Pediatr Blood Cancer* (2014), 61, 369–72.
Pro et al.	II	Brentuximab vedotin	ALCL	58	52(14–76)	86% (objective response = CR+PR, 57% (CR), 29% (PR))	*J Clin Oncol* (2012), 30, 2190–6.
Yu et al.	III	Dinutuximab	Neuroblastoma	226	96% <18 months	86% ± 4% (2-year OS), 66% ± 5% (2-year EFS)	*N Engl J Med* (2010), 363, 1324–34.
O'Hear et al.	III	Gemtuzumab ozogamicin alone	AML	17	No data	14 had a reduction in their MRD level and 13 became MRD-negative	*Cancer* (2013), 119, 4036–43.
		Gemtuzumab ozogamicin & chemotherapy		29		55% ± 13.9% (5-year OS), 50% ± 13.4% (5-year EFS)	
Ebb et al.	II	Trastuzumab	Osteosarcoma	41	13.8	59% ± 14% (30-month OS), 32% ± 14% (30-month EFS)	*J Clin Oncol* (2012), 30, 2545–51.
Malempati et al.	I/II	Cixutumumab	Solid tumours and Ewing sarcoma	47	15(4–28)	9% (PR Ewing sarcoma group)	*J Clin Oncol* (2012), 30, 256–62.
Mossé et al.	I	Crizotinib	Solid tumours and ALCL	79	10.1(1.1–21.4)	18% (RR)	COG Phase 1 Consortium, 2013.
von Stackelberg et al.	I/II	Blinatumomab	ALL	70	8(1–17)	39% ± 12% (CR) within the first two cycles	*J Clin Oncol* (2016), 34, 4381–9.
Merchant et al.	I	Ipilimumab	Solid tumours	33	13.4(2.3–21)	18% (SD), 0% (CR and PR)	*Clin Cancer Res* (2016), 22, 1364–70.
Blumenthal et al.	Retrospective analysis	Pembrolizumab	Brain tumour	5	5(3–7)	3.2 months (median OS), 100% (PD)	*J Neurooncol* (2016), 129, 453–60.

Abbreviations: NHL, non-Hodgkin lymphoma; AML, acute myelogenous leukaemia; ALCL, anaplastic large-cell lymphoma; ALL, acute lymphoblastic leukaemia; OS, overall survival; EFS, event-free survival; RR, response rate; SD, stable disease; PR, partial response; PD, progressive disease; PFS, progression-free survival

T-cell depletion of the graft. In haploidentical HSCT, the administration of cyclophosphamide post transplant, together with standard prophylaxis, reduces the incidence of GvHD to acceptable rates without the need for T-cell depletion of the graft. Interestingly, the timing of cyclophosphamide administration on the third to fifth day after transplant mirrors the timing predicted by preclinical models in which alloreactive T cells are activated.

As far as the selected T-cell depletion of the graft is concerned, the most novel approach consists of the selective removal of αβTCR(T-cell receptor)+CD3+ T cells, while preserving the γδTCR+CD3+ subset. Alloreactive precursors that mediate GvHD are confined to T cells expressing the αβTCR, which represent the great majority of T cells. Between 2% and 10% of T cells express the γδTCR and these cells do not cause GvHD, while maintaining protective effects against a wide range of pathogens. Administration of cyclophosphamide post transplant and selective removal of αβTCR+ T cells are both effective in controlling and preventing GvHD. However, the impact of these methodologies in promoting increased GvT effects require larger and controlled clinical studies.

Adoptive T-cell therapy after haematopoietic stem-cell transplantation

DLI continues to be used in the attempt to re-induce remission in patients relapsing after HSCT. While highly effective in patients with chronic myeloid leukaemia (CML), DLI is less efficient in controlling other malignancies and also increases the rate of GvHD.

Donor lymphocyte infusion with safety switches

To control GvHD associated with DLI and to improve GvT effects, T cells can be manipulated *ex vivo* to include safety switches or suicide genes. Insertion of the herpes simplex virus-derived enzyme thymidine kinase (HSV-tk) and the inducible human caspase9 (iCasp9) have been tested clinically as DLI after allogeneic HSCT. In particular, iCasp9 has been safely administered in paediatric patients. The iCasp9 is a human-derived, chimeric caspase9 that activates the cell's physiological apoptotic pathway when a specific small molecule, known as chemical inducer of dimerization (CID) (AP1903/Rimiducid), binds to the FK-binding portion of the chimeric caspase9. In a small group of patients, iCasp9-based DLI produced improved immune reconstitution, elimination of opportunistic pathogens, and effective control of acute GvHD in paediatric patients. Larger studies are currently ongoing and should provide definitive conclusions concerning the impact of iCasp9-based DLI in controlling GvHD and promoting GvL effects.

Natural killer cells as donor lymphocyte infusion

The adoptive transfer of NK cells is also an attractive option. The administration of these cells after HSCT does not cause GvHD. As NK cells recognize self MHC Class I molecules to prevent their activation, Rubnitz et al. investigated, in a pilot study, the safety and feasibility of haploidentical NK cell infusions in children or young adolescents with AML. Ten patients who had completed chemotherapy and were in first complete remission (CR) of AML were enrolled. They received cyclophosphamide and fludarabine, followed by KIR-HLA mismatched NK cells and interleukin-2 (IL-2) to support NK-cell expansion *in vivo*. All patients had transient engraftment and expansion of KIR-mismatched NK cells. Non-haematological toxicities were limited, with no GvHD. However, the efficacy of this approach remains to be determined. In another study, haploidentical NK cells obtained from parental donors were infused in 29 paediatric patients with relapsed or refractory leukaemia. Objective leukaemia regression was observed and patients successfully proceeded to a second HSCT.

Gene-modified donor lymphocyte infusion

The most innovative modified DLI is however represented by the infusion of donor T cells genetically modified to specifically target tumour-associated antigens via either chimeric antigen receptors (CARs) or conventional T-cell receptors (TCRs). These technologies are described in specific sections of this chapter. However, relevant for this section, in clinical studies so far reported using donor-derived T cells genetically manipulated *ex vivo* to express the CD19-specific CAR, no GvHD has occurred. In one of them, the lack of GvHD upon infusion of these cells was expected, since the specific CAR was engrafted on virus-specific cytotoxic T cells, which are well known to not cause GvHD. Importantly, when donor polyclonal T cells were used as the CAR vehicle in another study, anti-tumour activity was confirmed without the occurrence of GvHD. The mechanisms responsible for these effects remain elusive. However, a recent mouse model suggests that alloreactive T cells experience enhanced stimulation due to the engrafted CAR, resulting in the progressive loss of both their effector function and proliferative potential, which likely prevents the development of GvHD.

Monoclonal-based antibody therapies

Monoclonal antibodies (mAbs) recognize antigens expressed on the tumour cell surface and cause anti-tumour activity via either antibody-dependent cell-mediated cytotoxicity (ADCC), complement-dependent cytotoxicity (CDC), or delivery of toxic agents upon internalization of the antigen/mAb complex. ADCC occurs when the fragment crystallizable (Fc) domains of the mAb engage the Fc receptors on the surface of immune effector cells.

Antibodies targeting B-cell antigens

Rituximab, a CD20-directed chimeric mAb, is the most validated and effective mAb, and is currently included in many clinical protocols to treat B-cell lymphomas in adults. Safety and tolerability of rituximab have been reported for paediatric patients with high-risk mature B-cell lymphomas in a pilot study conducted by the Children's Oncology Group (COG). In this study, rituximab was used in association with conventional chemotherapy. An ongoing international Phase III trial will determine the efficacy of rituximab in paediatric B-cell lymphoma and B-cell ALL (NCT01595048 and NCT01516580).

Following promising results in Phase I/II studies, epratuzumab, a humanized IgG1 mAb that targets CD22 (a B-lineage restricted antigen expressed on B-precursor ALL), recently entered a Phase III clinical trial in paediatric patients with standard-risk relapsed ALL (NCT01802814). CD22 has also been targeted with inotuzumab (CMC-544), in which the mAb is conjugated to ozogamicin, with promising results in a small pilot study.

Antibodies targeting non-classical B-cell antigens

Brentuximab vedotin is a highly successful example of conjugated mAb. Brentuximab targets CD30 and is conjugated to the toxin monomethyl auristatin E (vedotin). After binding via CD30 mAb, the toxin binds to tubulin and disrupts the microtubule network with consequent cell-cycle arrest and apoptosis. Brentuximab is used in patients with Hodgkin's lymphoma and CD30+ anaplastic large-cell lymphoma (ALCL). CR rates in adults with relapsed/refractory CD30+ ALCL receiving brentuximab vedotin as a single agent are in the 57% range. Currently, an ongoing international Phase III trial is determining the efficacy of brentuximab vedotin in CD30+ ALCL and Hodgkin's lymphoma (NCT01979536, NCT01780662, and NCT02166463).

Antibodies targeting gangliosides

Dinutuximab is a chimeric anti-disialoganglioside-2 (GD2) CAR in Chimeric antigen receptor T cell section mAb, validated in a COG Phase III trial of post autologous HSCT in paediatric patients with neuroblastoma (NB). Patients were randomly assigned to receive dinutuximab administered with granulocyte macrophage colony-stimulating growth factor (GM-CSF) and IL-2 in conjunction with isotretinoin, versus isotretinoin alone. Immunotherapy combined with isotretinoin (event-free survival (EFS), 66%) was superior to standard isotretinoin maintenance therapy (EFS, 46%). As a result, immunotherapy with dinutuximab after autologous HSCT is currently considered the standard of care for high-risk NB.

Antibodies targeting myeloid antigens

Gentuzumab ozogamicin is an anti-CD33 mAb conjugated to the drug calicheamicin and designed to target AML. Upon initial encouraging Phase I studies, gentuzumab was withdrawn due to liver toxicity and lack of significant clinical benefit in a Phase III trial conducted in adult patients with AML. However, O'Hear et al. reported more promising results in paediatric patients. In a multicentre trial, paediatric patients with AML received gentuzumab, either alone or in combination with chemotherapy, and achieved molecular remission in both cohorts. All patients subsequently safely received HSCT, without significant increase in treatment-related mortality after transplantation. Furthermore, this study showed that lower doses of gentuzumab could be safely administered.

Antibodies targeting growth factors

Vascular endothelial growth factor (VEGF) is a signalling protein that is critical for solid tumour vascular proliferation. Bevacizumab, a VEGF inhibitor, has shown activity both as a single agent and in combination with other chemotherapy drugs for several tumours. Modak et al. reported a Phase II study that evaluated the combination therapy with bevacizumab, irinotecan, and temozolomide for refractory/relapsed NB. Although objective responses were achieved, the addition of bevacizumab did not improve response rates in resistant NB.

Antibodies targeting growth factor receptors

Cetuximab is an mAb directed against epidermal growth factor (EGF) receptors and, although approved for the treatment of several adult malignancies, its role in paediatric patients remains unclear. In a Phase I trial to determine the dose of cetuximab that can be safely combined with irinotecan in children and adolescents with refractory solid tumours, stable disease was reported, especially in patients with brain tumours (38.5%), granting further investigation.

The expression of human epidermal growth factor receptor 2 (HER2) has been associated with poor outcome in osteosarcoma, suggesting that targeting this antigen may have a clinical impact. Ebb et al. reported a Phase II trial of the anti-HER2 mAb trastuzumab in combination with cytotoxic chemotherapy in patients with metastatic HER2+ osteosarcoma. Forty-one patients were treated with chemotherapy and trastuzumab for 34 consecutive weeks, but no significant differences in EFS and overall survival (OS) rates were observed compared to patients receiving chemotherapy only.

Insulin-like growth factor-1 receptor (IGF-1R) promotes tumour growth, especially in sarcomas. Cixutumumab, a fully human IgG1 mAb against IGF-1R was used in a Phase I/II trial in paediatric patients with refractory solid tumours and Ewing sarcoma. The drug was well tolerated, but the number of responses observed did not meet the statistical criteria for single-agent activity in Ewing Sarcoma.

Antibodies targeting tumour-specific mutation

Various human cancers, including NB and ALCL, have gene translocations, amplifications, or oncogenic mutations of the anaplastic lymphoma kinase (ALK) tyrosine kinase receptor. The anti-ALK mAb Crizotinib was tested in a Phase I study in children with refractory solid tumours and ALCL. Objective tumour responses were documented in 14 of the 79 patients, including eight CR and five partial remission (PR). Responses were more evident in patients with ALK aberrations.

Bispecific T-cell engager antibodies

Bispecific T-cell engager (BiTE®) antibodies use a technology that capitalizes on T-cell cytotoxicity with direct cell-killing capability. These bispecific mAbs bridge surface antigens on target cells with the αβTCR of effector T cells to facilitate targeted cytotoxic T-cell-mediated cytolysis. The prototype of this new class of mAbs is blinatumomab, which is a bispecific CD19-directed CD3 T-cell engager. Blinatumomab has produced durable responses in patients with various B-cell malignancies. Von Stackelberg et al. reported a Phase I/II clinical trial which validated safety and efficacy of blinatumomab in paediatric patients with relapsed/refractory B-ALL. They treated 49 patients in Phase I and 44 patients in Phase II. Four patients had dose-limiting toxicities during cycle 1 (Phase I); three experienced grade 4 cytokine-release syndrome (one attributed to grade 5 cardiac failure); and one had fatal respiratory failure. Among the 70 patients who received the recommended dosage, 27 (39%) achieved CR (including molecular remission) within the first two cycles with 14 (52%) achieving molecular remission. These results demonstrated anti-leukaemic activity of blinatumomab as a single agent, endorsing additional studies for the approval of this drug. New BiTE®s, such as CEA/CD3 bispecific antibody (MEDI-565) and EpCAM/CD3 bispecific antibody (MT110) have also been developed and are being evaluated for safety and efficacy in clinical trials.

Immune checkpoint blockade

While endogenous immune responses to cancer cells are often detected in patients, their anti-tumour effects are usually insufficient to prevent cancer progression. This immune tolerance of tumours is induced through the expression of ligands by the tumour or tumour-infiltrating cells that ultimately hamper T-cell functions within the tumour microenvironment. To break these immune-inhibitory pathways, immune checkpoint blockades using anti-programmed cell death protein -1 (PD-1) mAb, anti-programmed death ligand (PD-L1) mAb, and anti-cytotoxic T lymphocytes-associated protein 4 (CTLA-4) mAb have been developed.

Anti-CTLA-4

CTLA-4 was the first immune checkpoint receptor to be clinically targeted. After T-cell activation, CTLA-4 is upregulated, to specifically inhibit effector function through a variety of mechanisms, including preventing co-stimulation by outcompeting CD28 for its ligand, B7, and also by inducing T-cell cycle arrest. Two antibodies targeting CTLA-4, ipilimumab and tremelimumab, entered clinical evaluation. A Phase I clinical trial of ipilimumab in paediatric patients with advanced solid tumours showed more toxicities than in adults.

Anti-PD-1 and anti-PD-L1

By interacting with its two ligands PD-L1 or PD-L2, PD-1 is also a negative regulator of T-cell activity. When engaged by its ligand, PD-1 inhibits kinase signalling pathways that normally lead to T-cell activation. PD-1 is expressed on many immunological cells, including B cells and NK cells, and blocking anti-PD-1 mAb and anti-PD-L1 mAb influences the function of these cells. Anti-PD-1 and PD-L1 mAbs have demonstrated unprecedented clinical efficacy in more than 15 cancer types in adults, with very good safety profiles. In paediatric cancer, Phase I or II clinical trials are currently under way. Blumenthal et al. retrospectively described outcomes in children with pontine gliomas, but no responses were documented. To enhance anti-tumour efficacy of the immune checkpoint blockade, combination therapy such as chemotherapy, targeted therapy, radiotherapy, and other immunotherapy may be required.

Chimeric antigen receptor T cells

Chimeric antigen receptors (CARs) are fusion proteins where the binding site of a monoclonal antibody is linked to intracellular signalling molecules of the TCR and co-stimulatory molecules. These molecules are expressed in T cells via viral or non-viral vector delivery. When CAR molecules bind to the specific antigen expressed on target cells through their single-chain variable fragment (scFv) segment, they activate the lytic and co-stimulatory pathways of the T cells, ultimately promoting MHC-independent cytotoxic activity and cell expansion. While first-generation CAR T cells rely on the exclusive intracellular CD3ζ chain-signalling domain, second- and third-generation versions have included one and two co-stimulatory molecules to improve activation and persistence of engineered T cells.

Cytokine release syndrome (CRS) is the most severe complication following the adoptive transfer of CAR T cells and is considered to occur following a dysregulated activation of the immune system driven by the activated CAR T cells. CRS ranges from mild and self-limiting symptoms such as high temperature and myalgia, to severe and life-threatening scenarios characterized by multi-organ failure. Corticosteroid and the interleukin-6 receptor-blocking mAb tocilizumab are useful for controlling CRS.

Clinical trials with chimeric antigen receptors for haematological malignancies

Thus far, the most successful example of CAR T-cell-based therapy is achieved by targeting CD19. Clinical trials of CD19-CAR T cells have shown remarkable outcomes in B-cell ALL, with CR rates of 70–90% in relapsed/refractory cases. Greater efficacy and tolerability is observed in children. The Children's Hospital of Philadelphia reported a 90% CR rate in 30 patients with relapsed/refractory ALL (25 treated on the paediatric trial) in Phase I trials with CTL019, a CD19-targeted CAR T-cell product containing the 4-1BB molecule as a co-stimulatory domain. EFS and OS at six months were 67% and 78%, respectively. The National Cancer Institute (NCI) Pediatric Oncology Branch performed an intent-to-treat analysis of 21 children and young adults with ALL treated with CD19-CAR T cells expressing the CD28 domain as a co-stimulatory molecule, and reported a 70% CR rate. At a median follow-up of ten months, OS was 51.6%. EFS in the 21 patients achieving molecular emission was 17.7 months, with all but three receiving subsequent HSCT. Despite high initial response rates, some patients had however relapsed. Antigen escape (loss of CD19 by tumour blasts) and short CAR T-cell persistence have been implicated as causes for failure. Up to 60% of the relapsed cases after CD19-CAR T cells have indeed shown loss of CD19 antigen expression, which renders the malignant cells invisible to CD19-specific immunotherapies. To overcome this tumour escape mechanism, CAR T cells targeting alternative antigens are being tested of which CAR T cells targeting the CD22 molecule are the most advanced. Concerning issues related to the limited persistence of CAR T cells, current clinical outcomes suggest that CAR co-stimulated through the 41BB endodomain have prolonged survival (up to two years) over CD28 co-stimulated CAR T cells (two to three months).

Clinical trials with chimeric antigen receptors for solid tumours

In addition to ALL, NB is another paediatric disease treated with CAR T cells. Actually, NB is the first paediatric solid tumour in which CAR T cells have been tested in clinical trials. The NB-specific GD2 molecule was targeted in the first trial with CAR T cells. Although challenges from the tumour microenvironment in solid tumours are expected to hinder CAR T cells, results were encouraging, with three of the 11 patients with active disease achieving a complete response.

Paediatric patients with osteosarcoma also underwent CAR T-cell therapy using HER2-specific CAR. In a Phase I/II trial, 19 patients with HER2+ tumours received escalating doses of autologous HER2-CAR T cells. Of the 17 evaluable patients, four had stable disease for 12 weeks to 14 months. Three of these patients had their tumour removed, with one showing extensive necrosis . The median OS of all 19 infused patients was 10.3 months (range, 5.1 to 29.1 months) (Figure 8.1).

Natural-killer-cell immunotherapy

NK cells are innate lymphoid cells dedicated to the clearance of malignant cells via direct cytotoxicity and production of immunoregulatory cytokines. Although cytokine stimulation promotes NK-cell activation and greater cytotoxicity against malignant targets *in vitro*, clinical trials based on the infusions of autologous NK cells have shown limited clinical efficacy. Suboptimal results are likely to be found in NK-cell dysfunctions produced by multiple rounds of chemotherapy that these patients undergo and in the expression of inhibitory receptors by tumour cells. On the other hand, clear benefits are reported in patients with AML and ALL receiving allogeneic KIR-mismatched NK-cell infusion (see the section 'Adoptive T-cell therapy after haematopoietic stem-cell transplantation'). To overcome the KIR-KIRL-mediated inhibition and increase the anti-leukaemic effects of NK cells, different strategies are being evaluated, including blocking of KIR-KIRL interactions with a monoclonal antibody, using bispecific killer engagers and a trispecific killer engager to activate NK cells via the Fc-receptor against antigens expressed on leukaemia cells and via expression of CARs.

Tumour vaccines and dendritic-cell immunotherapy

Active vaccination of patients with cancer, including paediatric patients, has been extensively explored, although the rate of clinical responses remains extremely low. Paediatric patients should in theory be more responsive to vaccination, since their immune system is largely composed of naive T cells. However, clinical studies based on cancer vaccines remain limited in paediatric patients, likely reflecting the scepticism in the field due to the poor outcome of clinical studies in adult patients. Kushner et al. reported a Phase I trial targeting GD2 and GD3 antigens with OPT-821 adjuvant in combination with oral β-glucan for high-risk NB in second or later remission. Vaccine and β-glucan were well tolerated, with 80% EFS at 24 months. Antibody responses against GD2 and/or GD3 were observed in patients achieving clinical responses. These data should encourage the use of cancer vaccines in other malignancies in paediatric patients, also taking into account that several candidate antigens have been identified and characterized.

Vaccination using dendritic cells (DCs) generated from peripheral monocytes following exposure to granulocyte macrophage colony-stimulating factor (GM-CSF) and IL-4 is the most advanced type of cancer vaccine. Sipuleucel-T (Provenge®) is an American Food and Drug Administration-approved autologous DC-based immunotherapy for metastatic hormone-refractory prostate cancer. In the paediatric setting, DC-based vaccines have been used in Phase I/II trials. Krishnadas et al. combined decitabine and DCs targeting MAGE-A1, MAGE-A3, and NY-ESO-1, and, although feasible and safe, this strategy produced only modest anti-tumour activity. Objective responses were documented in only one of the ten patients treated, and in two patients who had no evidence of disease at the time of treatment, one remained disease-free two years post therapy, while the other relapsed ten months post therapy. Mackall et al. reported a pilot study

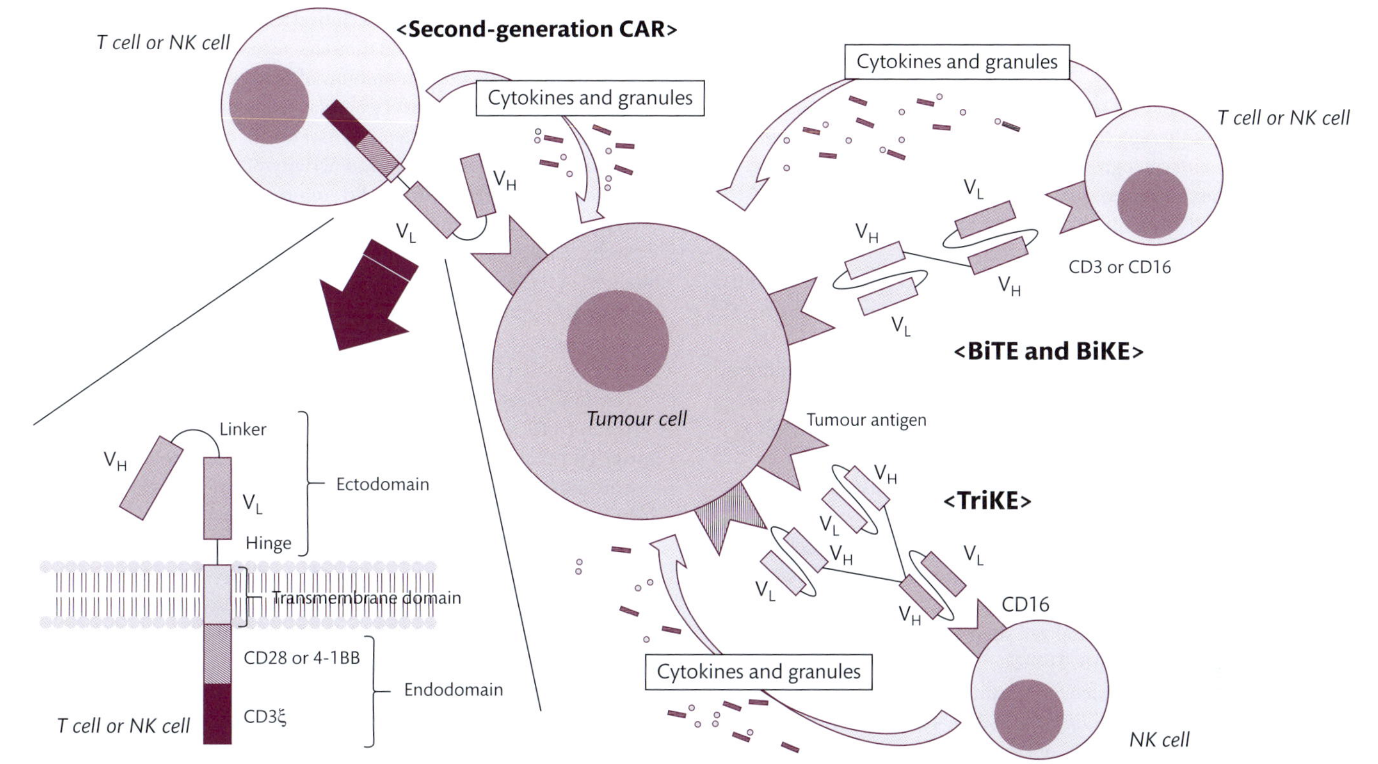

Figure 8.1 Cellular immunotherapy for tumours utilizing T cell/NK cells. Chimeric antigen receptors (CAR) are recombinant proteins composed of an extracellular single-chain variable fragment (scFv) derived from an antibody, joined to a hinge and a transmembrane domain, further linked to the intracellular signalling molecules of the T-cell receptor complex (CD3ζ) and co-stimulatory (CD28 or 4-1BB) endodomains. CAR T cells combine the specificity of an antibody with the cytotoxic and memory functions of T cells. Bispecific/trispecific T-cell/NK-cell engagers (BiTE/BiKE or TriKE) are unique bispecific/trispecific antibodies that have two/three linked scFv constructed to be flexible and have a 1+1 antigen-binding valence. They bind CD3 on T cells or CD16 on NK cells, and one and two antigens on tumour cells, to activate T cells/NK cells for effective elimination of tumour cells.

of consolidative DC vaccines in patients with high-risk paediatric sarcomas. Thirty patients with recurrent or metastatic Ewing's sarcoma had an initial cell harvest to collect autologous cells, and then received chemotherapy, radiation therapy, and/or surgery, followed by infusion of autologous T cells and DCs pulsed with tumour-specific peptides derived from tumour-specific breakpoints and the E7 antigen. Treatment was well tolerated and induced immune responses in 39% of patients vaccinated with the translocation breakpoint peptides. Nevertheless, the clinical benefits of the treatment are difficult to ascertain. The recent introduction in the cancer arena of immune checkpoint inhibitors may reinvigorate the interest in vaccine approaches.

Summary

HSCT has been refined for over 60 years by incorporating the latest clinical/preclinical findings. Consequently, it represents the best curative option for many diseases. New methods aimed at reducing the rate of malignant relapse, preventing and treating GvHD, further reducing infectious complications, as well as increasing the availability of HSCT, continue to be investigated.

There have been several new developments in cancer immunotherapy over the past decade which have dramatically altered standard cancer therapy mainly in adults. In addition to mAbs, immune checkpoint blockade, administered for a variety of cancers in adults, is one of the most promising drugs for paediatric patients. Considering the astonishing results of anti-CD19 CAR T-cell therapy for ALL, CAR T cells have also the potential to radically change conventional cancer treatment. As conventional and high-dose chemotherapy regimens maintain high toxicities, novel immune-based strategies validated in adults should be promptly moved to applications in children, who urgently require effective anti-tumour control with diminished toxicities.

FURTHER READING

Ahmed N, et al. (2015) Human epidermal growth factor receptor 2 (HER2)—specific chimeric antigen receptor-modified T cells for the immunotherapy of HER2-positive sarcoma. *J Clin Oncol* **33**, 1688–96.

Appelbaum FR (2007) Hematopoietic-cell transplantation at 50. *N Engl J Med* **357**, 1472–5.

Blumenthal DT, et al. (2016) Pembrolizumab: first experience with recurrent primary central nervous system (CNS) tumours. *J Neurooncol* **129**, 453–60.

Ciceri F, et al. (2007) Antitumour effects of HSV-TK-engineered donor lymphocytes after allogeneic stem-cell transplantation. *Blood* **109**, 4698–707.

Copelan EA (2006) Hematopoietic stem-cell transplantation. *N Engl J Med* **354**, 1813–26.

Cruz CR, et al. (2013) Infusion of donor-derived CD19-redirected virus-specific T cells for B-cell malignancies relapsed after allogeneic stem cell transplant: a phase 1 study. *Blood* **122**, 2965–73.

Daniele N, et al. (2012) Transplantation in the onco-hematology field: focus on the manipulation of αβ and γδ T cells. *Pathol Res Pract* **208**, 67–73.

Ebb D, et al. (2012) Phase II trial of trastuzumab in combination with cytotoxic chemotherapy for treatment of metastatic osteosarcoma with human epidermal growth factor receptor 2 overexpression: a report from the children's oncology group. *J Clin Oncol* **30**, 2545–51.

Geldres C, et al. (2016) Chimeric antigen receptor-redirected T cells return to the bench. *Semin Immunol* 28, 3–9.

Ghosh A, et al. (2017) Donor CD19 CAR T cells exert potent graft-versus-lymphoma activity with diminished graft-versus-host activity. *Nat Med* **23**, 242–9.

Goldman S, et al. (2014) Rituximab with chemotherapy in children and adolescents with central nervous system and/or bone marrow-positive Burkitt lymphoma/leukaemia: a Children's Oncology Group Report. *Br J Haematol* **167**, 394–401.

Holtan SG, et al. (2014) Acute graft-versus-host disease: a bench-to-bedside update. *Blood* **124**, 363–73.

Huang MA, et al. (2015) Cellular and antibody based approaches for pediatric cancer immunotherapy. *J Immunol Res* **2015**, 675269.

Jenq RR, van den Brink MR (2010) Allogeneic haematopoietic stem cell transplantation: individualized stem cell and immune therapy of cancer. *Nat Rev Cancer* **10**, 213–21.

Kantoff PW, et al. (2010) Sipuleucel-T immunotherapy for castration-resistant prostate cancer. *N Engl J Med* **363**, 411–22.

Klingemann H (2015) Challenges of cancer therapy with natural killer cells. *Cytotherapy* **17**, 245–49.

Krishnadas DK, et al. (2015) A phase I trial combining decitabine/dendritic cell vaccine targeting MAGE-A1, MAGE-A3 and NY-ESO-1 for children with relapsed or therapy-refractory neuroblastoma and sarcoma. *Cancer Immunol Immunother* **64**, 1251–60.

Kushner BH, et al. (2014) Phase I trial of a bivalent gangliosides vaccine in combination with β-glucan for high-risk neuroblastoma in second or later remission. *Clin Cancer Res* **20**, 1375–82.

Lee DW, et al. (2015) T cells expressing CD19 chimeric antigen receptors for acute lymphoblastic leukaemia in children and young adults: a phase 1 dose-escalation trial. *Lancet* **385**, 517–28.

Louis CU, et al. (2011) Antitumour activity and long-term fate of chimeric antigen receptor-positive T cells in patients with neuroblastoma. *Blood* **118**, 6050–6.

Luznik L, et al. (2008) HLA-haploidentical bone marrow transplantation for hematologic malignancies using nonmyeloablative conditioning and high-dose, posttransplantation cyclophosphamide. *Biol Blood Marrow Transplant* **14**, 641–50.

Mackall CL, et al. (2008) A pilot study of consolidative immunotherapy in patients with high-risk pediatric sarcomas. *Clin Cancer Res* **14**, 4850–8.

Malempati S, et al. (2012) Phase I/II trial and pharmacokinetic study of cixutumumab in pediatric patients with refractory solid tumours and Ewing sarcoma: a report from the Children's Oncology Group. *J Clin Oncol* **30**, 256–62.

Mallhi K, et al. (2015) Hematopoietic cell transplantation and cellular therapeutics in the treatment of childhood malignancies. *Pediatr Clin North Am* **62**, 257–73.

Maude SL (2017) Future directions in chimeric antigen receptor T cell therapy. *Curr Opin Pediatr* **29**, 27–33.

Maude SL, et al. (2014) Chimeric antigen receptor T cells for sustained remissions in leukemia. *N Engl J Med* **371**, 1507–17.

Meinhardt A, et al. (2010) Phase II window study on rituximab in newly diagnosed pediatric mature B-cell non-Hodgkin's lymphoma and Burkitt leukemia. *J Clin Oncol* **28**, 3115–21.

Merchant MS, et al. (2016) Phase I clinical trial of ipilimumab in pediatric patients with advanced solid tumours. *Clin Cancer Res* **22**, 1364–70.

Modak S, et al. (2017) Combination of bevacizumab, irinotecan, and temozolomide for refractory or relapsed neuroblastoma: results of a phase II study. *Pediatr Blood Cancer* **64**(8). doi: 10.1002/pbc.26448

Mossé YP, et al. (2013) Safety and activity of crizotinib for paediatric patients with refractory solid tumours or anaplastic large-cell lymphoma: a Children's Oncology Group phase 1 consortium study. *Lancet Oncol* **14**, 472–80.

Mussetti A, et al. (2017) Post-transplant cyclophosphamide, a promising anti-graft versus host disease prophylaxis: where do we stand? *Expert Rev Hematol* **10**(5), 479–92.

O'Hear C, et al. (2013) Gemtuzumab ozogamicin can reduce minimal residual disease in patients with childhood acute myeloid leukemia. *Cancer* **119**, 4036–43.

Porter DL, et al. (2011) Chimeric antigen receptor-modified T cells in chronic lymphoid leukemia. *N Engl J Med* **365**, 725–33.

Postow MA, et al. (2015) Immune checkpoint blockade in cancer therapy. *J Clin Oncol* **33**, 1974–82.

Pro B, et al. (2012) Brentuximab vedotin (SGN-35) in patients with relapsed or refractory systemic anaplastic large-cell lymphoma: results of a phase II study. *J Clin Oncol* **30**, 2190–6.

Pule MA, et al. (2008) Virus-specific T cells engineered to coexpress tumour-specific receptors: persistence and antitumour activity in individuals with neuroblastoma. *Nat Med* **14**, 1264–70.

Pulsipher MA, et al. (2014) New frontiers in pediatric allo-SCT: novel approaches for children and adolescents with ALL. *Bone Marrow Transplant* **49**, 1259–65.

Raetz EA, et al. (2015) Re-induction chemoimmunotherapy with epratuzumab in relapsed acute lymphoblastic leukemia (ALL): Phase II results from Children's Oncology Group (COG) study ADVL04P2. *Pediatr Blood Cancer* **62**, 1171–5.

Rashidi A, et al. (2016) Post-transplant high-dose cyclophosphamide after HLA-matched vs haploidentical hematopoietic cell transplantation for AML. *Bone Marrow Transplant* 51, 1561–4.

Rubnitz JE, et al. (2015) Natural killer cell therapy in children with relapsed leukemia. *Pediatr Blood Cancer* **62**, 1468–72.

Rubnitz JE, et al. (2010) NKAML: a pilot study to determine the safety and feasibility of haploidentical natural killer cell transplantation in childhood acute myeloid leukemia. *J Clin Oncol* **28**, 955–9.

Rytting M, et al. (2014) Initial experience with CMC-544 (inotuzumab ozogamicin) in pediatric patients with relapsed B-cell acute lymphoblastic leukemia. *Pediatr Blood Cancer* **61**, 369–72.

Sharma P, Allison JP (2015) The future of immune checkpoint therapy. *Science* **348**, 56–61.

Shimasaki N, et al. (2016) Expanded and armed natural killer cells for cancer treatment. *Cytotherapy* **18**, 1422–34.

Suck G, et al. (2016) Natural killer cells for therapy of leukemia. *Transfus Med Hemother* **43**, 89–95.

Tey SK, et al. (2007). Inducible caspase 9 suicide gene to improve the safety of allodepleted T cells after haploidentical stem cell transplantation. *Biol Blood Marrow Transplant* **13**, 913–24.

Trippett TM, et al. (2009) Phase I and pharmacokinetic study of cetuximab and irinotecan in children with refractory solid tumours: a study of the pediatric oncology experimental therapeutic investigators' consortium. *J Clin Oncol* **27**, 5102–8.

von Stackelberg A, et al. (2016) Phase I/Phase II Study of blinatumomab in pediatric patients with relapsed/refractory acute lymphoblastic leukemia. *J Clin Oncol* **34**, 4381–9.

Yu AL, et al. (2010) Anti-GD2 antibody with GM-CSF, interleukin-2, and isotretinoin for neuroblastoma. *N Engl J Med* **363**, 1324–34.

9

Supportive Care During Treatment

Marianne van de Wetering and Robert S. Phillips

Introduction

Reducing the toxic and unpleasant effects of cancer therapies is a critical component of cancer management in children. As the intensity of primary treatment has escalated, so have side effects such as myelosuppression and infection. Improved outcomes are dependent on skilled supportive care, and advances in supportive care have paralleled advances in cancer therapy. In this chapter we will highlight a few key aspects, evidence-based if possible.

Infection

Infection remains a common cause of hospital admission during cancer therapy and is the commonest cause of death after disease relapse/progression. Children are at increased risk of bacterial, viral, protozoal, and fungal infections, and the prevention and treatment of infection are central to supportive care.

Many factors influence the frequency and severity of infection in cancer patients. These include myelosuppression or immunosuppression as a result of disease or therapy, and disruption of natural barriers to infection. Neutropenia (often defined as an absolute neutrophil count of less than 500 cells/mm^3) is the most important risk factor, with both the depth and duration of neutropenia influencing infection risk. Death has been reported in 1–3% of episodes of febrile neutropenia (FN) in children, with adolescent/young adult patients at greater risk.

Around 15–20% of all episodes of FN in children are associated with positive blood-culture isolates. Gram-positive organisms cause up to 70% of proven bloodstream infections, Gram-negative infections cause 28%, and fungal infections, mainly yeasts, cause 2%. The commonest Gram-positive organisms are coagulase-negative *Staphylococci*, but enterococci and viridans group streptococcal species have the potential for severe disease and antibiotic resistance. Among Gram-negative organisms, the most frequent are *Escherichia coli, Klebsiella* species, *Pseudomonas aeruginosa, Serratia* species, and *Proteus* species. Infections with Gram-negative bacteria producing extended spectrum beta-lactamases are of increasing concern in hospitals and the community, but are not yet widely reported in children with cancer. As with antibiotic resistance in other groups of patients, the nature of the local resistance pattern is very geographically varied. Infections with fungal organisms such as *Candida* yeasts, *Aspergillus* moulds, or other opportunistic fungi, and with viruses such as cytomegalovirus (CMV), varicella zoster virus (VZV), adenovirus, and infections with *Pneumocystis jirovecii* (pneumocystis pneumonia, PCP) may occur.

Prevention of infection

A number of strategies are commonly used to reduce the risk of infection, although the evidence for some of these is lacking.

The environment

Neutropenic patients are at increased risk of hospital-acquired infections and the hospital environment should be avoided where possible. Children are encouraged to continue their normal lifestyle, including school and hobbies. Teachers should be informed of the risks to the child with cancer and asked to alert the child's parents when there is VZV or measles in the school.

The hospital environment

If hospitalized during neutropenia, children are often cared for in protective isolation in general hospitals, although many specialist paediatric oncology units manage neutropenic children on the open oncology ward, with isolation being reserved for those with clearly transmissible infections (e.g. respiratory viral infections, diarrhoea). Careful handwashing is essential and prevents the spread of infection.

Nutrition/diet

There are data refuting the role of special measures concerning food products during neutropenia, but sensible food hygiene rules and avoiding potentially contaminated products such as unpasteurized milk or cheese, seafood, and pâté should be followed. A Cochrane review was performed (with an update in 2016) summarizing the evidence concerning this topic. As the evidence is very poor, no definite recommendation could be given for clinical practice. Intensive dietary restrictions often apply to patients undergoing haematopoetic stem-cell transplantation (HSCT), though with little supportive data.

Invasive procedures

The requirement for any procedure that can disrupt the normal mucosa or skin barriers during neutropenic periods (e.g. dental procedures) should be carefully balanced against the increased possibility of infection.

Antibiotic prophylaxis

Oral antibiotics may be used to preserve beneficial anaerobic organisms while preventing colonization of the gut by pathogenic aerobic organisms. Historically, trimethoprim/sulfamethoxazole (TMP/SMZ) was used but, more recently, quinolones have been employed. Selective decontamination of the digestive tract (SDD) is effective in preventing (mainly Gram-negative) bacteraemia during neutropenic episodes, and reduces deaths from infective causes. Quinolones are slightly more effective than TMP/SMZ. Some groups support the use of antibiotic prophylaxis in selected patients, such as those with acute leukaemia, HSCT patients, and relapsed patients. The risk of emergence of resistant organisms as the result of routine prophylaxis has not been significant to date, but requires ongoing study.

Fungal prophylaxis

The need for fungal prophylaxis is less clear than for bacterial prophylaxis, but is recommended by many as standard of care in high-risk patients (i.e. HSCT patients, high-risk phases of acute leukaemia therapy). Early diagnosis of invasive fungal infection is expected to improve outcomes, but prevention remains the ultimate goal. The nature of the prophylactic agent chosen remains under considerable debate. Fluconazole provides effective prophylaxis against most *Candida* infections, although some species such as *Candida krusei* may be resistant. *Aspergillus* prophylaxis requires a mould-active, agent and co-administration of azoles. Monitoring of children at increased risk for *Aspergillus* infection is essential.

Viral prophylaxis

Aciclovir is used in patients at high risk of CMV and VZV activation, namely patients on very intensive protocols and those undergoing HSCT. Clinical VZV (shingles) is common after viral prophylaxis is discontinued in HSCT patients, and it is currently recommended to continue for up to a year post HSCT.

Children should be tested for VZV IgG at diagnosis, and VZV-negative patients should be given prophylaxis with varicella zoster immune globulin or aciclovir after significant contact. Little data is available to suggest which is better.

Prevention of *Pneumocystis jirovecii* pneumonia

TMP/SMZ is highly effective in preventing PCP and is important for all patients undergoing treatment for leukaemia, lymphoma, or HSCT, and for patients with solid tumours with prolonged neutropenic episodes. An alternative to TMP/SMZ prophylaxis is aerosolized or intravenous pentamidine. Dapsone can be given if patients cannot tolerate pentamidine.

Granulocyte colony-stimulating factor

Granulocyte colony-stimulating factor (G-CSF) is widely used in adult and paediatric practice to reduce the depth and duration of chemotherapy-associated neutropenia. Data support its use in preventing hospitalization, but not episodes of confirmed infection or death. The choice to give colony-stimulating factors is usually determined by protocol, to support the administration of dose-intense chemotherapy, or in the setting of progenitor cell mobilization. Secondary prophylactic G-CSF may be used if previous episodes of neutropenia have led to severe infections, delay, or dose reduction of chemotherapy. If given, G-CSF should be started 24–72 hours after chemotherapy and continued until the neutrophil count is greater than 1000/mm^3 on two occasions.

Immunization in prevention of infection

Some aspects of vaccine-acquired immunity are lost during cancer therapy. Booster vaccinations are recommended for all children six months after completing therapy, and a complete re-vaccination programme is recommended for children at a year or more after HSCT (Table 9.1). Off-treatment immunization with HPV (human papilloma virus) vaccines is recommended, at an appropriate age. There is a balance between the most significant time for infection risk and the likelihood of response to therapy. Live attenuated vaccines should not be administered until at least six months after stopping chemotherapy, but if herd immunity for measles is low,

Table 9.1 Vaccination recommendations during and after chemotherapy treatment (not applicable to children during/after autologous or allogeneic bone-marrow transplant)

Timing in relation to chemotherapy	Vaccination*	Recommendation
During chemotherapy	MMR	If low-herd immunity, then use single-antigen measles vaccine
	OPV	Not allowed. If needed, then eIPV
	DTaP	Prefer to wait until stopping chemotherapy
	Hepatitis B	High-risk areas—Recombivax HB
After chemotherapy	DTaP/MMR/HiB/pneumococcal/HPV (age-related)	Restart schedule 6 months after stopping chemotherapy
Special considerations	Influenza vaccine	Not contraindicated during chemotherapy
	Varicella zoster	Degree of protection uncertain
	Pneumococcal	No evidence-based recommendation
		In maintenance chemotherapy, safe and immunogenic, not registered yet for use in children with cancer. Indicated for splenic dysfunction e.g. splenectomy in Hodgkin lymphoma, post radiotherapy (radiation spleen)

* DTaP: diptheria, tetanus, acellular pertussis vaccine; eIPV: enhanced inactivated polio vaccine; HiB: haemophilus influenzae b conjugate vaccine; MMR: measles, mumps, rubella vaccine; OPV: oral polio vaccine; HPV: human papilloma virus

single-antigen measles vaccine may be given during or soon after chemotherapy, with measles vaccination repeated six months after stopping chemotherapy. Ideally, hepatitis B vaccination is given after completing chemotherapy, but in high-risk groups or areas it can be given during chemotherapy, with reduced immunogenic response. Periodic booster doses are usually necessary, with the timing determined by serological testing at 12-month intervals. There are no data on changes in immune status or re-vaccination against HPVs after chemotherapy or HSCT.

Most countries recommend yearly influenza vaccination of household contacts and patients during chemotherapy and after HSCT. A Cochrane systematic review emphasized the paucity of data on this vaccine. Serological responses are lower than expected in healthy controls, and antibody levels considered protective in healthy individuals may not prevent clinical infection in an immunocompromised individual. There are no data on whether vaccination of paediatric cancer patients protects against clinical infection. However, as the vaccine is well tolerated, it is not contraindicated.

Active VZV vaccination has been given to VZV IgG negative patients during leukaemia maintenance therapy. The vaccine is immunogenic, but some patients develop vaccine-related infection requiring aciclovir treatment. In addition, chemotherapy must be omitted for one week before and one week after the time of vaccination, and steroids should not be given for two weeks after vaccination. The vaccine has not been widely studied in other groups of children with malignancy. For these reasons, geographical differences in practice exist with respect to VZV vaccination of susceptible children with cancer.

Live or attenuated vaccines such as measles, mumps, rubella (MMR), or oral polio are contraindicated during cancer therapy. Siblings or household contacts may safely receive MMR, but enhanced inactivated polio vaccine (eIPV) should be given in place of oral polio vaccine (see **Table 9.1**).

Treatment of infection

FN is defined differently across the world but usually includes a neutrophil count of less than 500 cells/mm^3 (or above 500 cells/mm^3 and expected to fall) and significant fever. Fever definitions vary but include a single temperature of more than 38.5°C, or a temperature of more than 38°C twice in 12 hours. Defining the optimal limits is subject to ongoing study. Management is a medical emergency because of the potential risk of overwhelming sepsis. An international group has published evidence-based guidelines on the topic. Children who are neutropenic and significantly unwell, but without fever, should also be managed as for FN; occasionally, Gram-negative sepsis presents with abdominal pain and diarrhoea, but without fever, especially in children receiving steroid therapy.

Febrile, neutropenic children with cancer require careful assessment. Treatment is divided into empirical therapy and 'planned progressive therapy' stages.

Assessment

A careful history and thorough physical examination is needed, including emphasis on the mucosal membranes, the chest, soft tissues, central venous catheter site, and perianal area. The assessment phase is ongoing: careful and repeated evaluation for specific symptoms and signs or a focus of infection is critical, but there may be minimal signs of inflammation at an infected site during neutropenia. Laboratory evaluation should include a complete blood count, liver enzymes, renal function, and blood cultures from both central lines and peripherally. Urine culture is routinely advised, as dipstick screening and symptoms are less prevalent in this population. Stool culture testing for *Clostridioides (formely known as Clostridium)* toxin, cerebrospinal fluid examination, and chest X-ray should be done only if clinically indicated. Based on the patient history and initial clinical findings, patients may be assessed as at low or high risk of complications of FN. Multiple risk-assessment tools have been used in paediatric FN; geographical variation in their performance means local validation should be undertaken prior to their use in practice.

Empirical antibiotic therapy

The progression of infection in neutropenic patients can be rapid, so empirical intravenous antibiotic therapy should be started promptly. The initial goal is to provide broad-spectrum cover against both Gram-negative and Gram-positive organisms. In areas with appropriate resistance patterns, this is best accomplished with monotherapy with an extended-spectrum beta-lactam, fourth-generation cephalosporin, or carbapenem such as meropenem or imipenem. Through resistance, either prior isolation from the patient or knowledge of the local pattern, it may be that an aminoglycoside is required. Low-risk patients should be treated as part of a clinical trial or according to an established institutional low-risk protocol, which may recommend commencement of oral antibiotics instead. However, we should realize that this is not routine practice. The empirical antibiotic regimen should be reviewed regularly in each institution, taking account of changes in the spectrum of infections, antimicrobial susceptibility patterns, and the underlying aetiology of the neutropenia.

'Planned progressive' therapy

The therapeutic plan should be modified according to clinical response and microbiological findings. Children who are clinically well, lack a significant clinical focus of infection other than upper respiratory tract infection, have no positive cultures, and whose fever settles quickly, can discontinue antibiotics once afebrile after 24–48 hours. Some protocols allow for step down to oral antibiotics in patients at low risk of significant complications. If the patient without a positive clinical focus or cultures has persistent fever after three to five days of treatment, reassess carefully, take further cultures, and look for a focus. If the child is clinically well, the same antibiotics can be continued. If the child is deteriorating clinically, consider changing antibiotics and/or adding anaerobic cover. In patients with a high risk of fungal infection, empirically add antifungal therapy after five days of persistent fever where there is no other explanation, and consider early computed tomography (CT) of the chest and abdominal ultrasound scan, along with directed investigation if other symptoms suggest localized disease.

The duration of therapy for patients with positive blood cultures is not well defined, with many clinicians choosing to give seven to ten days of intravenous antibiotics. If fever settles quickly, therapy for the isolated organism should be optimized, but maintain broad-spectrum antibiotic cover to prevent breakthrough bacteraemia. It is not usually necessary to continue antibiotics until the neutrophils recover. Invasive fungal infection requires a prolonged course of antifungal therapy.

If fever persists in a child with a positive culture, optimize antibacterial therapy before making any other changes, and consider adding antifungal therapy after four to five days of fever. Rarely, fever may be due to the medication, but stopping antibiotics can be dangerous and should only be considered after a very careful, thorough exclusion of other causes of fever.

Central venous catheter infections

Complications related to the long-term use of central venous catheters are minimized by recommended protocols for catheter placement and care, but there is the potential for infection of the bloodstream and/or device, the subcutaneous pocket, and the tunnel or exit site. The overall incidence of catheter-related infections is approximately 2 in 1,000 catheter days. Decreasing the number of infections using preventative techniques with ethanol lock or taurolidine lock is promising but not implemented as standard care yet.

Most infections are with Gram-positive organisms (mainly coagulase-negative *Staphylococcus*), but cover for Gram-negative organisms is necessary until an organism is identified. More than 80% of documented catheter-related infections can be treated successfully by giving antibiotics through the catheter, but treatment failures may result from infections with multiple organisms, fungi, *Pseudomonas aeruginosae*, resistant Gram-negative organisms, and tunnel infections. In *Staphylococcus aureus* infection, antibiotics should be administered for at least two weeks if the catheter is left in place. Persistent bacterial catheter infections and most fungal (*Candida*) catheter infections require catheter removal. Catheter removal should also be considered early in the acutely unwell, septic patient whose condition is not responding rapidly to broad-spectrum antibiotics and fluid resuscitation.

Fever without neutropenia

The non-neutropenic, febrile child should be evaluated very carefully. Laboratory evaluation includes a blood count and blood cultures from the central venous catheter. Management is dictated by the clinical findings. If the child is clinically well other than fever, with no clinical focus of infection, blood-culture results can be awaited before starting antibiotics. If there is a clinical focus of bacterial infection (e.g. ear, throat, skin), consider appropriate oral antibiotics such as amoxicillin or co-amoxiclav until the blood-culture result is known. If the non-neutropenic child is unwell with fever, commence empirical antibiotics as for a neutropenic child and give appropriate supportive care, pending further results.

Viral infections

The most common viral pathogens that affect the immunocompromised child are the herpes viruses including herpes simplex virus (HSV), VZV, CMV, and Epstein–Barr virus (EBV). Herpes viruses can result in mucosal lesions, skin lesions, and neurological symptoms. Systemic treatment with aciclovir is needed for at least five days. Aciclovir is not routinely indicated for chemotherapy-induced mucositis.

Primary infection with VZV results in chickenpox. In the immunocompromised child, severe complications may be seen, leading to a fulminating illness with visceral dissemination of the virus. Untreated VZV pneumonitis can be fatal in up to 7% of affected children. In unwell children, treatment should be intravenous acyclovir. For those without significant illness, who have a rash but no fever, respiratory, or other symptoms, and without severe lymphopenia (less than 100 cell/mm^3), an oral treatment may be used.

CMV can result in fever, rash, hepatosplenomegaly, pneumonia, neurological symptoms, and retinitis. Treatment is with ganciclovir intravenously or foscarnet. Prolonged courses of therapy are necessary to eradicate the infection.

Blood-product transfusion

Anaemia and thrombocytopenia can occur as a consequence of chemotherapy or the underlying disease.

Red-cell transfusion

The haemoglobin concentration should be maintained at safe levels but normal physiological levels are not required. There is little evidence to guide the transfusion threshold but most centres choose a level of less than 7 g/dl and, with radiotherapy, an even higher level of more than 10 g/dl is maintained because of the theoretical benefit of cellular oxygenation during radiotherapy. Leukodepleted, packed red cells are given. Leukodepletion reduces the chance of human leukocyte antigen (HLA) sensitization and infection with prions and CMV. Irradiated products are not routinely required but important exceptions are before HSCT, after HSCT until lymphocytes have recovered (six months after transplant), in severe combined immunodeficiencies, in neonates, and in Hodgkin lymphoma. The volume requirement can be calculated variably, with some using 10–15 ml/kg and others using Target – Current Hb (in g/dL) × weight (kg) × 5. There are insufficient data to recommend the routine use of erythropoetin in paediatric oncology.

Platelet transfusions

Platelet transfusions are indicated if a thrombocytopenic patient is actively bleeding. Prophylactic platelet transfusions are indicated in patients who are septic, have a known bleeding disorder, or are undergoing an invasive procedure such as central venous catheter insertion or lumbar puncture. There is little evidence about the appropriate transfusion threshold. Platelets are usually kept more than 10×10^9/l, except for brain tumour patients (where levels of 20–40 × 10^9/l are often used) and for invasive procedures (where the level is kept more than 50×10^9/l). If patients develop allo-immunization, which reduces the therapeutic effect of transfused platelets, single-donor transfusions can be used.

Nausea and vomiting

Nausea and vomiting remain an important concern in cancer treatment but adequate control can often be achieved. Techniques such as relaxation, distraction, and explanation of procedures should be considered along with antiemetic medication. Paediatric-specific guidelines have been developed to guide practitioners.

A validated nausea and vomiting tool such as the PENAT score (comparable with the face pain rating scale for assessment of pain) should be used to assess the severity of nausea and vomiting at regular intervals. Management is adjusted according to findings.

Chemotherapeutic agents can be grouped into four classes: minimal (less than 10% of patients experience nausea and vomiting), low emetogenicity (10–30% of patients experience nausea and vomiting), moderate emetogenicity (30–90% of patients experience nausea and vomiting), and high emetogenicity (more than 90% of patients experience nausea and vomiting). Starting medication is tailored to the drug of highest emetogenicity within the chemotherapy combination (Table 9.2). In minimal emetogenic chemotherapy, no antiemetic therapy is needed. In low emetogenic chemotherapy, a serotonin receptor antagonist, usually ondansetron, is indicated; in moderate emetogenicity, corticosteroids can be added as the drugs work synergistically. In highly emetogenic chemotherapy, the combination of a serotonin receptor antagonist plus steroids plus an NK1 antagonist (e.g. aprepitant) should be used unless there are contraindications. Radiotherapy, especially of the abdomen, can also lead to nausea and vomiting, and a serotonin receptor antagonist is often given 30 minutes before treatment. Steroids can also be useful, especially for radiotherapy of the brain.

Those with breakthrough or refractory nausea or vomiting may be difficult to manage. Increasing the intensity of medication is recommended and, if necessary, olanzapine, levomepromazine, or metoclopramide may be used. An aggressive antiemetic plan at the start of therapy minimizes the initial experience of nausea and probably reduces the risk of anticipatory nausea and vomiting. If anticipatory vomiting does occur, hypnotherapy, cannabinoids, or banzodiazepines may be effective.

Table 9.2 Antiemetic therapy in relation to different types of chemotherapy

Emetogenic potential	Drug	Antiemetic therapy	Delayed emesis
Minimal	Asparaginase Bleomycin Bevacizumab Mercaptopurin Methotrexate (<50 mg/m^2) Rituximab Vinca alkaloids (except vinoralbine)	None	None
Low	Busulphan (oral) Cytarabine <1 g/m^2 Doxorubicin (liposomal) Etoposide Topotecan	5 HT3 antagonist (e.g. ondansetron/ granisetron)	None
Moderate	Busulfan Cyclophosphamide < 1g/m^2 Doxorubicin Irinotecan Ifosfamide Epirubicin Idarubicin Methotrexate >1 but <12 g/m^2	5 HT3 antagonist (e.g. ondansetron/ granisetron) Dexamethasone	None
High	Carboplatin Carmustine Cisplatin Cyclophosphamide >1 g/m^2 Cytarabine >3 g/m^2 Actinomycin Dacarbazine Doxorubicin >60 mg/m^2 Melfalan (iv) Methotrexate >12 g/m^2 Mitoxantrone >15mg/m^2 Procarbazine	5 HT3 antagonist (e.g. ondansetron/ granisetron) *and* dexamethasone (adjusted dose) *and* NK1 antagonist (aprepitant) If an NK1 antagonist is not used, usual dose of dexamethasone	Continue ondansetron for 72 hours

Source: data from Dupis L. et al., *Guideline for Classification of the Acute Emetogenic Potential of Antineoplastic Medication in Pediatric Cancer Patients*. Guideline release date: 11 August 2010. Pediatric Oncology Group of Ontario (POGO). Available from: https://www.pogo.ca/healthcare/practiceguidelines/ pogoemetogenicitycla/

Nutrition support

Good nutrition is important during cancer therapy. Patients may present undernourished at diagnosis and cancer treatment may profoundly impact their nutritional status.

Children with malnutrition or at high risk of developing malnutrition should be reviewed by a paediatric dietician for advice about healthy eating and vitamin supplementation. For children requiring nutritional intervention, enteral nutrition is the management of choice if gut function is maintained. Patients may be offered nutritional supplements such as high-calorie, nutritional drinks, if able to swallow normally and tolerate such supplements. Alternatively, nasogastric tube feeding or gastrostomy feeding may be indicated. Gastrostomy feeding is particularly suited to older children or young people who wish to avoid the cosmetic associations or irritation of a nasogastric tube or children who cannot safely tolerate a nasogastric tube. When gut function is poor for a prolonged period or where nasogastric feeds cannot be tolerated, intravenous total parenteral nutrition is used.

Mouth care

Good mouth care plays an important role in the prevention of infection and is essential for children developing complications such as mucositis, oral candidiasis, xerostomia, or herpes simplex infections. The evidence for mouth-care interventions is incomplete but guidelines based on available evidence are now available.

At diagnosis, an assessment of the mouth and teeth is essential, and children should be referred to a dentist or dental hygienist promptly. During cancer therapy, children should brush their teeth twice daily using a soft toothbrush and fluoride toothpaste, or clean the mouth with oral sponges moistened with water or diluted chlorhexidine. Regular assessment of the oral mucous membranes during inpatient therapy using one of the available scoring systems will allow early detection of, and intervention for, mucositis and other problems. Children who develop mucositis need ongoing basic mouth care and adequate analgesia.

Constipation

Constipation is a common problem in children and young people with cancer, and appropriate therapeutic intervention can greatly improve quality of life. The aetiology is mostly multifactorial: these patients have reduced activity, reduced oral fluid and food intake, and take medications such as opioids, vinca alkaloids, carboplatin, and ondansetron which contribute to constipation. There are no randomized controlled studies performed in this age group to inform laxative choice, so management is directed towards the most likely cause of constipation in the individual child. Stool softeners and osmotic laxatives (such as polyethelene glycol sachets) are most often used, and bowel evacuants are rarely needed.

Tumour lysis syndrome

Tumour lysis syndrome (TLS) is a set of complications that can arise from treatment of rapidly proliferating, drug-sensitive neoplasms. These are typically haematological malignancies (particularly Burkitt lymphoma and the acute leukaemias) but, rarely, also solid tumours. Chemotherapy causes rapid destruction of tumour cells leading to release of intracellular substances into the bloodstream. Metabolic disturbances include hyperuricaemia, hyperphosphataemia, hypocalcaemia, and hyperkalaemia. Clinical manifestations occur 12–72 hours after initial start of therapy and can include renal failure (from precipitation of uric acid crystals and calcium phosphate salts), seizures, and cardiac arrhythmias.

Prevention of TLS relies on identification of at-risk patients. Such patients should have laboratory and clinical TLS parameters monitored every 4–6 hours until stabilized. Therapy is best commenced in a unit with paediatric intensive-care facilities and nephrology input for advice and, potentially, dialysis.

Standard supportive care to prevent TLS consists of vigorous hyperhydration (2–3 L/m^2/day) and avoidance of hyperuricaemia. The primary treatment for hyperuricaemia has been allopurinol (50–100 mg/m^2 every eight hours orally, maximum 300 mg/m^2/day) combined with hyperhydration. The use of rasburicase (recombinant urate oxidase dose 0.2 mg/kg IV once a day) is preferred for high-risk patients, and alkalinization becomes unnecessary. Urate oxidase catalyses conversion of uric acid to water-soluble allantoin which is readily excreted in urine. It decreases uric acid levels more than allopurinol, with a rapid drop occurring within four hours of administration.

Management is tailored according to risk of TLS. Low-risk patients (solid tumours and AML with white blood-cell count (WCC) less than 25×10^9/l) only need monitoring and hyperhydration. ALL with WCC less than 100×10^9/l, AML with WCC more than 25×10^9/l, and large-cell anaplastic lymphoma are classified as intermediate-risk disease for which monitoring, hyperhydration, and allopurinol is given. High-risk disease (ALL WCC more than 100×10^9/l, bulky Burkitt lymphoma, and other stage IV lymphomas) should be managed in specialized paediatric oncology units where patients need careful monitoring, hyperhydration, and rasburicase.

Conclusion

This chapter highlights the most important physical aspects of supportive care for the child with cancer. Pain management is discussed in Chapter 11 ('Palliative Care for Children with Advanced Cancer'). Other aspects, such as psychological support, social interventions, and clinican–family–patient communication, have not been discussed here. The critical importance of supportive care continues to be the relief of cancer and treatment-related symptoms, less morbidity, and reduced mortality.

FURTHER READING

Baskin JL, et al. (2009) Management of occlusion and thrombosis associated with long-term indwelling central venous catheters. *Lancet* **374**, 159–69.

Cairo MS, et al. (2010) Recommendations for the evaluation of risk and prophylaxis of tumour lysis syndrome (TLS) in adults and children with malignant diseases: an expert TLS panel consensus. *Br J Haematol* **149**, 578–86.

Dupuis LL, et al. (2006) Development and validation of the pediatric nausea assessment tool for use in children receiving antineoplastic agents. *Pharmacotherapy* **26**, 1221–31.

Dupuis LL, et al. (2013) Guideline for the prevention of acute nausea and vomiting due to antineoplastic medication in pediatric cancer patients. *Pediatr Blood Cancer* **60**, 1073–82.

Dupuis LL, et al. (2013) Guideline for the prevention and treatment of anticipatory nausea and vomiting due to chemotherapy in pediatric cancer patients. *Pediatr Blood Cancer* **61**, 1506–12.

Dupuis LL, et al. (2017) Updated MASCC/ESMO consensus recommendations: prevention of acute chemotherapy-induced nausea and vomiting in children. *Support Care Cancer* **25**(1), 323–31.

Flank J, et al. (2016) Guideline for the treatment of breakthrough and the prevention of refractory chemotherapy-induced nausea and vomiting in children with cancer. *Pediatr Blood Cancer* **63**, 1144–51.

Gafter-Gvili A, et al. (2012) Antibiotic prophylaxis for bacterial infections in afebrile neutropenic patients following chemotherapy. *Cochrane Database Syst Rev* **18**(1), CD004386.Gaynor EP, Sullivan PB (2015) Nutritional status and nutritional management in children with cancer. *Arch Dis Child* **100**, 1169–72.

Gibson BE, et al. (2004) Transfusion guidelines for neonates and older children. *Br J Haematol* **124**(4), 433–53.

Glenny AM, et al. (2010) The development of evidence-based guidelines on mouth care for children, teenagers and young adults treated for cancer. *Eur J Cancer* **46**, 1399–1412.

Goossen GM1, et al. (2013) Influenza vaccination in children being treated with chemotherapy for cancer. *Cochrane Database Syst Rev* **1**(8), CD006484.

Jones L, et al. (2010) Nutritional support in children and young people with cancer undergoing chemotherapy. *Cochrane Database Syst Rev* **7**(7), Review. [2015 update in *Cochrane Database Syst Rev* **8**, CD003298]

Lehrnbecher T (2015) Antifungal prophylaxis in pediatric patients undergoing therapy for cancer: drugs and dosing. *Curr Opin Infect Dis* **28**(6), 523–31.

Lehrnbecher T, et al. (2012) Guideline for the management of fever and neutropenia in children with cancer and/or undergoing hematopoietic stem-cell transplantation. *J Clin Oncol* **30**, 4427–38.

Loeffen EAH, et al. (2017) The importance of evidence-based supportive care practice guidelines in childhood cancer—a plea for their development and implementation. *Support Care Cancer* **25**, 1121.

Mermel LA, et al. (2001) Guidelines for the management of intravascular catheter-related infections. *Clin Infect Dis* **32**, 1249–72.

Patel SR, et al. (2008) Vaccinations in children treated with standard-dose cancer therapy or hematopoietic stem cell transplantation. *Pediatr Clin North Am* **55**, 169–86, xi.

Phillips RS, Gibson F (2008) A systematic review of treatments for constipation in children and young adults undergoing cancer treatment. *J Pediatr Hematol Oncol* **30**, 829–30.

Pittiruti M, et al. (2016) Evidence-based criteria for the choice and the clinical use of the most appropriate lock solutions for central venous catheters (excluding dialysis catheters): a GAVeCeLT consensus. *J Vasc Access* **17**(6), 453–64.

Rheingans JI (2007) A systematic review of nonpharmacologic adjunctive therapies for symptom management in children with cancer. *J Pediatr Oncol Nurs* **24**, 81–94.

Robenshtok E, et al. (2007) Antifungal prophylaxis in cancer patients after chemotherapy or hematopoietic stem-cell transplantation: systematic review and meta-analysis. *J Clin Oncol* **25**, 5471–89.

Sartori AM (2004) A review of the varicella vaccine in immunocompromised individuals. *Int J Infect Dis* **8**, 259–70.

Sung L, et al. (2007) Meta-analysis: effect of prophylactic hematopoietic colony-stimulating factors on mortality and outcomes of infection. *Ann Intern Med* **147**, 400–11.

van Dalen EC, et al. (2016) Low bacterial diet versus control diet to prevent infection in cancer patients treated with chemotherapy causing episodes of neutropenia. *Cochrane Database Syst Rev* **4**, CD006247.

10

Psychosocial Care

Martha Grootenhuis, Momcilo Jankovic, Esther van den Bergh, and Femke Aarsen

Introduction

The diagnosis of cancer in a child is one of the most stressful events that can happen to a family. It confronts the child and parents with a range of stressors, including the most feared: the death of the child. Although treatment has greatly improved over the last decades and survival rates have increased dramatically, parents and children still face an extensive period of intensive treatment which fundamentally impacts their lives. The whole family has the difficult task of adjusting to a situation dominated by the stresses of long-lasting uncertainty and uncontrollability, in a situation with a risk for experiencing medical traumatic stress.

Children differ from adults. From birth until adulthood, children are in a process of physical, cognitive, emotional, and social development. In developing their abilities to cope with their environment, children are dependent on adults. Together they are in a child-rearing relationship, in which an important role is given to their parents. Younger children need their parents to help them cope with basic fears and basic desires, and also with the demands of socialization. Older children need their parents in learning to cope with questions related to physical and cognitive growth, development of personal identity, and difficulties of functioning in peer groups. Children also differ from adults in their understanding and experience of health, illness, and medical care. Depending on the child's developmental level, special needs have to be met in the context of the family (parents, siblings), education, and the enlarged social environment (friends, school, healthcare workers). Each phase of treatment has its own characteristics that contribute to the reactions of parents and children. In this chapter, psychosocial care in these different phases will be described, focusing on both children and parents.

Acute phase

For all children and their parents, the diagnostic phase and start of treatment is very stressful. It commences with invasive medical procedures necessary to obtain a diagnosis. The child has to endure pain and the parents have to witness their child in pain and fear. The challenge is to accomplish a realistic and, for the child, an age-appropriate understanding of diagnosis and treatment implications. This is especially necessary for decisions to be made at the beginning of treatment (e.g. study randomization). Children may anxiously ask 'Am I going to die?' in a phase where their parents are in emotional turmoil and experiencing loss of control. In the past, it was not common to communicate frankly with children about cancer, survival, and death. Fortunately, it is now argued that enabling children to assimilate information and feelings allows them to cope better. Research has shown that providing information to the child with cancer about diagnosis and prognosis is beneficial for the child's emotional experience of their situation. In this phase, parents may feel guilty about late identification of symptoms related to the disease. Parents may also be angry about delay in referral to the hospital. Learning to cope with these feelings takes time. Furthermore, parents have to cope with the reactions of other family members (e.g. siblings, grandparents), which sometimes can give a profound extra burden.

A second stressor at this stage is learning to deal with the effects of medical treatment. Chemotherapy usually starts shortly after diagnosis. The child rapidly comprehends what cancer treatment is about: painful medical procedures (e.g. port-a-cath, lumbar punctures, bone marrow aspirations), sickness because of chemotherapeutic agents (nausea, vomiting, mycosis), or fatigue because of radiotherapy, and side effects such as hair loss. As well as the chemotherapeutic treatment in the hospital, parents have to administer cancer treatment to their child at home (e.g. dexamethasone). Managing this is challenging and makes parents feel extremely responsible. After a tumour resection, children have to cope with physical disabilities, and for those with a brain tumour, they must also deal with neuropsychological deficits.

A third stressor, especially at the beginning of treatment, is informing the social environment (other family members, school, employers). Ensuring social support is of major importance because of the long duration of treatment. It is well known that social support is a protective factor in adaptation to the disease. Families need ongoing support and to stay in touch with everyday life as much as possible. Many families receive social support (e.g. for the care of siblings, household), but it is also important for a social worker to support the family in all the emotional, practical, or financial consequences of the disease and treatment (including contact with employers or welfare insurance companies). Special care is needed for non-native families. Both language and cultural background can make it very difficult to communicate properly about the cancer and its treatment. Using an interpreter in breaking the bad news, but also in subsequent conversations about changes in the course of treatment, contributes to their understanding.

To help parents adjust to the circumstances after diagnosis can be demanding (e.g. administering medication, timing of routine hospital visits, learning to evaluate symptoms and to decide whether or not it is necessary to go and see the doctor, maintaining balance inside the family). Thus, to help parents adjust, psychological intervention programmes can be useful in teaching them both practical and emotional problem-solving skills.

During treatment

Modern childhood cancer treatment, in spite of tremendous improvements in supportive care, still has many unwanted side effects. Especially older children have difficulties with losing their hair and changes in their physical appearance. These can be reversible changes such as the use of a feeding tube and substantial weight loss, but also irreversible changes such as stretch marks due to rapid increase in weight because of corticosteroid medication. Adolescents typically suffer from feelings of shame and inconvenience. The child or adolescent should be given information about the side effects of medication and treatment. Good psychosocial support may include teaching the child what he or she can do to cope with pain and other negative feelings. Cognitive behavioural techniques such as relaxation, visualization, distraction, and the use of 'helping thoughts' are beneficial.

In the first months after diagnosis, many children show adjustment towards treatment and being ill, but they also start to realize the impact of the cancer experience on their daily lives. Reactions to this adjustment can involve grief and mourning over the fact that their life as it was before being diagnosed is 'lost' or the development of a negative self-image due to changed appearance or loss of cognitive abilities. The way a child deals with his/her illness and treatment has a major impact on psychological well-being.

Most studies in this field indicate that children with cancer, as a group, are not very different to control groups or comparison groups in terms of adaptation or adjustment and psychopathology in all stages of the disease and treatment. However, there are children who are at risk for difficulties in adapting to the disease, such as those who react with withdrawal or social isolation, or those with premorbid psychopathology. These children need intensive psychological support during and after treatment. Possible types of treatment, to help them get their life back on track, include contact with fellow patients (through special camps or meetings), group training, or individual therapy aimed at dealing with the disease and its consequences. For younger children, play therapy is a common way to work through emotions, while older children are often treated with cognitive behavioural therapy techniques. Another group at risk for severe negative (neuro)psychological sequelae are the children treated with global central nervous system irradiation.

Children with cancer often feel anger and disappointment because of restrictions on their participation in important areas of life, such as going to school or engaging in sports and other social activities. Sometimes it is difficult to stay in touch with friends due to poor clinical conditions. Children who attend school during treatment often feel 'different'because of their changed appearance or decline in health or cognitive functions. As a group, however, they hardly seem different from their healthy peers in terms of their classroom behaviour and social acceptance. Research shows that children with cancer who receive social support from their teachers, parents, and friends report fewer psychosocial problems and have higher self-esteem.

A common problem in childhood cancer treatment is the reduced immunity due to therapy. This means that parents must be especially alert for risk of infections. Guidance in the realistic management of these risks and of not becoming too obsessive and frightened is one of the issues in which psychological care can make a firm contribution. Unscheduled hospital visits due to reduced immunity problems (e.g. fever) are largely disruptive for everyday family life. Daily life becomes unpredictable and difficult to plan.

Overall, parents also experience many stress reactions during treatment. Studies on parental stress indicate that both fathers and mothers, six and twelve months after diagnosis, report increased feelings of anxiety and depression which only return to 'normal' levels after about 20–24 months. It is important to deal with the parental stress and adaptation to the illness and treatment, because of the relationship of parental functioning with the adjustment of the child. For some parents, additional guidance is needed from either a social worker or a psychologist. Other parents turn to their own social network for help.

Parents of children in treatment for cancer may find it hard to set limits on their sick child or to be separated from their child. One reason is that the stress of parenting a child can be enhanced by the effects of certain medications, including dexamethasone, which may cause behavioural, mood, or cognitive problems in the child. Furthermore, in this stage, often one of the parents needs to go back to work. This can increase the burden on the other parent. Going to school is often encouraged and promoted by the hospital staff, but often parents are reluctant, as they are scared about the risk of infections. For the cognitive and social-emotional development of children, however, it is very important to stay in touch with the school. It is essential that a psychosocial approach is integrated in care, in terms of systematic attention to all quality-of-life domains (physical, emotional, social, and cognitive functioning). Multidisciplinary meetings with all team members involved (physician, nurses, psychologists, social worker, teacher)is of utmost importance.

After treatment

The end of the treatment in paediatric oncology can be considered a tremendous transition in care and can be very stressful. Children and parents are supported during the entire treatment by the multidisciplinary team. When treatment ends, this multidisciplinary guidance quickly diminishes and families must regain their own lives. In this phase, studies show that children of different ages report problems with physical functioning as a consequence of loss of general condition and strength or ongoing tiredness. In this new phase, returning to school, picking up the 'ordinary life', and being released from hospital care are the main goals for the children, but these goals might become hampered because of physical impairments. Next to physical functioning, adolescents often experience a sense of distance towards their peers, which sometimes makes it difficult to reintegrate. Individual counselling can help children and adolescents to express feelings of loneliness or of being misunderstood, and help them to bridge the gap to 'normal life'.

When chemotherapy or radiotherapy ends, parents typically realize that cure only lasts if there is no relapse, and that there are less treatment options if the disease recurs. In this period, parents have to deal with feelings of immense uncertainty and with diminishing social support, which can be very stressful. Besides the fear of relapse, parents are being informed about late effects of the cancer treatment, which also can give rise to post-treatment stress. At the same time, they have to pick up their lives, or are confronted with demands of the outside world such as employers who expect them to return to work quickly. This increases the pressure on parents at a time when they need to pay some attention to themselves after such a long and exhausting period. Parents often describe this as the first period in which they pay attention to their own functioning. Physicians should be sensitive to symptoms of severe exhaustion in parents and refer them to psychologists or social workers if needed.

Early monitoring of psychosocial distress and pre-existing problems is an important first step to identify families at risk for problems, and this is internationally endorsed by paediatric oncology psychosocial standards of care.

Long-term follow-up

Almost all children and adolescents who have been successfully treated for cancer have to deal with negative health outcomes. They may develop health problems as a result of treatment (e.g. second cancers, cardiac conditions, leukoencephalopathy, endocrine problems, infertility), but may also suffer cognitive or social disadvantages in terms of academic achievement, finding a job or a partner, getting insurance. Regular screening of survivors concerning all the important areas of functioning, in so-called 'late-effects clinics', is very important. Apart from screening for late effects, prevention is another issue that needs attention in paediatric survivorship programmes and should be aimed at addressing lifestyle issues such as smoking, sunbathing, and diet.

Neuropsychological consequences as a result of the treatment for childhood cancer can be severe and long-lasting. Children treated for brain tumours, treated with high-dose chemotherapy or with cranial radiotherapy, are especially at risk. Treatment has both short-term and long-term impact on neuropsychological functioning due to acquired brain injury. Early brain damage has a cumulative effect on brain development, with increasing deficits in skills that have yet to emerge. Common cognitive deficits are in the domains of intelligence, attention, speed, and memory. Long-term neuropsychological deficits for survivors of childhood acute lymphoblastic leukaemia (ALL) after treatment with chemotherapy appear only to be subtle. These mainly involve processes of attention and executive functioning, while global intellectual function is relatively preserved. Younger age at diagnosis, female sex, and treatment intensity have emerged as risk factors for ALL survivors.

With the replacement of prednisolone in many recent treatment protocols by dexamethasone, the interest in the long-term side effects of this treatment has increased. Studies report more neuropsychological side effects with dexamethasone than with prednisonolone, but randomized controlled trials do not reveal a significant difference. A dose of hydrocortisone seems to reduce the serious side effects of dexamethasone on sleep, mood, and cognition.

Survivors who have been treated for brain tumours are more likely to have neuropsychological and learning difficulties as well as psychosocial difficulties. Important risk factors for brain-tumour patients are hydrocephalus, dose of irradiation, time since cranial irradiation, effects of multiple treatments, female sex, and also younger age at diagnosis. Improvements of the understanding of the exact neuropsychological deficits that accompany both disease and treatment factors remain important goals. Prolonged intensive rehabilitation and monitoring of neuropsychological functioning is needed for this subgroup of patients to offer timely treatment interventions for neuropsychological sequelae.

Studies on the long-term psychosocial consequences of treatment on survivors show mixed results. Several studies report a reduced quality of life in physical and social functioning. Young adult survivors of childhood cancer achieve less developmental milestones, or at a later age, than their peers. They value their functioning lower in the areas of independence, and social and psychosexual development. In comparison with healthy controls, survivors are less likely to be married or living together, and seem to have problems finding a job that provides financial independence. Some of the survivors report mood swings or post-traumatic stress disorder (PTSD), a cluster of symptoms related to trauma such as intrusions, hypervigilance, and avoidance. However, the numbers of survivors with these problems are considerably fewer than for their parents.

Parents of survivors can suffer from anxiety, tension, and uncertainty. Also a large percentage of parents report PTSD symptoms, including intrusions and avoidance behaviour. Sometimes these avoidance behaviours compromise the follow-up of the child (parents are reluctant to revisit the hospital) and can be considered a risk factor. Raising a child who has had cancer is a challenging task for parents. It is sometimes difficult to modify habits consolidated during treatment, but that now limit the child's functioning. Finding a balance in caring for and protecting the child and, at the same time, promoting healthy development towards young adulthood is a very hard task.

End-of-life issues

Despite the increased survival and progress in treating children with cancer, about one quarter of parents and children have to face the fact that cure is not possible. The treatment goal shifts from cure to quality of life and dying, as quoted by Veronica, aged 13: 'What really matters in life is not so much being able to value it. What really counts, is being able to "embrace" the moment when it finishes.'

What is a terminally ill child? It is not a dying person; it is a child who has arrived at a phase of life where death is close and cure is no longer possible. This phase could last for months. The approach to it does not need to be either 'therapeutically renouncing' or display 'ruthless obstinacy'. It is essential to build up the most appropriate modality to assist a child and the family in the palliative and terminal phase. The main purpose in this phase is to keep control over both physical and psychological pain and discomfort, either with medical, psychological, or spiritual interventions, and to turn any experience into something positive.

Today, many children who die of cancer die at home, although this is highly variable between countries even within Europe. Psychosocial care should be focused on helping the family with their daily life, supporting parents in dealing with the dying child, their own emotions, and also with any siblings. The hospital psychologist can play an important role in this situation, either in an advisory or consultative role for the professionals visiting the families at home (e.g. general practitioner, palliative nursing team) or as caregiver. The paediatric oncologist can have an important role as well, although again, this differs from country to county.

For some children, talking about death and the fear of death is easier with a professional than a parent. The way in which children think about death, and their understanding of it, depends on their age and cognitive and psychological development. Young children do not yet have a fully developed sense of death. They are cognitively unable to grasp the sense of irreversibility and permanence of death. On the contrary, older schoolchildren have greater awareness of the irreversibility of death, and teenagers generally have a fully developed awareness. Teachers and classmates at the child's school should be informed about the child's impending death. In this phase, the classmates and the school will be an important help to the teacher. The continuous participation of the child in school activities can be of great importance. Most children want to participate in normal life, including school life, for as long as possible, and being with their peers distracts them from being sick. Siblings of the sick child need good guidance as well.

Many parents struggle with whether or not they should tell their child that he/she is dying. In a large Swedish study, parents of deceased children were asked retrospectively whether or not they told their child about their impending death, and how they experienced and looked back on their decision. This study included a group of 500 parents: 34% of the parents talked with their child, and none of these parents had regretted it afterwards. In the other group, where parents did not talk to the child, the majority (73%) also did not regret this afterwards. The main criterion was the age of the child. Most parents chose to talk in terms of 'not getting better' or used metaphors, thus creating space for the child to ask questions. This study shows that the perception and appreciation of the situation by parents themselves should be included in the guidance for these end-of-life matters. For many parents, it is confusing, after the fatal news, to see that their child wants to continue living as if nothing has changed. Children often want to go to school and play in spite of their impending death.

Communication remains the basic issue when the diagnosis of cancer has to be reported to the patient and the family. How best to do it becomes the first step in a communicative process that involves the medical team and the family, and allows for growth and change over time until the final stage. Parents most often manage what and how their children are told about cancer. Adolescents or young adults vary in their preferences as to how much information should be disclosed to them. Some adolescents and young adults with cancer prefer to be fully informed about their disease, but approximately one third among those who survived preferred not to know.

Many parents find it difficult to talk to young children about issues as serious as the diagnosis of cancer or impending death. Without proper communication, starting at diagnosis, the child's reaction to the disease, treatment, and new or altered life situation can cause additional stress for the parents at any time. Parental wishes may not always be in the best interest of the child. The parents may wish to shield the child, which may only make the patient's fear worse. Also, a conflict may arise when the family wishes to continue pursuing an unrealistic possibility of cure or, on the contrary, when the family wishes to stop curative treatment prematurely. If members of the healthcare team take time to try to understand and discuss the reasons for the family's wishes, the inevitably painful conflicts can usually be overcome. Advanced Care Planning guidelines (ACP) could be helpful in overcoming these difficulties. The continuation of curative treatment beyond the point when cure is no longer possible, the so-called 'ruthless obstinacy' treatment, should be avoided.

In their desperation to avoid the upcoming death, parents often look for alternative treatments. This can be interpreted as a way of dealing with what is perceived as unacceptable. Many complementary treatments give parents feelings of control and the perception that they can contribute to the quality of life of their child. Many parents experience anticipatory grief in the shape of depressive reactions or anger. The identification of these feelings as normal reactions to abnormal circumstances can be helpful. Once a child is deceased, parents often seek assistance from professionals such as a psychologist or grief counsellor. Furthermore, after a child dies, that individual child's medical history should be evaluated. This evaluation should be made by the healthcare team as a group. It is critical to reflect on all events, even minor ones, that occurred during the course of the child's treatment, and also on the choices that were made and why. This will help the staff come to terms with their own grieving and to learn from the experience in order to help future families. Furthermore, this could help parents to better understand and clarify conflicting final decisions, and to start to work through their bereavement.

Conclusion

Even with the increased survival rates of children with cancer, uncertainties about the nature and extent of late effects remain. To achieve optimal support for children and adolescents who grow up with childhood cancer, physicians should have knowledge about their developmental trajectory and pay attention to this during treatment and follow-up. Therefore, periodical evaluation of their ongoing psychosocial, educational, neuropsychological, and vocational needs during their development should be an integral component of the comprehensive care of children and adolescents with cancer.

FURTHER READING

Aarsen FK, et al. (2009) Cognitive deficits and predictors 3 years after diagnosis of a pilocytic astrocytoma in childhood. *J Clin Oncol* **27**, 3526.

Annet RD, et al. (2015) Monitoring and assessment of neuropsychological outcomes as a standard of care in pediatric oncology. *Pediatr Blood Cancer* **62**, S460.

Barakat LP, et al. (1997) Families surviving childhood cancer: a comparison of posttraumatic stress symptoms with families of healthy children. *J Pediatr Psychol* **22**, 843.

Eiser C, et al. (2000) Examining the psychological consequences of surviving childhood cancer: systematic review as a research method in pediatric psychology. *J Pediatr Psychol* **25**, 449.

Geenen MM, et al. (2007) Medical assessment of adverse health outcomes in long-term survivors of childhood cancer. *JAMA* **297**, 2705.

Hinds PS, et al. (2007) Dexamethasone alters sleep and fatigue in pediatric patients with acute lymphoblastic leukemia. *Cancer* **110**, 2321.

Hoekstra-Weebers JE, et al. (2001) Psychological adaptation and social support of parents of pediatric cancer patients: a prospective longitudinal study. *J Pediatr Psychol* **26**, 225.

Jankovic M, et al. (1994) Association of 1800 cGy cranial irradiation with intellectual function in children with acute lymphoblastic leukaemia. *Lancet* **344**, 224.

Kars MC, et al. (2010) Factors influencing parental readiness to let their child with cancer die. *Pediatr Blood Cancer* **54**, 1000.

Kazak AE, et al. (2006) An integrative model of pediatric medical traumatic stress. *J Pediatr Psychol* **31**, 343.

Kreicbergs UC, et al. (2007) Parental grief after losing a child to cancer: impact of professional and social support on long-term outcomes. *J Clin Oncol* **25**, 3307.

Landolt MA, et al. (2003) Incidence and associations of parental and child posttraumatic stress symptoms in pediatric patients. *J Child Psychol Psychiatry* **44**, 1199.

Langeveld NE, et al. (2002) Quality of life in young adult survivors of childhood cancer. *Support Care Cancer* **10**, 579.

Last BF, et al. (2007) Positive effects of a psycho-educational group intervention for children with a chronic disease: first results. *Patient Educ Counsel* **65**, 101.

Lotz J, et al. (2013) Pediatric advance care planning: a systematic review. *Pediatrics* **131**(3), e873–880.

Martel D, et al. (2005) Use of alternative and complementary therapies in children with cancer. *Pediatr Blood Cancer* **44**, 660.

Moore BD (2005) Neurocognitive outcomes in survivors of childhood cancer. *J Pediatr Psychol* **30**, 51.

Nazemi KJ, Butler RW (2011) Neuropsychological rehabilitation for survivors of childhood and adolescent brain tumors: a review of the past and a vision for a promising future. *J Pediatr Rehab Med* **4**, 37.

Patenaude AF, Kupst MJ (2005) Psychosocial functioning in pediatric cancer. *J Pediatr Psychol* **30**, 9.

Sahler OJ, et al. (2005) Using problem-solving skills training to reduce negative affectivity in mothers of children with newly diagnosed cancer: report of a multisite randomized trial. *J Consult Clin Psychol* **73**, 272.

Skinner R, et al. (2007) Long-term follow-up of children treated for cancer: why is it necessary, by whom, where and how?. *Arch Dis Child* **92**, 257.

Stam H, et al. (2005) The course of life of survivors of childhood cancer. *Psycho-Oncology* **14**, 227.

Stam H, et al. (2001) Social and emotional adjustment in young survivors of childhood cancer. *Support Care Cancer* **9**, 489.

Temming P, Jenney ME (2010) The neurodevelopmental sequelae of childhood leukaemia and its treatment. *Arch Dis Child* **95**, 936.

Trask PC, et al. (2003) Parent and adolescent adjustment to pediatric cancer: associations with coping, social support, and family function. *J Pediatr Oncol Nurs* **20**, 36.

Van der Geest IM, et al. (2013) Emotional distress in 652 Dutch very long-term survivors of childhood cancer, using the Hospital Anxiety and Depression Scale (HADS). *J Pediatr Hematol/Oncol* **35**, 525.

Varni JW, et al. (1994) Perceived social support and adjustment of children with newly diagnosed cancer. *J Develop Behav Pediatr* **15**, 20.

Vrijmoet-Wiersma CM, et al. (2008) Assessment of parental psychological stress in pediatric cancer: a review. *J Pediatr Psychol* **33**, 694.

Warris LT, et al. (2016) Hydrocortisone as an intervention for dexamethasone-induced adverse effects in pediatric patients with acute lymphoblastic leukemia: results of a double-blind randomized controlled trail. *J Clin Oncol* **34**, 2287.

Wiener L, et al. (2015) Standards for the psychosocial care of children with cancer and their families: an introduction to the special issue. *Pediatr Blood Cancer* **62**, S419.

Zebrack BJ, et al. (2002) Psychological outcomes in long-term survivors of childhood leukemia, Hodgkin's disease, and non-Hodgkin's lymphoma: a report from the Childhood Cancer Survivor Study. *Pediatrics* **110**, 42.

11

Palliative Care for Children with Advanced Cancer

Michelle Koh, Finella Craig, and Joanne Wolfe

Introduction

The World Health Organization (WHO) defines palliative care for children as 'the active, total care of the child's body, mind and spirit, and also involves giving support to the family' and recommends that:

- It begins when illness is diagnosed, and continues regardless of whether or not a child receives treatment directed at the disease.
- The child's physical, psychological, and social distress should be addressed.
- It requires an interdisciplinary approach which includes the family and utilizes available community resources.
- It can be provided in tertiary-care facilities, in community settings (school, respite care, primary care), and in the child's home.

Generalist palliative care involves care delivered by the interdisciplinary paediatric oncology team. Specialist palliative care is delivered by interdisciplinary clinicians with additional training and expertise in palliative care. All children with cancer should receive generalist palliative care from the time of diagnosis. Specialist palliative care is especially important for children with more complex symptom and/or quality-of-life needs and at more advanced stages of the illness. At any illness stage, palliative care is delivered alongside disease-directed therapy in concordance with family goals of care.

In this context, the palliative care team can be involved in symptom management and provide outreach home support for the family. The level of support provided by the service should be flexible, according to the child and family's requirements, which, to some extent, depends on the child's diagnosis, treatment, and prognosis. At times of crises (such as relapse) or when cure is no longer possible, the palliative care team may take a more active lead in the child's care and management, as a seamless continuation of the care they have already been receiving.

Communication and decision making

When a child with cancer relapses, it is typical for a family to fluctuate between hoping for a cure and contemplating death as they face the uncertainty that surrounds their child's prognosis. This uncertainty impacts the child and family's experience, their decision making on how intensively to pursue cancer-directed therapy, care planning, and prognostic communications. Acknowledging the uncertainty of prognosis and developing an awareness of the child and family's hopes and fears may lead to a greater understanding of the challenges faced and promote more open and honest communication at this critical period.

For many families, maintaining their belief that there might be a 'miracle round the corner' is crucial, yet can coexist alongside emotional and practical preparation for their child's death. Healthcare professionals tend to view hope as primarily related to a positive outcome, many finding it difficult to maintain hope in the face of a poor prognosis. Parents are more likely to report that physician communication always makes them feel hopeful when they are receiving more prognostic information and high-quality communication. Therefore, contrary to how many professionals may feel, an open discussion about prognosis can support hope, even when the prognosis is poor.

Palliative care services in this situation can often help in the following ways:

- Assessing physical and psychosocial symptoms
- Supporting patients and families in establishing goals of care and with decision making with regards to ongoing treatment
- Coordinating patient care based on the individual needs of the patient.

Decision making about cancer-directed therapies

Bluebond-Langner et al. studied parental decision making regarding further cancer-directed treatments for children when standard cancer treatment was unsuccessful. Parents bring to these discussions both the knowledge they have acquired throughout their child's illness as well as their emotions as parents. They sought meetings with the oncologist regarding further investigative procedures, and about half the parents looked for options beyond what was offered. No parent initiated discontinuation of cancer-directed or symptom-directed therapies.

Parents do not see cancer-directed therapy and symptom-directed care as mutually exclusive. Physicians and parents negotiate care throughout the child's treatment regardless of whether it is directed. Indeed, experience suggests that labels such as 'curative' or 'palliative intent' establish a false dichotomy, since ultimately parents hope that their child lives as long as possible.

Advanced-care planning

End-of-life care planning requires effective communication to guide parents through clarifying the goals of care and establishing agreement on what treatments are appropriate to achieve these goals, including resuscitative and palliative measures. Providing choice for place of end-of-life care is crucial and may impact on family decisions about hospital-based interventions. Among families who felt they had time to plan where their child would die, an overwhelming majority of parents preferred to have their child die at home.

Advanced-care planning requires time and often needs to be done in stages, with discussions around the appropriate level of cardio-pulmonary resuscitation, life-sustaining treatment, and intensive care, and about the child and family's preferred place of care and place of death. This should be accompanied by assurance that symptom management and supportive care will be proactive in whichever setting they choose.

There should be an understanding and acknowledgment of the past experiences as well as the cultural values and social set-up of the child and family. There must be clarity on the practicalities of what the different options of home, hospice (also called palliative care unit), or hospital care entail, so that the families have realistic expectations to inform their decision making.

The care plan must be communicated to the wider multidisciplinary team, including out-of-hours services and the ambulance service. Patient-held records of discussions, decisions, and contacts are useful communication tools.

Cancer-directed therapy

The purpose of ongoing cancer-directed treatments is to improve the quality of life, relieve symptoms, and prolong the symptom-free period. As a principle, side effects and toxicities must be minimal and manageable, but long-term toxicity is unlikely to be an issue. Decisions around these treatments are taken by the oncologist, in conjunction with the palliative care team, child, and family (Box 11.1).

Box 11.1 Features of ongoing oncological treatments

Chemotherapy

- Low-toxicity oral, intravenous, or intrathecal chemotherapy to halt or slow disease progression and manage symptoms of disseminated disease.
- Examples:
  - Oral etoposide in children with metastatic solid tumours, or oral temozolamide in children with relapsed brain cancers.
  - Intrathecal methotraxate for symptoms due to CNS leukaemia.
- Monitor the efficacy of treatment closely as treatment needs to be reconsidered or stopped if symptoms progress or side effects outweigh potential benefits for quality of life.

Radiotherapy

- Useful for controlling distressing symptoms from a focal site and can prophylactically treat sites of disease before they cause symptoms (e.g. radiation to bulky bony disease before the bone fractures).
- Given as hypofractionated regimens (i.e. fewer fractions with bigger doses per fraction).
- Symptomatic gain should be greater than the burden of any side effects or negative impact on quality of life (e.g. attending hospital, need for anaesthetic).
- Examples:
  - Pain caused by bulky disease, nerve compression, bone pain.
  - Obstruction of any hollow passage or viscus (e.g. spinal cord compression, SVC or airway obstruction).
  - Bleeding from rupture or breakdown of tumour: haemoptysis, vaginal or gastrointestinal bleeding, haematuria.
  - Fungating or disfiguring tumours, which can cause immense distress by their appearance and discharge. Tumour-volume reduction can help the surrounding skin and soft tissues to heal.

Surgery

- Considered early in situations where symptoms can be anticipated, as the child needs to be well enough to tolerate surgery.
- Examples:
  - Debulking of tumour can help with pain control.
  - Drains for effusions/ascites.
  - Decompression (e.g. for spinal cord compression, relief of bowel obstruction).
  - Stenting of intraluminal lesions can often be done endoscopically (e.g. biliary stents, nephrostomy stents, urinary catheterization).
  - Stabilization of fractures, prophylactically or post fracture.

Common and difficult symptoms

Many studies have shown that children with advanced cancer experience substantial suffering from symptoms amenable to palliation. Increased availability of palliative care services is associated with improvement in symptom control. The approach to symptom management involves:

- Assessment of the child's symptoms
- Evaluation of potentially reversible causes of the symptoms
- Planning and initiation of treatment
- Reassessment following intervention.

This is an ongoing process as the disease progresses and symptoms change over time.

Although the parents often provide vital information regarding the child's symptoms, it is important to focus on what the child may be able to tell us, as well as clinical signs. This is crucial for managing subjective symptoms such as pain, nausea, and breathlessness. It validates the child's symptom experience, and builds trust between the child, family, and professionals.

The child's symptom experience is affected by the pathophysiological processes, and other biological and psychosocial factors (Box 11.2).

Pain

It is crucial to elicit what the cause of pain is so that targeted oncological treatments may be considered. Assessment of the possible pain mechanism (nociceptive or neuropathic) will inform the treatment approach and drug selection. Nociceptive pain is caused by superficial and/or deep-tissue injury (somatic pain), or organ damage (visceral pain). Neuropathic pain is caused by nerve injury,

Box 11.2 Principles of symptom management

- Symptom management should be planned in advance.
- It requires a holistic approach, not just drug management.
- Parents and patients should be empowered to have some control over the situation. They should:
  - Know what to expect
  - Know how to deal with it
  - Know who to call for help.
- Assessment should include the use of developmentally appropriate instruments when available. Uncontrolled distressing symptoms constitute a medical emergency and should be managed intensively.

either in the peripheral nerves or the central nervous system. Pain may arise from a combination of nociceptive and neuropathic mechanisms, and a combined management approach is often required.

In assessing pain, as much information as possible should be derived directly from the child. Self-reporting using pain scales remain the 'gold standard' in measuring pain, but the child needs to be competent in using these. Parents and familiar carers can be good surrogates as they know the child's normal baseline behaviour and will be familiar with the child's pain behaviour. However, there is a risk that they may under-report pain, for fear of acknowledging a symptom that suggests disease progression. Physiological changes such as heart rate and blood pressure may help in identifying pain, but in a dying child these are likely to be affected by many confounding factors.

The WHO three-step analgesic ladder introduced in 1986 has now been modified for children to a two-step approach. The principles of dosing at regular intervals ('by the clock'), administering by the appropriate route ('by the mouth'), and individualizing treatment to each child ('by the child') remain central.

For **Step 1—mild pain**—paracetamol and ibuprofen are the medicines of choice. Other non-steroidal anti-inflammatory drugs (NSAIDs) may be considered if appropriate to the clinical situation. NSAIDs (e.g. ibuprofen, diclofenac) have analgesic, antipyretic, and anti-inflammatory properties. They are especially useful for musculoskeletal and liver pain. NSAIDs may cause gastric irritation, so their regular use should be accompanied by gut protection (e.g. Ranitidine, Omeprazole). As they cause platelet dysfunction, their potential benefit must be balanced against the child's risk of bleeding.

For **Step 2—moderate to severe pain**—an opioid should be administered in addition to paracetamol and ibuprofen. Morphine is the first-line opioid but alternative opioids may be needed in the event of poor analgesic response or significant side effects. Codeine was previously part of the recommendations but as a significant proportion of children are unable to effectively convert codeine to its active metabolites or may be hypermetabolizers, its use in children is restricted in many countries. Furthermore, codeine has a high toxicity-to-efficacy ratio; children experience substantial side effects even at very low doses. It is preferable to initiate lower doses of safer, more effective opioids such as morphine, and titrate as appropriate.

Opioids: morphine, oxycodone, fentanyl, methadone

The aim in using opioids is to obtain a dose that provides adequate analgesia with a minimal or acceptable degree of side effects. A short-acting form of opioid, usually morphine, may be started on an 'as needed' basis or, if the pain is severe, on a regular basis. The dose is then gradually increased until effective. If regular background analgesia is required, the use of a long-acting opioid preparation is preferable. It is important to continue the use of short-acting morphine as needed, to manage any breakthrough pain. There is no upper dosage limit for opioid analgesics because there is no 'ceiling' analgesic effect. The appropriate dose is the dose that produces pain relief for the individual child.

Morphine is currently the first-line opioid of choice as it is inexpensive and a wide range of formulations are available. Its efficacy, pharmacokinetics (caution in renal or hepatic impairment), and side effects (constipation, nausea, urinary retention, itch, drowsiness) are well understood. Oxycodone's efficacy and side-effect profile are similar to that of morphine. It has a different molecular structure and, therefore, can be an effective alternative to morphine in patients with intolerable side effects or inadequate analgesia from morphine.

Fentanyl is a synthetic opioid, useful in patients in renal failure as it metabolizes to inactive metabolites in the liver and has a shorter half-life. It is available in transdermal or transmucosal preparations. It can simplify analgesic management in patients with poor, deteriorating, or even absent renal function, but is not suitable for the initiation or titration phases in managing escalating pain because of the time lag to achieve steady state of the transdermal patch.

Methadone is an opioid with N-methyl-D-aspartate (NMDA) antagonistic properties and, therefore, effective in difficult pain with neuropathic qualities. Methadone should only be commenced by practitioners experienced in its use. This is due to wide inter-individual variation in response, variable conversion ratios with other opioids, complex pharmacokinetics (long half-life, large volume of distribution, and risk of accumulation), and side effects (prolongation of QT interval). It is available as a liquid and can be very useful in countries where liquid long-acting morphine is not available.

Routes of administration

Medications should always be given by the most acceptable route for the child. Practical considerations, such as place of care and ease of administration, as well as patient preference, may also influence route of administration and, as a consequence of this, drug of preference. The intramuscular route is to be avoided in children.

- **Oral medications:** the route of choice as long as the child is able to take and tolerate it. Enteral medications can often be continued throughout the child's terminal phase, particularly if they already have a nasogastric or gastrostomy tube.
- **Transdermal opioid patches:** appropriate for use in patients who are unable to take or comply with oral medications and who have stable pain. They are unsuitable for patients with escalating pain as the onset of effect of a higher-dose patch is too slow.
- **Continuous intravenous infusion:** may be the preferred route of choice for a child who already has a central line and cannot manage oral medications.
- **Continuous subcutaneous infusion:** should be considered in preference to intravenous medication if the child does not have pre-existing venous access.
- **Buccal/sublingual preparations:** useful in children who cannot manage oral medications, particularly for breakthrough symptoms. Most, however, will have a short duration of action, so are not ideal for sustained symptom relief.

Neuropathic pain

When nerves are invaded or compressed by tumour, it results in changes to normal pain transmission, causing neuropathic pain. Often, there is considerable overlap between neuropathic and nociceptive pain. Some children report sharp pain associated with tingling and numbness or a burning sensation or a deep ache. Others may not be able to articulate this type of pain clearly. Knowledge of the disease pathology, location, and invasive nature should alert physicians to the potential for neuropathic pain. It should be considered when the patient has a poorer than expected response to escalating doses of opioids.

As neuropathic pain is mostly mediated through NMDA receptors, a single class of analgesic is not usually adequate; a combination of opioids and adjuvant analgesics benefit patients most.

Adjuvant analgesics

Adjuvant analgesics can be opioid-sparing, and it is important to consider if the child's pain is likely to be neuropathic in origin, or if it is not responding to escalating opioid therapy. Although there is no evidence for the use of these drugs for pain management in children, there is a large body of clinical experience. The following are the most commonly used adjuvant neuropathic analgesics:

- Antidepressants: amitriptyline, nortriptyline
- Anticonvulsants: gabapentin, carbamazepine
- NMDA antagonists: ketamine, methadone

Other alternative agents may also be helpful for specific situations, such as bisphosphonates in the management of pain associated with metastatic bone disease.

Any patient with intractable pain despite optimal management of systemic analgesia should be discussed with an anaesthetics team, for consideration of an appropriate intervention such as epidural analgesia or a nerve block. Patients most likely to benefit include patients with significant locally advanced disease, neuropathic pain, or marked movement-related pain.

Breathlessness

Breathlessness may be secondary to disease, causing airway obstruction, pulmonary metastases, pleural effusion or infection, and pooling of secretions. This may be compounded if there is bone marrow disease causing anaemia.

Breathlessness is a subjective symptom: its severity is what the patient says it is. It can be frightening. General measures such as reassurance, optimizing the child's position, and, in older children, relaxation techniques, may help. A stream of cool air on the face (e.g. by opening a window or having a fan on) stimulates the trigeminal nerve and can reduce the perception of breathlessness. Oxygen may be recommended if it reduces the child's sensation of breathlessness, rather than aiming to improve the child's oxygen saturation levels.

As the child becomes less conscious, they become less able to clear their secretions effectively. Glycopyrronium or a hyoscine hydrobromide patch reduces the volume of secretions, but can also make them thicker and cause anti-cholinergic side effects (e.g. dry mouth or eyes). They should be used judiciously, with appropriate suctioning, gentle chest physiotherapy, and mouth care.

Opioids reduce the sensation of breathlessness by reducing the ventilatory response to hypercapnia and hypoxia. Oral morphine preparations can be tried in the first instance, although some patients respond better to a continuous infusion of morphine. A benzodiazepine can be used in conjunction as an anxiolytic.

Nausea and vomiting

The following simple, practical measures can often improve nausea significantly:

- The child should be given small, manageable amounts of food they enjoy, at the time they feel most able to eat. Several small meals are preferable to three large meals a day.
- Strong smells should be avoided, such as cooking smells and perfumes.
- Constipation must be actively managed.
- The number of medications and drug volumes should be reduced as much as possible. Medication should be timed so that large amounts are not being given together.

The key to successful management of nausea and vomiting is to elicit the causes, as this informs the antiemetic choice (Table 11.1).

Constipation

Constipation in children with advanced cancer may be secondary to decreased mobility and oral intake, as a direct result of tumour obstruction or as a side effect of opioids or anti-cholinergic drugs. As a general rule, a laxative should be prescribed when prescribing any opioid for a patient. Constipation should be proactively prevented as it is often difficult to manage once established; it is usually multifactorial and a combination of laxatives is often required. Three classes of laxatives are commonly used:

- Osmotic laxatives (macrogol)
- Softening agents (lactulose, docusate sodium)
- Stimulant agents (senna, sodium picosulphate, bisacodyl)

Table 11.1 Choice of antiemetics for different causes of vomiting

Cause (site of action)	Drug	Class/Action
Raised intracranial pressure (vomiting centre)	Cyclizine Hyoscine Levomepromazine	Antihistamine Antimuscurinic $5HT_2$-antagonist
Decreased intestinal motility or dysmotility	Metoclopramide Domperidone Erythromycin	D_2-antagonist D_2-antagonist Motilin-receptor agonist
Metabolic or drug-induced (chemoreceptor trigger zone)	Haloperidol Metoclopramide	D_2-antagonist D_2-antagonist
Chemotherapy-induced (gut wall/chemoreceptor trigger zone)	Ondansetron	$5HT_3$-antagonist
'Broad-spectrum' agent for resistant nausea (vomiting centre)	Levomepromazine	$5HT_2$-antagonist
Chemotherapy-induced nausea and vomiting	Aprepitant (used in combination with a corticosteroid or $5HT_3$-antagonist)	NK_1-antagonist

Rectal enemas (phosphate enemas) and suppositories (glycerine suppositories) can be tried if laxatives are ineffective but may only empty the rectum, and can cause significant pain if the stool is not softened. Their use should be limited in children with profound neutropenia.

For patients with opioid-induced constipation, when the response to laxatives is inadequate, methylnaltrexone (a peripheral opioid receptor antagonist) may be helpful. It acts on the bowel but does not reverse the central analgesic effects of opioids. It is contraindicated in bowel obstruction and is available as a subcutaneous or intravenous bolus injection.

Fatigue

Fatigue is the most common symptom experienced by children with terminal cancer and is often under-recognized and undertreated. It is an overwhelming tiredness, out of proportion to activity and exertion, and not adequately relieved by rest. It is important to address underlying aetiologies (e.g. pain, nutrition, anaemia) including psychological symptoms such as depression and anxiety. Increasingly, methylphenidate or dextroamphetamine is recommended for symptomatic relief of fatigue, regardless of the suspected aetiology. Physiotherapy and sports activities may be effective in relieving fatigue for children, even near the end of life.

Agitation

Agitation and restlessness are common at the end of life and can be distressing for parents and carers. Symptomatic causes of agitation, such as pain or vomiting, should be assessed and treated. Fear and unaddressed anxieties can be a major factor and early, open discussion with the child, allowing them to express their fears and concerns, may reduce agitation as death approaches. Calm reassurance is crucial, and other measures, such as careful attention to lighting, particularly at night or if a child's vision is failing, as well as relaxation techniques, may be helpful. If medication is necessary, a short-acting benzodiazepine such as buccal midazolam or sublingual lorazepam is often effective. For more severe agitation, haloperidol or levomepromazine can be very effective.

Gastrointestinal complications: malignant ascites/ intestinal obstruction

These complications are less common in children than adults, and tend to happen late and close to end of-life. They can be very difficult to manage.

Malignant ascites most commonly occurs in patients with liver involvement or peritoneal disease. Although, in children, draining ascites will usually require sedation or a general anaesthetic, it is an effective way to relieve the pain and distension. Importantly, the ascites is likely to recur, requiring repeated procedures unless a catheter is left *in situ*. The risk of hypoalbuminaemia and hypovolaemia from the draining of the peritoneal fluid also needs to be considered. Intestinal obstruction can be caused by intraluminal, intramural, or extramural obstruction, motility disorders, or severe constipation.

Surgery should only be considered if there is clear benefit. Medical management with antisecretory and antiemetic medication should aim to control nausea and reduce the frequency and severity of vomiting to an acceptable level. The route of drug delivery will need to be parenteral, and a nasogastric tube would only be recommended to decompress the stomach if there is faeculant vomiting or gastric outlet obstruction. 'Broad-spectrum' antiemetics should be used: cyclizine as the first line, with haloperidol or levomepromazine added in if required. Laxatives (combination of senna and docusate) should be used to maintain a comfortable stool without colic. Octreotide can be effective in reducing the amount of gastrointestinal secretions in children with severe outlet obstruction.

Parenteral hyoscine butylbromide can be rapidly effective for colic. If the coeliac or superior mesenteric plexus is involved, there may be severe neuropathic pain that will require opioids and an anti-neuropathic pain agent.

Bone marrow failure

Decisions surrounding the appropriate use of transfusions need to be addressed sensitively as families who have been through intensive oncological treatments will be used to having anaemia or thrombocytopenia managed aggressively. Continued transfusions are usually warranted when the child with advanced cancer remains active. In the context of end-of-life care, transfusions are recommended only if the child's symptoms are likely to be ameliorated by the transfusion. The burden of transferring the child and spending several hours in hospital must be considered, as well as the potential fluid shifts the transfusion will cause.

Bleeding is a major distressing symptom of bone marrow failure. The child may bleed from fungating tumours, nose and gums, and pressure areas. Management includes:

- Preparing the family adequately; dark towels and sheets can help moderate the anxiety of the child and witnesses.
- Positioning the child: for example, in acute haemoptysis or a severe nose bleed, lie them on their bleeding side, or upright/reclined with head tilted forward.
- Topical adrenaline 1:1000 or tranexamic acid intravenous preparation, soaked in gauze, applied to bleeding point. A mouthwash preparation of tranexamic acid is also available.
- An anxiolytic such as buccal midazolam can help calm the distressed child.

Anxiety and depression

Anxiety and depression are common emotions in children with life-limiting conditions. It is important to assess if the symptoms are appropriate reactions to the difficult situation, or more severe and entrenched emotions that require intervention.

The child psychiatry team should be consulted on the medical management of psychological symptoms. Serotonin-reuptake inhibitors such as fluoxetine can be effective; however, they require several weeks to achieve maximum benefit. When indicated, such medications should be started early. Psychostimulants (dextroamphetamine and methylphenidate) deserve special consideration in treating depression near the end of life, because they take effect quickly. Non-medical interventions, such as counselling, cognitive behavioural therapy, drama, art, or play therapy, are also important. Acute anxiety can be managed with a short-acting benzodiazepine such as buccal midazolam or sublingual lorazepam.

Use of steroids for symptomatic relief

The rationale for the use of steroids in relieving symptoms of raised intracranial pressure is the effect of reducing tumour-associated oedema. There are also other indications for the use of steroids in cancer management, such as spinal cord and/or nerve compression, bone pain, superior vena caval obstruction, and airway obstruction.

The initiation of steroids must be carefully considered and the benefits be weighed against the many potential side effects. For example, steroids frequently stimulate appetite but, if the tumour has caused the patient to have a poor or unsafe swallow, they may become highly distressed, being unable to satisfy their hunger. Other side effects include gastritis or peptic ulceration, behavioural problems, agitation, and extreme exacerbation and lability of mood (tearfulness, physical aggression). Longer-term side effects such as diabetes, osteoporosis, and muscle wasting may or may not be relevant. The use of steroids should always be accompanied by gastric protection such a proton-pump inhibitor.

If the patient is on a short course of steroids (less than seven days), the treatment can be stopped abruptly. If the course is longer, a weaning regimen may help prevent rebound symptoms.

Issues around feeding at the end of life

Loss of appetite and loss of interest in food is common in children who are dying. Fluid and caloric requirements decrease as their underlying illness deteriorates and activity levels decrease. Artificial hydration and feeds need to be given judiciously. If the child is already on artificial hydration, reassess the child's likely fluid requirement and reduce the amount given appropriately. If the child had previously been feeding orally, it is not usually beneficial to start artificial hydration. Close attention should also be paid to mouth care and care of pressure areas.

At the end of life, artificial hydration could alleviate signs of dehydration but worsen peripheral oedema, ascites, pleural effusions, respiratory distress, and frequency of urination. The potential benefits of artificial hydration therapy need to be considered against the distress of worsening fluid retention.

Spiritual distress

Healthcare professionals often feel uncomfortable and inadequate in addressing the spiritual needs of the dying child and their family. It is important to access the spiritual and faith leaders in the interdisciplinary team or in the child's community. Often, a multi-faith chaplain will be expert in exploring spiritual distress in a non-religious context with families who may not have a specific religious belief.

The main spiritual need described by parents is maintaining connection with their child. Parents maintain connection at the time of death by physical presence and, after the death, through memories, mementos, memorials, and altruistic acts such as organ donation and charitable work. The other spiritual needs include the need for truth, compassion, prayer, and ritual; connection with others; bereavement support; meaning and purpose; anger, blame, and dignity. Professionals can support parents by ensuring that the child and family remain a unit at the time of death, able to create memories and say their goodbyes.

Family support and bereavement care

The child and family face a series of losses even before the child approaches the terminal stages of the illness. These include the physical loss of skills and abilities; social losses such as social isolation and pressures on the parents' marriage; financial losses as parents often have to reduce or give up their jobs to care for their child, in addition to the financial cost of care; and the emotional loss of the parents' hopes and dreams for their child.

Families need to be allowed to grieve and adapt to these changes at their own pace. Siblings have to cope with different relationships with their parents and the unwell child; grandparents grieve not only for their grandchild, but also the heartbreak that their child is enduring.

Support for the children may be available through schools and hospices, music, drama, or play therapy; voluntary sector organizations such as children's hospices provide sibling support; and adults and older children may find pre-bereavement counselling valuable, with therapy continuing through and after their bereavement. Social-work input is invaluable in helping the family obtain their financial entitlements and funding for extra care or home adaptations. In the UK, there are voluntary organizations (e.g. Rainbow's Trust) which provide practical help with such as household chores or care of the other children.

The sick child should be encouraged to maintain their interests and have things to look forward to. This often includes continuing access to an appropriate level of educational input, play, and social interaction with their peers. It is frequently useful, with the family's permission, to provide relevant information for the school.

After the child's death, the family may need to be supported through the activities of mourning, be given information about the sources of support, and referred to specialist bereavement counselling if needed.

FURTHER READING

Bennett M (2010) Palliative medications: drugs for neuropathic pain. *Eur J Palliat Care* **17**(4), 167–9.

Bluebond-Langner M, et al. (2007) Understanding parents' approaches to care and treatment of children with cancer when standard therapy has failed. *J Clin Oncol* **25**(17), 2414–19.

Bruera E, et al. (2003) Patient-controlled methylphenidate for the management of fatigue in patients with advanced cancer: a preliminary report. *J Clin Oncol* **21**, 4439–43.

De Graves S, Aranda S (2008) Living with hope and fear--the uncertainty of childhood cancer after relapse. *Cancer Nurs* **31**(4), 292–301.

Dussel V, et al. (2009) Looking beyond where children die: determinants and effects of planning a child's location of death. *J Pain Symptom Manage* **37**(1), 33–43.

Friedrichsdorf SJ, et al. (2015) Improved quality of life at end of life related to home-based palliative care in children with cancer. *J Palliat Med* **18**(2), 143–50.

Goldman A (1998) ABC of palliative care: special problems of children. *BMJ* **316**, 49–52.

Jalmsell L, et al. (2006) Symptoms affecting children with malignancies during the last month of life: a nationwide follow-up. *Pediatrics* **117**(4), 1314–20.

Jennings A (2010) Palliation of breathlessness: a combined approach is needed. *Eur J Palliat Care* **17**(4), 162–6.

Kreicbergs UC, et al. (2007) Parental grief after losing a child to cancer: impact of professional and social support on long-term outcomes. *J Clin Oncol* **25**(22), 3307–12.

Meert KL, et al. (2005) The spiritual needs of parents at the time of their child's death in the pediatric intensive care unit and during bereavement: a qualitative study. *Pediatr Crit Care* **6**(4), 420–7.

Ripamonti C, et al. (2000) Role of octreotide, scopolamine butylbromide, and hydration in symptom control of patients with inoperable bowel obstruction and nasogastric tubes: a prospective randomized trial. *J Pain Symptom Manage* **19**(1), 23–34.

Rosenberg AR, et al. (2016) Quality of life in children with advanced cancer: a report from the PediQUEST Study. J Pain Symptom Manage **52**(2), 243–53.

Temel JS, et al. (2010) Early palliative care for patients with metastatic non-small-cell lung cancer. *N Engl J Med* **363**, 733–42.

Thompson A, et al. (2006) Feeding in palliative care. In: A Goldman, et al. (eds) *Oxford Textbook of Palliative Care for Children*, pp. 374–86. Oxford: Oxford University Press.

Twycross R, Wilcock A (2007) Anti-emetics. In: R Twycross (ed.) *Palliative Care Formulary* (3rd edn), pp. 175–9. Nottingham: palliativedrugs.com.

Ullrich CK, et al. (2010) Fatigue in children with cancer at the end of life. *J Pain Symptom Manage* **40**(4), 483–94.

Wolfe J et al. (2000) Understanding of prognosis among parents of children who died of cancer: impact on treatment goals and integration of palliative care. *JAMA* **284**(19), 2469–75.

Wolfe J, et al. (2008) Easing of suffering in children with cancer at the end of life: is care changing? *J Clin Oncol* **26**(10), 1717–23.

Wolfe J, et al. (2015) Symptoms and distress in children with advanced cancer: prospective patient-reported outcomes from the PediQUEST Study. *J Clin Oncol* 10(33:17), 1928–35.

World Health Organization (2012) *WHO Guidelines on the Pharmacological Treatment of Persisting Pain in Children with Medical Illnesses*. Geneva: World Health Organization.

Yee JD, Berde CB (1994) Dextroamphetamine or methylphenidate as adjuvants to opioid analgesia for adolescents with cancer. *J Pain Symptom Manage* **9**,122–5.

12

Cancer Treatment in Low- and Middle-Income Countries

Elizabeth Molyneux, Trijn Israels, and Scott C. Howard

Introduction

The World Bank divides economies (according to their gross national income per capita in US dollars) into low income ($1,025 or less), lower middle income ($1,026–$4,035), upper middle income ($4,036–$12,475), and high income ($12,476 or more), calculated using the World Bank Atlas method (http://data.worldbank.org/about/country-classifications/world-bank-atlas-method). Cancer treatment in low- and middle-income countries, referred to hereafter as LMIC, differs substantially from that in high-income countries (HIC), and these differences are the focus of this chapter.

Healthcare disparities between low- and middle-income countries and high-income countries

Cure rates for children with cancer differ greatly between LMIC and HIC. Cancer cure depends on a series of steps which can be conceptualized as links in the chain of care, from suspicion by the patient and family to primary care, secondary care, tertiary care, and, finally, correct diagnosis and treatment (Figure 12.1). The cure rate is the product of access to diagnosis, treatment, and event-free survival, each of which can be problematic in LMIC. Late diagnosis and misdiagnosis are common in healthcare systems with inadequate infrastructure for early referral, inadequate pathology laboratories that often lack even basic tools like immunohistochemistry, and high costs of cancer diagnosis and staging. These and other obstacles decrease access to diagnosis in many LMIC. For example, in Mali and Malawi, the reported incidence of acute leukaemia is less than 10% of the incidence in HIC (Table 12.1).

Poverty and inadequate public health infrastructure prevent or delay access to even primary care for many of the world's children, and many LMIC have few or no paediatric cancer units (PCUs), so that patients must sometimes travel long distances for cancer care. For example, only an estimated 55% of children with cancer in Guatemala are referred to the National Pediatric Oncology Unit (the only PCU in the country). However, all patients who reach the PCU in Guatemala City have access to treatment, since the costs of care are paid by a non-profit foundation, Ayúdame a Vivir (Help Me to Live, www.ayuvi.org.gt). In many other countries, the greatest barrier to cure is the lack of access to treatment, because families must cover the costs of diagnosis, staging, treatment, and follow-up in addition to the non-medical costs associated with missed work, travel, and lodging.

Even patients who attain access to diagnosis and treatment may not survive, since socioeconomic and cultural factors in LMIC make abandonment of treatment a common occurrence and death rates due to the toxicity of chemotherapy are frequently high. For example, in the 1980s in Recife, Brazil, 8.4% of children with acute lymphoblastic leukaemia (ALL) died of toxicity and 16% abandoned treatment, versus 1.5% toxic death and no abandonment with the same chemotherapy regimen in Memphis, USA. Similarly, in Honduras a decade ago, 21% of children with ALL died of toxicity and 23% abandoned treatment.

Government spending on healthcare per capita is the strongest predictor of childhood cancer survival, because it is associated with healthcare infrastructure at all levels (Figure 12.2), and correlates strongly with access to diagnosis, treatment, and event-free survival since well-funded health systems are more likely to have tertiary care centres equipped with immunohistochemistry and flow cytometry, access to necessary chemotherapy and supportive care, and to be staffed with trained pathologists, surgeons, oncologists, radiation therapists, and nurses. Unfortunately, most paediatric oncologists have little influence over public health infrastructure, so the focus of their efforts must be to establish functional PCUs and to progressively develop them into centres of excellence, as discussed in the section 'Importance of paediatric cancer units'. Fortunately, there are many proven strategies to overcome each cause of preventable treatment failure.

Importance of paediatric cancer units

A PCU is a centre at which children with cancer can receive services necessary to make a correct diagnosis of cancer, perform a staging evaluation, and deliver protocol-based therapy. Establishing a unit

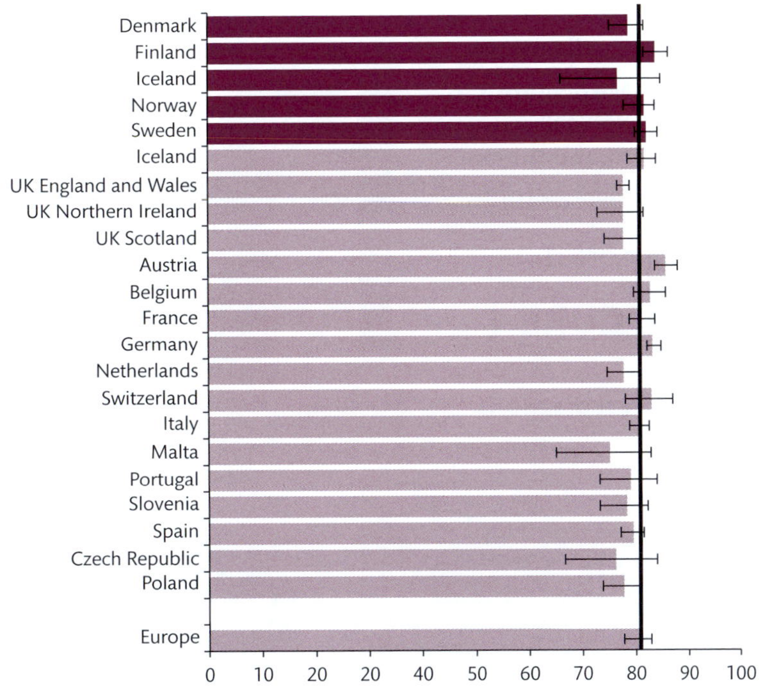

Figure 12.1 Links in the chain of care for children with cancer.

SES, socioeconomic status

Reproduced with permission from Howard SC et al. 'Improving outcomes for children with cancer in low-income countries in Latin America: a report on the recent meetings of the Monza International School of Pediatric Hematology/Oncology (MISPHO)–Part I'. *Pediatric Blood Cancer*, Volume 48, Issue 3, pp. 364–9, Copyright © 2007, John Wiley and Sons. DOI: https://doi.org/10.1002/pbc.21003

with its own physical space, dedicated personnel, and self-contained administrative structure allows the multidisciplinary team of doctors, nurses, pharmacists, social workers, psychologists, physical therapists, and data managers to work together to improve all aspects of patient care.

Recruitment, training, and retention of personnel

Delivery of anti-cancer therapy requires trained personnel, but healthcare providers with expertise in paediatric oncology in LMIC are far fewer per capita than in HIC. In some cases, no paediatric oncologist is available and medical oncologists with little paediatric experience or paediatricians with little oncology experience manage children with cancer. Oncology nurses in LMIC are rare, and in many hospitals, nurses are required to rotate among all the hospital services, such that none gains expertise in oncology nursing and the effect of training programmes is limited. Even if trained personnel are recruited, they must have a stable salary in the PCU to develop professionally and feel they have a future career path.

Education and training of healthcare professionals at all levels is paramount to developing and improving a PCU, and many professional organizations have made educational materials and training scholarships available on their websites (e.g. International Society of Pediatric Oncology www.siop.nl, American Society of Pediatric Hematology/Oncology www.ASPHO.org, International Network for Cancer Treatment and Research www.inctr.org, American Society of Hematology www.hematology.org). Online meetings can provide not only education but also a forum to discuss individual patients, adapted protocols, and quality-improvement initiatives with local, regional, and global collaborators.

Until recently there were few training opportunities in oncology for clinicians and nurses working in low-income settings. Those that were available often took the applicant away from home for long periods of time to study and gain experience in settings very

Table 12.1 Determinants of cure for children with cancer: estimated access to diagnosis, treatment, and event-free survival by country-income category

Country or region	Approximate rate of access to diagnosis	Approximate rate of access to treatment	Approximate event-free survival of treated patients	Estimated cure rate
High-income countries	100%	100%	83%	83%
Upper middle-income countries	95%	95%	75%	68%
Lower middle-income countries	80%	70%	50%	28%
Low-income countries	60%	40%	30%	7%

Reproduced courtesy of Scott C. Howard, University of Tennessee College of Health Sciences, USA.

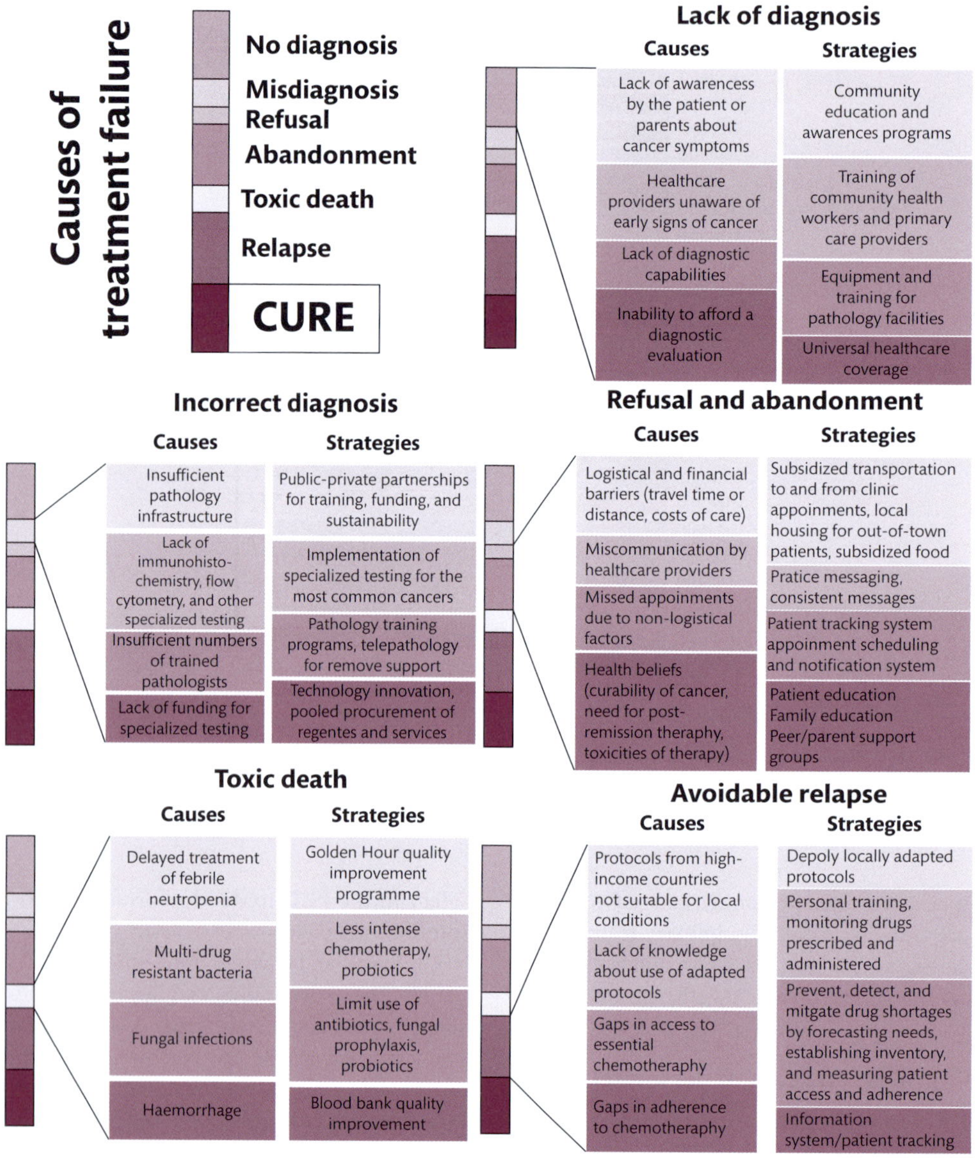

Figure 12.2 Strategies to reduce each cause of preventable treatment failure for children with cancer in low- and middle-income countries.
Reproduced courtesy of Scott C. Howard, University of Tennessee College of Health Sciences, USA.

different from his/her own. On returning, it was difficult to align what had been taught with what was feasible and locally appropriate. Now there are several opportunities to train appropriately on short courses, and on Master's, Bachelor's, and Certificate courses that are designed for busy people working in less resourced parts of the world. Some courses are taught by distance learning (online), others by rotations in countries with well-developed educational programmes, and others are a combination of the two, with short periods of training away from home and work. Many are open to nurses and clinicians, while others are specifically for one healthcare cadre.

Table 12.2 highlights some useful websites to help find appropriate training. For (paediatric) radiotherapy, the International Atomic Energy Agency (IAEA) supports LMICs in the development of infrastructure and training of human resources needed to provide high-quality radiation treatment.

Continuous quality improvement

The process of continuous quality improvement requires a data management programme, which consists of a data manager, a database, and data analysis. Training for data managers can be conducted online, and participation in patient discussion meetings with the supervising doctor can improve collegiality, data quality, and the utility of data collection for improving patient care. Many free software tools are available, including spreadsheets (www.OpenOffice.org, Google documents) and EpiInfo (www.cdc.gov/epiinfo/), which allow the user to quickly configure databases with any type of data for any purpose. EpiInfo includes security features, double-data entry to improve accuracy, and analytical tools. Both are easy to use and ideal for single-centre research. For centres with reliable internet access, that work within multi-centre groups, the Resonance Patient Center (http://rpcprod.manuhsolutions.com:9090/RPC/ or www.ResonanceOncology.org) is available at no cost. It includes

Table 12.2 Training opportunities for paediatric oncology professionals from low- and middle-income countries

Programme	Description
Cure4Kids (www.cure4kids.org)	Excellent online resource for healthcare professionals worldwide, which includes disease- and treatment-specific seminars, articles, image-based instruction, and online education and collaboration tools. Funded by St Jude Children's Research Hospital
CancerPointe (www.cancerpointe.com)	POINTE has compiled information about clinical and research training courses in paediatric oncology for healthcare workers from resource-limited locations. This excellent website was developed and is maintained by the Pediatric Oncology in Developing Countries (PODC) group of the International Society of Pediatric Oncology (SIOP).
Groupe Franco-Africain d'Oncologie Pédiatrique (GFAOP; French–African Paediatric Oncology Group) (www.gfaop.org)	GFAOP offers a one-year intensive course for nurse educators, a one-year diploma in paediatric oncology for paediatricians, and an intensive course in paediatric surgical oncology. There are many Francophone courses developed through the GFAOP. These are listed on the POINTE website.
The African Pediatric Fellowship Program	The Program offers training opportunities to African paediatricians seeking subspecialty training. The Red Cross Children's Hospital in Cape Town offers this programme through recognized institutions in several African countries.
Uganda training programmes (www.fredhutch.org/en/labs/vaccine and www.oncology/uganda/training.html)	The Uganda Cancer Institute in Kampala and University of Washington offers a wide range of training opportunities including PhDs and Masters degrees to Ugandan scientists and doctors. Funded by the Fred Hutchinson Cancer Research Center.
Hospice training (www.hospice-africa.merseyside.org/Internat.html)	Training in palliative care is offered by Hospice Africa International Programmes which are based in Kampala and run distance learning courses open to all.
International Paediatric Oncology Society (SIOP) Asia Continental Branch (www.siop.asia.com)	The website provides information about training opportunities in Asia including www.siop.asia.com/index.php/information/fellowship.html, which describes the SIOP international outreach fellowships scheme.
CaseHippo (www.CaseHippo.com)	Paediatric oncology content, connection to paediatric professional societies, and networking capabilities.

customizable data-entry forms and reports, anonymized data sharing among sites that choose to do so, high-level security, automated off-site back-ups, and an integrated clinical trials management system for sites that wish to conduct clinical research. It also has a large base of existing users with whom new users can collaborate.

Data analysis to improve patient care is the most important component of any data-management programme, the utility of which depends far more on the quality of the data collected, regular and critical analysis of results, and the quality-improvement strategies implemented than on the software tool selected. The top priority in LMIC (after prompt and correct diagnosis) is to prevent toxic deaths, reduce abandonment, and monitor compliance with therapy and, thus, reduce relapse. This clinical research is best undertaken with the support and encouragement of regional colleagues in the context of regional and global networks, as discussed in the next section.

Development of paediatric cancer units and national paediatric oncology programmes

Some PCUs began as pilot projects, the goal of which was to simply demonstrate that some children with cancer can be cured with simple therapy that can be delivered locally, like the simplified Burkitt lymphoma treatment used in Malawi. A successful pilot project can lead to development of a PCU, which can be further developed into a centre of excellence, eventually with its own satellite centres for shared care, and, finally, into a regional or national network of PCUs (Figure 12.3). For example, the Pediatric Oncology Unit of Guatemala began as a pilot unit, developed into a centre of excellence, and recently launched its first satellite in an effort to eventually provide national coverage and to improve event-free survival by promoting early diagnosis and referral for locally-adapted protocol-based care. Implementing such care is discussed in the next section.

Protocol-based care

Protocol-based care standardizes treatment regimens and improves results for every cancer in which its effect has been measured. However, clinicians who apply protocols in LMIC face uncertainties about disease stage and risk classification, medication shortages, excess toxicity from comorbid illnesses, and preventable deaths due to poor transportation or other social factors. Furthermore, doctors in LMIC manage large numbers of patients with little time, rarely have the luxury of specializing in a subset of childhood cancers, and often lack access to experts. Information systems provided at no cost to centres in LMIC, like Resonance Oncology (www.ResonanceOncology.org), facilitate adherence to the protocol by

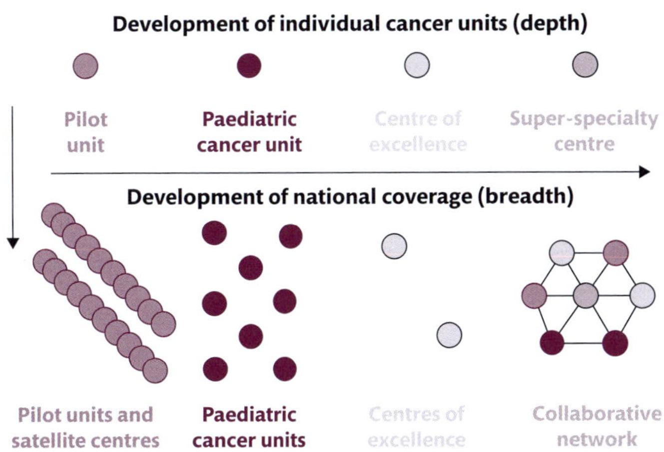

Figure 12.3 Phases of development of paediatric oncology and the central role of paediatric cancer units.

Reproduced courtesy of Scott C. Howard, University of Tennessee College of Health Sciences, USA.

providing patient-specific chemotherapy roadmaps, patient treatment diaries, and automated calculation of drug doses based on the patient's height and weight. Such systems can also reduce abandonment by including a scheduling system with call-back functionality for patients who miss appointments and are at risk to abandon. Finally, information systems form the backbone of any quality-improvement effort designed to address specific causes of preventable treatment failure (**Figure 12.2**).

Adapted-treatment regimens and clinical research

Protocols that work well in HIC may cause disastrous toxicity in LMIC, as occurred when a regimen developed at St Jude Children's Research Hospital in Memphis, USA, was adopted in El Salvador without modification. Regimens must be adapted for use in LMIC, and the rate of toxic death monitored to determine whether the supportive care in the hospital is adequate to support the proposed treatment regimens and to identify preventable causes of treatment failure. If toxic death occurs too frequently, the regimen must be further adapted pending improvements in supportive care and hospital infrastructure. Practical research to address causes of treatment failure in the local setting is best conducted with colleagues who practice in similar circumstances. For example, centres in Central America (AHOPCA) and Latin America (MISPHO) have shared protocols and compared results for the past two decades, with great benefits to all. Collaborating centres in French-speaking Africa, India, Malaysia, and elsewhere have also developed adapted-treatment regimens and locally feasible supportive-care guidelines.

In addition to local adaptation and implementation of protocol-based care, adapted-treatment regimens have been developed for Burkitt lymphoma, Wilms tumour, Kaposi sarcoma, low-grade glioma, Hodgkin lymphoma, medulloblastoma, and acute lymphoblastic leukaemia (ALL). In the case of ALL, the regimens establish a backbone of therapy with low toxicity and cost that will cure a large proportion of children with ALL while minimizing toxic death. If there are less than two toxic deaths among the first 25 patients, the PCU is ready to 'step up' to a more intense treatment regimen to try to reduce the rate of relapse. If two or more patients die of toxicity, the PCU can 'step down' to a safer, less intense regimen and work to improve supportive care. Rational movement between steps requires monitoring of patient outcomes in real time, so a data-management programme is a prerequisite to successful implementation of an adapted-treatment strategy. The adapted treatment for Wilms tumour is currently being field-tested in many centres in Africa with prospective data collection and practical support including training for pathologists, sonographers, and surgeons.

Regional and global networks

Twinning partnerships between centres in HIC and LMIC can greatly speed the development of PCUs and centres of excellence, but such partnerships are even more effective when associated with other PCUs in the same region. Interaction with colleagues who practice in a similar setting and face similar problems affords an opportunity to learn from each other's mistakes, share guidelines, and optimize adapted-treatment regimens for each centre. In this regard, cooperating centres in Argentina, Brazil, India, Colombia, and many other LMIC have developed shared protocols and joint advocacy programmes to improve outcomes at the national and regional level.

Improving outcomes for children with cancer by developing and improving PCUs has proven effective all over the world, and regional and global networks of collaborators have kept the momentum by sharing protocols, projects, funding sources, and supportive-care guidelines. Online meetings via www.Cure4Kids.org have transformed twinning programmes and regional collaborations. For example, since 2005 professionals from centres in Morocco, St Jude Children's Research Hospital, and guests from several continents have been meeting weekly to discuss patients, review supportive care issues, and develop and implement treatment protocols adapted to local conditions. An Asia Pacific Leukemia Lymphoma meeting held every other Friday, via Cure4Kids, currently draws healthcare providers from 5–10 countries to present and discuss patients, protocols, and supportive-care issues. The Global Neuroblastoma Network (www.globalneuroblastoma.net) meets weekly on Thursdays to improve care for this disease.

Treatment challenges in low- and middle-income countries

Toxicity of treatment

Chemotherapy is especially toxic in malnourished children with advanced disease. In HIC, more intense and toxic therapies, matched by intense and costly supportive therapy, have achieved good outcomes. In LMIC, children present with advanced cancers and large tumour loads. For example, in children with Burkitt lymphoma in Africa, the tumour burden is high, with frequent kidney involvement and high risk of tumour lysis syndrome even with low-intensity chemotherapeutic regimens. The risk to the patient is increased even more by lack of rasburicase and inadequate access to laboratory testing to follow potassium levels and prevent cardiac dysrhythmias. Malnutrition and underlying infections must also be managed prior to starting chemotherapy (to the extent possible) to minimize treatment toxicity. HIV-infected children can be expected to have more episodes of fever, neutropenia, and treatment delays.

Malnutrition has been shown to be associated with more chemotherapy-induced neutropenia and fever episodes with consequent delays in therapy, but few PCUs in LMIC can provide parenteral feeding, which is unacceptable to many parents who equate it with death. Nausea and vomiting, and especially mucositis, become difficult to manage when oral feeding is required. Pre-treatment fluids (oral or intravenous) and allopurinol (in children with haematological cancers) should be given, as well as an antiemetic such as metoclopromide, which is inexpensive and widely available. Enriched milk (F100) or ready-to-use therapeutic foods such as Plumpynut or Chiponde can rapidly improve nutritional status.

Nursing staff should be empowered to act quickly and independently to initiate a fever protocol and start antibiotics as soon as fever is recorded and malaria (in malaria-endemic areas) is ruled out. Treatment should be modified to suit local facilities and expertise, to use doses and drugs that can be safely given to achieve the best outcome possible. As experience is gained with protocols and as local health provision improves, the protocols can be intensified in a stepwise fashion.

Abandonment of treatment

When treatment is initiated but not completed, it is described as abandonment. In children with cancer, abandonment significantly decreases the probability of cure. The reasons for abandonment of treatment are various and individual, but there is an overarching pattern of causes reported from LMIC. The most commonly cited reason for abandonment is financial. Families from LMIC cannot afford transportation to a distant care centre. The long stays in the hospital drain family funds and keep them away from any gainful employment they had previously. In Recife, Brazil, a social support programme for children with ALL and their families included transportation, accommodation, financial support, and job training. This reduced the number who abandoned treatment from 16% to 0.5%. Patient and family education are essential, in addition to logistical and financial support. Keeping an open ward or providing accommodation for those who live far away and cannot easily get to and from home between courses of chemotherapy is necessary.

Assisting on the ward with extra food and basic necessities such as soap and laundry detergent also helps prevent abandonment. The hospital is a bewildering place to people new to the city, so a system to welcome newcomers and provide amenities such as washing lines and cooking facilities is essential. In Blantyre, Malawi, the mothers are given a small amount of money to spend in the market every weekend on simple foodstuffs and firewood so that they can cook in a shelter close to the ward. This programme improves nutritional status, and also bonds the women together in a shared and enjoyable task. Other reasons for abandonment of therapy include an extended family's reluctance or inability to help with home chores while the mother is absent in the hospital with one child; death or illness in other close relatives; anxiety about leaving the remaining children in inadequate care at home; and concerns about the fidelity of a spouse during long absences at the hospital.

Palliative care

Sometimes pragmatic decisions must be made. Surgical options may be unavailable, and if chemotherapy does not improve the patient's disease, palliative care may be the only way to help a child. Palliative care offers symptom control and emotional and spiritual support. One of the most significant recent advances in LMIC is the recognition that pain control is a fundamental human right and that oral morphine must be made available for children with cancer who experience pain.

Advocacy

Given the rarity of cancer in children compared to infectious diseases and other health problems, it is not surprising that cancer is not a priority for health systems in LMIC. Therefore, other ways must be found to support cancer care. Twinning between PCUs in HIC and LMIC has been very successful. The gain is bilateral. Funds, expertise, drugs, and specialized diagnostic tests flow from high-income to low-income centres, while experience, thinking outside the box, valuing what is possible, and using what is available are lessons learned by those who work in HIC centres.

Charitable organizations and professional organizations can support PCUs in LMIC with expert advice, assistance with modifying protocols, and moral support. World Child Cancer (www.worldchildcancer.org and www.worldchildcancer.us) was formed to channel support to cancer units in low-income countries. It offers long-term support to PCUs to help them get established and gradually develop their own support networks. The International Society of Pediatric Oncology (SIOP), with its regional organizations in Africa, Asia, Oceania, and Latin America, provides professional support and expertise. The Children's Oncology Group (COG, www.childrensoncologygroup.org) collaborates with South American centres for training and shared protocols, and the Groupe Franco-Africaine d'Oncologie Pediatrique (GFAOP, www.igr.fr/gfaop) has a long tradition of international collaboration between PCUs in France and those in Africa.

The World Health Organization (WHO) has increasingly become involved in improving paediatric cancer care, and has joined forces with SIOP, Childhood Cancer International, St Jude Children's Research Hospital, World Child Cancer, and others to strengthen local health systems and support cancer planning and strategy development in selected LMIC. It has endorsed an essential drug list for paediatric cancer treatment, which should be made available to all children in all countries (http://www.who.int/selection_medicines/committees/expert/17/second_children_list_en.pdf). Parent support organizations can provide a strong voice to influence political decisions and raise the profile of cancer in LMIC. Wherever we work and however meagre our tools, there is always something that we can do to improve the lives of children with cancer.

FURTHER READING

Arora RS, et al. (2007) The problem of treatment abandonment in children from developing countries with cancer. *Pediatr Blood Cancer* **49**, 941–6.

Arya LS, et al. (2010) Pattern of relapse in childhood ALL: challenges and lessons from a uniform treatment protocol. *J Pediatr Hematol Oncol* **32**, 370–5.

Cavalli F (2008) The World Cancer Declaration: a roadmap for change. *Lancet Oncol* **9**, 810–11.

Gupta S, et al. (2009) Incidence and predictors of treatment-related mortality in paediatric acute leukaemia in El Salvador. *Br J Cancer* **100**, 1026–31.

Harif M, et al. (2008) Treatment of B-cell lymphoma with LMB modified protocols in Africa—report of the French-African Pediatric Oncology Group (GFAOP). *Pediatr Blood Cancer* **50**, 1138–42.

Hesseling P, et al. (2005) The 2000 Burkitt lymphoma trial in Malawi. *Pediatr Blood Cancer* **44**, 245–50.

Hesseling P, et al. (2009) Endemic Burkitt lymphoma: a 28-day treatment schedule with cyclophosphamide and intrathecal methotrexate. *Ann Trop Paediatr* **29**, 29–34.

Howard SC, et al. (2004) Establishment of a pediatric oncology program and outcomes of childhood acute lymphoblastic leukemia in a resource-poor area. *JAMA* **291**, 2471–5.

Howard SC, et al. (2007) Improving outcomes for children with cancer in low-income countries in Latin America: a report on the recent meetings of the Monza International School of Pediatric Hematology/Oncology (MISPHO)-Part I. *Pediatr Blood Cancer* **48**, 364–9.

Howard SC, et al. (2008) Childhood cancer epidemiology in low-income countries. *Cancer* **112**, 461–72.

Hunger SP, et al. (2009) Treatment strategies and regimens of graduated intensity for childhood acute lymphoblastic leukemia in low-income countries: a proposal. *Pediatr Blood Cancer* **52**, 559–65.

Israels T, et al. (2008) The guardians' perspective on paediatric cancer treatment in Malawi and factors affecting adherence. *Pediatr Blood Cancer* **51**, 639–42.

Israels T, et al. (2009) Malnutrition and neutropenia in children treated for Burkitt lymphoma in Malawi. *Pediatr Blood Cancer* **53**, 47–52.

Israels T, et al. (2010) Strategies to improve care for children with cancer in Sub-Saharan Africa. *Eur J Cancer* **46**, 1960–6.

Leander C, et al. (2007) Impact of an education program on late diagnosis of retinoblastoma in Honduras. *Pediatr Blood Cancer* **49**, 817–9.

Magrath I, et al. (2005) Treatment of acute lymphoblastic leukaemia in countries with limited resources; lessons from use of a single protocol in India over a twenty year period. *Eur J Cancer* **41**, 1570–83.

Masera G (2009) Bridging the childhood cancer mortality gap between economically developed and low-income countries. *J Pediatr Hematol Oncol* **31**, 710–12.

Masera G, et al. (1998) North-South twinning in paediatric haemato-oncology: the La Mascota programme, Nicaragua. *Lancet* **352**, 1923–6.

Metzger ML, et al. (2003) Outcome of childhood acute lymphoblastic leukaemia in resource-poor countries. *Lancet* **362**, 706–8.

Mostert S, et al. (2010) Comparing childhood leukaemia treatment before and after the introduction of a parental education programme in Indonesia. *Arch Dis Child* **95**, 20–5.

Norman K, et al. (2008) Prognostic impact of disease-related malnutrition. *Clin Nutr* **27**, 5–15.

Ribeiro RC, et al. (2008) Baseline status of paediatric oncology care in ten low-income or mid-income countries receiving My Child Matters support: a descriptive study. *Lancet Oncol* **9**, 721–9.

Sinfield RL, et al. (2007) Spectrum and presentation of pediatric malignancies in the HIV era: experience from Blantyre, Malawi, 1998–2003. *Pediatr Blood Cancer* **48**, 515–20.

Sitaresmi MN, et al. (2010) Treatment refusal and abandonment in childhood acute lymphoblastic leukemia in Indonesia: an analysis of causes and consequences. *Psycho-oncology* **19**, 361–7.

Wilmshurst JM, et al. (2016) The African Pediatric Fellowship Program: Training in Africa for Africans. *Pediatrics* **137**(1). doi: 10.1542/peds.2015-2741.

13

Cancer in Adolescents and Young Adults

Lucy J.W. Jones, Emmanouil Saloustros, Andrea Ferrari, and Dan Stark

Epidemiology and outcomes

Incidence

Cancer in the adolescent and young adult (AYA) population is uncommon: 2–4% of all invasive malignancies overall depending upon precise definitions. However, the annual incidence of cancer in the 15- to 39-year age group is estimated to be 50–70,000 in Europe, and one million worldwide. The incidence of cancer increases with age, from childhood to adulthood; between the ages of 15 and 30, cancer is 2.7 times more frequent than in the under 15 age group.

The overall incidence of cancer in the AYA population is increasing. Testicular cancer has seen substantial increases in the recent era, while in the USA, increasing diagnosis of early thyroid cancers may be partly responsible. The incidence of some cancers seen in AYAs is decreasing in the Western world (such as Kaposi's sarcoma, melanoma, lung carcinoma, cervical carcinoma) as a result of public health measures directed at young people.

The spectrum of cancer types diagnosed in AYAs aged 15–39 is distinct from children and older adults. The most frequently occurring cancers in the AYA population are:

- carcinomas (in particular breast, melanoma, gynaecological, and thyroid carcinomas, but also colorectal tumours),
- haematological malignancies, notably Hodgkin and non-Hodgkin lymphoma (HL and NHL),
- germ-cell tumours.

In contrast to children under 12, embryonal tumours are much rarer in the AYA population. Within AYAs, the incidence of certain cancers varies with age, and some cancer types, such as osteosarcoma, peak in incidence. The incidence of carcinomas gradually increases with age, while HL and germ-cell tumours peak at ages 15–24 years and 20–29 years respectively. The incidence of acute lymphoblastic leukaemia (ALL) declines with increasing age.

The causes of cancer in AYAs are poorly understood, and appear to differ from adults and children. Fewer than 5% of all cancers in the AYA population are attributed to currently known inherited cancer syndromes, although AYA-specific studies of this are planned, such as SPECTA-AYA across Europe and INFORM specifically in Germany. While prenatal factors may have some effect on the occurrence of AYA malignancies, in contrast to childhood cancer, environmental factors appear more significant; increased age increases individual risk of exposure to pathogens, such as ultraviolet sunlight, smoking, viruses (e.g. HPV, HIV, EBV), and iatrogenic causes, such as the treatment of childhood cancers (see the section 'Late effects'). However, the aetiology for the majority of cancers in this age group remains unknown, and unrelated to environmental exposures or inherited genetic disorders.

Outcome

Cancer is the most common cause of disease-related death in the 15- to 24-year age group in high-income countries, accounting for 10% of deaths in AYAs annually in Europe. Survival varies with the specific cancer diagnosed. Malignancies with the highest survival rates include thyroid carcinoma, Hodgkin lymphoma, germ-cell tumours, malignant melanoma, chondrosarcomas, and fibrosarcomas. Conversely, poorer outcomes are associated with liver and lung carcinomas, rhabdomyosarcomas, astrocytomas, Ewing's sarcoma, and acute myeloid leukaemia (AML), whose relative five-year survival is less than 55%.

In high-income countries, the overall five-year survival rate of all cancers in the AYA population is now greater than 80%. Survival outcomes in AYA malignancies are improving after a prolonged period of stagnation or deterioration going back to the 1990s when there was little if any focus upon the field. A recent study of five-year survival trends in the UK demonstrated an overall increase in five-year survival from 75.5% in 1992–1996, to 82.2% in 2002–2006. An improvement was observed in all cancer types, except for osteosarcoma, rhabdomyosarcoma, non-gonadal and ovarian germ-cell tumours, and thyroid carcinomas; comparable with that observed in other countries. However, despite this improvement in survival outcomes, in comparison to younger age groups, AYAs still have worse outcomes. In Europe, between 2000 and 2007, patients under 15 years had a better five-year relative survival compared to AYAs for ALL (85.8% versus 55.7%), AML (60.5% versus 49.7%), NHL (83% versus 77.4%), Ewing's tumours (66.6% versus 49.3%), rhabdomyosarcoma (66.6% versus 37.7%), and astrocytomas (61.9% versus 46.5%). Some differences can be understood to some extent by examining the detail; astrocytoma is associated with a higher proportion of pilocytic pathology in children (25%) and adolescents (35%) than at 20–24 years (17%), 25–29 years (8%), or 30–39 years (4%). The reason for each of these poorer outcomes is not clearly elucidated but is undoubtedly multifactorial and should be subject to more research.

The five-year relative survival in all cancers is 78% in men, compared to 83% in women. There is some data suggesting this may relate in part to clinical management choices and drug pharmacology during chemotherapy treatment administration in AYA cancers. There are also differences in cancer biology (see the section 'Biology').

These disparities highlight the need to better understand and characterize what it is that makes AYA cancer management distinct from other age groups. Throughout this chapter we will explore some of these differences in terms of characteristic biology, patient factors, and the methods of treatment delivery within current healthcare institutions, and how we can work towards improving outcomes.

Biology

There is growing evidence that the biology of AYA cancers is distinct from children and older adults, enabling physicians to target therapy more specifically. Examples to highlight the clinical importance of this include:

- ALL: the TEL-AML1 translocation is favourable for response to therapy, and occurs in only 10% of AYA cases, compared to 50% of childhood cases. In contrast, the poor prognostic indicator, Ph-1, peaks in incidence in the AYA age group.
- Malignant melanoma: BRAF-positive disease is much commoner in AYAs than in older adults. This increases treatment options.
- Breast cancer: more younger women have tumours that are 'triple negative' for hormonal and epithelial growth factor receptors compared to older women, therefore making them resistant to many targeted systemic therapies.
- Rhabdomyosarcoma (RMS): outcomes are also significantly worse in the AYA population, with more young people found to have the alveolar subtype, which is associated with a worse survival outcome. Additionally, the incidence of MYOD1, a recently identified mutation associated with an aggressive and more advanced form of embryonal RMS, peaks at age 25.

Access to care and delay in diagnosis

A credible causal candidate for poorer outcomes in AYA cancer patients is that AYA patients frequently report a prolonged period with symptoms (before presenting for care) and then after presenting (before receiving a cancer diagnosis and treatment). Such prolonged time to diagnosis may impact the chance of cure. However, the impact of this, clinically, may not be uniform between cancer types, appearing to be particularly important in sarcomas and germ-cell tumours.

In many countries, the general practitioner (GP) is the first healthcare professional to see these patients, and therefore plays a key role in the diagnostic pathway. It has been suggested that AYAs may be 'embarrassed' to discuss their bodily symptoms, and therefore might avoid seeing their GP in the first place. However, this is not the case—AYAs do consult. A retrospective study investigating the use of primary care by AYA patients preceding their cancer diagnosis reported a significant increase in GP attendance across all cancers in the interval proceeding a cancer diagnosis. This time period varied according to malignancy: 17 months for central nervous system (CNS) tumours, 12 months for sarcoma, nine months for lymphomas, five to six months for leukaemia, bone tumour, or germ-cell tumour, and three months for malignant melanoma. Researchers also observed an increase in the number of blood tests performed by the GP, which began on average 11 months before a cancer diagnosis.

It has been hypothesized that young people's cancers result in them reporting non-specific symptoms. However, pain and lumps are the most prevalent in population-based studies of presenting symptoms in primary care. If reassured initially, some believe AYAs may be more loathe to return for a further review than older people or the parents of a symptomatic small child. The challenge is to differentiate patients with malignancy from the majority with a benign illness. The comparatively rare occurrence of AYA malignancies also may result in a high threshold (and therefore low likelihood) for investigation for cancer in this age group. This highlights the need to improve awareness and understanding of cancer in the AYA population among both the general public and healthcare professionals, as well as establishing clear diagnostic pathways. A number of countries, including the UK and Denmark have implemented a fast-track service for suspected cases of cancer, in order to facilitate prompt diagnosis and treatment.[1] These pathways may require particular attention in making them optimal for AYA.

Age-specific psychosocial aspects

While the biology and range of malignancies in the AYA population is distinct from that of children and older adults, there are many other age-specific issues that can form barriers for AYAs. The large, distinct, and very specific impact of cancer at this age can affect patients' experience, quality of life, adherence to treatment, and survival outcomes. Many of the developmental goals of life in this phase are not just impaired but directly placed into reverse by cancer: independence, financially and personally, already being delayed in many modern Western societies, can go into 'reverse gear'.

AYAs are in the process of developing their own thoughts and perceptions of the world, forming new relationships, and pushing boundaries. This stage of life is often formative in terms of education, career planning, and for some, family planning. There is often a desire to challenge the rules set by their parents, and experiment with risk-taking behaviours such as smoking, alcohol consumption, or recreational drug use. With cancer, there are commonly periods of returning to reliance on parents, and moving away from independent thinking and decision making.

During adolescence, many young people also begin to explore sexual activity. Sexual identity development may regress, due to physical and psychological challenges, and issues relating to body image, psychosexual identity, and fertility (see the section 'Late effects'). Young people have to find their own 'new normal'.[2] These issues, therefore, must be addressed during their treatment by health professionals skilled at delivering clear, sensitive, and age-appropriate information, which is not what AYAs frequently report they experienced. Preserving fertility or safe menstrual periods with low platelets may require medically-induced amenorrhea. This is also a physiological regression towards childhood.

Throughout their diagnosis and treatment, AYA patients should be empowered to live as normal a life as possible, and be able to achieve as many developmental milestones as possible, despite their disease. Even when life is short, young people often benefit from a project or some personal development. While this may require treating teams to demonstrate focus, creativity, and flexibility, the frequent result is the development of a trusting rapport with the patient, better treatment adherence, and the best chance of the best outcome.

Maintaining normality includes the importance of peer support, which is easily lost during long periods of treatment and hospitalization. This can be facilitated by a welcoming, age-appropriate environment, with flexible visiting times, and opportunities for young people to connect with both healthy peers and fellow AYA patients. Social isolation is a problem, but work on quality of life specifically for AYAs also indicates that simple boredom is a large but remediable problem during their cancer treatment. Providing support is a key component of any AYA cancer service, from the point of diagnosis to beyond the completion of treatment, and not only in relation to care for individual patients but also as one considers the design of AYA-specific services and models of care.

Therefore, healthcare professionals caring for these patients need to have not only expert clinical knowledge about AYA malignancies but also of the broad and varied psychosocial needs and the fight by some young people against a return to childhood. This knowledge is acquired through regular experience of 'walking with patients' throughout their cancer journey, and also through national and international forums where experiences and ideas can be shared, and current practices reviewed and developed.[3]

Models of care

The clinical interface

Historically, and still in many parts of the world, AYAs were either treated by paediatric oncologists or adult specialists, neither of which had specific expertise in their age group. This resulted in young people feeling isolated from their peers, at a time of life when friendship with those of a similar age is particularly important. Both the model of care tailored to children's services and the model of care adopted in adult services fail to cater to the complex specific needs of the AYA group. This was also the period when clinical outcomes stagnated.

- Paediatric services are often based on a 'family-centred model': information shared with the patients is limited to what is considered by parents to be essential, and much of the decision making is done by their parents/carers. Both medical and non-medical specialists in the multidisciplinary team (MDT) work to ensure that all the needs of the patient and their family are addressed, but the patient's personal involvement may be less than they want (to 'protect' them), increasing problems with challenge to authority and poor treatment concordance.
- Adult services aim to be patient-centred (not family-centred), and clinical management is structured according to disease site. Again, AYAs are isolated by this from other young people, and communication channels to their peers and family may not be used with authenticity and at the ideal frequency. The adult MDT is focused upon clinical diagnosis and decision making, and there is less access to non-medical specialists such as psychological, social, and educational support.
- An AYA model of care must be patient-centred, and support fragile patient autonomy and informed decision making. There is also a need to adapt the involvement of parents and other significant parties, depending on the maturity and life stage of the patient.

A broad MDT is required to meet the holistic needs of these patients. Experience of working as a team with AYAs enables, for example, any challenges of concordance to be managed proactively, using flexibility but also clear, consistent information. Then, 'battlegrounds' between young people and their carers (such as over nutrition or the balance between social and clinical priorities) should be expected, identified, and minimized.

AYAs have been described as existing in a 'no man's land' between children and adult services. A key aspect of AYA care is the integration of paediatric and adult oncologists and haematologists. Fundamental to providing quality, personalized care to AYA cancer patients is the bringing together of paediatric and adults services. However, clinically, departments operate in dissimilar ways; for example, they apply different staging and grading of diseases. The challenge of AYA healthcare providers is to act as a bridge between these interfaces.

Table 13.1 describes the models of care currently adopted by various counties, and the projects that are currently in place. At present, no 'one-size fits all' model of care for AYA oncology services has been agreed, although there are detailed descriptions of several effective models. The collaborative work of national and international professional, government, and charitable organizations over the last ten years has seen much development in the design and implementation of specialist oncology services for AYAs. The variation may be a good thing, enabling the services to meet the needs of young people in their local healthcare and societal context.

Age range

There is much variation between countries as to the age at which AYAs reach this interface between children and adult care. In some southern European countries, this starts at age 14, while in other countries, such as Germany, it does not begin until age 18. In the UK, AYA patients are teenagers (13–18 years) and young adults (19–24 years). Different age ranges are also applied depending on the purpose. In general, the upper age limit for clinical facilities is in the mid-twenties. This extends to age 29 or 30 for epidemiology, and 39 or 40 years for clinical follow-up. European Network for Teenagers and Young Adults with Cancer (ENTYAC) guidance for AYA care suggests that rather than defining specific age ranges, departments should treat according to the needs of the community they serve, ensuring that those who fall in the interface between children and adult service have their needs met.

Care environment

Hospitals in many countries now have specified care environments for AYA cancer patients. These comprise inpatient wards and/or outpatient facilities which provide an environment, staff, and facilities

Table 13.1 The models of adolescent and young adult care currently adopted by various countries, and the projects that are currently in place

	UK	France	Germany	Italy	Spain	The Netherlands	Denmark	The Czech Republic
Model of care	Collaboration between paediatric and adult services; specalization in AYA care.	National integrated cooperative programme, joining paediatric and adult oncology/ haematology. National cancer plans have an AYA element.	Inpatient treatment of adolescent cancer patients < 18 years takes place within a German Society for Paediatric Oncology and Haematology (GPOH)-certified unit.	Developed within the national paediatric oncology community. Currentlydeveloping a national programme, through collaboration between paediatric and adult oncologists.	Developed by local paediatric oncologists.	Health professionals from regional centres started a national cooperative AYA project in 2013, initiated by medical oncology, focused on those in the 18-35 age range.	No nation model	
Age range	15–24 years (13–24 years in several departments)	15–25 years	>18 years	15–29 years	14–30 years	18–35 years	Not defined	15–19 years
Local projects	25 AYA units	8 AYA programmes, with 3 AYA units	4 centres with interdisciplinary programmes	2 TYA units, 1 regional project	1 TYA unit and local initiatives in paediatric centres	2 AYA centres	2 AYA units	Collaboration on leukaemia trials

Adapted with permission from Stark D et al. 'Teenagers and young adults with cancer in Europe: from national programmes to a European integrated coordinated project'. *European Journal Cancer Care*, Volume 25, Issue 3, pp. 419–427, Copyright © 2015, John Wiley and Sons. DOI: https://doi.org/10.1111/ecc.1236

tailored to the holistic needs of AYA patients. These also raise the profile and act as physical focal points for the AYA MDT. Often these environments display colourful, contemporary, and creative décor, and cater for the variable needs of AYAs. This may include games areas, music facilities, study zones, relaxation areas, and places to socialize and spend time with other young people. AYAs have emphasized the importance of access to youth workers, psychologists, and therapists. These environments are fundamental in facilitating peer support, which is hugely important in this age group, and have a positive effect on patient experience and engagement in their healthcare. They also bring their own specific challenges, such as bereavement of other patients, although on balance they are reported by young people to be highly beneficial in overcoming some of the social stigma of cancer.

Centralization of services versus local hospital care

In order to provide experienced, specialized teams, treating a large number of patients with the variety of AYA malignancies, the care of these patients needs to be led from larger centres. Related to this is the challenge of conducting AYA-friendly clinical trials (see the section 'Accrual in clinical trials'). However, the negative consequence of this is the requirement for some patients and their families to travel significant distances in order to receive care. This also affects the patient's social and vocational development, as they may be moved far from their social network, educational institution, or workplace.

In 2005, the UK National Institute of Clinical Excellence (NICE) Improving Outcomes Guidance for Cancer in Children and Young People specified the need for all AYA cancer patients to be overseen by the regional principal treatment centre (PTC) team. Patients may request to receive their care at their local designated hospitals. More recently, some AYA PTCs have provided specialist AYA outreach services in local hospitals.[4] This requires robust healthcare professional networks across different care centres, and may also be helpful in managing the late effects of cancer.

France has an established national cooperative programme, integrating paediatric and adult oncology/haematology services. The national cancer plans involve AYA malignancies, and describe the establishment of regional care pathways and an increased amount of research in AYA oncology. The Institut National du Cancer (INCa) has set out clear guidelines for how each of their eight AYA centres and teams should be structured, including the integration of medical and nursing staff with psychologists and social workers. In the USA, the number of specialist centres is growing.

The need for adolescent and young adult-specific professional training

The distinct population and needs highlights a training gap in both paediatric and adult oncology. Professionals need to be educated in the distinct biology and clinical management of AYA cancers, as well as the psychosocial and interpersonal issues. AYAs have commented on the importance of personal qualities, and the ability to communicate effectively with young people and to be able to develop a good rapport. Some of this ability is cancer-specific and some is generic to staff working with young people with any chronic disease. This training is reflected in adolescent health programmes created through collaboration between the Royal Colleges of Paediatrics and Child Health, Nursing, General Practice, and Obstetricians and Gynaecologists in the UK, and intended for all health professions working with children aged 12–18 years. It is openly available as an online e-learning module.[5]

There is a growing recognition of the need for professional training and qualifications for staff working specifically in AYA oncology. The aim is that, in collaboration with universities and professional societies, healthcare staff will be able to achieve an accredited qualification in AYA oncology. International courses include:

- http://www.coventry.ac.uk/study-at-coventry/faculties-and-schools/health-and-life-sciences/nursing-midwifery-and-health/teenager-young-adults-cancer-care/
- http://university.asco.org/focus-under-forty
- https://www.youtube.com/playlist?list=PLD962FF429F3E4F4A
- http://mdhs-study.unimelb.edu.au/degrees/graduate-certificate-in-adolescent-health-and-wellbeing/overview
- http://oncologypro.esmo.org/Tumour-Portal/Cancer-in-Young-Adults

Some have suggested the establishment of the 'AYA oncologist'. Currently, systems are not mature enough for specific training schemes and whole departments for AYA. More achievable, however, is the formation of further AYA-specialized MDTs, in which all have expertise and qualifications.

Accrual in clinical trials

The best possible access to care remains a challenge for AYA with cancer; in particular, it has been variously reported that patients in this age category are enrolled in clinical protocols at far lower rates than children. The accrual rate gap has been suggested as one of the possible reasons why AYAs with certain tumour types have worse survival rates than children with the same disease. On the one hand, there is no question that clinical trials are a fundamental part of cancer research, benefitting subsequent generations of patients and furthering the scientific knowledge; meanwhile, on the other hand, it is difficult to demonstrate whether participating in clinical trials improves survival on an individual level. However, there is indirect evidence suggesting a positive effect of trials on participants' outcome. Participation in trials may be associated with a better quality of care thanks to the involvement of a broader group of highly-specialized professionals and/or to the stricter organization and process control demanded by clinical protocols.

A review of various studies showed that the rates of AYAs entering clinical trials ranged from 5% to 34%. For example, a French population-based study underlined that most teenagers (82%) were treated on adult units, and only a small proportion of them (27%) were recruited in clinical trials. A study conducted by the Italian national paediatric oncology society AIEOP (Associazione Italiana Ematologia Oncologia Pediatrica) demonstrated that only 10% of 15- to 19-year-old cancer patients were treated at AIEOP-affiliated paediatric oncology centres (between 1989 and 2006), as opposed to 77% of children (0–14 years); in addition, only half of adolescents were enrolled in clinical trials. However, the proportion of 15-19 yearolds treated at Italian paediatric oncology referral centres thankfully improved significantly in the subsequent years, reaching 28% for the years 2007–2012. Improvement in the adolescent accrual rate was also recently observed in the UK (from the 25% reported in the 2005–2007 period, with variations across cancer types), as a result of a global healthcare policy including a strategic approach to improve AYAs' recruitment to clinical trials based on five key words: 'available, accessible, aware, appropriate, and acceptable'.

A comprehensive, multi-level, coordinated strategy specifically addressing the poor clinical trial enrolment among AYAs is necessary to overcome barriers: for example, regulatory and practice-related challenges; that in some trials, regulatory guidelines are implemented to protect 'minors'; the fact that AYAs with cancer are not referred to institutions where clinical trials are offered; the age eligibility criteria of protocols or the age cut-off for the admission to paediatric or adult medical wards; and the insufficient collaboration between paediatric and adult medical oncology cooperative groups. But there are also patient-related challenges that can affect an adolescent's decision to enrol and adhere to a clinical trial: young people may feel shocked at the diagnosis, can experience denial, and might be overwhelmed by a long-term commitment to adhering to a protocol.

The low referral rate of adolescents as compared to children has been discussed in a recent study developed by the European paediatric Soft-Tissue Sarcoma Study Group (EpSSG), that compared the number of 15–19 year olds (and 0–14 year olds) treated in EpSSG trials with the number of cases expected to occur in European countries according to the incidence rates estimated through population-based cancer registries. The 'observed to expected' ratio (in the period 2008–2015) was 0.64 for children and 0.30 for adolescents (with differences according to sarcoma subtypes and the different countries considered). That study emphasizes that the AYA-dedicated national programmes developed across Europe should increase the exchanges with the disease-specific cooperative groups running clinical trials.

Late effects

Cancer and its treatment are toxic, and AYAs are potentially exposed to a wide range of chemotherapy agents, surgery, radiotherapy, and other systemic agents such as immunological or hormonal therapies, each with distinct toxic effects that may occur acutely but also disrupt health and well-being many years after completion of cancer treatment. Some of these effects are distinct in AYAs compared to older or younger patients. These result in significant burden upon young people and health services. Most late effects are linked to the therapy received, so AYAs should be specifically informed as soon as they are receptive to this complex information; this may benefit from the expertise found in AYA centres in counselling young people.

Cardiovascular disease

Chemotherapy is associated with delayed cardiovascular complications including hypertension, accelerated atherosclerosis, coronary artery disease, and heart failure. In a Danish cohort of more than 43,000 AYA cancer survivors, an absolute excess risk of up to 400 extra hospitalizations due to cardiovascular disease per 100,000 person years in survivors was found. The mediastinal radiotherapy commonly used for the treatment of lymphomas and anthracycline chemotherapy have been linked to increased risk. Regardless of therapy received, all AYA survivors should be offered lifestyle advice to reduce their risk of cardiovascular disease.

Second malignant neoplasms

AYAs are at greater risk of developing new, secondary cancers due to predisposition or treatment, when compared to older survivors. AYAs should be supported to follow the appropriate evidence-based cancer screening guidelines applicable to themselves as members of the general population, but also additional procedures. For example, young women who had thoracic radiotherapy should receive mammogram and magnetic resonance imaging (MRI) due to their excess breast-cancer risk. In all AYA survivors it is essential to support the young person to undertake lifestyle modifications that reduce cancer risk—smoking cessation, alcohol moderation, moderate sun exposure, a balanced diet, and regular exercise.

Fertility

Treatment-induced reduction in fertility, either in terms of lowered immediate fertility or reduction in the duration of fertility after treatment, is primarily due to dose-dependent gonadal toxicity, although disruption of reproductive endocrine or reproductive anatomy should also be considered. The risk depends on the age at treatment (higher with older age) and the treatment selected. Those containing radiotherapy and/or alkylating agents such as cyclophosphamide and procarbazine are considered as the most toxic to the gonad. In all AYA patients planning to receive any treatment that may impact upon future fertility, expert discussion regarding fertility preservation early in treatment planning is recommended, in both men and women, followed by referral to specialized services if the patient wishes.

Fatigue

Fatigue is prevalent in AYA cancer survivors; Spathis et al. define it as a 'distressing, persistent, subjective sense of physical, emotional, and/or cognitive tiredness or exhaustion related to cancer or cancer treatment that is not proportional to recent activity and interferes with usual functioning' (see 'Further reading'). When reversible medical causes have been excluded (such as anaemia or depression), structured aerobic exercise routines (such as moderate walking exercise) may be helpful, as may educational interventions.

Psychosocial late effects

Anxiety, depression, and stress are more prevalent in AYAs than some other patient groups living after cancer, particularly soon after treatment. Financial issues, difficulties with work or education, and maintaining or forming close or sexual relationships with peers and life partners are common issues reported by AYAs over a prolonged period. It is important to offer support, to highlight reliable sources of information to ameliorate these adverse effects of cancer and its treatment, and also to manage AYAs in a multi-professional team with occupational health and social services that have expertise in managing these specific issues in AYAs.

Transition

Cancer care services can only provide expert specialist care for subgroups of the population. Therefore, as children living with or after cancer grow up into young people, it can be very good practice to transition their care to AYA services who specialize in that aspect of care. Later, they will move on to adult services and, eventually, if care has been successful, elderly care services. These transition processes will not succeed if they are not carried out proactively and expertly.

Future national and international priorities in this area

Internationally, various recent priorities have been set in this field. In the USA, in 2013, an update meeting was held to review evidence, scientific data, and priorities for AYAs aged 15–39 at cancer diagnosis. A group of 60 experts identified the large increase in published research in seven years and prioritized next steps, including:

- Epidemiology—subgroup analyses in incidence and outcomes, population-based data, and treatment data
- Biology—translational studies on 'difference' in AYA cancer biology, tissue banking, and data sharing
- Trials—population trial-entry data, age of eligibility, trial intergroups and collaborations, and consent processes
- Health services—place of care, pathways to care, financial toxicity, protocols, adherence, and insurance coverage
- Patient-reported outcomes—prospective, comparative, intervention, and psychometric study designs

In Canada, a group in Toronto have prioritized symptom management, return to work, and other aspects of survivorship such as fatigue. Fernandez et al. identified, as priorities, age-specific psychosocial, survivorship, palliative, and cancer care, and research to redress inequities in care for both the younger and older cancer patient. A pan-European group, funded by the European Union, prioritized work on professional networks and professional education, clinical trials, international comparative epidemiology, health lifestyles for young people to minimize cancer risk, and public and patient involvement in cancer services and research.

Globally, the importance of collaborative working and a network approach, bringing together the patient, charities, professionals, and their organizations is growing in the AYA field, including:

- Professional societies with specific groups working on AYAs through SIOPE ESMO and ASCO
- Professional networking groups such as CPAC (Canada), ENTYAC (EU), Go-AJA (France), AjeT (Germany), SIAMO (Italy), Space4AYA (Netherlands), AAA (Spain), TYAC (UK), and Critical Mass (USA)
- Charities such as Teenage Cancer Trust (UK), CanTeen (Australia), Canteen (Eire), and Teen Cancer America (USA)

Working together, the next few years appear promising for further improvements in outcomes for young people living with and after cancer.

NOTES

1. See http://www.sst.dk/~/media/A7052DCF93A641508A48A5B60A933A7D.ashx
2. See http://www.cancerworld.org/Articles/Issues/66/May-June-2015/e-Grand-Round/719/Teenagers-and-young-adults-with-cancer-addressing-the-most-important-care-needs.html
3. See https://www.teenagecancertrust.org/about-us/what-we-do/professional-leadership/international-conference and http://criticalmass.org/.
4. See https://www.teenagecancertrust.org/about-us/what-we-do/support-outside-our-units
5. See http://www.e-lfh.org.uk/programmes/adolescent-health/

FURTHER READING

Abrams AN, et al. (2007) Psychosocial issues in adolescents with cancer. *Cancer Treat Rev* **33**, 622–30.

Abrams AN, et al. (2007) Psychosocial issues in adolescents with cancer. *Cancer Treat Rev* **33**, 622–30.

Ahrensberg JM, et al. (2016) Primary care use before cancer diagnosis in adolescents and young adults—a nationwide register study. *PLoS One,* **11**, e0155933.

Barnett M, et al. (2016) Psychosocial outcomes and interventions among cancer survivors diagnosed during adolescence and young adulthood (AYA): a systematic review. *J Cancer Surviv* **10**(5), 814–31.

Barr RD, et al. (2016) Cancer in adolescents and young adults: a narrative review of the current status and a view of the future. *JAMA Pediatr* **170**(5), 495–501.

Barr RD, et al. (2016) Incidence and incidence trends of the most frequent cancers in adolescent and young adult Americans, including 'nonmalignant/noninvasive' tumors. *Cancer* **122**, 1000–8.

Bennett S, et al. (2016) Educational interventions for the management of cancer-related fatigue in adults. *Cochrane Database Syst Rev* **11**, CD008144.

Bleyer A, Barr R (2009) Cancer in young adults 20 to 39 years of age: overview. *Semin Oncol* **36**, 194–206.

Bleyer A, et al. (2005) National survival trends of young adults with sarcoma: lack of progress is associated with lack of clinical trial participation. *Cancer* **103**, 1891–7.

Bleyer A, et al. (2006) Cancer in 15- to 29-year-olds by primary site. *Oncologist* **11**, 590–601.

Bleyer A, et al. (2012) Children, adolescents, and young adults with leukemia: the empty half of the glass is growing. *J Clin Oncol* **30**, 4037–38; author reply 4038–9.

Bleyer WA, et al. (eds) (2006) *Cancer Epidemiology in Older Adolescents and Young Adults 15 to 29 Years of Age, Including SEER Incidence and Survival, 1975–2000.* Bethesda: National Cancer Institute.

Bleyer WA, et al. (1997) National cancer clinical trials: children have equal access; adolescents do not. *J Adolesc Health* **21**, 366–73.

Butow P, et al. (2010) Review of adherence-related issues in adolescents and young adults with cancer. *J Clin Oncol* **28**, 4800–9.

Campbell F, et al. (2016) Transition of care for adolescents from paediatric services to adult health services. *Cochrane Database System Rev* **4**, CD009794.

Chiavari L, et al. (2015) Difficult choices for young patients with cancer: the supportive role of decisional counseling. *Support Care Cancer* **23**, 3555–62.

Coccia PF, et al. (2014) Adolescent and young adult oncology, version 2. *J Natl Compr Canc Netw* **12**, 21–32; quiz 32.

Collins M, et al. (2013) Benefits and adverse events in younger versus older patients receiving neoadjuvant chemotherapy for osteosarcoma: findings from a meta-analysis. *J Clin Oncol* **31**, 2303–12.

Desandes E, Stark DP (2016) Epidemiology of adolescents and young adults with cancer in Europe. *Prog Tumor Res* **43**, 1–15. doi: 10.1159/000447037

Desandes E, et al. (2012) Pathways of care for adolescent patients with cancer in France from 2006 to 2007. *Pediatr Blood Cancer* **58**, 924–9.

Dieluweit U, et al. (2011) Educational and vocational achievement among long-term survivors of adolescent cancer in Germany. *Pediatr Blood Cancer* **56**, 432–8. doi: 10.1002/pbc.22806.

Dommett RM, et al. (2013) Features of cancer in teenagers and young adults in primary care: a population-based nested case-control study. *Br J Cancer* **108**, 2329–33.

Felgenhauer J, Hooke MC (2014) Regulatory barriers to clinical trial enrollment of adolescent and young adult oncology patients. *Pediatrics* **133**, S119–22. doi: 10.1542/peds.2014-0122H

Fern L, et al. (2008) Rates of inclusion of teenagers and young adults in England into National Cancer Research Network clinical trials: report from the National Cancer Research Institute (NCRI) Teenage and Young Adult Clinical Studies Development Group. *Br J Cancer* **99**, 1967–74.

Fern LA, et al. (2013) Why can't we improve the timeliness of cancer diagnosis in children, teenagers, and young adults? *BMJ* **347**, f6493.

Fern LA, et al. (2014) Available, accessible, aware, appropriate, and acceptable: a strategy to improve participation of teenagers and young adults in cancer trials. *Lancet Oncol* **15**, e341–50.

Fernandez C, et al. (2011) Principles and recommendations for the provision of healthcare in Canada to adolescent and young adult-aged cancer patients and survivors. *J Adolesc Young Adult Oncol* **1**, 53–9.

Ferrari A, et al. (2012) Upper age limits for accessing pediatric oncology centers in Italy: a barrier preventing adolescents with cancer from entering national cooperative AIEOP trials. *Pediatr Hematol Oncol* **29**, 55–61.

Ferrari A, Bleyer A (2007) Participation of adolescents with cancer in clinical trials. *Cancer Treat Rev* **33**, 603–8.

Ferrari A, et al. (2009) Adolescents with cancer in Italy: entry into the national cooperative paediatric oncology group AIEOP trials. *Eur J Cancer* **45**, 328–34.

Ferrari A, et al. (2010) Starting an adolescent and young adult program: some success stories and some obstacles to overcome. *J Clin Oncol* **28**, 4850–7.

Ferrari A, et al. (2015) Clouds of oxygen: adolescents with cancer tell their story in music. *J Clin Oncol* **33**, 218–21.

Ferrari A, et al. (2016) The sooner the better? How symptom interval correlates with outcome in children and adolescents with solid tumors: regression tree analysis of the findings of a prospective study. *Pediatr Blood Cancer* **63**, 479–85.

Ferrari A, et al. (2016) Adolescents with cancer in Italy: improving access to National Cooperative Pediatric Oncology Group (AIEOP) centers. *Pediatr Blood Cancer* **63**, 1116–19.

Ferrari A, et al. (2017) Access to clinical trials for adolescents with soft tissue sarcomas: enrollment in European pediatric Soft tissue sarcoma Study Group (EpSSG) protocols. *Pediatr Blood Cancer* **64**(6). doi: 10.1002/pbc.26348

Frazier AL, et al. (2008) Application of the adult international germ cell classification system to pediatric malignant non-seminomatous germ cell tumors: a report from the Children's Oncology Group. *Pediatr Blood Cancer* **50**, 746–51.

Frazier AL, et al. (2015) Revised risk classification for pediatric extracranial germ cell tumors based on 25 years of clinical trial data from the United Kingdom and United States. *J Clin Oncol* **33**, 195–201.

FREYER DR, Brugieres L (2008) Adolescent and young adult oncology: transition of care. *Pediatr Blood Cancer* **50**, 1116–19.

FUNG C, et al. (2013) Solid tumors after chemotherapy or surgery for testicular nonseminoma: a population-based study. *J Clin Oncol* **31**, 3807–14.

Gatta G, et al. (2014) Childhood cancer survival in Europe 1999–2007: results of EUROCARE-5—a population-based study. *Lancet Oncol* **15**, 35–47.

Geraci M, et al. (2007) Cancer mortality in 13 to 29-year-olds in England and Wales, 1981–2005. *Br J Cancer* **97**, 1588–94.

Gibson F, et al. (2012) A scoping exercise of favourable characteristics of professionals working in teenage and young adult cancer care: 'thinking outside of the box'. *Eur J Cancer Care (Engl)* **21**, 330–9.

Gupta AA, et al. (2010) Clinical outcome of children and adults with localized Ewing sarcoma: impact of chemotherapy dose and timing of local therapy. *Cancer* 116, 3189–94. doi: 10.1002/cncr.25144

Gupta AA, et al. (2012) Patterns of chemotherapy-induced toxicities in younger children and adolescents with rhabdomyosarcoma: a report from the Children's Oncology Group Soft Tissue Sarcoma Committee. *Cancer* **118**, 1130–7.

Gupta AA, et al. (2016) Reimagining care for adolescent and young adult cancer programs: moving with the times. *Cancer* **122**, 1038–46.

Hayes-Lattin B, et al. (2010) Adolescent and young adult oncology training for health professionals: a position statement. *J Clin Oncol* 28, 4858–61.

Hollis R, Morgan S (2001) The adolescent with cancer—at the edge of no-man's land. *Lancet Oncol* **2**, 43–8.

Jakes AD, et al. (2014) Critical review of clinical practice guidelines for fertility preservation in teenagers and young adults with cancer. *J Adolesc Young Adult Oncol* **3**, 144–52.

Jones LJ, et al. (2016) How do teenagers and young adults with cancer experience their care? A European survey. *J Adolesc Young Adult Oncol* **17**, 17.

Keegan TH, et al. (2016) Comparison of cancer survival trends in the United States of adolescents and young adults with those in children and older adults. *Cancer* **122**, 1009–16.

Kelly D, et al. (2004) 'Being in the same boat': ethnographic insights into an adolescent cancer unit. *Int J Nurs Stud* **41**, 847–57.

Kohsaka S, et al. (2014) A recurrent neomorphic mutation in MYOD1 defines a clinically aggressive subset of embryonal rhabdomyosarcoma associated with PI3K-AKT pathway mutations. *Nat Genet* **46**, 595–600.

Kondryn HJ, et al. (2011) Treatment non-adherence in teenage and young adult patients with cancer. *Lancet Oncol* **12**, 100–8.

Kumar A, et al. (2005) Are experimental treatments for cancer in children superior to established treatments? Observational study of randomised controlled trials by the Children's Oncology Group. *BMJ* **331**(7528), 1295.

Kwak M, et al. (2013) Trajectories of psychological distress in adolescent and young adult patients with cancer: a 1-year longitudinal study. *J Clin Oncol* **31**, 2160–6.

Lambertini M, et al. (2016) Cancer and fertility preservation: international recommendations from an expert meeting. *BMC Med* **14**, 1.

Lee JS, et al. (2016) Increased risk of second malignant neoplasms in adolescents and young adults with cancer. *Cancer* **122**, 116–23.

Michelagnoli MP, et al. (2003) Adolescent oncology—a homeland for the 'lost tribe'. *Eur J Cancer* 39, 2571–2.

Moricke A, et al. (2005) Prognostic impact of age in children and adolescents with acute lymphoblastic leukemia: data from the trials ALL-BFM 86, 90, and 95. *Klin Padiatr* 217, 310–20.

Mulder RL, et al. (2013) Recommendations for breast cancer surveillance for female survivors of childhood, adolescent, and young adult cancer given chest radiation: a report from the International Late Effects of Childhood Cancer Guideline Harmonization Group. *Lancet Oncol* **14**, e621–9.

Munhoz RR, et al. (2016) Gonadotropin-releasing hormone agonists for ovarian function preservation in premenopausal women undergoing chemotherapy for early-stage breast cancer: a systematic review and meta-analysis. *JAMA Oncol* **2**, 65–73. doi: 10.1001/jamaoncol.2015.3251

NICE(UK) (2005) *Improving Outcomes in Children and Young People with Cancer. Cancer Service Guidance*. London: NICE.

O'Hara C, et al. (2015) Trends in survival for teenagers and young adults with cancer in the UK 1992–2006. *Eur J Cancer* **51**, 2039–48.

Partridge AH, et al. (2016) Subtype-dependent relationship between young age at diagnosis and breast cancer survival. *J Clin Oncol* **34**, 3308–14. doi: 10.1200/JCO.2015.65.8013

Peccatori FA, et al. (2013) Cancer, pregnancy and fertility: ESMO Clinical Practice Guidelines for diagnosis, treatment and follow-up. *Ann Oncol* **24**(Suppl 6), vi160–70.

Peppercorn JM, et al. (2004) Comparison of outcomes in cancer patients treated within and outside clinical trials: conceptual framework and structured review. *Lancet* **363**, 263–70.

Pini S, et al. (2013) The impact of a cancer diagnosis on the education engagement of teenagers—patient and staff perspective. *Eur J Oncol Nurs* **17**, 317–23. doi: 10.1016/j.ejon.2012.08.005

Pini S, et al. (2012) What effect does a cancer diagnosis have on the educational engagement and school life of teenagers? A systematic review. *Psycho-oncology* **21**, 685–94. doi: 10.1002/pon.2082

Richardson DP, et al. (2015) Hospitalization rates among survivors of young adult malignancies. *J Clin Oncol* **33**, 2655–9.

Robert C, et al. (2015) Improved overall survival in melanoma with combined dabrafenib and trametinib. *N Engl J Med* **372**, 30–9. doi: 10.1056/NEJMoa1412690

Robison LL, Hudson MM (2014) Survivors of childhood and adolescent cancer: life-long risks and responsibilities. *Nat Rev Cancer* **14**, 61–70.

Rosen DS, et al. (2003) Transition to adult health care for adolescents and young adults with chronic conditions: position paper of the Society for Adolescent Medicine. *J Adolesc Health* **33**, 309–11.

Rugbjerg K, Olsen JH (2016) Long-term risk of hospitalization for somatic diseases in survivors of adolescent or young adult cancer. *JAMA Oncol* 2(2), 193–200.

Rugbjerg K, et al. (2014) Cardiovascular disease in survivors of adolescent and young adult cancer: a Danish cohort study, 1943–2009. *J Natl Cancer Inst* **106**(6), dju110.

Smith AW, et al. (2013) Unmet support service needs and health-related quality of life among adolescents and young adults with cancer: the AYA HOPE Study. *Front Oncol* **3**, 75.

Smith AW, et al. (2016) Next steps for adolescent and young adult oncology workshop: An update on progress and recommendations for the future. *Cancer* **122**, 988–99.

Spathis A, et al. (2015) Teenage and young adult cancer-related fatigue is prevalent, distressing, and neglected: it is time to intervene. A systematic literature review and narrative synthesis. *J Adolesc Young Adult Oncol* **4**, 3–17.

Stark D, et al. (2015) Teenagers and young adults with cancer in Europe: from national programmes to a European integrated co-ordinated project. *Eur J Cancer Care (Engl)* **25**(3), 419–27.

Stiller CA, et al. (2012) Population survival from childhood cancer in Britain during 1978–2005 by eras of entry to clinical trials. *Ann Oncol* **23**, 2464–69. doi: 10.1093/annonc/mds183

Sultan I, et al. (2009) Comparing adult and pediatric rhabdomyosarcoma in the surveillance, epidemiology and end results program, 1973 to 2005: an analysis of 2,600 patients. *J Clin Oncol* **27**, 3391–7.

Tai E, et al. (2014) Understanding and addressing the lack of clinical trial enrollment among adolescents with cancer. *Pediatrics* **133**, S98–103. doi: 10.1542/peds.2014-0122D

Taylor RM, et al. (2013) Developing a conceptual model of teenage and young adult experiences of cancer through meta-synthesis. *Int J Nurs Stud* **50**, 832–46.

Teenage Cancer Trust (2016) The *Blueprint of Care: For Teenagers and Young Adults with Cancer* (2nd edn). London: Teenage Cancer Trust.

Tian L, et al. (2016) Effects of aerobic exercise on cancer-related fatigue: a meta-analysis of randomized controlled trials. *Support Care Cancer* **24**, 969–83.

Trama A, et al. (2016) Survival of European adolescents and young adults diagnosed with cancer in 2000–07: population-based data from EUROCARE-5. *Lancet Oncol* **17**, 896–906.

Tricoli JV, et al. (2016) Biologic and clinical characteristics of adolescent and young adult cancers: acute lymphoblastic leukemia, colorectal cancer, breast cancer, melanoma, and sarcoma. *Cancer* **122**, 1017–28.

Veal GJ, et al. (2010) Clinical pharmacology in the adolescent oncology patient. *J Clin Oncol* **28**, 4790–9.

Warner EL, et al. (2016) Social well-being among adolescents and young adults with cancer: a systematic review. *Cancer* **122**(7), 1029–37.

Weller D, et al. (2012) The Aarhus statement: improving design and reporting of studies on early cancer diagnosis. *Br J Cancer* **106**, 1262–7.

Woodward E, et al. (2011) Late effects in survivors of teenage and young adult cancer: does age matter? *Ann Oncol* **22**, 2561–8.

Zebrack B, et al. (2010) To foster healing among adolescents and young adults with cancer. What helps? What hurts? *Support Care Cancer* **18**, 131–5.

Zebrack B, Isaacson S (2012) Psychosocial care of adolescent and young adult patients with cancer and survivors. *J Clin Oncol* **30**, 1221–6. doi: 10.1200/JCO.2011.39.5467

14

Late Effects of Therapy and Survivorship Issues

Lars Hjorth, Riccardo Haupt, Gisela Michel, Maria Luisa Garrè, Leontien C.M. Kremer, and Rod Skinner

Introduction

The high survival rate in children and adolescents with malignancy is accompanied by a substantial risk of late adverse events (LAEs). Treatment may interfere with physiological growth and psychosocial development in children and adolescents, and have an important impact on health status later in life, whilst some late toxicities may even cause premature death.

One study in the USA revealed that 62% of adult survivors of childhood malignancy have at least one treatment-induced chronic health condition (and 38% have two or more), whilst 28% have a severe or life-threatening problem. Similar data were reported in a Dutch study. Survivors of central nervous system (CNS) tumours or haematopoietic stem-cell transplantation (HSCT) are at particularly high risk. Much of the survivorship data has come from the North American Childhood Cancer Survivor Study (CCSS), the British Childhood Cancer Survivor Study (BCCSS), the Dutch Childhood Oncology Group LATER (DCOG LATER), and the Nordic Adult Life after Childhood Cancer in Scandinavia (ALiCCS) study.

In general, frequently recognized risk factors include patient age at treatment, site and type of the tumour, type and cumulative dose of chemotherapeutic agents, as well as dose and site of radiotherapy. In addition, the patient's pre-existing clinical status and previous or concurrent exposure to other toxic treatments may predispose to greater late toxicity.

The importance of moving from cure at any cost to cure at least cost is now well recognized, especially for patients with high cure rates. For all patients, higher cure rates and the risk of late complications make long-term follow-up (LTFU) a vital component of care (Figure 14.1).

Epidemiology

Recent estimates from several western countries put the proportion of long-term childhood cancer survivors (CCSs) at 0.10–0.15% of the general population, implying that one in every 650–1,000 persons is a CCS. It has been estimated that there are now about 400,000 CCSs in the USA, and 300,000–500,000 in Europe. Based on a conservative estimate that 75% of those treated on current protocols for childhood cancer will become long-term survivors (more than5 years), each year about 8,000 new CCSs are added to each of the USA and European populations. Their median age is estimated at 29 years, some are already more than 50 years old, and more than 20% have already survived more than 30 years since cancer diagnosis. These data demonstrate the need for adult physicians to be interested in the care of CCSs.

Late mortality

Cumulative mortality rates rise amongst CCSs as the duration of their follow-up continues. The BCCSS recently showed that CCSs had a 9.1-fold increased risk of dying prematurely, which equals 64.2 excess deaths per 10,000 person years. Similar data have been reported by the Swiss population-based registry, with an 11.0 times increased risk of premature death and 45 excess deaths per 10,000 person years. However, a decline in late mortality has been observed with more recent treatment periods. Data from the CCSS found 15-year cumulative mortality for CCSs diagnosed between 1970 and 1979 to be 10.7%, while it was 5.8% for those diagnosed between 1990 and 1999. A Nordic study found the overall standardized mortality ratio (SMR) to be 8.3, with an absolute excess risk of 6.2 per 1,000 person years. This study also found that after ten years, the mortality changed very little with time period. During the first 10–15 years after diagnosis, excess mortality is mainly due to the primary cancer, but beyond this point there is increasing mortality from second malignant neoplasms (SMNs) and circulatory and pulmonary causes.

There is good evidence that exposures to radiotherapy, alkylating agents, or epipodophyllotoxins carry the greatest relative risks (RRs) for late mortality from SMNs. The risk factors for long-term circulatory and cardiovascular risk have been less well determined. A French and UK study evaluated this in the context of data on

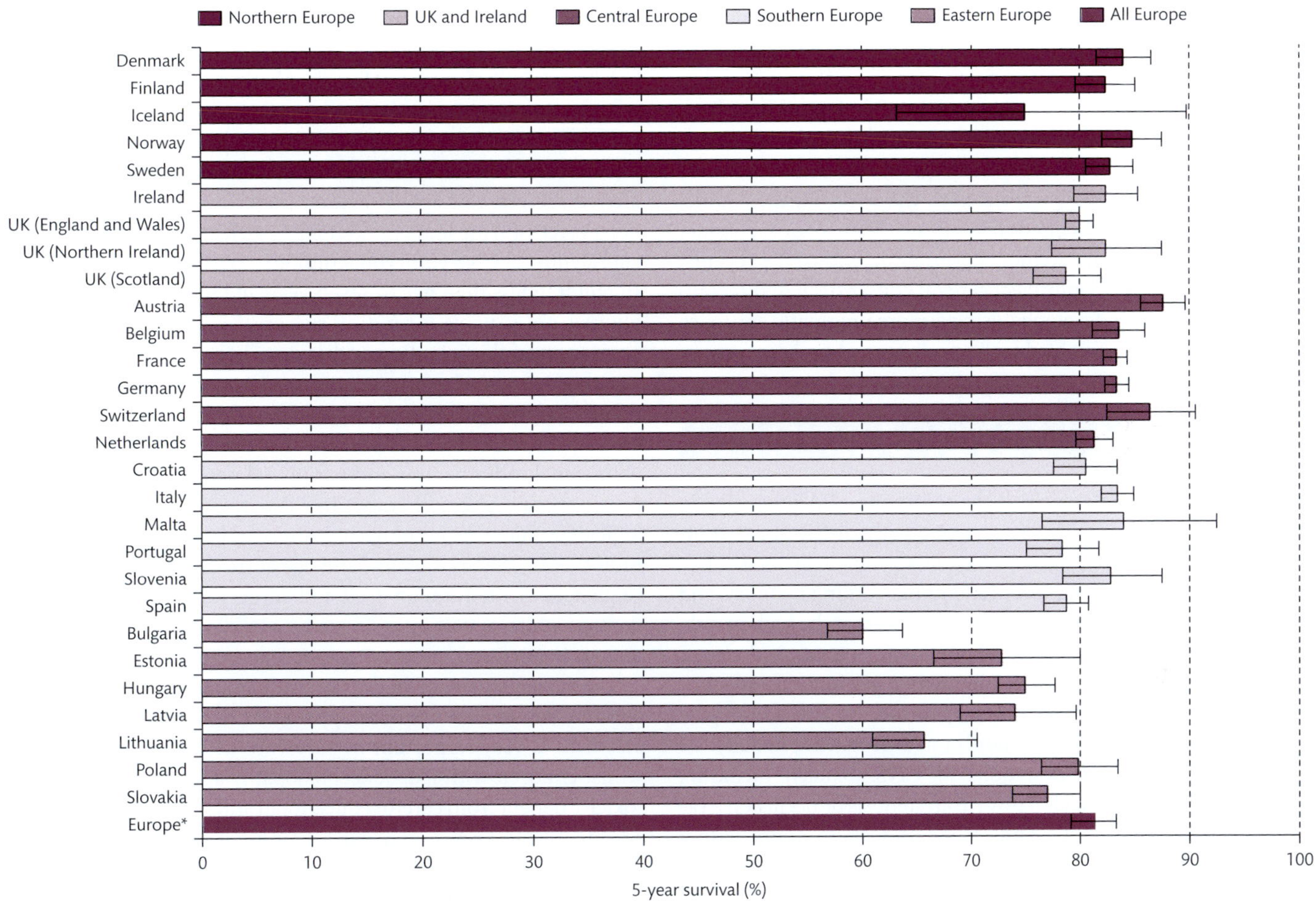

Figure 14.1 Five-year survival for all cancers combined (CNS tumours excluded) diagnosed in 2000–2007, by country, in European children (0–14 years) of both sexes. The data are adjusted by age, sex, case mix, and period of diagnosis using a Cox proportional hazards model.

Reproduced with permission from Gatta G. et al. 'Childhood cancer survival in Europe 1999-2007: results of EUROCARE-5—a population-based study', *Lancet Oncology*, Volume 15, Issue 1, pp. 35–47. Copyright © 2014 Elsevier Ltd. DOI: https://doi.org/10.1016/S1470-2045(13)70548-5

both chemotherapy exposure and radiation dose to the heart. The overall SMR for survivors was 8.3-fold higher in relation to the general populations in France and the UK, and there was a five-fold increase in death from cardiovascular disease. The risk of dying was significantly higher in individuals who had received a cumulative anthracycline dose greater than 360 mg/m^2 and in individuals who received an average cardiac radiation dose that exceeded 5 Gy. The largest analysis of late mortality yet is being performed by the PanCareSurFup Consortium and includes 77,279 five-year survivors with a mean follow-up of 23 years.

These findings highlight the need for adult healthcare providers to understand the risks confronting CCSs and for strategies to detect serious complications early in an attempt to prevent excess late deaths. Screening for secondary breast cancer is one example of such an approach.

Secondary malignant neoplasms

Several studies have shown that CCSs have an increased risk of developing SMNs. The RR is high (5–10) but, in absolute numbers, the individual risk is low, ranging from one to three additional cancers per 1,000 person years. After 20 years' follow-up, the cumulative risk is 3–7%. The risk remains elevated even in the fifth and sixth decades of life. A recent study from the CCSS found that the risk of a second cancer remained higher for CCSs diagnosed in the 1990s than for the age-matched general population, but that the scale of increased risk was lower than that observed in CCSs diagnosed in the 1970s. Use of lower treatment doses was considered to be the likeliest reason for this reduction in risk.

The most common SMNs are breast cancer, myelodysplasia/acute myeloid leukaemia (MDS/AML), bone and soft-tissue sarcoma, CNS tumours (e.g. meningiomas), and thyroid cancer. The latency period varies greatly, with an average of 12 years between first and second malignancies, with leukaemia occurring earlier and solid tumours later. Patients with a genetic tumour predisposition have an increased risk of developing a SMN. Radiotherapy, even at doses of less than 1 Gy, is the main risk factor for developing SMNs, whilst alkylating agents and epipodophyllotoxins are the most commonly implicated cytotoxic drugs. Recently, the LATER study showed that doxorubicin exposure increases the risk of subsequent solid cancers and breast cancer, whereas cyclophosphamide increases the risk of subsequent sarcomas.

Measures that CCSs can take to decrease their risk of developing SMNs include avoidance of tobacco smoking and protection from excessive exposure to sunlight. The International Guideline Harmonization Group (IGHG) has been developing evidence based guidelines concerning surveillance for SMNs as well for other clinical relevant late complications. So far recommendations have been published for secondary breast cancer screening in female survivors treated with radiotherapy in the breast region, as well for secondary thyroid cancer in survivors irradiated to the neck. Further guidelines are under development addressing surveillance for secondary CNS tumours and colon carcinoma. Moreover, within the recently granted PanCareFollowUp project general consensus based recommendations are being developed using a more pragmatic approach to address secondary skin, bladder, bone, lung, and oral cancers.

Neurological and neuropsychological toxicity

Long-term neurological toxicity is the commonest LAE reported in the CCSS, occurring in 27% of survivors, with an RR of 3.3 compared to a sibling control group. Cognitive impairments are frequently found in processing speed, attention, working memory, and executive function. Survivors of CNS tumours are at the highest risk, followed by survivors of Hodgkin lymphoma or acute leukaemia. However, not only tumour and treatment type, but also psychological distress, social support, and long absences from school play an important role in the development of neurocognitive toxicity.

There are several manifestations of CNS toxicity, including leucoencephalopathy, vasculopathy (from stenosis or occlusion), radiation necrosis, myelopathy, and secondary CNS tumours, with a wide variety of clinical sequelae threatening life or greatly impairing the survivor's quality of life. In contrast, peripheral nervous system toxicity has fewer manifestations, usually presenting as peripheral neuropathy, although long-term functional difficulties are increasingly recognized in CCSs treated with vincristine (e.g. for acute lymphoblastic leukaemia (ALL)) or cisplatin.

Leucoencephalopathy may present with focal motor signs, spasticity, seizures, and ataxia. Neuropsychological dysfunction may occur, being apparent by cognitive impairment with considerable adverse impact on intelligence, attention and learning skills, memory, and verbal and visual–spatial skills. Vasculopathy may cause seizures, stroke, and dementia. Radiation necrosis may result in neurocognitive and/or neuropsychological dysfunction, whilst myelopathy may lead to paraplegia or quadriplegia, as well as sphincter dysfunction. A variety of secondary CNS tumours are reported including malignant gliomas, neuroectodermal tumours, and meningiomas.

Most neurological/neuropsychological toxicity is related to CNS radiotherapy and/or CNS-directed chemotherapy (i.e. intrathecal chemotherapy, or certain chemotherapy regimens such as high-dose methotrexate or cytarabine). Leucoencephalopathy and neuropsychological toxicity occur predominantly in survivors of CNS tumours or acute leukaemia treated with CNS radiotherapy or CNS-directed chemotherapy, and are commoner and more severe in patients treated at a younger age.

Cranial radiotherapy (CRT) can decrease the white-matter volume and has been associated with reduced cognitive abilities across domains including global intelligence, attention, working memory, and executive dysfunction, translating into a higher risk of educational and social difficulties. Intrathecal chemotherapy has been associated with reduced academic achievement, deficits in attention and working memory, and slower processing speed, perhaps due to disruption of white-matter circuitry in the developing brain.

Alternative options to CRT, such as high-dose chemotherapy or intensification of systemic chemotherapy (with or without intrathecal chemotherapy), have been investigated in young children with malignant brain tumours, in order avoid irradiation or to delay it until after three years of age. However, these treatment strategies have been successful for some tumour types such as medulloblastoma and supratentorial CNS embryonal tumours, but not for ependymomas. In children less than five to seven years old with midline low-grade gliomas not suitable for radical surgery, 'gentle chemotherapy' has been successful in avoiding or delaying CRT.

Other aspects of neurotoxicity are related more to specific treatment components. For example, vasculopathy and radiation necrosis are associated with previous CNS radiotherapy, myelopathy with spinal radiotherapy, and peripheral neuropathy with cisplatin or vincristine chemotherapy. In CNS tumour survivors, neurological and neuropsychological status can be impaired not only by radiotherapy, chemotherapy, and age at treatment, but also by consequences of the tumour itself and surgery. Surgical resection can damage white-matter integrity, reduce intellectual ability, and cause deficits in attention, processing speed, and memory.

The management of neurotoxicity comprises both general and specific measures. Physiotherapy and/or occupational therapy assessment is very important in survivors with physical disabilities, whilst children with leucoencephalopathy and neuropsychological toxicity benefit from careful educational and neuropsychological assessment, with provision of extra support at school and subsequent employment guidance. Psychotherapy and specific drug therapy can be used to treat depression and anxiety, resulting in a better quality of life. Surgery may be considered in selected cases of vasculopathy and drug treatment may be beneficial in painful neuropathy.

In recent years, the doses of radiotherapy used in the treatment of several childhood malignancies have been reduced (especially those used in CRT), as have the volumes of normal brain treated. Radiotherapy has been omitted in many malignancies (especially ALL) or delayed until the child is older (e.g. in infants with brain tumours). Improvement of CRT techniques has been obtained with intensity-modulated radiotherapy (IMRT), intensity-modulated arc therapy (IMAT), and proton therapy. These techniques allow sparing of normal brain with the aim of minimizing neurocognitive sequelae.

Endocrine toxicity

Endocrine complications are the second commonest group of chronic conditions in CCSs, occurring in 20–50% of survivors followed into adulthood. They include hypothalamic–pituitary, thyroid, and gonadal dysfunction, bone disease, and metabolic disorders.

Sequelae may be associated both with the tumour type and location, and with treatment. In addition to the effects of surgery, direct endocrine gland involvement by the malignancy (e.g. germinal tumours, CNS tumours involving the hypothalamic–pituitary axis (HPA)), and hydrocephalus caused by some brain tumours, both radiotherapy and chemotherapy may increase the risk of endocrine complications. Survivors treated with radiotherapy to the head, neck, or pelvis, and those treated with total body irradiation (TBI) or with alkylating agents, are at increased risk.

Hypothalamic-pituitary dysfunction

The total dose of CRT is the strongest risk factor for anterior pituitary dysfunction. However, the threshold dose for specific endocrine dysfunction varies for different pituitary hormones.

Growth hormone

Growth hormone (GH) deficiency is the most common anterior pituitary deficiency observed after CRT, and if it occurs, it is usually permanent. It may become manifest after a CRT dose ≥18 Gy; after more than 24 Gy, the deficiency usually becomes apparent within five years, while for doses in the range of 18–24 Gy, GH deficiency may develop ten years or even later after treatment, with increased risk persisting throughout adult life.

Patients treated for brain tumours, sarcomas, or ALL are at higher risk of GH deficiency. The frequency of GH deficiency in CCSs treated in the last two decades has fallen since leukaemic patients treated with recent protocols are less likely to have received CRT.

Growth and pubertal development should be monitored closely in children at risk of GH deficiency to facilitate early diagnosis and treatment. Untreated GH deficiency will impair growth velocity and eventually final height. However, other factors such as spinal radiotherapy (which may impair vertebral growth), age at treatment, and timing of puberty contribute to the individual's final height. Importantly, precocious puberty (see below) may mask GH deficiency, which then becomes evident only after cessation of the growth spurt. CNS tumour survivors are at higher risk of developing precocious puberty, thus careful examination of such individuals may maximize their potential to achieve adequate final height.

The most sensitive and specific test to diagnose GH deficiency is the insulin tolerance test (ITT). If abnormal, another stimulation test (either with GNRH-arginine or glucagon) should be performed to confirm the diagnosis. Measurement of insulin-like growth factor (IGF-1) and IGFBP-3 alone is not a good predictor of GH deficiency.

If GH deficiency is confirmed, GH replacement therapy should be considered. Concerns have arisen about the potential impact of GH treatment on tumour recurrence, but the available data do not demonstrate a significantly increased risk of tumour relapse in children treated with GH compared to those with the same type of tumour not treated with GH. Although a small but significant increased risk of SMNs seems to exist for survivors during GH treatment, the second tumours observed are the same as those occurring in those CCSs not treated with GH.

Gonadotrophins

Timely and appropriate gonadotrophin release from the HPA triggers hormonal release from the testis or ovary. This allows a linear growth spurt, development of secondary sexual characteristics, fertility, and maintenance of gonadal function during adulthood. Except in a few cases of CNS tumours directly affecting the HPA, CRT is the main risk factor for altered gonadotrophin release. In these cases, gonadotrophins may be secreted either earlier or later (precocious or delayed puberty, respectively) than the usual physiological timing.

Precocious puberty has been associated with intracranial tumours, raised intracranial pressure, cranial surgery, or radiation doses to the HPA as low as those given for CNS prophylactic treatment in ALL (range 18–24 Gy), in particular in females treated at a younger age. However, delayed puberty is more common. The risk of developing gonadotrophin deficiency is dose-related, especially with CRT doses of more than 30 Gy.

Patients at risk should be closely monitored during the peripubertal years (from nine years in females and ten years in males) or even before in survivors at risk for precocious puberty. Growth and pubertal status assessed by Tanner scoring should be monitored at least yearly until completion of puberty; follicle-stimulating hormone/luteinizing hormone (FSH/LH) and 17β-oestradiol or testosterone should be evaluated in children with suspected early or delayed onset of puberty. This allows identification of hypo- or hypergonadotrophic hypogonadism, or precocious puberty, and the initiation of appropriate replacement (delayed puberty) or antagonist (precocious puberty) treatment.

Other hypothalamic trophins

Both thyroid-stimulating hormone (TSH) and adrenocorticotropic hormone (ACTH)deficiency may occur after radiotherapy doses to the brain of more than 30 Gy in up to 10% of patients at risk. Hyperprolactinaemia is rare and usually subclinical, occurring only in women treated with high-dose radiotherapy.

Hypothalamic obesity syndrome

Hypothalamic obesity may occur in patients with tumours infiltrating the medial hypothalamic region, like craniopharyngiomas. Severe obesity is seen in about 50% of patients, leading to a high rate of cardiovascular mortality. Structural damage to the hypothalamic nuclei may lead to hyperphagia, rapid weight gain, central insulin and leptin resistance, decreased sympathetic activity, low energy expenditure, and increased energy storage in adipose tissue.

Gonadal dysfunction

Pubertal growth and reproductive function are controlled by hormones secreted by the testis or ovary. The main difference between males and females is that in males, two distinct testicular cell types control sexual development (Leydig cells) and fertility (Sertoli cells), while in females, the oocyte controls both pubertal development and fertility.

Ovarian dysfunction

Germ-cell failure and loss of ovarian endocrine function occur concomitantly in females. They may be due either to pelvic, abdominal, or spinal radiotherapy, TBI, or alkylating-agent chemotherapy. There is no clear threshold dose for either radiotherapy or alkylating agents, but there is evidence that women exposed to higher doses have a higher risk of premature ovarian insufficiency. Doses above 20 Gy to the ovaries will almost always lead to permanent hormonal deficit. Age at treatment is important in predicting ovarian failure; females treated at a younger age are less likely to develop ovarian failure, probably because of the higher number of primordial follicles at the time of treatment.

The clinical picture depends on the age at onset and severity of the ovarian damage. In pre- or peripubertal girls, delay, arrest, or failure of pubertal onset may occur; in post-pubertal women, the clinical picture may comprise secondary amenorrhoea, irregular menstrual periods, or premature menopause. Laboratory testing demonstrates elevated gonadotrophins and reduced or absent 17β-oestradiol. Replacement oestro-progestogen therapy should be considered in order to induce puberty in females without onset and/or maintenance of regular periods. Ovarian insufficiency may be permanent or transient, thus replacement treatment should be discontinued at intervals to determine if spontaneous periods occur. Most of these females are infertile or at high risk of premature menopause, thus appropriate counselling should be given concerning the likely need for assisted reproduction.

Uterine morphology (shape, dimensions, and structure, e.g. fibrosis or reduced endometrial thickness) should be evaluated in females treated with pelvic or abdominal radiotherapy to assess the likelihood of embryonal implantation or successful completion of foetal development.

Testicular dysfunction

The testis is sensitive both to chemotherapy and radiotherapy. Among chemotherapeutic agents, cumulative doses of alkylating agents and timing of treatment influence the risk of oligo/azoospermia. Damage to germinal epithelium is estimated to occur after a testicular radiotherapy dose of more than 2–3 Gy (and occasionally even lower doses) either as direct testicular radiotherapy or during abdominal or spinal radiotherapy or an inverted Y field for Hodgkin lymphoma treatment. Leydig cells are much more radioresistant and only doses ≥20 Gy or TBI are likely to cause complete primary hypogonadism. In contrast to females, age at treatment has minimal impact on testicular function.

The clinical picture of testicular insufficiency depends on the severity and timing of damage. Low testosterone levels with high gonadotrophins indicate decreased Leydig cell function, resulting in delayed or absent pubertal onset in younger patients, or clinical symptoms of testosterone deficiency such as reduced muscle strength, irritability, and decreased libido in post-pubertal survivors.

CCSs with evidence of testosterone deficiency should be referred to an appropriate specialist for consideration of testosterone replacement treatment. This should be given for delayed or absent pubertal onset, or in adults with documented testosterone deficiency (less than 250 ng/dl; less than 8.7 nmol/l) with or without symptoms. Damage to the Sertoli cells is more frequent and it is nearly always permanent. A definitive diagnosis of male infertility may only be made after semen analysis. For pre-pubertal boys, studies of testicular tissue cryopreservation are ongoing.

Thyroid toxicity

The thyroid gland is sensitive to radiotherapy given either externally to the neck (as in Hodgkin lymphoma treatment, CRT, or TBI) or targeted via thyroid metabolism (^{131}I treatment for thyroid diseases like carcinoma or hyperthyroidism, sometimes after metaiodobenzylguanidine (MIBG) treatment in neuroblastoma due to uncoupling of ^{131}I from ^{131}I-MIBG). The functional changes after external-beam radiotherapy sometimes occur as early as six months after treatment, but may only become evident up to 20 years later, and comprise clinical or subclinical hypothyroidism with a combined incidence of 20–30%. Hyperthyroidism and autoimmune manifestations (Hashimoto thyroiditis) have been described in a smaller proportion. The morphological changes consist of benign lesions (primarily adenomas), multinodular goitre, and malignant lesions, with an average 5–69-fold increased risk compared to the normal population, depending on the radiotherapy dose. The effect of radiotherapy on the thyroid gland seems to be both dose- and age-dependent, with younger children at higher risk. A linear relationship with radiotherapy doses and thyroid late complications has been observed, but after doses of more than 30 Gy, the cancer risk decreases, probably because of a cell-killing effect.

Thyroid hormones and TSH should be measured routinely in patients at risk. Overt (clinical) primary hypothyroidism results in low thyroid hormone values with high TSH concentrations, whilst subclinical hypothyroidism is characterized by normal thyroxine but high TSH levels. Replacement therapy must be prescribed in case of overt hypothyroidism and should be considered in case of multinodular goitre.

Surveillance for thyroid cancer should be recommended to all patients at risk. Careful clinical examination of the neck to detect nodules or lumps should be performed regularly, and some centres supplement this with ultrasound imaging, although it is uncertain which, if any, strategy is superior in terms of reducing morbidity and mortality from thyroid cancer. Therefore no strong recommendation can be made about the type and timing of screening modalities. This aspect has been summarized by the IGHG, addressing the balance between benefits and harms of each screening modality. Needle biopsy may be considered for suspicious abnormalities.

Metabolic syndrome

Metabolic syndrome (MS) is characterized by a clustering of hypertension, dyslipidaemia (low HDL cholesterol, hypertriglyceridaemia, hypercholesterolaemia), type 2 diabetes, or preclinical conditions (insulin resistance or glucose intolerance) and obesity. This condition is associated with a pro-inflammatory and pro-thrombotic state that may lead to atherogenic dyslipidaemia. There is evidence that survivors exposed to CRT, prolonged steroid treatment, TBI, or abdominal irradiation, and those with hypogonadism or limitations in physical performance (e.g. due to cardiac or pulmonary toxicity or functional impairments caused by major surgery) are at increased risk of glucose intolerance and MS.

Diagnosis of MS in adults is defined (International Diabetes Federation) by the presence of central obesity (waist circumference ≥94 cm in males, ≥80 cm in females), and at least two of the following:

- Raised blood pressure: more than 130/85 mmHg
- Raised triglycerides: more than 150 mg/dl (1.7 mmol/l)
- Reduced HDL cholesterol: less than 40 mg/dl (1.03 mmol/l) in males, or less than 50 mg/dl (1.29 mmol/l) in females
- Raised fasting glucose: ≥100 mg/ml (5.6 mmol/l).

The International Diabetes Federation does not recommend the diagnosis of MS in children under ten years, but the criteria for the diagnosis of MS in children from 10 to 16 years of age are broadly similar to those used in adults. Survivors, and in particular those with predisposing or treatment-related risk factors for MS, should be monitored with waist circumference and markers of MS, and counselled about appropriate diet and/or physical activity and avoidance of smoking.

Other toxicities

Cardiac toxicity

Cardiovascular disease, including heart failure, coronary artery disease, pericarditis, arrhythmia, and valvular disease, is an important health problem for CCSs. Survivors have a three- to seven-fold increased risk of premature death due to cardiac causes. Van der Pal et al. concluded that one in eight survivors treated with anthracyclines and radiotherapy to the heart region will develop a life-threatening cardiovascular event by 30 years after treatment.

Heart failure is the most common cardiovascular disease. The risk factors for heart failure are treatment with anthracyclines, mitoxantrone and/or radiotherapy to the heart region, and younger age at treatment. However, there is an individual variability for heart failure which may be caused by genetic susceptibility, although it is too early to use genetic assessment in clinical practice. Radiotherapy to the heart is a major risk factor for coronary artery disease, myocardial infarction, pericardial disease, and valvular abnormalities. At doses ≥15 Gy, the CCSS study found a two- to six-fold increased risk for the above complications in CCSs compared to healthy siblings.

Early detection of cardiovascular disease in CCSs is important. Surveillance recommendations exist for early detection of heart failure. Echocardiography is widely used to identify asymptomatic cardiac dysfunction before symptoms occur in survivors treated with cardiotoxic chemotherapy or radiotherapy to the heart. Routine surveillance is recommended for survivors at high risk for cardiomyopathy, defined as those with anthracycline exposure ≥250 mg/m^2, or ≥35 Gy chest radiotherapy, or a combination of ≥100 mg/m^2 of anthracyclines and ≥15 Gy chest radiotherapy. It may also be reasonable for survivors treated with lower doses, as is the case in more recent years. Although some studies have shown elevated levels of blood biomarkers (troponin and NT-proBNP), monitoring of biomarkers during follow-up is not recommended due to insufficient evidence for added diagnostic value. For the other cardiovascular diseases, no routine surveillance is recommended currently in the follow-up of survivors.

Prevention of cardiovascular diseases for patients treated for childhood cancer is essential. Primary prevention (before and during treatment) can include limiting anthracycline and radiotherapy doses. Other strategies include liposomal encapsulated doxorubicin or longer infusion time of anthracyclines. However, data in children are lacking. Concomitant treatment with a cardioprotective agent, such as dexrazoxane, has also been suggested for primary prevention. Randomized controlled trials (RCTs) in children and adults showed a cardioprotective effect. One observational study suggested an association between dexrazoxane and a higher risk of secondary malignancies, but these concerns have not been substantiated. Secondary prevention strategies include treatment with angiotensin-converting-enzyme (ACE) inhibitors and beta-blockers, and studies have suggested this may prevent or delay deterioration of cardiac function in survivors of cancer, although this remains to be confirmed in CCSs. Furthermore, it is important for survivors to have a healthy lifestyle and to seek early treatment of comorbidities.

Pulmonary toxicity

A recent Swiss study looked at self-reported pulmonary disease compared to siblings and found an increased risk of pneumonias and chest-wall abnormalities, with a cumulative incidence of 21% after 35 years. Chronic pulmonary health conditions were reported in 11.8% (RR 2.8) of survivors in the overall CCSS population. In survivors of CNS malignancies, the CCSS found rates of pulmonary fibrosis, chest-wall abnormalities, chronic cough, and the need for extra oxygen to be increased compared to siblings. There was a strong correlation between craniospinal irradiation and these adverse outcomes.

Both restrictive and obstructive lung disease may occur, whilst bronchiectasis may result from previous infections of the lower respiratory tract. Restrictive pulmonary disease may be subclinical, manifest only by abnormalities in pulmonary function tests (PFTs), or may present with progressive dyspnoea and respiratory failure due to pulmonary fibrosis, and is usually a consequence of either chemotherapy (particularly busulfan, carmustine, or lomustine) or radiotherapy that includes large volumes of normal lung, which is less and less the case with current techniques. Obstructive lung disease occurs most commonly in survivors of HSCT and is associated with chronic graft-versus-host (GvH) disease. Previous thoracic surgery may also impair lung function.

PFTs should be performed at the completion of treatment in at-risk patients and at regular intervals thereafter in symptomatic patients or those with abnormal test results. It is advisable to recommend pneumococcal and annual influenza immunization in patients with established lung disease.

Renal toxicity

Nephrotoxicity may be due to glomerular or tubular damage, or both. Chronic kidney disease (CKD) or the requirement for dialysis is an uncommon but serious late complication, occurring in 0.5% of survivors in the CCSS (RR 8.9). Glomerular toxicity is commonly subclinical and revealed only by a high-serum creatinine concentration, but may occasionally lead to CKD or, rarely, end-stage renal failure. Likewise, tubular damage may be subclinical, but clinically overt proximal tubulopathy may occur in 25–30% of children treated with potentially nephrotoxic chemotherapy. Chronic tubular toxicity after ifosfamide may result in hypophosphataemia and even hypophosphataemic rickets (HR), whilst cisplatin (and less commonly carboplatin) nephrotoxicity may cause hypomagnesaemia, which when severe may lead to convulsions, tetany, or cardiac arrhythmias. Ifosfamide may also rarely cause nephrogenic diabetes insipidus (NDI) due to distal tubular damage, or proximal or distal renal tubular acidosis (RTA). Renal damage may also cause hypertension and proteinuria in CCSs.

The main risk factors for nephrotoxicity are the specific chemotherapy drugs received and their doses, radiotherapy including renal tissue, and previous nephrectomy, whilst tumour-related urinary tract obstruction or pre-existing renal dysfunction may exacerbate renal impairment. Ifosfamide nephrotoxicity is more common in patients treated with a cumulative dose of more than 80 g/m^2. The increased frequency and severity of ifosfamide nephrotoxicity in children younger than five years old at treatment reported in several studies is not a universal finding, especially with longer follow-up. Platinum nephrotoxicity is more common in children treated with a higher cisplatin dose rate (more than 40 mg/m^2/day) or higher cumulative carboplatin doses, and those treated at an older age. Other cytotoxic drugs that may cause or contribute to nephrotoxicity in children include melphalan and high-dose methotrexate (both of which usually present with acute kidney injury which may not recover completely, leading to CKD), and the nitrosoureas (carmustine, lomustine, semustine) which may cause CKD. In addition, supportive-care drugs including aminoglycoside antibiotics and amphotericin, or immunosuppressive agents such as ciclosporin, may contribute to or represent a primary cause of renal damage.

Patients with suspected or established nephrotoxicity should undergo regular surveillance including measurement of blood pressure (especially also for those who received radiotherapy on the kidneys) and growth, urinalysis for proteinuria, and biochemical monitoring. Electrolyte supplementation or specific treatment of HR, RTA, and NDI may be required.

Lower urinary tract toxicity

Chronic lower urinary tract toxicity may manifest as haemorrhagic cystitis (HC) which may follow either radiotherapy or oxazaphosphorine (cyclophosphamide or ifosfamide) chemotherapy. Although most acute episodes of HC resolve fully, a few patients suffer from persistent or recurrent urinary symptoms, including frequency, dysuria, irritability and/or urgency, incontinence, and, occasionally, retention due to bladder fibrosis and dysfunction. Bladder damage due to the original malignancy or its treatment (with surgery or radiotherapy) may result in a small-volume bladder or sometimes a urethral stricture. Bladder malignancy is an uncommon but well recognized late complication of HC.

Urinary tract symptoms in CCSs should be evaluated by urinalysis, microscopy, and culture, and referral to a urologist may be required for cytoscopy or urodynamic studies. Regular urine cytology has been recommended in patients with a history of previous severe HC.

Visual toxicity

A wide variety of late ocular and visual toxicities may occur, ranging from dry eyes due to impaired lacrimal gland tear production, which predisposes to corneal ulceration and scarring, to visual impairment due to posterior subcapsular cataracts. Severe visual impairment was reported in 3% of survivors in the CCSS (RR 5.8) and may also be a consequence of the underlying disease (e.g. by direct invasion of optic structures or by intracranial hypertension) in survivors of CNS tumours, 13% of whom reported legal blindness in one or both eyes in the CCSS. Rarer adverse effects include keratitis, uveitis, chorioretinopathy, and optic neuritis.

Lacrimal gland dysfunction and cataract are related to radiotherapy including the eye or the use of TBI in children with haematological malignancies, up to a third of whom may develop later cataracts. Prolonged steroid treatment may also lead to cataract formation even in the absence of radiotherapy. Very rarely, chemotherapy may cause severe visual toxicity (e.g. visual loss related to high-dose fludarabine).

Treatment of ocular/visual toxicities includes artificial tear replacement for dry eyes and surgical removal of the lens affected by cataract (with insertion of a lens implant), but established visual loss is usually irreversible.

Auditory toxicity

Chronic hearing loss not corrected by a hearing aid was noted in 2% of CCSS survivors (RR 6.3), and any hearing impairment in 12% of CNS tumour survivors. The consequences of deafness in children include delayed speech development and impaired educational/social functioning, especially in younger children.

The major cause of chronic deafness in survivors of childhood malignancy is platinum chemotherapy, particularly cisplatin and, less commonly, high-dose carboplatin. Both higher cumulative cisplatin dose and younger age at treatment predict a higher risk of deafness, with a total dose of more than 400 mg/m^2 and an age of under five years being associated with development of bilateral sensorineural hearing loss in 40% of children. High-dose radiotherapy to the middle ear may cause mixed sensorineural and conductive hearing loss, but clinically significant deafness is uncommon in children who have not also received platinum treatment. Hearing loss may also be exacerbated or caused by other ototoxic treatment (e.g. aminoglycosides). Finally, CNS surgery, in particular for posterior fossa or brainstem tumours, may cause hearing problems.

Children who may have hearing loss should be assessed by pure-tone audiography, or by behavioural audiometry or otoacoustic emissions (or occasionally auditory brainstem responses) in younger children, and referred for ear, nose, and throat (ENT) or audiometric/speech-therapy assessment if hearing loss is identified. Education and community paediatric services should be alerted to children with significant hearing impairment. Early evaluation, even before confirmation of hearing loss, is important in infants treated with cisplatin or high-dose carboplatin.

Craniofacial and dental toxicity

Craniofacial and dental complications are more prevalent in patients treated at a young age. The most important risk factor is radiotherapy to the face or brain, although chemotherapy may be an added risk factor. Radiotherapy to the growing skull and face will lead to hypoplasia of the irradiated area; the younger the child and the higher the radiotherapy dose, the more pronounced the growth impairment. As normal growth occurs, the deformity becomes progressively more pronounced.

Correction of skeletal complications may be problematic due to the nature of the irradiated bone which can make surgery difficult. Damage to rudimentary teeth may result in the absence of permanent teeth, whilst that occurring later in dental development may result in small, brittle teeth. Damage to dental roots may lead to tooth loss, and caries is accelerated by xerostomia from radiation effect on salivary glands.

Due to these potential dental problems, preventive measures are very important when receiving radiotherapy and/or chemotherapy, and guidelines for this have been published.

Gastrointestinal and hepatic toxicity

Surgery (including permanent stomas) and radiotherapy to the gastrointestinal tract may cause late complications including strictures, malabsorption, and vitamin B_{12} deficiency. Large radiotherapy volumes and/or high doses are associated with a higher incidence of gastrointestinal problems. Hepatitis due to viral infection after blood transfusion remains a problem, although the frequency is now much lower due to better blood-product surveillance. Long-term follow-up (LTFU) for those at risk should include liver function tests and examination for signs of liver disease, such as hepatosplenomegaly or jaundice.

Skin toxicity

Late skin complications after treatment for childhood cancer include non-melanomatous skin cancer (NMSC) (most commonly basal cell carcinoma, but also squamous cell carcinoma), melanoma, alopecia and sparse/patchy hair, scarring, atrophy, and pigmentation disorders. Although rarely fatal, NMSC can cause substantial cosmetic problems if not treated in a timely fashion. These tumours also occur at a much younger age in CCSs than in the rest of the population, sometimes even below the age of ten.

Radiotherapy is the main culprit (RR 4–6); 90% of these tumours occur within the irradiated skin area and young age at treatment confers increased risk. Higher radiotherapy dose is a risk factor for malignant melanoma, as is treatment with alkylating agents and vinca alkaloids. Chemotherapy may also increase the frequency of pigmented naevi which may be precursors to a more malignant transformation. Avoiding excess ultraviolet (UV) radiation and careful examination of irradiated areas is of vital importance during follow-up.

Skeletal toxicity

Bone growth involves both linear growth and increase in width and density. The process is controlled by a complex interaction between many endocrine signals including GH, IGF-1, thyroid hormone, oestrogens, androgens, glucocorticoids, parathyroid hormone, and vitamin D, and other factors such as nutrition and physical activity. In cancer patients, disease itself or reduced physical activity or inadequate nutrition, as well as radiotherapy or chemotherapy, may interfere with normal bone metabolism.

The most evident effect on linear growth is that of radiotherapy when given before bone maturation has completed. Bone irradiation of more than 20 Gy (although there is no consensus on a clear threshold), especially when long bone growth plates are included, leads to reduced bone growth and potentially to asymmetric limb growth. If the spine is involved, vertebral bodies will display impaired growth leading to a reduced final height with disproportion between standing and sitting height. Scoliosis may result from soft-tissue fibrosis secondary to radiotherapy to paravertebral tissues/organs and surgery in that area. Finally, facial asymmetry may result from radiotherapy including the facial bones.

It is vital to maximize the peak bone mineral density (BMD), which normally occurs on completion of puberty, with subsequent physiological decay over decades. Dual X-ray absorptiometry (DXA) is used to assess BMD.

CRT may indirectly affect BMD by interfering with GH and sex hormone secretion; in addition, prolonged steroid treatment and antimetabolites may have a dose-dependent adverse effect on BMD. Survivors of HSCT are at increased risk of skeletal late complications due to the multiple effects of TBI and high-dose chemotherapy on the neuroendocrine and gonadal systems, and the effects of impaired physical activity. After treatment discontinuation, recovery usually occurs but cumulative prednisone-equivalent doses of more than 9 g/m^2 or methotrexate doses of more than 40 g/m^2 are associated with a higher risk of failure to regain normal BMD. Finally, bone metabolism may be indirectly affected in case of urinary calcium and/or phosphate wasting in patients with ifosfamide-induced tubulopathy.

DXA examination should be performed two years after treatment completion and at the end of puberty in at-risk survivors. Vitamin D supplementation and appropriate dietary calcium intake should be advised. After puberty, and in severe cases, treatment with bisphosphonates may also be considered.

Avascular necrosis of bone may occur either during or after therapy, particularly with radiotherapy and/or prolonged steroid treatment, and usually effects joints in long bones, causing pain and functional impairment.

Immunological dysfunction

Immunological function usually recovers satisfactorily within 6–12 months of standard chemotherapy but is slower after HSCT (possibly up to 18 months after mismatched or unrelated donor allogeneic transplants), especially in the presence of chronic GvH disease.

Patients who have undergone splenectomy or received high-dose splenic radiotherapy (more than 40Gy), and survivors of HSCT (especially those with functional hyposplenism following conditioning with TBI), are at increased lifelong risk of potentially life-threatening encapsulated bacterial infections. These individuals should be immunized with conjugate haemophilus influenzae type b (Hib), meningococcal and pneumococcal vaccines, and given antibiotic prophylaxis with phenoxymethylpenicillin or amoxicillin.

Survivors of haematopoietic stem-cell transplantation

Survivors of HSCT are at particularly high risk of LAEs, with more than 90% suffering from at least one and more than 70% from at least three. Patients conditioned with TBI are at the highest risk of late toxicity, and high-dose conditioning chemotherapy is an additional potent risk factor. Additive and potentially synergistic damage results from numerous other factors, including previous treatment given before transplant, the development of other serious complications after HSCT, potentially toxic supportive-care drugs, and especially chronic GvH disease which may affect any organ, tissue, or body system.

It is important to undertake regular and detailed surveillance in view of the wide range, frequency, and severity of potential complications. For example, SMNs are reported in up to 10–15% of HSCT survivors 15 years post HSCT (skin, oral, thyroid, and CNS tumours and post-transplant lymphoproliferative disease being amongst the commonest diagnoses), whilst reproductive toxicity with germ-cell failure (leading to azoospermia in males and ovarian failure in females) is virtually inevitable after TBI and occurs in at least 90% after busulfan/cyclophosphamide.

Chronic GvH disease occurs in up to 30% of HSCT patients, with multiple potential sequelae including organ and tissue damage (e.g. pulmonary, gastrointestinal, hepatic, renal, musculoskeletal, skin, serosal effusion), as well as functional impairment (e.g. immune-mediated cytopenias, delayed immune reconstitution) and the potential adverse effects of immunosuppressive drugs.

Survivors of central nervous system tumours

LAEs are reported with higher frequency and usually higher severity among survivors of CNS tumours as compared to CCSs from other tumour types. The reported frequencies vary between studies due to methodological differences and length of follow-up. Neurological and neuropsychological toxicity, hypothalamic–pituitary dysfunction, and visual and auditory toxicity can occur after treatment of other tumour types, but also occur frequently in survivors of CNS tumours. They have already been discussed earlier in this chapter; this section deals with some other toxicities and deficits that are more specific in survivors of CNS tumours.

More than one functional deficit often occurs in the same survivor and these may be due either to the tumour itself (e.g. seizures, focal nerve palsies, hemiparesis, hemiplegia, visual impairment, cerebellar dysfunction, endocrine deficits) or to treatment. Surgery may cause cerebellar mutism and posterior fossa syndrome (usually regressing in the months after surgery), shunting sequelae, stroke, oculomotor deficits, ataxia, vision and hearing loss, and hypothalamic damage. Radiotherapy may lead to stroke, leucoencephalopathy, neurocognitive impairment, radiation necrosis, endocrinopathies, and secondary tumours. Chemotherapy may be associated with ototoxicity, peripheral neuropathy, and gonadotoxicity. Recently introduced novel biological agents (e.g. bevacizumab and mTOR inhibitors) have also been associated with complications such as chronic hypertension and amenorrhoea, and their long-term toxicity (currently only partially known about) requires further investigation.

Age at treatment and irradiation remain the most relevant independent risk factors for neurocognitive, endocrine, and hearing changes. Late neurological impairment can also occur because of tumour recurrence, secondary CNS tumours, or bleeding of cavernous angiomas (cavernomas).

Neurocognitive and neuropsychological impairment has been reported, with frequencies ranging between 8% and 57% depending on the measured skill. Endocrine late effects have been reported at frequencies ranging between 43% and 61%, and in up to 95% of children treated for a midline tumour. Other complications are reported with different frequencies: seizures in 27% of subjects, motor deficits in 20–35%, stroke in 29.3% of irradiated cases, social impairment in 50%, hearing loss in 9–14%, visual changes in up to 40%, and SMNs in 10.7% of cases at 25 years from diagnosis. As mentioned earlier, the tumour itself may also be responsible for these problems, next to the consequences of treatment. Patients and parents should be given a fair appraisal of all factors involved, including to what extent recovery may be expected or not.

Cancer predisposition syndromes are associated with a higher frequency of CNS tumours, which occur in 15% of patients with these syndromes. This is particularly the case in infants with medulloblastoma (20% of cases with Gorlin syndrome) and in children with choroid plexus tumours (40% of cases with Li Fraumeni syndrome). Furthermore, patients with these syndromes have an increased risk of chemotherapy- or radiotherapy-related organ damage or SMNs, and should be followed up carefully.

Strategies to improve the quality of survival of CNS tumour survivors and to prevent LAEs as far as possible are mandatory in planning treatment for these patients, and an increasing number of clinical trials are including quality of survival as one of the main outcome measures.

The management of CNS tumour survivors requires LTFU, with appropriate imaging and a multidisciplinary approach including specialists not always involved with other childhood solid tumours (e.g. (paediatric) endocrinologists, ophthalmologists, ENT specialists, neuropsychologists, social workers). The transition to adult life may require special facilities and collaborations with adult specialists, as already mentioned, and the adoption of rehabilitation programmes or specific support measures through adult life. Survivors of CNS tumours may require additional help in finding an appropriate job and for independent living or support to live semi-independently. The way social and governmental services deal with these problems may differ from country to country, but all specialists involved should be aware of the possibilities that are available.

Surgical complications

Surgical complications and late physical effects may be obvious, and although the quality of life of these patients in domains other than physical functioning may be rated as high as that in controls, there is a lifelong need for many patients to have continued contact with health services (e.g. for prosthetic reasons after limb-salvage surgery or for post-surgical complications). Other complications vary in location and may be subtle, depending on the anatomy and physiology of the affected part of the body. Spinal and neurological surgery may lead to complications affecting the central and peripheral nervous and musculoskeletal systems. Thoracic surgery may affect cardiac and pulmonary function. Abdominal surgery may affect the gastrointestinal system (adhesions, strictures, and obstruction), liver, or kidneys, and this risk is, as for most of the surgical complications, increased with additional radiotherapy. Surgery to the head and neck may lead to facial deformities and thyroid disease.

Although surgeons always try to avoid mutilating or functional damage, this may be unavoidable for some diagnoses and tumour locations when cure is the ultimate aim. Late complications that may require surgical intervention later on include prosthetic surgery for osteonecrosis of major joints and the occurrence of SMNs.

Psychosocial outcomes

In addition to medical complications, CCSs may also suffer psychological or social consequences. Survivors may go through contrasting experiences: on the one hand, enhancing their appreciation of life (post-traumatic growth) by promoting maturity and resilience, while at the same time increasing psychological vulnerability because of the previous cancer history or the presence of chronic health conditions. While many survivors fare well, a considerable number report psychological distress such as depression or anxiety, post-traumatic stress symptoms, and fatigue. Psychological and social problems are often interrelated: distress may lead to problems in school, employment, or relationships, and problems in the social field may, in return, influence psychological well-being. The provision of medical, psychological, and social care to survivors in need is therefore paramount. The term 'Damocles syndrome' has been used to illustrate their psychological condition of aiming to achieve full integration as active members of the society whilst living with the fear that possible treatment complications or cancer recurrence may interfere with their aspirations.

It is important that the general public recognizes and accepts the reality of cure of childhood cancer, and ensures that survivors have equal access to education, jobs, insurance, and medical care.

Follow-up care

LTFU of CCSs is essential to identify and treat LAEs early, increase knowledge about specific groups at higher risk of long-term morbidity and mortality, and improve patient care. Research indicates that chronic LAEs increase in frequency and severity with time, and may interact adversely with the normal ageing process, resulting in increasing and clinically significant impairment of vital organ systems during adulthood at a younger age than normal and an increased risk of premature major illness or death. This highlights the need to develop effective models of LTFU care which will optimize efficient use of health-service resources to deliver maximal benefit to survivors.

LTFU should be lifelong and transition programmes should be organized to successfully transfer survivors from paediatric to adult healthcare. Furthermore, care should be based on surveillance guidelines. The IGHG (www.ighg.org) is a collaboration of paediatric late-effect guideline groups, the PanCare network (www.pancare.eu), and other professionals to formulate harmonized recommendations.

Each CCS should be provided with a paper or electronic document providing information on their cancer-related medical history, including treatment received, and offering risk-adapted suggestions for LTFU care which can then be tailored to each survivor, based on the type and dose of treatment received, and age at treatment and at follow-up. Survivors should be able to decide if, when, and where they would like their LTFU to be conducted, and the treating centre should be able to respond to any queries that may arise over time.

The future

Increased understanding of the pathogenesis of LAEs of treatment should ultimately reduce their frequency and severity. In particular, it should inform the design of newer and less toxic agents or protocols and facilitate the development of protective drugs to reduce or prevent damage to normal tissues. Genetic risk factors may be identified that predict a higher risk for the development of LAEs in individual patients, hence explaining why some patients develop severe LAEs whilst others, with apparently similar clinical risk factors, do not.

Finally, newer agents may have as yet unknown LAEs, so clinical research is vital to document the nature of and risk factors for such toxicities. In particular, it is important that phase III randomized trials should evaluate LAEs of treatment. The knowledge gained from LTFU of CCSs should be used not only to facilitate design of new treatment protocols but also to provide important information for survivors and their families to enable them to become advocates for their own health.

FURTHER READING

Ajithkumar T, et al. (2017) Prevention of radiotherapy-induced neurocognitive dysfunction in survivors of paediatric brain tumours: the potential role of modern imaging and radiotherapy techniques. *Lancet Oncol* **18**, e91–100.

Allodji RS, et al. (2019) Risk of subsequent primary leukaemias among 69,460 five-year survivors of childhood cancer diagnosed from 1940 to 2008 in Europe: A cohort study within PanCareSurFup. *Eur J Cancer* **117**, 71–83.

Armstrong GT (2009) Long-term survivors of childhood central nervous system malignancies: the experience of the Childhood Cancer Survivor Study. *Eur J Paediatr Neurol* **14**, 298–303.

Armstrong GT, et al. (2016) Reduction in late mortality among 5-year survivors of childhood cancer. *N Engl J Med* **374**, 833–42.

Bass JK, et al. (2016) Hearing loss in patients who received cranial radiation therapy for childhood cancer. *J Clin Oncol* **34**(11), 1248–55. doi: 10.1200/JCO.2015.63.6738

Bhakta N, et al. (2016) Cumulative burden of cardiovascular morbidity among pediatric, adolescent and young adult Hodgkin lymphoma survivors: an analysis from the St Jude Lifetime Cohort Study. *Lancet Oncol* **17**, 1325–34. doi:10.1016/S1470-2045(16)30215-7.

Bitsko MJ, et al. (2016) Psychosocial late effects in pediatric cancer survivors: a report from the Children's Oncology Group. *Pediatr Blood Cancer* **63**, 337–43.

Bright CJ, et al. (2018) Risk of Soft-Tissue Sarcoma Among 69 460 Five-Year Survivors of Childhood Cancer in Europe. *J Natl Cancer Inst* **110**, 649–660.

Brown MC, et al. (2015) The views of European clinicians on guidelines for long-term follow-up of childhood cancer survivors. *Pediatr Blood Cancer* **62**, 322–8.

Byer L, et al. (2016) Clinical trials in pediatric neuro-oncology: what is missing and how we can improve. *CNS Oncol* **5**, 233–9.

Clement SC, et al. (2018) Balancing the benefits and harms of thyroid cancer surveillance in survivors of childhood, adolescent and young adult cancer: recommendations from the International Late Effects of Childhood Cancer Guideline Harmonization Group in collaboration with the PanCareSurFup Consortium. *Cancer Treat Rev* **63**, 28–39.

El-Fayechh C, et al. (2017) Cerebrovascular diseases in childhood cancer survivors: role of the radiation dose to Willis circle arteries. *Int J Radiat Oncol Biol Phys* **97**, 278–86.

Essig S, et al. (2012) Follow-up programs for childhood cancer survivors in Europe: a questionnaire survey. *PLoS One* **7**, e53201.

Fidler MM, et al. (2016) Long term cause specific mortality among 34,489 five year survivors of childhood cancer in Great Britain: population based cohort study. *BMJ* **354**, i4351. doi: 10.1136/bmj.i4351

Fidler MM, et al. (2018) Risk of subsequent bone cancers among 69 460 five-year survivors of childhood and adolescent cancer in Europe. *J Natl Cancer Inst* **110**, 183–194.

Friedman DL, et al. (2010) Subsequent neoplasms in 5-year survivors of childhood cancer: the Childhood Cancer Survivor Study. *J Natl Cancer Inst* **102**, 1083–95.

Garwicz S, et al. (2012) Late and very late mortality in 5-year survivors of childhood cancer: changing pattern over four decades—experience from the Nordic countries. *Int J Cancer* **131**, 1659–66.

Gawade PL, et al. (2014) A systematic review of dental late effects in survivors of childhood cancer. *Pediatr Blood Cancer* **61**, 407–16.

Geenen MM, et al. (2007) Medical assessment of adverse health outcomes in long-term survivors of childhood cancer. *JAMA* **297**, 2705–15.

Gibson TM, Robison LL. (2015) Impact of cancer therapy-related exposures on late mortality in childhood cancer survivors. *Chem Res Toxicol* **28**, 31–7.

Glenny AM, et al. (2010) The development of evidence-based guidelines on mouth care for children, teenagers and young adults treated for cancer. *Eur J Cancer* **46**, 1399–412.

Gunn ME, et al. (2016). Use of endocrinological and neurological medication among 5-year survivors of young onset brain tumours. *J Neurooncol* **128**, 473–9.

Henderson TO, Nathan PC. (2015) Childhood cancer survivors: considerations for surgeons in the transition from pediatric to adult care. *Semin Pediatr Surg* **24**, 93–9.

Huang TT, et al. (2014) Pulmonary outcomes in survivors of childhood central nervous system malignancies: a report from the Childhood Cancer Survivor Study. *Pediatr Blood Cancer* **61**, 319–25.

Hutchinson AD, et al. (2017) Cancer-related cognitive impairment in children. *Curr Opin Support Pall Care* **11**, 70–5.

Lund LW, et al. (2011) A systematic review of studies on psychosocial late effects of childhood cancer: structures of society and methodological pitfalls may challenge the conclusions. *Pediatr Blood Cancer* **56**, 532–43.

McCurdy D, et al. (2016) Associations among treatment-related neurological risk factors and neuropsychological functioning in survivors of childhood brain tumor. *J Neurooncol* **127**, 137–44.

Michel G, et al. (2019) Evidence-based recommendations for the organization of long-term follow-up care for childhood and adolescent cancer survivors: a report from the PanCareSurFup Guidelines Working Group. *J Cancer Surviv* **13**(5), 759–772.

Mulder RL, et al. (2009) Prevalence and risk factors of radiation-induced growth hormone deficiency in childhood cancer survivors: a systematic review. *Cancer Treat Rev* **35**, 616–32.

Mulrooney DA, et al. (2009) Cardiac outcomes in a cohort of adult survivors of childhood and adolescent cancer: retrospective analysis of the Childhood Cancer Survivor Study cohort. *BMJ* **339**, b4606.

Oeffinger KC, et al. (2006) Chronic health conditions in adult survivors of childhood cancer. *N Engl J Med* **355**, 1572–82.

Olsen JH, et al. (2009) Lifelong cancer incidence in 47,697 patients treated for childhood cancer in the Nordic countries. *J Natl Cancer Inst* **101**, 806–13.

Pierson C, et al. (2016) A meta-analysis of the neuropsychological effects of chemotherapy in the treatment of childhood cancer. *Pediatr Blood Cancer* **63**, 1998–2003.

Reulen RC, et al. (2010) Long-term cause-specific mortality among survivors of childhood cancer. *JAMA* **304**, 172–9.

Roth CL (2015) Hypothalamic obesity in craniopharyngioma patients: disturbed energy homeostasis related to extent of hypothalamic damage and its implication for obesity intervention. *J Clin Med* 4(9), 1774–97. doi: 10.3390/jcm4091774

Shah SS, et al. (2015) Long-term psychiatric outcomes in pediatric brain tumor survivors. *Childs Nerv Syst* **31**, 653–63.

Sharma D, et al. (2017) Need for improved skin cancer surveillance in pediatric cancer survivors. *Am J Clin Dermatol* **18**, 165–8.

Skinner R. (2018) Late renal toxicity of treatment for childhood malignancy—risk factors, long-term outcomes and surveillance. *Pediatr Nephrol* **33**(2), 215–25. doi: 10.1007/s00467-017-3662-z

Skinner R, Leiper AD. (2004) Bone marrow transplantation. In: WHB Wallace, DM Green (eds) *Late Effects of Childhood Cancer*, pp. 304–20. London: Arnold.

Taiwo Z, et al. (2017) The Neurological Predictor Scale: a predictive tool for long-term core cognitive outcomes in survivors of childhood brain tumors. *Pediatr Blood Cancer* **64**, 172–9.

Tallen G, et al. (2015) Strategies to improve the quality of survival for childhood brain tumours survivors. *Eur J Paediatr Neurol* **19**, 619–39.

Tukenova M, et al. (2010) Role of cancer treatment in long-term overall and cardiovascular mortality after childhood cancer. *J Clin Oncol* **28**, 1308–15.

Turcotte LM, et al. (2017) Temporal trends in treatment and subsequent neoplasm risk among 5-year survivors of childhood cancer, 1970–2015. *JAMA* **317**, 814–24.

Turcotte LM, et al. (2015) Risk of subsequent neoplasms during the fifth and sixth decades of life in the CCSS. *J Clin Oncol* **33**, 3568–75.

Wells EM, et al. (2017) Longitudinal assessment of late onset neurologic conditions in survivors of childhood central nervous system tumors: a Childhood Cancer Survivor Study report. *Neuro Oncol* **20**(1), 132–42. doi: 10.1093/neuonc/nox148

Whelan KF, et al. (2010) Ocular late effects in childhood and adolescent cancer survivors: a report from the Childhood Cancer Survivor Study. *Pediatr Blood Cancer* **54**, 103–9.

15

Acute Lymphoblastic Leukaemia

Denis Schewe, Mignon Loh, Rob Pieters, and Martin Schrappe

Epidemiology

Acute lymphoblastic leukemia (ALL) is the most common type of cancer in childhood. It accounts for 20–25% of all childhood cancers. The peak incidence is at 2–5 years of age, which is mainly due to a peak of ALL cases with hyperdiploid ALL and *ETV6/RUNX1* gene-rearranged ALL. The incidence rate is higher in high-income countries and in Hispanic children, and lower in black children as compared to white children. Males are affected more often than females, except in infants.

The aetiology of ALL is characterized by the fact that immature lymphoid cells acquire different consecutive genetic lesions of which the first lesion can occur before birth. For example, the most common translocation that occurs in childhood ALL, the *ETV6/RUNX1* translocation, can be traced back in the Guthrie cards of the patients. However, only few children born with this translocation will develop ALL, suggesting that leukemogenesis is multifactorial and depends on multiple consecutive genetic events. Less than a few percent of children with ALL have an underlying genetic predisposition, such as Down syndrome, even though germline variants in certain driver genes such as *PAX5* or *p53* can lead to leukaemia development. Leukaemia initiation by environmental exposures or common infectious pathogens is frequently hypothesized but cannot yet be confirmed based on the available data.

Clinical presentation

Most symptoms at diagnosis are secondary to leukaemic infiltration of the bone marrow: pallor, petechiae, and haematomas. General symptoms such as fatigue and fever often occur. Bone or musculoskeletal pain is sometimes misinterpreted as a rheumatological condition. Refusal to walk in young children is always an alarming symptom. Physical examination may show hepatosplenomegaly and lymphadenopathy. In rare cases, especially in T-ALL, dyspnoea or signs of vena cava superior compression can be found due to the presence of an anterior mediastinal mass. Other rare symptoms are one-sided testicular enlargement, headaches, or focal neurological abnormalities due to leukaemic involvement of the testes or the central nervous system. Often, ALL is diagnosed upon peripheral blood abnormalities (cytopenias, atypical cells) detected in a blood draw for workup of non-specific symptoms.

Diagnosis

The blood-cell counts often show anaemia and/or thrombocytopenia and granulocytopenia. The leucocyte count is increased to more than 10e9/l in 50% of cases. Hyperleukocytosis more than 50e9/l is seen in more than 50% of infants, 15–20% of children, and 20–30% of adolescents, and occurs in T-ALL more frequently. Leukocyte counts may also be normal or even leukopenic. Morphological examination of peripheral blood smears shows lymphoblasts in the majority, but not all, cases.

Nowadays, the diagnosis of ALL is made by a combination of morphology, immunophenotyping, cytogenetics, and molecular genetic techniques in bone marrow and peripheral blood samples. Even though the French–American–British (FAB) classification has become historical due to a lack of information regarding treatment decisions or prognosis, classic cytomorphology still plays an important role for the differential diagnosis with other diseases such as myelodysplastic syndrome, aplastic anaemia, or cytopenias due to infections. Although most protocols still require the classic cut-off level of 25% or greater lymphoblasts in the bone marrow for the diagnosis of ALL, lower percentages will be accepted in some clinical trials if this is confirmed by immunophenotyping or the presence of typical genetic abnormalities.

Immunophenotyping by flow cytometry is considered standard of care and is used to determine the type of ALL (B-lineage or T-lineage) and the differentiation stage of the leukaemic cells. B-cell precursor ALL is usually CD79a+, CD10+, or CD19+, and often CD22+ and CD20+. Mature B-cell ALL cases are usually CD19+, CD20+, CD22+, or CD25+, and express surface immunoglobulin. Co-expression of myeloid markers (e. g. CD13 and CD33) is common. T-lineage ALL is positive for CDs 2, 3, 4, 5, 7, and 8, unless they express a CD5dim, CD8- profile typical for early T-cell precursor ALL (ETP-ALL). Genetic or fluorescence *in situ* hybridization (FISH) techniques are used for the detection of recurrent chromosomal or molecular abnormalities, the most common of which are the *ETV6/RUNX1* translocation in 20–25%, hyperdiploidy in 20–25%, rearrangements involving the *KMT2A (MLL)* gene in 5%, and the *BCR/ABL1* and *TCF3/PBX1* translocations, each in 3–4% of BCP-ALL cases.

Recently, the molecular features of *TCF3/HLF*-positive BCP-ALL have been described, which occurs in less than 1% of the cases and is a disease that is almost always fatal. Roughly 2% of patients have hypodiploid BCP-ALL, encompassing near-haploid (24–31 chromosomes) and low-hypodiploid (32–39 chromosomes) cases. The former is characterized by alterations in *IKZF3* while the latter very frequently harbours *TP53, RB1,*and *IKZF2* mutations. In low-hypodiploid ALL, the *TP53* mutations are germline in nearly half of patients, indicative of Li Fraumeni syndrome. Both entities can have activated RAS and PI3K signalling and are associated with a very poor prognosis. Ten to fifteen percent of children with BCP-ALL suffer from '*BCR/ABL*-like' or 'Ph-like' ALL, which has a gene-expression profile similar to *BCR/ABL1*- positive ALL but lacks the *BCR/ABL1* fusion. This disease entity is characterized by deletions in B-cell development genes such as *IKZF1, TCF3,* or *PAX5*, and has been associated with a poor prognosis. However, when therapy was stratified based on minimal residual disease (MRD), these patients had survival rates comparable to other BCP-ALL patients in a small cohort and with the use of allogeneic haematopoetic stem cell transplantation.

'*BCR/ABL1*-like' patients partly harbour ABL1-class translocations which are targetable. The therapeutic targeting of *JAK2* and *CRLF2* abnormalities in '*BCR/ABL1*-like' patients is the subject of further investigation. Recurrent chromosomal or molecular abnormalities in T-ALL such as *TAL/LMO, TLX1/HOX11, TLX3/HOX11L2*, and *HOXA* are usually present in only small patient subgroups, and their effect on patient prognosis is less pronounced.

Central nervous system (CNS) involvement is present in less than 5% of children at the onset of ALL. It is diagnosed when more than five WBC/μL cerebrospinal fluid (CSF) are measured upon cytospin and lymphoblasts are morphologically identifiable (CNS3 status), or if focal neurological symptoms are present due to leukaemic infiltration. CNS2 status is defined as the presence of leukaemic cells upon microscopy but ≤five WBC/μl in the CSF. CNS1 means that neither leukaemic cells nor leukocytes are detected. Traumatic lumbar puncture (TLP) potentially leads to leukaemic contamination of the CSF and, similar to CNS3 status, has been associated with an inferior prognosis. In the case of TLP, some protocols advocate extra intrathecal chemotherapy.

Table 15.1 Most important prognostic factors currently used for therapy stratification (prevalence in % of all cases)

Risk factor	Favourable	Less favourable
Gender	Female (~45%)	Male (~55%)
White blood-cell count	Low (e.g. <50e9/L) (~80%)	High (e.g. >50e9/L) (~20%)
Age	1-9.99 years (~75%)	<1 year (~4%) 15–18 years (~7%)
Central nervous system	CNS1 (~75%) TLP- (~90%)	CNS3 (~3–5%) TLP+ (~10%)
Immunophenotype	Common/preB ALL (~80%)	ProB ALL (~4%) T-ALL (~15%)
Genetic abnormalities	*ETV6/RUNX1* (~25%) Hyperdiploidy (~25%) *E2A/PBX1* (~3%)	*KMT2A* translocations (~5%) *BCR/ABL* (~3%) Hypodiploidy (1%) *TCF3/HLF* (<1%) *IKZF* del (~12%) *BCR-ABL*-like (~13%)
Response to therapy		
Day 8 prednisone response in peripheral blood	<1×10e9 blasts/l (~90%)	≥1×10e9 blasts/l (~10%)
Day 15 bone marrow response	M1 marrow <5% blasts (~60%)	M3 marrow >25% blasts (~15%)
Morphological complete remission after induction therapy	Yes (~98%)	No (~2%)
Bone marrow minimal residual disease by PCR	<10e-4 after 5 weeks (~25–40%)	≥10e-3 after 12 weeks (~5%)
Bone marrow minimal residual disease by FCM	<0.1% at day 15 of induction, or <0.01% at end of induction	≥10% at day 15, or ≥0.1% at the end of induction

Prognostic factors and risk classification

Many clinical and biological factors predict patient outcome. However, many of these factors are related to or dependent on each other, so that proper analyses establishing the independent and quantitative values of each factor are challenging. Moreover, therapy is often adjusted based on these factors influencing the contribution of a factor on outcome. Table 15.1 presents an overview of clinical and biological risk factors currently used for treatment stratification in paediatric ALL protocols.

In most protocols, early response to therapy is used for therapy stratification. Many European protocols use the absolute peripheral blast count after one week of systemic prednisone and one dose of intrathecal methotrexate. A classic parameter still used in all protocols is the achievement of morphological response after induction therapy which is defined as less than 5% blasts in the bone marrow and the absence of other evidence of leukaemia. Measurement of minimal residual disease (MRD) is incorporated as a major stratification factor in many protocols. MRD is measured by flow cytometry or by polymerase chain reaction (PCR) at the end of induction and during the first months of post-induction therapy.

Treatment

The backbone of every ALL treatment protocol consists of four phases: induction, consolidation, intensification (re-induction), and maintenance (continuation) therapy. All treatment phases contain CNS-directed therapy elements. Only a few patients receive CNS irradiation or allogeneic haematopoietic stem-cell transplantation (SCT) in addition to chemotherapy. Current treatment protocols result in five-year event-free survival (EFS) rates of up to 85% and five year overall survival rates of up to 90%. However, relapses and secondary malignancies may also occur more than five years after diagnosis. Also, a significant number of relapsed patients may be salvaged for many years before they ultimately die. Therefore, the final EFS and survival rate are lower than the five-year figures usually presented.

Induction

The goal of induction therapy is to achieve complete morphological remission and restore normal haematopoiesis. This is achieved after 4–6 weeks of chemotherapy in about 98% of all children. Almost all protocols use a glucocorticoid (prednisone or dexamethasone), vincristine, and L-asparaginase as a so-called three-drug backbone plus intrathecal chemotherapy for this course. The addition of an anthracycline as a fourth systemic drug is a matter of debate. Some studies have made clear that at least about 50% of children can be cured without the use of anthracyclines, but definitive answers to this question require further evidence from clinical trials. About 2% of patients do not achieve remission after induction therapy, which may be due to early death often caused by infection or bleeding or to chemotherapy-resistant leukaemic cells. In this latter group, very intensive treatment can result in improved survival and about 30–40% long-term survivorship.

Induction therapy involves therapy with asparaginase. Several studies have shown that patient outcome with low L-asparaginase doses or suboptimal L-asparaginase serum levels are unfavourable. L-asparaginase derived from E. coli has a longer half-life than the preparation derived from Erwinia chrysanthemi (Erwinase), which can result in differences in asparagine depletion. Erwinase is usually reserved for patients intolerant to these preparations or showing silent inactivation of L-asparaginase due to neutralizing antibodies. PEGylated L-asparaginase (PEG-asparaginase) is less immunogenic, results in longer periods of asparagine depletion due to its longer half-life, and has a comparable toxicity profile to other L-asparaginase preparations. The drug can be conveniently administered once every 2–4 weeks, instead of once every 2–3 days, to ensure complete continuous asparagine depletion.

Consolidation and intensification

Consolidation and intensification courses aim at eradicating residual leukaemic cells. Berlin–Frankfurt–Munster (BFM) protocols use a post-induction course consisting of low-dose cytarabine, 6-MP, and cyclophosphamide, which reduces the MRD load significantly. Other groups use different combinations of drugs in this phase with the same results. Many study groups use high-dose methotrexate (MTX) and 6-mercaptopurine (6-MP) in combination with frequent intrathecal therapy in the consolidation phase. The use of high-dose MTX significantly reduces the risk of bone marrow relapse, in particular if combined with dexamethasone.

Drugs used in intensification courses are the same as in induction therapy. Several randomized studies have proven the value of intensification treatment. Intensified and double-delayed intensification improves outcome for patients with a slow initial response to treatment. In patients with rapid early response, a more intensive (but not a longer) intensification treatment was of benefit. Omission of the intensification led to a significant rise in the relapse rate, although the same study showed that 50% of patients could be cured without the use of intensification.

Dexamethasone or prednisone?

Several, but not all, randomized studies have shown that the use of dexamethasone at a dose of 6 mg/m^2 results in a lower rate of bone marrow and CNS relapses than prednisone at a dose of 40 mg/m^2. This benefit of dexamethasone might be due to higher free plasma levels and better CNS penetration or to the fact that despite equivalent doses, dexamethasone is still more potent than prednisone, as some *in vitro* studies suggest. Unfortunately, dexamethasone also leads to more side effects. The largest study thus far examining this issue found that dexamethasone was superior to prednisone regarding five-year EFS rates, mainly due to improved prevention of extramedullary relapses, and a particularly good outcome of dexamethasone-treated T-ALL patients with good response to the prednisone pre-phase. However, this was at the expense of a significantly higher rate of induction-related deaths with dexamethasone.

Reduction of therapy intensity

Measurements of MRD during the first months of ALL treatment predict patient outcome. Five-year overall survival rates for MRD-negative patients come close to 100%, which raised the question of whether therapy intensity could safely be reduced in order to lower toxicity without jeopardizing outcome. A non-randomized trial recently showed that reduced-intensity delayed intensification was feasible in patients with undetectable MRD at the end of induction. It could also be demonstrated that in patients with undetectable MRD levels, one or two courses of delayed intensification therapy were equally effective, with lower rates of toxicity in patients receiving only one course. It is important to consider that the low number of relapses occurring in MRD-negative patients can be salvaged in a vast majority of the cases, especially if the patient has been exposed to only low levels of chemotherapy during initial treatment. It may thus be an alternative to accept slightly higher relapse rates in a few standard-risk patients, whilst sparing substantial toxicities for the majority, by reducing the intensity of chemotherapy protocols. Clinical studies on treatment reduction in the MRD-negative risk group are currently ongoing in various settings.

Maintenance

The aim of maintenance treatment is to further reduce residual disease and to suppress the outgrowth of these cells. The importance of maintenance therapy is illustrated by the fact that outcome depends on the intensity and duration of therapy. Most protocols continue the maintenance for up to two years after diagnosis or achievement of morphological remission. Other protocols include a time period of two years' maintenance treatment for girls and three years' maintenance for boys. A meta-analysis showed that longer maintenance leads to lower relapse rates but also increased toxic death rates. Reduction of the duration of maintenance to less than two years led to an increased relapse risk but also showed that a significant proportion of patients survive without two years of maintenance. It is yet completely unclear how to identify patients who profit from longer phases of maintenance or in whom therapy can be shortened without any risk.

The backbone of every maintenance course is weekly (oral or intravenous) methotrexate and daily oral 6-MP. Doses of these drugs are usually adapted according to leukocyte count or to lymphocyte, neutrophil, and platelet counts. At an international expert meeting, consensus was reached to use a target leukocyte count of 1.5–3× 10e9/L. There are large intra- and inter-individual differences in MTX and 6-MP doses that are tolerated or required to achieve the target leukocyte count. These may be due to infections or underlying pharmacogenetic factors such as polymorphisms in the thiopurine methyltransferase gene. Maintaining the highest dose of 6-MP and

MTX leads to a better outcome. Treatment adherence of doctors and patients (especially adolescents) therefore has an impact on outcome. 6-MP remains the drug of choice in maintenance as patients receiving 6-thioguanine (6-TG) may more frequently suffer from liver toxicity, with features of veno-occlusive disease.

The addition of steroid and vincristine pulses to maintenance is a matter of debate, and data from randomized studies and meta-analyses are conflicting. Taken together, the use of pulses in maintenance therapy is probably not beneficial but may contribute to a better outcome for specific risk groups or for patients treated on a protocol without an intensification course.

Central nervous system directed therapy

CNS-directed therapy is a prerequisite for successful treatment of ALL. In the 1960s, more than half of the patients suffered from CNS relapses. Several treatment elements were effective in reducing this high CNS recurrence rate to currently below 5%. First, cranial or craniospinal irradiation prevents CNS relapses, but has major side effects such as long-term neurocognitive deficits and secondary malignant neoplasms. Because secondary neoplasms often occur decades after radiation therapy, it is important to implement long follow-up into studies comparing the outcomes of radiation and other CNS-directed therapies. Second, intrathecal chemotherapy delivered at regular intervals reduces CNS relapse. Finally, systemic application of drugs that penetrate the blood brain barrier (dexamethasone, high-dose MTX, and cytarabine) all contribute to decreased CNS relapses.

Current data favours the omission of cranial radiotherapy in patients on contemporary treatment protocols. However, although the majority of CNS relapses can be prevented by adequate systemic and intrathecal chemotherapy, this does not exclude that specific high risk groups may benefit from radiation. Most clinical protocols still use radiation for a minority of high risk patients such as patients with a CNS3 status at diagnosis, and T-ALL patients with a high initial leukaemia burden. Elimination of cranial radiation in the latter group led to an increase in systemic but not CNS relapses. Most protocols advise extra intrathecal injections for patients with a CNS3 or CNS2 status or in case of a traumatic lumbar puncture at diagnosis. Finally, radiotherapy has still a role in CNS and testicular relapse.

Allogeneic haematopoietic stem-cell transplantation

Improved outcomes with more intense chemotherapeutic regimens has reduced the need for allogeneic haematopoietic stem-cell transplantation (alloHSCT) in childhood ALL. In addition, only a few studies have proven the efficacy of alloHSCT in specific high-risk groups. A collaborative study showed that *BCR/ABL*-positive ALL cases benefit from alloHSCT after having received intensive chemotherapy courses. However, even in this patient group, the role of alloHSCT has been debated since the introduction of ABL tyrosine kinase inhibitors. Another collaborative analysis showed that alloHSCT was of no benefit for children with *KMT2A*-rearranged ALL. A further publication made clear that only 25% of infant *KMT2A*-rearranged ALL cases, namely those that carry two other high-risk features (age younger that six months at diagnosis and WBC more than 300×10e9/L or poor prednisone response) may benefit from alloHSCT. Some evidence suggests a benefit from alloHSCT in patients with high-risk T-ALL, but contradictory data exists. Some patients not achieving morphological complete remission after induction therapy may also have a better outcome with alloHSCT, especially if they have T-ALL. As a stem-cell source, matched sibling or unrelated donors perform equally well in children with ALL. Given the serious acute and late risks of alloHSCT, its role in first-line treatment for childhood ALL is currently limited and offered to less than 5% of patients.

Immunotherapy

Antibody-based and cellular immunotherapy is increasingly implemented into current clinical study protocols in childhood BCP-ALL. CD19 and CD22, but also CD20, have been used as target antigens in preclinical and, partly, in clinical phase I/II trials. These include naked antibodies modified for improved effector-cell binding, immunotoxins/immunoconjugates, and the bispecific T-cell-engaging antibody blinatumomab. Blinatumomab recruits T-cells into close proximity of CD19-positive ALL cells, thereby causing cytotoxicity. It has been shown to be highly efficient in an MRD-positive situation in relapsed/refractory adult ALL patients, but evidence in children is scarce (Table 15.2). An alternative to blinatumomab is the use of autologous chimeric antigen receptor T-cells (CAR T-cells) engineered to express a CD19-specific T-cell receptor. CAR T-cells have been found to be efficient in several trials in relapsed/refractory ALL patients in the post-HSCT setting, including children (Table 15.2). Both therapeutic modalities bear the risk of acute cytokine-release syndrome and encephalopathy, as well as CD19-negative disease relapse. Inotuzumab ozogamicin, an anti-CD22 antibody conjugated to calicheamicin has been shown to outperform standard therapy in adult patients with relapsed/refractory BCP-ALL. This has, however, not been shown yet in paediatric patients, but trials are ongoing. The coming years will clarify how these therapies can further be developed so that they are most efficient and usable not only at relapse but also in the upfront setting.

Specific patient groups

Adolescents

The prognosis of paediatric ALL deteriorates with increasing patient age. Studies in four different countries have shown that outcomes for adolescents with ALL from the same age are better when these patients are treated on paediatric or paediatric-inspired rather than adult protocols, with approximately 30% higher EFS. This effect was mainly explained by differences in the dose intensity of the treatments. The paediatric protocols contained more glucocorticoids, vincristine, L-asparaginase, MTX, and 6-MP. Longer delays between courses in adolescents treated according to adult protocols might also have played a role. It is possible that adult haematologists are less used to glucocorticoid- and asparaginase-induced toxicities, and that delays between courses are due to the fact that they generally treat older patients who do not tolerate intensive therapy as well. In a Dutch study, for instance, use of the adult ALL treatment protocol resulted in both a significantly higher relapse rate and in a significantly higher toxic death rate for adolescents due to the use of alloSCT in many patients. Adolescents and young adults display ALL with the '*BCR-ABL*-like' gene-expression signature more frequently, while *ETV6/RUNX1* and hyperdiploidy are less common, which likely leads to an inferior prognosis in this population.

Table 15.2 Clinical trials using immunotherapeutic approaches (blinatumomab and CAR T-cells) including adult and paediatric BCP-ALL patients

Citation	Trial type	Patient number (adult/paediatric)	Therapy/Dosage	Response	Response duration	Severe toxicities requiring permanent therapy discontinuation*
Topp et al., *J Clin Oncol*, 2011	Single arm phase II	21/0 BCP-ALL with MRD persistence	Blinatumomab (15 µg/m² × 24 h × 4 w)	Complete 16/21 (MRD negativity)	RFS 78% @ 405 days RFS 61% @ 33 months Topp et al., *Blood*, 2012	1/21 (seizure)
Topp et al., *J Clin Oncol*, 2014	Single arm phase II + dose-finding cohorts	36/0 BCP-ALL, relapsed/refractory (>5% blasts in bone marrow)	Blinatumomab (5–30 µg/m² × 24 h × up to five 4-week cycles)	Complete 25/36 Partial 2/36 MRD response 22/36	Median RFS 7.6 months (7.9 months if censored at HSCT) Median OS 9.8 months 10/36 long-term survival >30 months, 6 of which were relapse-free Zugmaier et al., *Blood*, 2015	1/36 (death, possibly related to treatment) 2/36 (other CNS) 1/36 (cytokine release syndrome)
Topp et al., *Lancet Oncol*, 2015	Single arm phase II	189/0 BCP-ALL, relapsed/refractory (>10% blasts in bone marrow)	Blinatumomab (28 µg/m² × 24 h × up to 57 days), dose reduction to 9 µg/m² × 24 h × 7 days in the first cycle	Complete 81/189 MRD response 60/73	Median RFS 5.9 months Median OS 6.1 months	5/189 (death due to disease progression) 23/189 (death due to infection) 29/189 (seizure and other CNS)
Schlegel et al., *Haematologica*, 2014	Compassionate use programme	0/9 BCP-ALL, relapsed/refractory (>5% blasts in bone marrow)	Blinatumomab (5–15 µg/m² × 24 h × up to 18 4-week cycles)	Complete 6/9 MRD response 5/9 (MRD negativity at one point)	EFS/OS 30% at 243 and 398 days, respectively	4/9 (death due to disease progression and relapse) 2/9 (death due to infection)
Cruz et al., *Blood*, 2013	Phase I	6/2 BCP-ALL, 4 adults with CLL, variable disease remission stages	Autologous CD19. CAR-VSTs, 1or 2 infusions	Complete 3/8 (1 of which is causally uncertain) Partial 1/8 Stable disease 1/8	n/a	Not reported
Grupp et al., *N Engl J Med*, 2013	Phase I	0/2 BCP-ALL, relapsed/refractory in remission	Autologous CTL019	Complete 2/2 MRD response 2/2 (<0.01% by FACS and deep sequencing)	1/2 continuous molecular remission for 9 months 1/2 CD19-negative relapse after 2 months	1/2 (severe CRS) 1/2 (encephalopathy)
Brentjens et al., *Science Transl Med*, 2013	Phase I	5/0 BCP-ALL, relapsed/refractory, variable disease remission stages	Autologous 19-28z CAR	Complete 5/5 MRD response 5/5 (negative by deep sequencing)	4/5 received alloHSCT, 3/4 are in continuous remission for variable times 1/5 CD19-positive relapse after 90 days	4/5 (likely CRS and/or neurological side effects of varying degrees)
Davila et al., *Science Transl Med*, 2014	Phase I	16/0 BCP-ALL, relapsed/refractory, variable disease remission stages	Autologous 19-28z CAR	Complete 14/16 MRD response 12/16 (negative by FACS, PCR, and/or deep sequencing)	7/16 received alloHSCT	7/16 (severe CRS) 2/16 (seizure) 2/16 (other CNS)
Lee et al., *Lancet*, 2015	Phase I	6/15 BCP-ALL, relapsed/refractory, variable disease remission stages; adults were young adults <30 years	Autologous CD19-CAR	Complete 14/21 Stable disease 3/21 MRD response 12/21 (MRD negativity)	OS 51.6% at 9.7 months RFS of MRD-negative patients 78.8% at 4.8 months 2/12 CD19-negative relapses after 3 and 5 months	6/21 (severe CRS) 1/21 (cardiac arrest with successful resuscitation) 1/21 (other CNS)
Brudno et al., *J Clin Oncol*, 2016	Phase I	20/0 mixed B-cell malignancy, mainly B-NHL, some BCP-ALL	Allogeneic CD19-CAR from donor-derived T-cells	Complete 6/20 Partial 2/20 Stable disease 8/20 MRD response 4/6 CR patients (MRD negativity)	CR durations 3–30 months SD durations 1–31 months	12/20 (grade 3 or 4 toxicities) No severe GVHD

*Discontinuation in case of blinatumomab; Grade 3/4 SAE for CAR T-cells

Infants

Infants have an inferior outcome mainly due to the fact that around 80% of them have an aggressive type of ALL characterized by the presence of *KMT2A* gene rearrangements. Several specific treatment protocols are used by the Children's Oncology Group (COG), Japan, and the Interfant Collaborative Study Group. The survival rate with current treatment is 50–60%. Infant ALL cells have been shown to be relatively resistant to glucocorticoids and L-asparaginase but highly sensitive to cytarabine, which is therefore more intensively used in these protocols. Within infant ALL, all types of *KMT2A*-rearrangements are associated with the same poor prognosis, and MRD diagnostics is equally important to predict prognosis as in childhood ALL. The younger the infant, the worse the outcome, with the survival rate of congenital ALL being only 20%. AlloHSCT in infant ALL causes many late side effects and its efficacy is uncertain. Its role may be limited to a small, very high-risk group of infant ALL.

BCR/ABL-positive acute lymphoblastic leukaemia

The translocation t(9;22) fuses the *BCR* gene on chromosome 22 to the *ABL* gene on chromosome 9 causing an abnormal ABL tyrosine kinase activity. The incidence of *BCR/ABL* increases with age and is seen in ~3% of children with ALL but in more than 25% of adult ALL. Overall, children with *BCR/ABL* ALL have a survival rate of about 60% with intensive chemotherapy and alloHSCT. Initial good responders to therapy have a better outcome, and outcome is worse in initial poor responders. In the last decade, targeted therapy of the ABL tyrosine kinase has become available. Data from two study groups suggest that the incorporation of imatinib into the backbone of intensive chemotherapy improves patient outcome. In the near future, favourable therapy response will lead to a further reduction in the use of alloHSCT in these patients.

Relapse

Treatment outcome for relapsed patients mainly depends on the time and the site of relapse as well as biological characteristics. Poor prognostic features include a short duration of initial remission, bone marrow involvement at relapse, a T-cell phenotype, the presence of *BCR-ABL* or *KMT2A* abnormalities in infancy, and, of course, MRD response measured after the first courses of chemotherapy. Genetic risk factors such as *TP53* alterations or *Ras* pathway mutations can be predictive of outcome in the relapsed setting. Overall, about one third of patients with relapsed ALL will be cured. Paediatric patients with favourable characteristics (e.g. late relapse or isolated CNS relapse) can even be cured without alloHSCT, especially those initially defined as standard-risk patients.

Toxicity and late effects

Almost all side effects of treatment are temporary. The most important cause of toxic death are infections: 0.5% to 1.5% of patients die from infections during induction therapy, and between 1% and 3% while in complete remission. The most frequent drug-specific toxicities include neuropathy and constipation caused by vincristine; mucositis caused by MTX; diabetes, behaviour disturbances, Cushingoid appearance, osteoporosis, and avascular necrosis of bone caused by glucocorticoids; and allergic reactions, pancreatitis, and thrombosis caused by asparaginase. Older patients (i.e. older than ten years) experience more toxicities (e.g. avascular necrosis of bones, hyperglycaemia, thromboembolic complications, liver function disturbances) than younger patients. Late effects include cardiomyopathy due to anthracyclines, neurocognitive deficits and secondary brain tumours due to cranial radiation, and avascular necrosis of bone (although often reversible) due to glucocorticoids. An increasing body of evidence suggests that ALL treatment is associated with a number of long-term neurobehavioural and neurocognitive deficits. Late effects of ALL treatment on fertility are subject to ongoing investigations.

Perspectives

Improvements in therapy are still being made by studying dose schedules of known drugs, especially glucocorticoids and L-asparaginase. Many groups study reductions (e.g. anthracycline dose) in specific risk groups (e.g. *ETV6/RUNX1* rearranged ALL), while other groups have intensified therapy with L-asparaginase and dexamethasone.

Genome-wide screening and molecular analyses have revealed genetic abnormalities with prognostic significance. Examples are the discovery of the '*BCR/ABL*-like' genetic subtype, *IKZF1* abnormalities, and CRLF2 overexpression that predict a poor outcome. In the coming years, we will learn how to implement these markers for risk stratification and discover novel molecular mechanisms that underpin the high-risk features of the disease. Immunotherapies with monoclonal antibodies, bispecific T-cell-engaging molecules, and 'living drugs' (chimeric antigen receptors) are exciting therapies with promising results. Considering the excellent survival rates currently obtained with traditional chemotherapy, it is always a challenge to investigate how new drugs and immunotherapy can be incorporated in existing paediatric treatment regimens in ALL.

FURTHER READING

Armstrong GT, et al. (2016) Reduction in late mortality among 5-year survivors of childhood cancer. *N Engl J Med* **374**, 833–42.

Biondi A, et al. (2012) Imatinib after induction for treatment of children and adolescents with Philadelphia-chromosome-positive acute lymphoblastic leukaemia (EsPhALL): a randomised, open-label, intergroup study. *Lancet Oncol* **13**, 936–45.

Boer JM, et al. (2017) Tyrosine kinase fusion genes in pediatric BCR-ABL1-like acute lymphoblastic leukemia. *Oncotarget* **8**, 4618–28.

Boissel N, et al. (2003) Should adolescents with acute lymphoblastic leukemia be treated as old children or young adults? Comparison of the French FRALLE-93 and LALA-94 trials. *J Clin Oncol* **21**, 774–80.

Cario G, et al. (2010) Presence of the P2RY8-CRLF2 rearrangement is associated with a poor prognosis in non-high-risk precursor B-cell acute lymphoblastic leukemia in children treated according to the ALL-BFM 2000 protocol. *Blood* **115**, 5393–7.

Cheung YT, et al. (2016) Leukoencephalopathy and long-term neurobehavioural, neurocognitive, and brain imaging outcomes in survivors of childhood acute lymphoblastic leukaemia treated with chemotherapy: a longitudinal analysis. *Lancet Haematol* **3**, e456–66.

Den Boer ML, et al. (2009) A subtype of childhood acute lymphoblastic leukaemia with poor treatment outcome: a genome-wide classification study. *Lancet Oncol* **10**, 125–34.

Fischer U, et al. (2015) Genomics and drug profiling of fatal TCF3-HLF-positive acute lymphoblastic leukemia identifies recurrent mutation patterns and therapeutic options. *Nature Gen* **47**, 1020–9.

Hof J, et al. (2011) Mutations and deletions of the TP53 gene predict nonresponse to treatment and poor outcome in first relapse of childhood acute lymphoblastic leukemia. *J Clin Oncol* **29**, 3185–93.

Holmfeldt L, et al. (2013) The genomic landscape of hypodiploid acute lymphoblastic leukemia. *Nature Gen* **45**, 242–52.

Hunger SP, Mullighan CG (2015) Acute lymphoblastic leukemia in children. *N Engl J Med* **373**, 1541–52.

Irving JA, et al. (2016) Integration of genetic and clinical risk factors improves prognostication in relapsed childhood B-cell precursor acute lymphoblastic leukemia. *Blood* **128**, 911–22.

Larsen EC, et al. (2016) Dexamethasone and high-dose methotrexate improve outcome for children and young adults with high-risk B-acute lymphoblastic leukemia: a report from Children's Oncology Group Study AALL0232. *J Clin Oncol* **34**, 2380–8.

Loh ML, et al. (2013) Tyrosine kinome sequencing of pediatric acute lymphoblastic leukemia: a report from the Children's Oncology Group TARGET Project. *Blood* **121**, 485–8.

Mann G, et al. (2010) Improved outcome with hematopoietic stem cell transplantation in a poor prognostic subgroup of infants with mixed-lineage-leukemia (MLL)-rearranged acute lymphoblastic leukemia: results from the Interfant-99 Study. *Blood* **116**, 2644–50.

Moricke A, et al. (2016) Dexamethasone vs prednisone in induction treatment of pediatric ALL: results of the randomized trial AIEOP-BFM ALL 2000. *Blood* **127**, 2101–12.

Mullighan CG, et al. (2009) Deletion of IKZF1 and prognosis in acute lymphoblastic leukemia. *N Engl J Med* **360**, 470–80.

Peters C, et al. (2015) Stem-cell transplantation in children with acute lymphoblastic leukemia: a prospective international multicenter trial comparing sibling donors with matched unrelated donors–the ALL-SCT-BFM-2003 trial. *J Clin Oncol* **33**, 1265–74.

Pieters R, et al. (2016) Successful therapy reduction and intensification for childhood acute lymphoblastic leukemia based on minimal residual disease monitoring: study ALL10 from the Dutch Childhood Oncology Group. *J Clin Oncol* **34**, 2591–601.

Pieters R, et al. (2007) A treatment protocol for infants younger than 1 year with acute lymphoblastic leukaemia (Interfant-99): an observational study and a multicentre randomised trial. *Lancet* **370**, 240–50.

Pui CH, et al. (2009) Treating childhood acute lymphoblastic leukemia without cranial irradiation. *N Engl J Med* **360**, 2730–41.

Pui CH, et al. (2002) Outcome of treatment in childhood acute lymphoblastic leukaemia with rearrangements of the 11q23 chromosomal region. *Lancet* **359**, 1909–15.

Roberts KG, et al. (2014) Targetable kinase-activating lesions in Ph-like acute lymphoblastic leukemia. *N Engl J Med* **371**, 1005–15.

Roberts KG, et al. (2014) Outcomes of children with BCR-ABL1-like acute lymphoblastic leukemia treated with risk-directed therapy based on the levels of minimal residual disease. *J Clin Oncol* **32**, 3012–20.

Schrappe M, et al. (2012) Outcomes after induction failure in childhood acute lymphoblastic leukemia. *N Engl J Med* **366**, 1371–81.

Schultz KR, et al. (2014) Long-term follow-up of imatinib in pediatric Philadelphia chromosome-positive acute lymphoblastic leukemia: Children's Oncology Group study AALL0031. *Leukemia* **28**, 1467–71.

Stork LC, et al. (2010) Oral 6-mercaptopurine versus oral 6-thioguanine and veno-occlusive disease in children with standard-risk acute lymphoblastic leukemia: report of the Children's Oncology Group CCG-1952 clinical trial. *Blood* **115**, 2740–8.

Vora A, et al. (2016) Influence of cranial radiotherapy on outcome in children with acute lymphoblastic leukemia treated with contemporary therapy. *J Clin Oncol* **34**, 919–26.

Vora A, et al. (2013) Treatment reduction for children and young adults with low-risk acute lymphoblastic leukaemia defined by minimal residual disease (UKALL 2003): a randomised controlled trial. *Lancet Oncol* **14**, 199–209.

16

Acute Myeloid Leukaemia

Gertjan Kaspers and Dirk Reinhardt

Introduction

Acute myeloid leukaemia (AML) is the second most frequent type of leukaemia in children, after acute lymphoblastic leukaemia (ALL). AML encompasses not only the myeloid leukaemias but also acute eythroblastic and acute megakaryoblastic leukaemia. Therefore, the term acute non-lymphoblastic leukaemia (as used formally in the past) is better, but AML is used in clinical practice. Improvement in the prognosis of AML in children came somewhat later than for ALL, but has definitely occurred. Applying contemporary chemotherapy, 70–75% of children with AML are cured in high-income countries. In contrast to ALL, treatment is relatively short and usually consists of four or five courses of very intensive combination chemotherapy given over four to six months. A subset of the patients may benefit from allogeneic haematopoietic stem-cell transplantation (HSCT). Experience with the intensive treatment and high-quality supportive care is of utmost importance in this setting. Therefore, the treatment of childhood AML should be centralized in a limited number of paediatric oncology centres.

Epidemiology and aetiology

The incidence of AML in children is about 7.6 per million children per year, and it accounts for about 20% of acute leukaemias in this age group and for about 5% of all types of childhood cancer. An increased frequency of AML, especially of acute monoblastic and megakaryoblastic leukaemia, occurs within the first two years of life (1.5 in 100,000). The incidence remains relatively low during childhood (0.5 in 100,000) and starts to increase during adolescence and in young adults (0.9 in 100,000). There is a very high concordance rate for leukaemia in monozygous twins, probably the result of a common prezygotic or intrauterine genetic event or transplacental passage of a single leukaemic clone. The incidence of AML seems rather similar all over the world, with one clear exception, which is acute promyelocytic leukaemia (APL). APL is a subtype of AML, and occurs more frequently among the Hispanic and Mediterranean populations, and genetic susceptibility seems to play a role. Occasionally it is suggested that AML is more frequent in certain Asian countries, but underreporting of other types of cancer such as ALL, as an explanation, cannot yet be excluded.

AML is the most frequent secondary malignancy in children treated for ALL, lymphomas, or other solid tumours, induced by intensified therapy with exposure to alkylating agents such as cyclophosphamide, ifosfamide, or melphalan, and to topoisomersase II inhibitors.

The cause of AML is unclear in most cases. Unlike ALL, there is no indication that infections play a role in the development of AML. In a minority of cases, a predisposing condition to develop AML is present, such as a chromosal breakage syndrome (e.g. Fanconi anaemia), a stem-cell disease (congenital neutropenia, also known as Kostmann syndrome), and, most frequently, Down syndrome. Nowadays, a clear causative factor such as ionizing irradiation, previous chemotherapy, and certain chemicals is evident in even fewer cases.

Although the aetiology is usually unknown, the pathophysiology of AML is becoming more and more clear. AML is a clonal disorder of haematopoietic stem cells, common myeloid-lymphoid or early myeloid progenitors. The hierarchical differentiation of AML in part resembles normal haematopoiesis. Like normal haematopoietic stem cells (HSC), the leukaemic stem cell (LSC) is characterized by the capacity of self-renewal, proliferation, remnant differentiation programmes, and maturation. Several stages of leukaemic blast differentiation could be defined.

One model for AML development describes the coincidence of type II and type I mutations as indispensable (**Figure 16.1**). The type II (or class II) mutations are typically recurrent translocations ((t(8;21), inv(16), t(15;17), etc.) which are involved in impaired differentiation and maturation of early haematopoietic progenitors. The isolated occurrence in a cell clone does not cause overt leukaemia directly; however, it may define a pre-leukaemic stem cell. Only if a second activating mutation (type I) occurs as an additional event, the uncontrolled proliferation and decreased rate of apoptosis cause the survival advantage of the leukaemic blasts, displace normal haematopoiesis, and result in a frank leukaemia. Type I mutations are typically related to cytokine receptors or other factors in signal transduction pathways such as FLT3-receptor, c-kit-receptor, *ras*, PTPN11, and WT1.

Although these events seem to be sufficient to cause leukaemia in some combinations, in most subtypes, additional events, specific conditions of the bone marrow microenvironment, or dysfunctions of the immunological system might contribute to the probability of

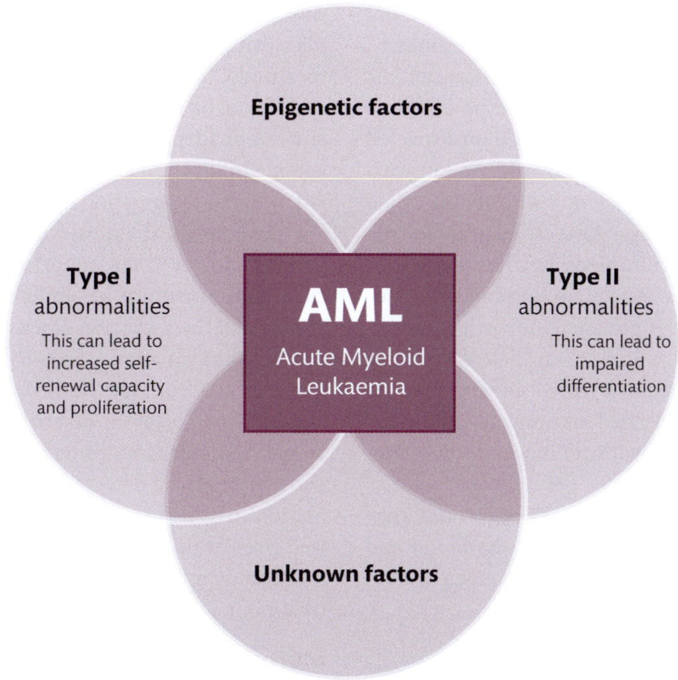

Figure 16.1 A model for leukaemogenesis in acute myeloid leukaemia involving type I abnormalities that lead to increased self-renewal capacity and proliferation, type II abnormalities that result in impaired differentiation, and other partly unknown factors.

leukaemia. These molecular abnormalities become more important in this era of targeted therapy, but they also provide opportunities for monitoring minimal residual disease during and after treatment. Recent studies, based on next-generation sequencing, revealed a more complex clonal hierarchy, with about three to seven subclones at diagnosis. Figure 16.2 illustrates current knowledge on chromosomal and molecular abnormalities in paediatric AML.

Symptoms and signs: clinical presentation

The presentation of a child with AML is not fundamentally different from a child with ALL, although children with AML tend be older (on average seven to eight years of age) and they more often have extramedullary disease. The children usually have malaise and often weight loss. Major symptoms are caused by the leukaemic infiltration of the bone marrow, resulting in reduced normal haematopoiesis. This translates into anaemia (resulting in paleness, fatigue, and headache) and to thrombocytopenia (resulting in skin bleeding, epistaxis, and sometimes other signs of increased bleeding tendency). Fever is a frequent symptom, either reflecting the inflammation caused by leukaemia or an infection as a consequence of the insufficient number of normal white blood cells. The bone marrow infiltration often gives bone pain, which can be very severe. Enlargement of the liver and/or spleen has been reported in about 50% of patients, and so is lymphadenopathy. A well-known extramedullary localization of AML is the central nervous system (CNS), most typically presenting as asymptomatic disease detected at routine examination of

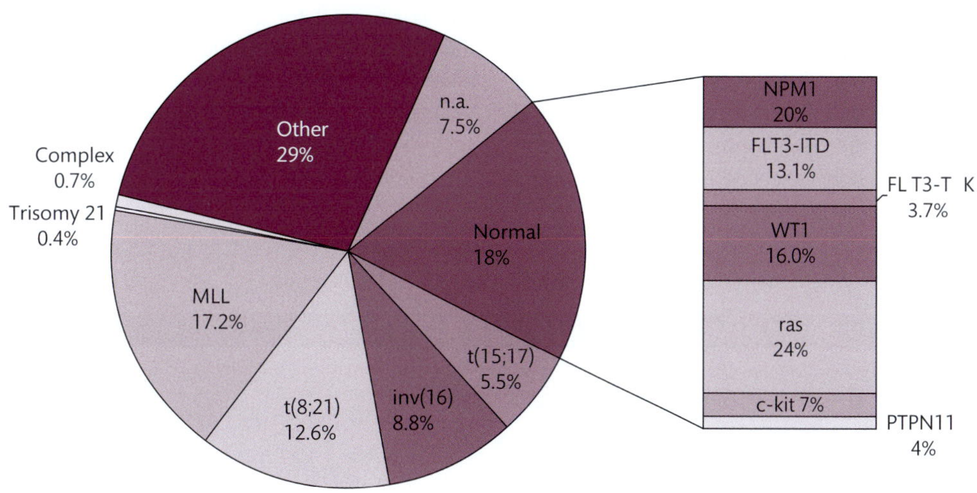

Figure 16.2 Percentages of acute myeloid leukaemia (AML) karyotypes; frequency of type I mutations.

the cerebrospinal fluid. However, CNS involvement can also present with, for example, headache, intracerebral bleeding, and seizures.

Certain subtypes of AML (discussed later) have characteristic clinical problems. In acute promyelocytic and acute monoblastic leukaemia, bleeding tendency is often more severe than expected as based on the platelet count. This is caused by diffuse intravascular coagulation. Acute myeloblastic leukaemia with the so-called t(8;21) is often associated with chloromas. Also called granulocytic or myeloid sarcomas, chloromas are extramedullary manifestations of AML presenting as solid masses. Acute myelomonocytic leukaemia in general, and especially the patient group with eosinophilia and the chromosal abnormality inv(16) in their AML cells, has a very high frequency of extramedullary involvement, in up to 60% of patients. Finally, acute monoblastic leukaemia is often characterized by skin involvement and gingival swelling, and sometimes with eye involvement.

A significantly increased white blood cell (WBC) count may result in so-called sludging, with hyperviscosity of the blood and leukostasis. This can give rise to, for example, dyspnoea and to confusion.

Diagnosis and biology

A correct and rapid diagnosis of AML is of utmost importance for optimal treatment. First, the presence of AML should be established without doubt, which occasionally is difficult when it resembles ALL or, for example, in case of a low blast count. Morphology and, if available, immunophenotyping are still the fastest methods for distinguishing between AML and ALL, or as an emergency means to identifying APL immediately. Next, the extent of the disease should be determined, as CNS disease especially has therapeutic consequences.

Initial work-up

Examinations required to determine the extent of AML are a chest X-ray, lumbar puncture for investigation of the cerebrospinal fluid, and an ultrasound of the abdomen. The chest X-ray should be done the same day a leukaemia is suspected, because of the possibility of mediastinal enlargement and compression on the trachea and upper airways. If that is the case, and depending on the severity, general anaesthesia may be contraindicated, as might investigations for which the patient must lie down flat. It also should lead to prompt treatment. A diagnostic lumbar puncture should only be done when there is no significant risk of bleeding and thereby introduction of peripheral leukaemic cells into the cerebrospinal fluid. If necessary, platelets should be transfused first. In case of APL, a lumbar puncture should be postponed because of the very high risk of bleeding complications. Another reason to withhold a lumbar puncture is when localized CNS disease is suspected, with the risk of herniation. The abdominal ultrasound should look not only for hepatosplenomegaly and lymphadenopathy, but also for renal enlargement caused by leukaemic infiltration. The latter should make the clinician aware of the risk of renal dysfunction in the first days of treatment.

Of course, the diagnosis of leukaemia requires laboratory investigations. However, the importance of a detailed history and physical examination cannot be underestimated. For example, the history may reveal the suspicion of a preceding myelodysplastic syndrome. Physical examination is important both to detect features compatible with syndromes such as Down syndrome and Fanconi anaemia, and also to correctly determine extramedullary disease. For example, testicular involvement, gingival hyperplasia, and leukaemia cutis will only be detected at physical examination. Physical examination may also reveal serious bleeding tendency and a compromised circulation because of anaemia or sludging, which should result in immediate and appropriate supportive care and anti-leukaemic treatment.

Morphology

For the diagnosis of leukaemia, bone marrow aspiration is always attempted. Abnormal cells may also be present in sufficient number in the peripheral blood. However, if this is not the case and if bone marrow aspiration does not provide enough cells ('dry tap'), a bone biopsy should be done and smears should be made, 'rolling' the biopsy over the slide. Normally, enough abnormal cells from bone marrow and peripheral blood are available for extensive characterization. First, this is done by morphological examination of the smears after staining. Additional enzymatic stainings are also helpful to diagnose AML (Table 16.1). It requires experience to distinguish leukaemic cells from normal precursors and, for example, from non-malignant blasts in case of an infection, to identify a low percentage of leukaemic cells, and to distinguish AML from ALL. Similarly, experience is required for diagnosing the correct FAB type according to the French–American–British (FAB) classification, described in Table 16.2.

Although the most recent World Health Organization (WHO) classification relies more on chromosomal abnormalities than on morphology, a correct morphological diagnosis remains the basis and is essential for correct initial treatment. This can be simply illustrated by two examples. First, it is essential to quickly distinguish AML from ALL in case of a high WBC count and the need to install anti-leukaemic treatment immediately. A glucocorticoid such as prednisone or dexamethasone is indicated in case of ALL, but is contraindicated in AML because it may actually increase the

Table 16.1 The usefulness of enzymatic staining in the diagnosis of acute myeloid leukaemia

	M0	M1-M3	M4	M5	M6	M7	ALL
MPO	–	+	+	–	–	–	–
ANAE	–	–	+	+	–	+/–	–
SB-B	–	+	+	–	–	–	–
PAS	–	–	+/–	+/–	+	–	+

MPO = myeloperoxidase, ANAE = acid alpha-naphthyl acetate esterase, SB-B = Sudan-Black B, PAS = Periodic Acid Schiff positive.

Table 16.2 Different types of acute myeloid leukaemia according to the French–American–British (FAB) classification, with percentage of the total number of cases per FAB type, and the relation with karyotypic abnormalities

FAB subtype	Full name (% of total number of cases)	Associated chromosomal abnormalities
M0	Acute myeloblastic leukaemia with minimal differentiation (3%)	
M1	Acute myeloblastic leukaemia without maturation (10–15%)	
M2	Acute myeloblastic leukaemia with maturation (25–30%)	t(6;9)
M2au+	AML M2 with auer rods	t(8;21)(q22;q22)
M3	Acute promyelocytic leukaemia (5–10%)	t(15;17)
M4	Acute myelomonocytic leukaemia (5–15%)	inv(16); del(16q)
M4Eo	Acute myelomonocytic leukaemia with abnormal eosinophils (5–15%)	inv(16); t(16;16)
M5	Acute monocytic leukaemia (15–25%)	t(9;11); t(11;19); del(11q)
M6	Acute erythroid leukaemia (1–3%)	
M7	Acute megakaryocytic leukaemia (5–10%)	t(1;22)

WBC count (especially if given without chemotherapy). Second, the early morphological recognition of AML FAB type M3 (APL) directs therapy. The diagnosis (or even the suspicion) of APL should prompt the clinicians to start all-trans retinoic acid (ATRA) and/or arsenic trioxide (ATO) immediately. ATRA and ATO are essential in the initial treatment of APL because these drugs quickly reduce the risk of bleeding complications. Early bleeding is life-threatening in patients with APL and fatal in 5–10% of children with APL. In addition, continued use of ATRA and ATO makes a very important contribution to the cure of most children with APL with contemporary treatment. Finally, sometimes additional investigations for immunophenotypical and chromosomal abnormalities fail or are not available. In these cases, morphology may indicate the presence of a specific chromosomal abnormality that is associated with a better prognosis. This is especially the case for AML FAB type M2 with auer rods, which is associated with t(8;21), and for AML FAB type M4 with eosinophilia, which is associated with inv(16). (The other example, AML FAB type M3 or APL which is associated with t(15;17), was described earlier.) Advantages of the WHO classification are that myeloid proliferations related to Down syndrome are now recognized entities, as well as that patients with specific recurrent genetic abnormalities are diagnosed with AML, even if the leukaemic blast percentage in the bone marrow is below 20%.

In conclusion, paediatric haemato-oncologists and those in training for that specialty should be capable of diagnosing AML based on morphological examination of bone marrow or peripheral blood smears. The official WHO classification requires at least 20% of leukaemic cells in the bone marrow for the diagnosis of AML. In addition, the presence of specific recurrent chromosomal abnormalities, independent from the percentage of leukaemic cells, already leads to the diagnosis of AML in the WHO classification, such as for t(8;21), inv(16), and t(15;17). It seems that many paediatric collaborative groups do not follow the WHO classification completely. Especially in case of 20–30% leukaemic cells in the bone marrow, additional features such as organ involvement and extramedullary disease are taken into account before the diagnosis of AML or, alternatively, myelodysplastic syndrome (MDS) is established (**Figure 16.3**). If no additional features are present and doubt remains about the diagnosis being AML or MDS, bone marrow aspiration and biopsy should be repeated after several weeks, to look for progressive disease resulting in clear AML. However, the presence of specific cytogenetic abnormalities, such as those mentioned here, leads to the diagnosis of AML independent from the blast percentage, even in children.

Immunophenotyping

Additional characterization of AML is based on immunophenotype and chromosomal abnormalities. Nowadays, immunophenotyping is done with multi-colour flow cytometry in high-income countries, but can be done on slides if such facilities are lacking. Immunophenotyping may profit from the asynchronous or aberrant

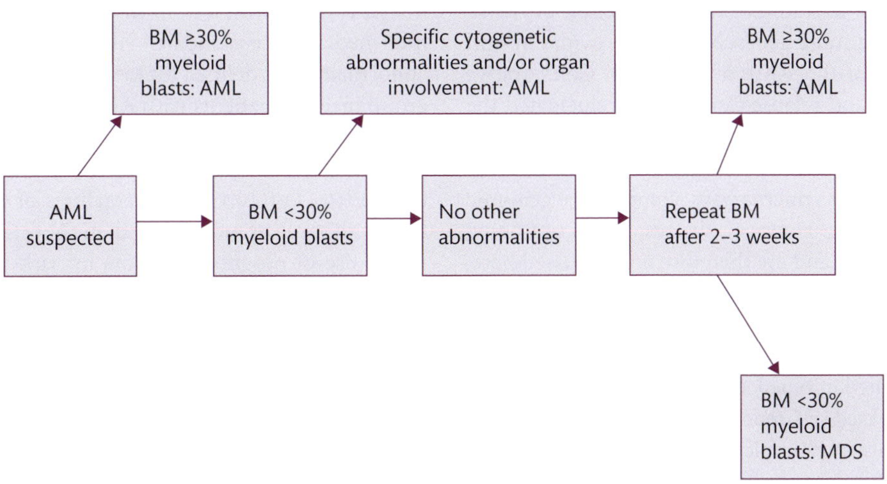

Figure 16.3 A systematic approach for dissecting acute myeloid leukaemia (AML) from myelodysplastic syndrome (MDS).

antigen expression on the leukaemic blasts. Asynchronous expression is the simultaneous expression of stem-cell antigens (CD34/CD117) and antigens indicating myeloid differentiation (CD13, CD14, CD15, CD33, myeloperoxidase (MPO)). Aberrant expression includes the simultaneous expression of myeloid antigen and lymphoid or natural killer cell antigens (CD2, CD7, CD19, CD56). Typical antigens indicative for AML are CD33, CD13, CD14, CDw41, CD15, CD11b, CD36, and CD61. In the diagnostic setting, immunophenotyping is especially important for the diagnosis of acute undifferentiated leukaemia (FAB type M0; no expression of MPO but reactivity with CD13 and/or CD33) and acute megakaryoblastic leukaemia (FAB type M7, expression of CD36, CD41, CD42b, or CD61)), because these subtypes are notably difficult to recognize and distinguish morphologically. Specific immunophenotypes could also be defined for acute erythoid leukaemia (FAB M6, expression of CD235a/glycophorin) and for acute monoblastic leukaemia (AML FAB M5; CD33/CD56/CD36). Some immunophenotypes are associated with genetic aberration, such as the combination of CD33/CD19/CD56 positivity that is indicative of t(8;21). Immunophenotyping is also instrumental in the measurement of minimal residual disease by the detection of leukaemic cells with a leukaemia-aberrant immunophenotype.

Cytogenetic and molecular diagnostics

Chromosomal abnormalities can be detected with a number of techniques. Conventionally, karyotyping is used, but, more and more, fluorescent *in situ* hybridization (FISH) is routinely applied as well, while polymerase chain reaction (PCR) techniques are additionally being used to detect molecular abnormalities. In the case of karyotyping, at least 20 metaphases are needed in order to reliably exclude an abnormal karyotype. If karyotyping and other techniques looking for chromosomal abnormalities fail, another attempt to obtain leukaemic cells should be considered, in view of the clinical relevance of these investigations. FISH is a reliable and robust technique to detect, for example, gene rearrangements. PCR techniques and other assays, such as the multiplex ligation polymerase assay, are useful for the detection of somatic molecular abnormalities occurring in the leukaemic cells exclusively.

Recently, next-generation sequencing (NGS), applied as targeted or whole-exome sequencing, has become routine in some laboratories. Targeted NGS analyses predefined genes known to carry AML-associated mutations. In addition to the detection of AML-specific mutations in one or more genes, NGS also provides insight into the clonal hierarchy of the AML at diagnosis. Comparative studies between diagnosis and relapse samples have elucidated the clonal evolution of the AML.

There are a wide range of other techniques being used to characterize leukaemic cells, such as microarrays, comparative genomic hybridization, and proteomics. However, the results are not being applied in clinical practice yet and are therefore not discussed here, except in relation to the detection of molecular abnormalities. Such abnormalities are detected mainly with PCR techniques (as already mentioned regarding leukaemogenesis). Often these molecular abnormalities are distinguished in type I and type II aberrations. Type I aberrations lead to increased self-renewal and increased proliferative capacity, and well-known examples are mutations in the *RAS, KIT, FLT3, WT1*, and *PTPN11* genes. Type II aberrations cause differentiation arrest, and often concern chromosomal rearrangements of transcription factors, including *PML-RARα* (t(15;17)(q22;q21)), *AML1-ETO* (t(8;21)(q22;q22)), *CBFB-MYH11* (inv(16)(p13q22)), *MLL* rearrangements, or mutations in *NPM1* or *CEBPA*. Aside from possibleinvolvement in leukaemogenesis, molecular abnormalities have other potential clinical applications. These include a prognostic significance (see the section 'Prognostic factors') and use for the detection of minimal residual disease. Perhaps most importantly, they have the potential to provide leukaemia-specific treatment targets.

Prognostic factors

The previously described characterization of AML and its extension has prognostic relevance. Chromosomal abnormalities dominate clinical features (e.g. age, sex, WBC count), disease extension, and morphology of the AML cells, as prognostic factors. In addition, early clinical response—as determined by either morphological examination of bone marrow one, two, or four weeks after the start of treatment, or by more sophisticated minimal residual disease measurements—is an important predictor of long-term outcome.

Clinically, a high WBC count remains an adverse prognostic factor. Otherwise, extramedullary involvement does not seem to impact prognosis with current intensive therapy, including high-dose cytarabine. If information on chromosomal abnormalities is lacking, morphological subtypes can be used to predict outcome. Favourable are FAB type M2 with auer rods, FAB type M3 (APL), and FAB type M4, especially (but not exclusively) if associated with eosinophilia. Moreover, myeloid leukaemia of Down syndrome (usually FAB type M7, occasionally M6) has a favourable prognosis and will be described later as a separate disease entity. Immunophenotype is not of significant prognostic relevance in AML.

More and more, cytogenetic abnormalities are being used as a prognostic factor, and most groups agree with three cytogenetic risk groups. The low-risk group has core-binding factor AML (i.e. either inv(16), t(16;16), or t(8;21)) or has APL with t(15;17). Patients with these low-risk cytogenetic features, but a less than favourable early treatment response, should most likely remain low-risk patients, if they achieve complete remission (CR) after two induction courses; and similarly for t(8;21)-positive patients, if there is no coinciding gain of chromosome 4. Patients with other molecular abnormalities, such as mutations in *NPM1* or *GATA1s* and double mutations in *CEPBA*, and with t(1;11), also qualify for the low-risk group. The intermediate- (i.e. standard) risk group has no specific cytogenetic abnormalities as defined for low- or high-risk groups. The high-risk group includes patients with AML cells that harbour FLT3-ITD but without a *NPM1* mutation, monosomy 7, an abnormal chromosome 5 (monosomy 5, 5q-), inv(3) or t(3;3)/t(6;9)/t(7;12)/t(9;22)/t(4;11)/t(5;11)/t(6;11)/t(10;11), abnormalities of 12p, or a complex karyotype with three or more cytogenetic aberrations.

The use of prognostic factors for risk-group-adapted therapy is described in the section 'Risk classification'.

Risk classification

According to the WHO classification, AML subgroups are defined by the history of the disease—a preceding myelodysplastic syndrome or treatment for a malignancy, by recurrent cytogenetic abnormalities such as t(8;21), inv(16), t(15;17), and MLL rearrangements, and by the lack of such features (not otherwise characterized). This last category largely reflects the former FAB classification, which is based on morphology and cytochemistry.

AML is a heterogeneous disease, and the prognosis of the subtypes varies widely. In addition, the prognostic relevance of an identified factor does not only depend on the biological characteristics but also on the applied therapy. The occurrence of balanced translocations—t(8;21)/inv(16)—affecting core-binding factors (CBF-AML) is associated with a relatively good prognosis. This has been shown in both children and adults. The event-free and overall survival in this particular group of children is more than 70% and 85%, respectively. Even in cases of relapse, these karyotypes remain a favourable prognostic factor, and these patients have achieved an overall survival of more than 60% from relapse. Further, APL can be treated successfully in most cases if the frequently occurring early complications such as severe bleedings or infections can be treated or, better, prevented. The introduction of ATRA and ATO therapy in particular has prevented early deaths and enables survival rates of about 90% in APL.

Nucleophosmin-1 (NPM1) mutations, occurring in about 8% of childhood AML, seems to be associated with a favourable prognosis. In the subgroup of AML with a normal karyotype, the incidence is up to 20%. Interestingly, the non-type A mutations are more frequent in children than in adults. Further, a correlation with increasing age has been observed.

A special entity is myeloid leukaemia of Down syndrome (ML-DS) with GATA1s mutation. If adapted treatment is applied, the prognosis is good. The intensity of the treatment schedule should be significantly reduced as compared to standard protocols. By contrast to other AML subtypes, the immediate continuation of treatment is not time-sensitive; a treatment element should be started only if the child is in a good general condition.

In the past, MLL rearrangements were generally recognized as a poor prognostic factor; however, at least two studies in children found the t(9;11) as a favourable marker. These results, based on a relatively low number of patients, have not been confirmed by larger study groups. The prognosis of childhood AML with t(9;11) seems to be insignificantly better than in other MLL-positive leukaemia; it is still within the range of intermediate- and high-risk patients. Several aberrations that are associated with a very poor prognosis in adults do not discriminate in children. For example, a complex karyotype (three or more aberrations) or 7q− do not predict a particularly poor outcome in children. However, isolated monosomy 7 is associated with an impaired CR rate and a poor outcome.

Several additional molecular events, mostly type I mutations, have been identified as a prognostic marker in childhood AML. Most data are available about the poor prognostic value of internal tandem duplications in the *FLT3* gene (FLT3-ITDs). Especially in children with normal karyotype, FLT3-ITD is associated with poor prognosis. While FLT3-ITD and NPM1 are frequently associated with AML with normal karyotype, the relevance of other aberrations such as *RAS* or *c-KIT* mutations remains unclear. Recently, *WT1* mutations have been identified as a poor prognostic factor in childhood AML.

Interestingly, there are recent reports that have described a possible prognostic relevance of certain polymorphisms in AML; however, this is probably dependent on age and treatment regimen. Indeed, treatment itself remains the most important prognostic factor. A lot of other prognostic factors have been proposed. These include the WBC count at diagnosis, age, the occurrence of extramedullary leukaemia, or the immunophenotype, although the prognostic relevance seems to be associated to intensity and schedule of therapy.

Apart from genetic characteristics, treatment response is an important prognostic factor. Assessed by bone marrow morphology, CR—defined as less than 5% blasts and sufficient haematological regeneration (neutrophils higher than 1000/μl; platelets higher than 80.000/μl)—is a strong predictor for outcome. More difficult is the measurement of early response. Morphology is impeded by a low sensitivity and specificity, but has been successfully used at day 14 or 15 and/or day 28, after the first induction course to stratify patients to risk groups. However, measurements of so-called minimal residual disease (MRD) have become more important.

Minimal residual disease

Several attempts have been made to establish more sensitive methods to measure response and MRD. Quantitative reverse transcription PCR (RT-PCR) allows the sensitive detection and quantification of known fusion genes such as *AML1/ETO* or *CBF/MYH11*. As the frequency of these aberrations is about 40%, only a minority of children can be monitored based on these leukaemia-specific abnormalities. More critical is the fact that a relevant portion of patients remains 'MRD-positive' throughout the complete course of the disease, with persisting cells with the fusion gene. Up to 40% of the children show detectable *AML/ETO1* even after intensive therapy without predicting relapse. By contrast, the monitoring of *PML/RARα* in APL has generally been shown to be very predictive and is used to stratify treatment intensity, if *PML/RARα* remains after several cycles of therapy. This even includes the recommendation to act upon molecular refractory disease and to treat a molecular relapse.

In *MLL*-gene rearranged AML the situation is even more complicated. Persistence of the rearranged *MLL* gene is clearly associated with a very high risk of relapse; however, in most cases the *MLL* arrangement is not detectable after the first or second chemotherapy induction course, which does not exclude relapse. Further, reoccurrence of the *MLL* rearrangement is strongly associated with relapse within two to four weeks. Whether this very short pre-warning phase has any clinical meaning is unclear.

Another approach to monitoring MRD is immunophenotyping. In almost all cases of AML, a leukaemia-associated immunophenotype (LAIP) can be defined based on an asynchronous expression of differential, stage-dependent antigens (simultaneous expression of stem-cell antigens and antigens of myeloid maturation) or based on lineage-aberrant antigen expression. Although some studies have demonstrated the possibility of monitoring the treatment response, the independent value of the MRD diagnostic is so far hampered by the limited specificity. First, the LAIP of the bulk of leukaemic blasts could differ from the immunophenotype of the leukaemic stem cell. Second, the expression pattern of leukaemic blasts changes during treatment and at relapse. Third, especially in a regenerating bone marrow, the leukaemic blasts may not be distinguishable from normal progenitors.

The discovery of a leukaemic stem-cell-specific antigen (CLL-1) within the CD34+/CD38− compartment might improve the specificity of immunophenotyping and provide a more reliable method in the future. This might also be achieved by improved techniques (8 colour-flow) and better methods of analysis. Indeed, nowadays, most collaborative groups have implemented MRD monitoring by flow cytometry to stratify consolidation treatment. Recently, MRD has also been evaluated by using NGS. This seems promising, especially because additional information about the residual clone might become available. However, the clinical and prognostic relevance of MRD monitoring by NGS have not yet been proven.

Treatment and prognosis

Over the last three decades, the prognosis of childhood AML has markedly improved (Figure 16.4). In children, the first approaches with intensive chemotherapy were initiated in the 1970s. These protocols were adapted from ALL treatment schedules. In the 1980s, the benefit of intensified elements, including cytarabine and anthracyclines, became obvious. Several other drugs such as etoposide (a topoisomerase II inhibitor), amsacrine, thioguanine, or cyclophosphamide have been combined. The mechanism of action of these drugs has been described elsewhere.

Most of the treatment protocols recommend four or five elements of intensive chemotherapy. At least with regard to children with favourable cytogenetics, the results of the UK Medical Research Council (MRC) group and the AML-BFM (Berlin–Frankfurt–Munster) group did not provide strong evidence that a fifth intensive element improves outcome. However, the subgroup of AML with t(8;21) might benefit from high-dose cytarabine during induction and/or consolidation.

In spite of the different treatment regimens of several different study groups, the final results for disease-free survival (DFS) and overall survival (OS) have been within similar ranges. The most relevant treatment differences concern the cumulative dose of anthracyclines and the percentage of patients that undergoes allogeneic HSCT. Table 16.3 summarizes the EFS and OS of several large clinical trials in paediatric AML.

Induction

Anthracycline- and cytarabine-based regimens are generally accepted to induce remission in AML. Sequential studies proved the efficacy of intensive, high-dose chemotherapy. Double-induction schedules are now used by all collaborative groups in high-income countries. Today, on average, 90% of the children with AML achieve CR after induction, although this does depend on the risk group.

Cytarabine is used in different dose regimens. Whereas in first induction 3×60 mg/m^2 daunorubicin is frequently administered in combination with lower-dose cytarabine (and often etoposide), in second induction, several studies schedule high-dose cytarabine, with 1–3 g/m^2 combined with mitoxantrone or an anthracycline. Newer analogues of cytarabine (such as fludarabine, cladribine, or clofarabine) are frequently used in re-induction in relapsed AML, but are rarely included in frontline protocols. The addition of chlor or fluor to the basic cytosine-arabinoside impairs the intracellular degradation by purine nucleoside phosphorylase or hydrolysis. The latest development in this field is clofarabine, which might combine the advantages of fludarabine and cladribine, and which has shown promising results in relapsed AML. However, a randomized comparison to currently used drugs is still lacking.

Post remission

In most studies, post-remission treatment includes intensive chemotherapy such as high-dose cytarabine-based regimens and, additionally, an anthracycline or etoposide. After two courses of induction, between two to four intensive post-remission courses have

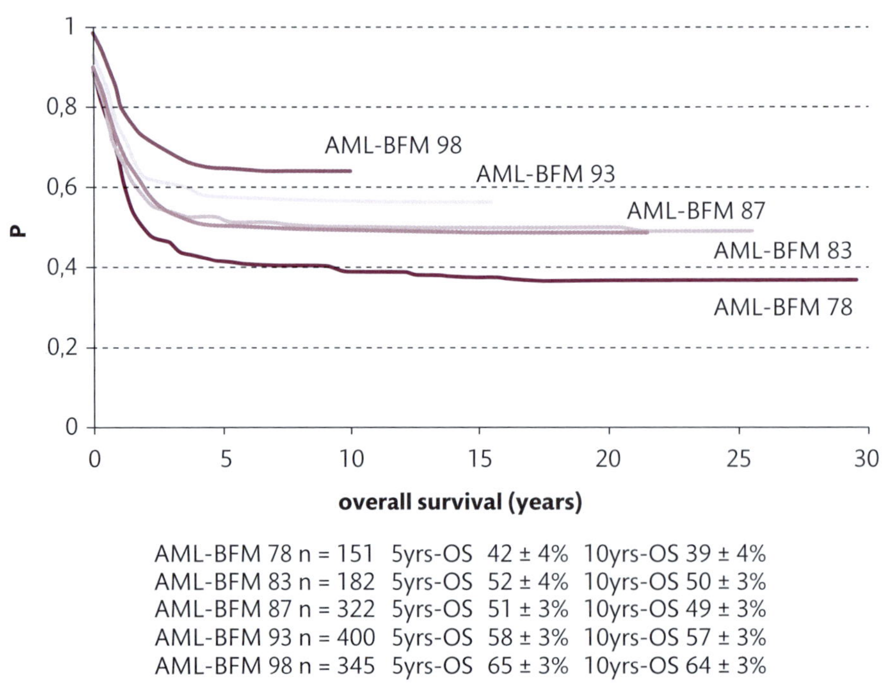

Figure 16.4 Improvement of overall survival in childhood acute myeloid leukaemia (AML): example, AML-BFM Studies 78 to 98.

Table 16.3 Results from paediatric acute myeloid leukaemia studies

Study group	Trial name (period)	Event-free survival (%)	Overall survival (%)
AIEOP	AML2002/01 (2002-2011)	8-yr (55±3)	8-yr (68±2)
AML-BFM	AML-BFM 2004 (2004-2010)	5-yr (55±2)	5-yr (74±2)
COG	AAML0531	3-yr (53±4)	3-yr (69±4)
DB	(2006–2010) DB-AML01 (2010–2014)	3-yr (50) (95%CI 40–59%)	3-yr (74) (95%CI 64–82%)
JPLSG	AML05 (2006-2010)	3-yr (54±2)	3-yr (73±2)
MRC	MRC AML12 (1995-2002)	10-yr (54)	10-yr (63)
NOPHO	NOPHO AML 2004 (2004–2009)	3-yr (57±5)	3-yr (69±5)
PPLLSG	PPLLSG AML-98 (1998-2002)	5-yr (47±5)	5-yr (50±5)
SJCRH	AML02 (2002-2008)	3-yr (63±4)	3-yr (71±4)

been scheduled in paediatric AML studies. Although not uniformly defined, at least one to two courses followed by allogeneic stem-cell transplantation (SCT), are given in high-risk AML.

Stem-cell transplantation

The value of allogeneic HSCT in first CR is controversial. Whereas some groups still recommend allogeneic HSCT for all AML subgroups (except for APL) if a matched sibling donor (MSD) is available, other groups have recently tended to restrict HSCT to intermediate- or high-risk AML patients. Children's Oncology Group (COG) studies, which previously recommended allogeneic HSCT, could not prove the advantage of allogeneic HSCT in patients with favourable or unfavourable cytogenetics.

Although, as confirmed in a recent meta-analysis, the relapse rate of intermediate- and high-risk AML could be lowered by allogeneic SCT in most studies, the higher treatment-related mortality counterbalanced this advantage. New specific prognostic factors need to be identified to define those patients who will benefit from allogeneic HSCT. Preliminary but yet unpublished results suggest that allogeneic SCT in high-risk patients, as defined by a poor early treatment response or specific biological features of the AML cells, might improve EFS and OS.

By contrast, there is a clear indication to perform allogeneic HSCT in refractory or relapsed AML, after the attempt to achieve a second CR with two cycles of intensive combination chemotherapy, usually including fludarabine, high-dose cytarabine, and liposomal daunorubicin or another anthracycline or mitoxantrone. Even more experimental approaches, such as haploidentical SCT or cord blood SCT, may be indicated in these cases, if a matched donor is lacking. Interestingly, recent data suggest that children with very late relapse and favourable prognostic features can also be rescued by chemotherapy only.

Maintenance

With the possible exception of APL, there is no evidence of a benefit of maintenance therapy in childhood AML. Only the AML-BFM group applied low-dose maintenance therapy until recently, adapted from adult AML studies, because the combination of thioguanine and cytarabine has shown improved results in some adult groups. However, this has not been prospectively proven in children. Even in APL, the recent introduction of ATO in addition to ATRA seems to have abolished the need for maintenance treatment.

Acute promyelocytic leukaemia

APL is the first subtype of acute leukaemia which nowadays can be cured without conventional cytostatic drugs, but with ATRA and ATO. The combination of these differentiating agents, which apparently also eliminates the leukaemic stem cells, has shown very favourable cure rates and, at the same time, reduced side effects and improved quality of life.

Side effects and late effects

Side effects

Each treatment option in childhood AML have considerable acute and long-term adverse effects, and almost all organ systems are involved. Of the acute side effects and toxicities, expected myelosuppression, mucositis, and the consecutive high risk of severe infections and septicaemia are the most relevant, since infections are responsible for most treatment-related deaths.

Improved supportive and intensive care can reduce early deaths by infections to less than 5%. This includes guidelines for supportive care that cover prophylactic and pre-emptive antibiotic and antifungal therapy, recent development of effective and orally applicable antifungal drugs, and the availability of antiviral compounds. Improved intensive care has also enabled the management of severe complications and continuation of treatment.

The most impressive effect has been achieved by the introduction of ATRA and/or ATO into the initial treatment of APL, which has reduced the early deaths in this particular subgroup substantially.

Efforts to reduce the duration of myelosuppression by administering the granulocyte growth factor G-CSF resulted in a limited shortening of neutropenia but did not change the rate of severe infections or the probability of survival. In fact, in those children treated with G-CSF, there is increased incidence of relapse in those with favourable cytogenetics and an increased expression of the G-CSF receptor isoform IV. In conclusion, G-CSF should not be administered routinely to children with AML. Other options, such as the application of supportive granulocyte infusions, are controversial and efficacy has not been proven.

Another open question concerns the management of hyperleukocytosis. It is undisputed that rasburicase and antiproliferative therapy should be started immediately; however, because of the risk of tumour lysis, the best starting dose cannot easily be defined. Children with severe hyperleukocytosis (more than 100,000 leukocytes/μl blood; APL more than 10,000 leukocytes/μl) should be treated on an intensive-care unit, especially if they show any additional abnormal parameters such as those related to coagulation, blood-gas analysis, renal parameters, and increased lactate. If severe tumour lysis is expected, the effect of the first dose of cytostatics should be carefully monitored. There is no consensus on whether such first doses should be lower than normal in patients with hyperleukocytosis above 50,000–100,000 WBC/μl blood.

Another option that is sometimes considered in the case of a critically ill child due to hyperleukocytosis, is an exchange transfusion or even leukapheresis, although the efficacy of this latter procedure is not proven.

Late toxicity

Late sequelae of therapy (see also Chapter 14) can be attributed to the initial disease and to the complications of its treatment. The literature offers a range of perspectives on the incidence of significant late effects in survivors of AML. In one retrospective study from the AML-BFM study group, only about 5% of all long-term survivors were reported to experience severe late toxicities (such as blindness/cataracts, severe osteonecrosis, cardiomyopathy, or secondary malignancies). In comparison to reports from other studies, this incidence is relatively low, and there is much greater morbidity in patients who undergo allogeneicHSCT. The importance of anthracycline drugs in schedules for the treatment of AML raises particular concern about the risk of cardiotoxicity.

Challenges and perspectives

Prognosis of paediatric AML has improved significantly, to even above 70% long-term survival in some recently published clinical studies. The biggest challenge is to further improve outcome to a cure rate of well above 90% and ultimately 100%, with acceptable side effects and limited late effects of treatment. Current conventional chemotherapy cannot be intensified further because of toxicity. Some novel but conventional (non-targeted) drugs, such as liposomal daunorubicin and clofarabine, will likely make an improvement, but main steps forward are more likely to be achieved with really novel drugs and novel treatment modalities. Novel agents are usually targeted, which has the implication that they will be used only in patients whose AML cells harbour the treatment target. An example is tyrosine kinase inhibitors targeting mutated *FLT3* or *c-KIT*. Another example is monoclonal antibodies that, either alone or by being linked to a cytotoxic agent, exert an anti-leukaemic effect. A good example of the latter is gemtuzumab ozogamicin—an anti-CD33 antibody linked to the highly toxic calcheamicin.

Studies on such novel agents in subgroups of paediatric AML will require international collaboration because of the rarity of these subgroups. An important challenge in such international collaborative studies is that, ideally, a common chemotherapeutic backbone is used. Although most paediatric groups worldwide are now using four or five courses of intensive chemotherapy, there are still many differences in drugs, doses, and schedules, and concerning the indications for allogeneic HSCT. Another main challenge is the performance of clinical trials under the EU directive and good clinical practice guidelines. Although this EU directive has had a positive effect on the number of clinical studies on new agents in children with cancer, it has become a very complicated process in which, unfortunately, not all countries apply it similarly. Investigator-initiated studies have become much more cumbersome and there is a risk that such studies will be done less often. That would be a major problem, because company-driven studies are still rare in children with cancer, including AML.

Despite these challenges, the paediatric community has always been able to improve the treatment and outcome of all types of malignancies. Techniques are rapidly improving to identify subgroups that should be treated differently. More and more novel drugs are emerging that could be used in different subgroups. Therefore, it seems realistic to expect long-term survival in more than 90% of paediatric AML patients, with an acceptable quality of life during treatment and with limited late effects.

FURTHER READING

Arber DA, et al. (2016) The 2016 revision to the World Health Organization classification of myeloid neoplasms and acute leukemia. *Blood* **127**(20), 2391–405. doi: 10.1182/blood-2016-03-643544.

Bonnet D, Dick JE (1997) Human acute myeloid leukemia is organized as a hierarchy that originates from a primitive hematopoietic cell. *Nat Med* **3**, 730–7.

Creutzig U, et al. (2006) Less toxicity by optimizing chemotherapy, but not by addition of granulocyte colony-stimulating factor in children and adolescents with acute myeloid leukemia: results of AML-BFM 98. *J Clin Oncol* **24**, 4499–506.

Creutzig U, et al. (2007) Longitudinal evaluation of early and late anthracycline cardiotoxicity in children with AML. *Pediatr Blood Cancer* **48**, 651–62.

Creutzig U, et al. (2012) Diagnosis and management of acute myeloid leukemia in children and adolescents: recommendations from an international expert panel. *Blood* **120**, 3187–205.

Creutzig U, et al. (2013) Randomized trial comparing liposomal daunorubicin with idarubicin as induction for pediatric acute myeloid leukemia: results from Study AML-BFM 2004. *Blood* **122**, 37–43.

Creutzig U, et al. (2017) First experience of the AML-Berlin–Frankfurt–Münster group in pediatric patients with standard-risk acute promyelocytic leukemia treated with arsenic trioxide and all-trans retinoid acid. *Pediatr Blood Cancer* **64**(8). doi: 10.1002/pbc.26461

Ehlers S, et al. (2010) Granulocyte colony-stimulating factor (G-CSF) treatment of childhood acute myeloid leukemias that overexpress the differentiation-defective G-CSF receptor isoform IV is associated with a higher incidence of relapse. *J Clin Oncol* **28**, 2591–7.

Gibson BE, et al. (2005) Treatment strategy and long-term results in paediatric patients treated in consecutive UK AML trials. *Leukemia* **19**, 2130–8.

Gibson BES, et al. (2011) Results of a randomized trial in children with acute myeloid leukemia: Medical Research Council AML12 trial. *Br J Haematol* **155**, 366–76.

Gilliland DG (2001) Hematologic malignancies. *Curr Opin Hematol* **8**, 189–91.

Greaves MF, Wiemels J (2003) Origins of chromosome translocations in childhood leukaemia. *Nat Rev Cancer* **3**, 639–49.

Harrison CJ, et al. (2010) Cytogenetics of childhood acute myeloid leukemia: United Kingdom Medical Research Council treatment trials AML 10 and 12. *J Clin Oncol* **28**, 2674–81.

Hasle H, et al. (2007) Monosomy 7 and deletion 7q in children and adolescents with acute myeloid leukemia: an international retrospective study. *Blood* **109**, 4641–7.

Hasle H, Kaspers GJL (2017) Strategies for reducing the treatment-related physical burden of childhood acute myeloid leukaemia—a review. *Br J Haematol* **176**, 168–78.

Jeha S, et al. (2004) Clofarabine, a novel nucleoside analog, is active in pediatric patients with advanced leukemia. *Blood* **103**, 784–9.

Kaspers GJ, Zwaan CM. (2007) Pediatric acute myeloid leukemia: towards high-quality cure of all patients. *Haematologica* **92**, 1519–32.

Kaspers GJL (2014) How I treat paediatric relapsed acute myeloid leukaemia. *Br J Haematol* **166**, 636–45.

Kaspers GJ, et al. (2013) Improved outcome in pediatric relapsed acute myeloid leukemia: results of a randomized trial on liposomal daunorubicin by the International BFM Study Group. *J Clin Oncol* **31**, 599–607.

Langebrake C, et al. (2006) Residual disease monitoring in childhood acute myeloid leukemia by multiparameter flow cytometry: the MRD-AML-BFM Study Group. *J Clin Oncol* **24**, 3686–92.

Lehrnbecher T, et al. (2007) Prophylactic human granulocyte colony-stimulating factor after induction therapy in pediatric acute myeloid leukemia. *Blood* **109**, 936–43.

Leung W, et al. (2000) Late effects of treatment in survivors of childhood acute myeloid leukemia. *J Clin Oncol* **18**, 3273–9.

Lipshultz SE, et al. (1995) Female sex and drug dose as risk factors for late cardiotoxic effects of doxorubicin therapy for childhood cancer. *N Engl J Med* **332**, 1738–43.

Perel Y, et al. (2002) Impact of addition of maintenance therapy to intensive induction and consolidation chemotherapy for childhood acute myeloblastic leukemia: results of a prospective randomized trial, LAME 89/91 for the group LAME of the French Society of Pediatric Hematology and Immunology. *J Clin Oncol* **20**, 2774–82.

Rubnitz JE, et al. (2002) Favorable impact of the t(9;11) in childhood acute myeloid leukemia. *J Clin Oncol* **20**, 2302–9.

Rubnitz JE, et al. (2010) Minimal residual disease-directed therapy for childhood acute myeloid leukaemia: results of the AML02 multicentre trial. *Lancet Oncol* **11**, 543–52.

Testi AM, et al. (2005) GIMEMA-AIEOPAIDA protocol for the treatment of newly diagnosed acute promyelocytic leukemia (APL) in children. *Blood* **106**, 447–53.

Zwaan CM, et al. (2003) FLT3 internal tandem duplication in 234 children with acute myeloid leukemia: prognostic significance and relation to cellular drug resistance. *Blood* **102**, 2387–94.

Zwaan CM, et al. (2010) Salvage treatment for children with refractory first or second relapse of acute myeloid leukaemia with gemtuzumab ozogamicin: results of a phase II study. *Br J Haematol* **148**, 768–76.

Zwaan CM, et al. (2015) Collaborative efforts driving progress. in pediatric acute myeloid leukemia. *J Clin Oncol* **33**, 2949–62.

17

Myelodysplastic Syndrome, Myeloid Leukaemia of Down Syndrome, and Juvenile Myelomonocytic Leukaemia

Henrik Hasle and Charlotte M. Niemeyer

Introduction

Myeloid malignancies in children are subdivided into four main groups: acute myeloid leukaemia (AML), myelodysplastic syndrome (MDS), juvenile myelomonocytic leukaemia (JMML), and the myeloid leukaemias of Down syndrome (TAM and ML-DS). The rarity of MDS in children and the lack of definite morphological and cytogenetic markers have contributed to the paucity of MDS in the paediatric literature. Most protocol-based studies on MDS and JMML have been performed by the European Working Group of MDS in Childhood (EWOG-MDS; www.ewog-mds.org).

Myelodysplastic syndrome

Classification

Starting in the early 1980s, the French–American–British (FAB) group developed the first widely accepted MDS classification, with five subgroups: refractory anaemia (RA), RA with ringed sideroblasts (RARS), RA with excess of blasts (RAEB), RAEB in transformation (RAEB-T), and chronic myelomonocytic leukaemia (CMML). The World Health Organization (WHO) classification of 2001 elaborated on this and prompted a paediatric approach. Myelodysplastic and myeloproliferative disorders in children were separated into three main groups: JMML, MDS, and ML-DS. MDS was further subdivided into refractory cytopenia (RC), RAEB, and RAEB-T. The change in nomenclature from RA to RC reflects that anaemia is not a prerequisite for the diagnosis. The revised WHO classification of 2008 recognized ML-DS as a unique group and describes refractory cytopenia of childhood (RCC) as a new provisional entity (Box 17.1). The most recent WHO classification of 2017 substitutes the term RAEB by MDS with excess of blasts (MDS-EB; Box 17.1).

Epidemiology

Incidence, sex, age, and subtype distribution

Combined population-based data from Denmark and British Columbia in Canada showed an annual incidence of MDS of 1.8 and of JMML of 1.2 per million children, corresponding to a total of 6% of all haematological malignancies in children, although data from the UK suggest a lower incidence of MDS of 0.8 per million. The UK study excluded secondary MDS, partly explaining the lower incidence. The male/female distribution in paediatric MDS is equal, with a median age at presentation of 6.8 years. The exclusion of Down syndrome from patient series of MDS has decreased the number of cases diagnosed as MDS-EB by almost 50%. Most paediatric MDS presents as RCC.

Associated abnormalities

MDS has been reported in a number of constitutional cytogenetic abnormalities other than Down syndrome, but there is only solid evidence for an association between trisomy 8 mosaicism and MDS. Reports of MDS and AML in patients with Klinefelter and Turner syndrome have appeared sporadically, but no increased risk has been documented in larger cohort studies.

With careful examination, the percentage of children with MDS and abnormalities of other organ systems (e.g. skeleton, heart, central nervous system) and urogenital tract malformations, or signs and symptoms of immunodeficiency, rises sharply. Besides the classical, inherited bone-marrow failure disorders, several autosomal dominant predisposition syndromes have recently been discovered which often display a non-haemological phenotype.

Myelodysplastic syndrome in inherited bone-marrow failure disorder

Inherited bone-marrow failure disorders (IBMFDs) have an increased risk of MDS/AML. The risk varies greatly and is highest in Fanconi anaemia and severe congenital neutropenia (SCN). Diagnosing low-grade MDS in a patient with IBFD is a challenge because cytopenia and dysplasia may be part of the bone-marrow

Box 17.1 Diagnostic categories of myelodysplastic and myeloproliferative diseases in children according to the paediatric approach to the World Health Organization (WHO) classification and revised classification

Myelodysplastic/myeloproliferative disease
- Juvenile myelomonocytic leukaemia (JMML)

Myeloid proliferations related to Down syndrome (DS)
- Transient abnormal myelopoiesis (TAM)
- Myeloid leukaemia of Down syndrome (ML-DS)

Myelodysplastic syndrome (MDS)
- Refractory cytopenia (RCC) (PB blasts <2% and BM blasts <5%)
- MDS with excess blasts (MDS-EB) (PB blasts 2–19% or BM blasts 5–19%)
- MDS-EB in transformation (PB or BM blasts 20–29%)/acute myeloid leukaemia (AML) with myelodysplasia-related changes (PB or BM blasts >20%)

PB: peripheral blood; BM: bone marrow

Source: data from Arber DA et al. 'The 2016 revision to the World Health Organization classification of myeloid neoplasms and acute leukemia'. *Blood*, Volume 217, Issue 20, pp. 2391–2405, (2016) American Society of Hematology.

failure, and cytogenetic or molecular aberrations marking small clones may be temporary. The hierarchy of clonal events indicating progression to MDS is quite specific for the individual IBMFDs.

In Fanconi anaemia, myeloid neoplasia develops in a large fraction of patients during childhood or early adult life. The risk varies according to genetic subgroup and associated abnormalities. Studies from the SCN International Register show a 15-year accumulated risk of MDS of 15%. Partial or complete loss of chromosome 7 is found in more than half the patients who develop MDS. There is no direct cause and effect relationship between the development of MDS and growth factor therapy using granulocyte colony-stimulating growth factor (G-CSF), but the risk of MDS is highest in patients with a poor response to G-CSF.

MDS/AML develops in approximately 30% of those with Shwachman–Diamond syndrome (SDS) and is often associated with chromosome 7 abnormalities of which isochromosome 7q may represent a separate entity with a long, stable clinical course and a low risk of progression. Most SDS patients can be diagnosed by clinical features: screening for *SBDS* gene mutations in children diagnosed with primary hypoplastic RCC identifies only very few (less than 1%) SDS patients.

Patients with dyskeratosis congenita (DC) carry mutations in genes encoding components of the telomerase complex like *DKC1*, *TERC*, or *TERT*. These mutations impair telomerase activity, causing excessive telomere shortening and eventually inducing cellular senescence and apoptosis. The cumulative incidence of MDS/AML in DC may be similar to what has been reported in Fanconi anaemia. Many patients with DC cannot be diagnosed by clinical features alone. Screening of a large cohort of patients with RCC indicates that up to 5% of children with RCC have unrecognized DC.

Other predisposition syndromes

While MDS in IBMFD is conventionally named 'secondary' MDS (like MDS following cytotoxic therapy), a number of predisposition syndromes have recently been identified among patients with 'primary' MDS. The most common of these conditions is GATA2 deficiency. The phenotype of germline *GATA2* mutations may lead to immunodeficiency with recurrent warts and monocytopenia (previously named MonoMAC syndrome), or congenital deafness and lymphoedema (described as Emberger syndrome), but also to urogenital malformation or autism-like psychological problems. GATA2 deficiency can be diagnosed in 7% of all paediatric MDS and 15% of MDS-EB. It is associated with monosomy 7 and present in 70% of adolescents with monosomy 7.

Most recently, germline mutations in the paralogue genes *SAMD9* and *SAMD9L* have been described in children with pancytopenia with ataxia or a complex developmental disorder. These patients frequently develop MDS with monosomy 7 or del(7q) which may be transient but can progress to advanced MDS. Germline *SAMD9/SAMD9L* mutations can also underlie MDS in children without syndromic features.

There is a group of predisposition syndromes with germline mutations in *RUNX1*, *ANKRD26*, or *ETV6* which present with isolated thrombocytopenia/bleeding tendency prior to MDS development. Like GATA2 deficiency and SAMD9/SAMD9L disease, the inheritance pattern is autosomal dominant with *de novo* mutations. Collectively, these disorders cause many but not all cases of familial MDS.

Clinical and laboratory features

The presenting features in MDS are those of pancytopenia. Single-lineage cytopenia may occasionally be the predominant characteristic. Foetal haemoglobin (HbF) is frequently moderately elevated, mean corpuscular volume (MCV) of red cells is high, white blood-cell (WBC) count is low to normal, and leukocytosis is generally not a feature of MDS. Some patients present with moderate hepatosplenomegaly, but most have no organomegaly. Extramedullary myeloid tumour may be the presenting feature of MDS, but blasts in the cerebrospinal fluid is not.

Bone-marrow features

The bone marrow is hypocellular in most cases of RCC but normocellular or hypercellular in most cases of MDS-EB. Both peripheral blood and bone marrow display characteristic dysplastic features with macrocytic and/or megaloblastic erythropoiesis, bizarre small or unusual large megakaryocytes, and dysgranulopoiesis (**Figure 17.1**). These characteristic dysplastic features are suggestive of MDS but not diagnostic. A diagnosis of MDS should be confirmed by a repeat bone-marrow examination after two to four weeks.

Cytogenetics

An abnormal karyotype is found in 55% of children with primary MDS-EB and in 76% with secondary MDS. The numerical abnormalities dominate, and structural abnormalities are frequently part of a complex karyotype with numerical abnormalities. This is in contrast to AML where structural abnormalities are by far the most frequent findings. Monosomy 7 is the most common cytogenetic abnormality in childhood MDS. It is seen in 25% of patients and not considered an unfavourable feature. Trisomy 8 and trisomy 21 are the most common numerical abnormalities after monosomy 7. AML specific translocations (e.g. t(8;21)(q22; q22), t(15;17)(q22;

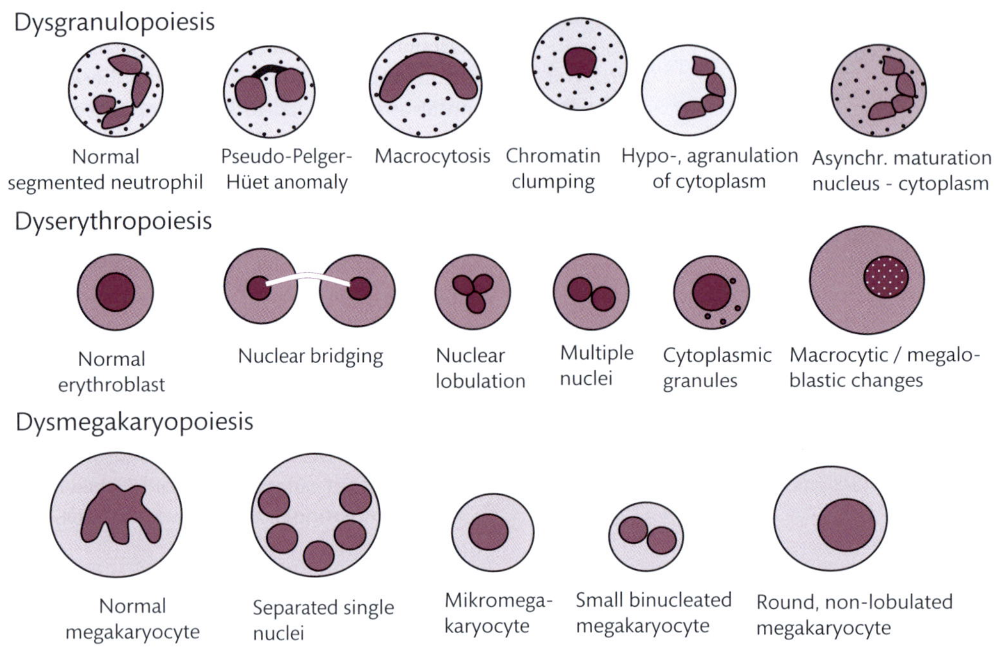

Figure 17.1 Cytological features of myelodysplasia.
Reproduced courtesy of Irith Baumann, Institute for Pathology Kaufbeuren-Ravensburg, Germany

q12), or inv(16)(p13q22)) should be considered as AML regardless of the blast count.

Molecular genetics

MDS is a clonal disease arising in a stem or progenitor cell giving rise to myelopoiesis, erythropoiesis, and megakaryopoiesis. The genes often mutated in adult MDS, such as *TET2, DNMT3A, TP53*,and the spliceosome complex, are not involved in the pathogenesis in children. Instead, somatic driver mutations in *SETBP1, ASXL1, RUNX1*, and the *RAS* oncogenes contribute to the genomic landscape of MDS in children. While one to four mutations are generally present in MDS-EB, most cases of RCC do not exhibit any of these somatic changes.

Immunophenotype

Immunophenotyping by flow cytometry has not the same diagnostic yield in MDS as in acute leukaemia, but may be of value in the quantitative and qualitative assessment of immature progenitor cells, especially when bone-marrow smears are of suboptimal quality. Flow-cytometry immunophenotyping may be a useful addition to histopathology in the diagnosis of RCC.

Differential diagnosis

The two main diagnostic challenges are to distinguish RCC from aplastic anaemia and other non-clonal disorders including IBMF syndromes, and also to differentiate MDS-EB from *de novo* AML. The traditional classification has been based on pure morphology, but a number of additional factors need to be considered.

Myelodysplastic syndrome versus non-clonal disorders

Dysplasia of haematopoietic cells can be present in a variety of disorders of very different aetiologies including infections, metabolic disorders and vitamin deficiencies, rheumatological and autoimmune disease, and drug therapy. It can usually be separated from the typical histological pattern of RCC by islets of immature red cells, dysplastic megakaryocytes, and hypoplastic granulopoiesis. Although dysplasia is essential for the diagnosis of MDS, it constitutes only one aspect of the morphological diagnosis and may be discrete. Since RCC cannot be distinguished from IBMFD, a diagnosis of MDS in IBMFD requires an increased blast count, a cytogenetic or molecular abnormality known to be indicative for disease progression, or an increase in bone-marrow cellularity despite persistent peripheral blood (PB) cytopenia.

Ringsideroblasts in hypoplastic bone-marrow disorders are extremely rare in children. They may indicate a diagnosis of congenital ringsideroblastic anaemia or mitochondrial disease like Pearson syndrome. In MDS, they can indicate the presence of spliceosome mutations.

Refractory cytopenia of childhood versus aplastic anaemia

As bone-marrow cellularity is decreased in most cases of RCC, a trephine biopsy is fundamental for the evaluation of a child with suspected aplastic anaemia or MDS. In contrast to aplastic anaemia, hypoplastic RCC shows scarcely scattered granulopoiesis, patchy islands of immature erythropoiesis and micromegakaryocytes, or absent megakaryopoiesis. Of note, the morphological picture of recovering aplastic anaemia (e.g. under immunosuppressive therapy) cannot be distinguished from RCC. The morphology group of EWOG-MDS have shown that after training of dedicated pathologists and consensus on dysplastic features, the inter-observer variation is very low.

Separating myelodysplastic syndrome from acute myeloid leukaemia

The major differential diagnosis of MDS-EB is AML. There are significant differences between MDS and AML in clinical features,

Table 17.1 Major differences between myelodysplastic syndrome (MDS) and acute myeloid leukaemia (AML) in children

Parameter	MDS	AML
WBC	Low-normal	Low-normal-high
Hepatomegaly	Infrequent	Common
Cytogenetic aberrations	Numerical (-7)	Structural
Dysplasia	Multi-lineage	Infrequent
Haematopoiesis	Clonal (including CR)	Non-clonal in CR
Cell of origin	Stem cell	Lineage-restricted
Response to chemotherapy	Poor	Moderate
Iatrogenic model	Alkylating agents	Epipodophyllotoxins

cytogenetics, and in response to therapy. The latter reflect fundamental biological differences, thus making the morphologically based classification a surrogate marker for the distinction between biological entities (Table 17.1). The morphologically defined MDS-EB-T group is heterogeneous and blast count in a single specimen is insufficient to differentiate MDS from AML. Biological features, rather than any arbitrary cut-off in blast count, may be more important in distinguishing MDS from (chemosensitive) AML.

In borderline cases, with bone-marrow blasts around 20% and no cytogenetic clues to the diagnosis, the bone-marrow examination should be repeated after about two weeks. The major diagnostic pitfall may be associated with undue haste in starting therapy. Significant organomegaly or increased WBC is suggestive of a diagnosis of AML. It should be emphasized that most children with myeloid malignancies have clear-cut AML, some have MDS with low blast count, and only a small percentage have borderline features.

Prognosis and natural course

Children with RCC and MDS-EB or even MDS-EB-T may show a long and stable clinical course without treatment. Blood transfusions may only be required infrequently and severe infections are rarely seen. The condition may smoulder, with unchanged cytopenia, for months or even years. RCC with monosomy 7 is associated with a higher risk of progression; once progression has occurred, the outcome is inferior.

The International Prognostic Scoring System (IPSS), or other scoring systems for adult MDS, weigh data on bone-marrow blasts count, cytopenia, and cytogenetics, to separate patients into prognostic groups. Overall, these scoring systems provide little diagnostic information in children, but presence of a complex karyotype is associated with a poorer outcome.

Spontaneous regression of MDS has occasionally been reported in the literature. The frequency of spontaneous remission is unknown, but estimated to occur in well below 5% of patients, and may be related to *SAMD9/SAMD9L* mutations.

Treatment

MDS is a clonal disorder of an early stem or progenitor cell with limited residual non-clonal stem cells. Therefore, haematopoietic stem-cell transplantation (HSCT) is the main curative therapy approach for children with all types of MDS. Hypermethylation may occur at a similar frequency in children and adults, thus making children potential candidates for epigenetic therapy, however, the response to azacitidine in paediatric MDS-EB is limited. Immunosuppressive therapy with antithymocyte globulin and cyclosporine in hypoplastic RCC has produced complete or partial response in 70%; the salvage rate for those who fail is high with HSCT.

Acute myeloid leukaemia-type chemotherapy

Conventional intensive chemotherapy without HSCT is unlikely to eradicate the primitive pluripotent cells involved in MDS, rendering the therapy non-curative in most patients. Induction chemotherapy is associated with significant morbidity and mortality, with a complete remission (CR) rate of less than 60%, treatment-related mortality rate of 10–30%, many relapses, and overall survival less than 30%. Children with monosomy 7, diagnosed as AML, have a poor response to induction chemotherapy as in MDS patients but, in contrast to MDS, those who respond well to chemotherapy have an outcome similar to AML patients. The EWOG-MDS experiences showed poor response to chemotherapy in MDS-EB and no benefit from chemotherapy before HSCT.

Haematopoietic allogeneic stem-cell transplantation

Children with hypoplastic RCC may be successfully treated with a reduced-intensity conditioning regimen, but for RCC with monosomy 7 or MDS-EB, a myeloablative regimen (e.g. with busulfan, cyclophosphamide, and melphalan) is necessary and has cured more than half of the children with MDS-EB, both after matched family donor (MFD) and matched unrelated donor (MUD) HSCT. Total body irradiation (TBI) has no superior anti-leukaemic effect compared with busulfan and is associated with more long-term effects in children. Data from EWOG-MDS on children with primary advanced MDS showed no benefit of intensive AML-type therapy preceding HSCT. Considering the significant morbidity and mortality of induction chemotherapy and the high rate of transplant-related mortality following HSCT, highest in adolescents, most children with MDS may benefit from HSCT as first-line therapy, sparing the toxicity related to induction chemotherapy. Updated guidelines for the HSCT procedure may be found at www.ewog-mds.org.

Relapse following HSCT for advanced MDS is associated with a very grave outcome. Successful donor leukocyte infusions have occasionally been reported. Especially early relapse, detected by increasing mixed chimerism, may benefit from withdrawal of immunosuppressive therapy and donor leukocyte infusion. Close analyses of chimerism status post HSCT may allow initiation of pre-emptive immunotherapy.

In contrast to advanced MDS, relapse following HSCT is rare in RCC. HSCT early in the course of the disease has therefore been recommended for all children and adolescents with MDS. However, in children with RCC and absence of profound cytopenia, postponement of HSCT, with a 'watch and wait' strategy, may be justified, especially in patients with a normal karyotype. A fludarabine-based reduced-intensity conditioning regimen has been piloted in a few children with RCC and normal karyotype, resulting in survival rates comparable to those of patients treated with myeloablative HSCT.

Myeloid leukaemia and Down syndrome

Neonates with Down syndrome (DS) may have transient abnormal myelopoiesis (TAM), and DS individuals later have a strongly age-related increased risk of myeloid leukaemia. The recognition of the unique biological features of *GATA1*-mutated diseases in DS is reflected in the inclusion in the WHO classification of TAM and myeloid leukaemia of Down syndrome (ML-DS).

Transient abnormal myelopoiesis

Increased WBC and circulating blasts with cell-surface antigens characteristic of megakaryoblasts, sometimes accompanied by anaemia and thrombocytopenia, are seen in up to 10% of neonates with DS. The percentage of blasts is often higher in blood than in bone marrow, and bone-marrow aspiration has limited additional diagnostic value. Clonal abnormalities are observed in 35%. The condition is referred to as transient abnormal myelopoiesis (TAM), transient leukaemic reaction, or transient myeloproliferative disorder. The presentation is indistinguishable from leukaemia and some have therefore favoured the name 'transient leukaemia'. TAM involves, selectively, the trisomic cells in individuals with DS mosaicism.

Life-threatening complications (mainly progressive hepatic dysfunction, coagulopathy, or pulmonary problems) may occur in 10–20% of patients with TAM, but spontaneous remission appears in the majority within one to three months. Generally, no chemotherapy is indicated in TAM. However, in those with progressive hepatic or pulmonary problems, a short course of low-dose cytarabine may be very effective and life-saving. Myeloid leukaemia develops one to three years later in 25% of children who recover from TAM.

Myeloid leukaemia of Down syndrome

ML-DS develops in 1% of the children with DS. A history of TAM is known in some 30%. The age distribution of ML-DS is very remarkable, with half being one year of age at diagnosis, one third being two years of age, and only 2% being more than four years of age. Only very few present before one year of age. There appears to be no age overlap between ML-DS and TAM.

ML-DS may have a smouldering presentation with thrombocytopenia and low blast count, and has been classified as MDS, while others presenting with higher blast counts have been labelled AML. However, in contrast to non-DS children, there are no biological or therapeutic differences between those presenting with a low or high blast count. Furthermore, the bone marrow in ML-DS is often fibrotic and assessment of the blast count may be difficult. ML-DS is preferred to acute megakaryoblastic leukaemia (AMKL) because other phenotypes in DS are observed sharing the same biological and clinical characteristics. It is not appropriate to use the terms MDS or AML (or acute megakaryoblastic leukaemia) in young children with DS. There may be rare cases of DS patients older than four years of age who present with spontaneous MDS and AML without *GATA1* mutation. These older patients have a worse prognosis.

Pathobiology

Leukaemia in children with trisomy 21 mosaicism selectively involves the trisomic cells, pointing at the aetiological role of the additional chromosome 21 as the first hit in the multistep process leading to leukaemia. An acquired mutation in *GATA1* is found in both TAM and ML-DS, and the identical mutation is found in TAM and ML-DS in the same patient. *GATA1* mutation is not found in AKML or other AML patients without DS. The *GATA1* gene encodes a transcription factor essential for the normal erythroid and megakaryocytic differentiation in accordance with the selective involvement of these two lineages in ML-DS.

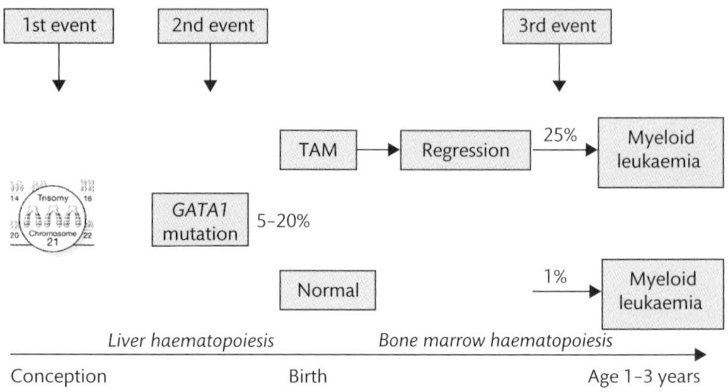

Figure 17.2 Pathogenetic model for myeloid leukaemia in Down syndrome.

A model of the pathogenic steps in ML-DS is presented in **Figure 17.2**. Trisomy 21 is the first event that may predispose the cells to a proliferative advantage or further mutations. *GATA1* mutation is found in TAM and is present in at least 5% of neonates with DS and normal haematology. With more sensitive methods, *GATA1* mutation is found in 20% of the neonates, in what may be called 'silent TAM'. The mechanisms of the spontaneous regression of TAM remain unexplained but may be associated with the natural switch of haematopoiesis from foetal liver to bone marrow.

Clinical and laboratory features

Isolated thrombocytopenia is often the presenting feature of ML-DS. At diagnosis, both platelet count and WBC are lower than in non-DS patients and in contrast to the very high WBC seen in TAM. The blast cells have, in most cases, morphological and antigen features of megakaryoblasts, although other morphological variants, especially erythroblasts, may occur. Many patients have a relatively indolent course, characterized by a period of thrombocytopenia and dysplasia, with relatively few symptoms and low blast count in the bone marrow.

Cytogenetics

Numerical aberrations, mainly trisomy 8 and an extra chromosome 21 (tetrasomy 21), are the most common acquired cytogenetic abnormalities. The recurrent structural aberrations seen in AML are not a feature of ML-DS. Karyotype has no strong prognostic impact.

Treatment

In contrast to TAM, ML-DS is fatal if untreated. The prognosis of ML-DS was considered very poor before 1990, when reports from the Nordic Society of Paediatric Haematology and Oncology (NOPHO) and the Pediatric Oncology Group (POG) showed a surprisingly high survival rate for DS patients receiving AML treatment. However, intensive induction therapy is associated with an increased risk of death during induction and consolidation. Less time-intensive therapy, allowing recovery prior to initiation of the next chemotherapeutic course, is fundamental. HSCT in first remission is not indicated in children with ML-DS. Several recent studies have successfully lowered the cumulated doses of chemotherapy and reported survival of 90%. Response evaluated by flow cytometry may help identify those with the highest risk of relapse. The outcome following relapse is also poor after HSCT.

DS myeloblasts are ten-fold more sensitive to cytarabine *in vitro* than non-DS cells. The increased sensitivity of DS blasts may be related to the expression of chromosome 21 localized genes like cystathionine-β-synthetase and superoxide dismutase.

Juvenile myelomonocytic leukaemia

JMML is a unique paediatric disorder previously named chronic myelomonocytic leukaemia (CMML) in childhood or juvenile chronic myeloid leukaemia (JCML), recognizing the distinction from CML occurring in older children and adults. JMML is considered a separate bridging disorder between MDS and myeloproliferative disorders in the WHO classification.

Epidemiology

Incidence studies from Denmark and British Columbia showed a similar JMML incidence of 1.2 per million children per year, corresponding to 2.4% of all haematological malignancies. However, an incidence of only 0.6 per million was reported from the UK. The median age at presentation is 1.8 years; 35% are below one year of age at presentation and only 4% are more than five years of age. JMML displays a male predominance, with a male:female ratio of 2:1.

Clinical and haematological features

Patients present with pallor, fever, infection, bleeding, or symptoms from the hepatomegaly, splenomegaly, or generalized lymphadenopathy. A macular-papular skin rash is seen in 35% of patients. An elevated WBC with absolute monocytosis, anaemia, and thrombocytopenia is almost universal. WBC at presentation exceeds 50×10^9/l in 30% of cases and is above 100×10^9/l in 7%. Blood film appearance with immature myeloid and/or erythroid precursors as well as monocytosis is characteristic, while bone-marrow monocytosis may be discrete. Blast count in the bone marrow is generally less than 20%. Increased HbF is one of the main characteristics of JMML, with the notable exception being those with monosomy 7, who generally have a normal HbF for their age.

Cytogenetics

Monosomy 7 (mostly as the sole abnormality) is present in about 25% of JMML; 10% have other aberrations, and 65% have a normal karyotype. Data from the EWOG-MDS did not show any major clinical differences between JMML in patients with and without monosomy 7.

Molecular diagnostics and pathophysiology

JMML is a clonal disorder that arises from a pluripotent stem cell. The pathophysiology is characterized by hyperactivation of the Ras/MAPK signal transduction pathway. Germline and somatic mutations that deregulate Ras signalling are implicated as key initiating events in JMML. Approximately 90% of patients have disease-initiating mutations in *PTPN11, NF1, CBL, NRAS*,or *KRAS*.

Ras

Members of the Ras family of signalling proteins regulate cellular proliferation by cycling between an active guanosine triphosphate bound state (Ras-GTP) and an inactive guanosine diphosphate bound state (Ras-GDP). Somatic point mutations in codons 12, 13, and 61 of *NRAS* or *KRAS*, impairing the intrinsic GTPase activity of RAS and thereby causing high constitutive Ras-GTP levels, are noted in leukaemic cells of about 25% of JMML patients.

In rare cases, a developmental disorder with germline *KRAS* or *NRAS* mutations is accompanied by a myeloproliferative disorder clinically indistinguishable from JMML which, however, spontaneously regresses. Interestingly, a few cases of JMML associated with acquired somatic *NRAS* mutations have also been reported to regress spontaneously over time.

Neurofibromatosis

Neurofibromatosis (NF1) is associated with a more than 200-fold increased risk of JMML. A clinical diagnosis of NF1 is made in 10–15% of children with JMML. NF1 is caused by mutations of the *NF1* tumour suppressor gene, which encodes the Ras-GTPase activating protein (Ras-GAP) neurofibromin. Children with NF1 and JMML have biallelic inactivation of the normal *NF1* allele by uniparental disomy, resulting in duplication of the mutant NF1 allele or compound heterozygous mutations.

SHP-2

Somatic mutations in *PTPN11*, the gene encoding for the non-receptor tyrosine phosphatase SHP-2, are noted in about 35% of children with JMML. SHP-2 relays growth signals from activated growth factor receptors to other signalling molecules, including Ras. Most *PTPN11* mutations are predicted to disrupt the auto-inhibition of the catalytic phosphatase (PTPase) domain by the N-terminal src-homology 2 (N-SH2) domain, thereby promoting the active conformation of the protein.

A transient myeloproliferative disorder is occasionally seen in young infants with Noonan syndrome (NS). NS is an autosomal dominant disorder characterized by short stature, distinct facial anomalies, a typical spectrum of congenital heart defects, and developmental delays. Approximately 50% of patients with NS carry germline mutations of *PTPN11*. In contrast to JMML with somatic mutations in *PTPN11*, most cases with myeloproliferation in NS resolve spontaneously. Normalization of myeloproliferation may take several months or even years, especially the monocytosis and splenomegaly, which may persist for more than ten years. Fatal progressive disease has only been reported in a few patients with NS.

CBL

CBL is an E3 ligase which promotes ubiquitylation and thereby degradation of a large number of tyrosine kinases. *CBL* mutations are acquired somatically in adults with myeloproliferative disorders. In JMML, 10–15% of the children have a developmental germline disorder with heterozygous *CBL* mutations and a high percentage of developmental delay, cryptorchidism, and impaired growth. *CBL* appears to function as a classic tumour suppressor, with loss of heterozygosity in leukaemic cells. Clinical data reveals that most patients with CBL syndrome and JMML experience spontaneous resolution of their disease but are at risk to develop vasculopathies.

Differential diagnoses

JMML may mimic infections like Epstein–Barr virus, cytomegalovirus, herpes virus-6 and parvovirus, Wiskott–Aldrich syndrome, leukocyte adhesion defects, or infantile malignant osteoscleosis. However, since the discovery of the underlying lesions, more than 80% of children with JMML can be diagnosed by a typical clinical picture and molecular markers.

Natural course and prognostic factors

For patients carrying somatic *RAS* and *PTPN11* mutations or NF1, JMML is a rapidly fatal disorder if left untreated. Blastic transformation is infrequent with JMML and most untreated patients die from organ failure due to infiltration of the leukaemic cells. Low platelet count, age above two years, and high HbF at diagnosis are the main factors predicting a short survival. Acquisition of secondary mutations in *SETPB1* and *JAK3*, or an additional acquired lesion of the RAS pathway, generally infers a poor outcome. Gene-expression studies and aberrant DNA methylation separate JMML into subgroups with distinct prognoses.

Patients with germline mutations in *PTPN11* often show spontaneous regression of their JMML-like myeloproliferation. Therefore, mutational studies have to be carried out in haematopoietic and non-haematopoietic tissue (fibroblasts or cells from hair bulbs).

Treatment

Intensive chemotherapy is mostly unsuccessful in JMML, resulting in long-term survival of less than 10%. While there is no evidence that cyto-reduction prior to HSCT increases long-term survival, some investigators propose high-dose ara-C and fludarabine for children with a large tumour burden. Purine analogues, etoposide, and cytarabine as single agents may produce short term clinical response and azacitidine seems to provide clinical benefits in a considerable number of patients pre HSCT.

Allogeneic HSCT is the only curative approach for children with JMML and somatic mutations in *PTPN11* or NF1, and most children with *KRAS* or *NRAS* mutations. It results in overall survival in more than half the patients after both MFD and MUD HSCT or cord blood transplantation. Busulfan-based myeloablative therapy offers similar or greater anti-leukaemic efficacy than TBI, which is to be avoided because of deleterious radiation-induced late effects in these young patients. The current EWOG-MDS study uses a preparative regimen with busulfan, cyclophosphamide, and melphalan, and has shown event-free survival (EFS) of around 50%, with no difference between related and unrelated donors. Splenectomy before HSCT, as well as spleen size at time of the allograft, did not appear to have an impact on post-transplantation outcome. Monosomy 7 is associated with an outcome comparable to or even better than that of patients with normal karyotype.

Disease recurrence, generally within the first year, remains the main cause of treatment failure. Age of above four years is the major significant risk factor for failure in multivariate analysis. Reduced intensity and duration of graft-versus-host (GvH) disease prophylaxis may significantly contribute to successful leukaemia control, and both acute and chronic GvH disease is associated with a lower risk of relapse. Early detection of donor cells by increasing mixed chimerism may be successfully eradicated by reducing ongoing immunosuppressive therapy. Donor lymphocyte infusion (DLI) in JMML relapse is largely unsuccessful, but a second or even third transplantation gives a relatively high chance of long-term survival.

FURTHER READING

Aalbers AM, et al. (2015) Bone marrow immunophenotyping by flow cytometry in refractory cytopenia of childhood. *Haematologica* **100**, 315–23.

Arber DA, et al. (2016) The 2016 revision to the World Health Organization classification of myeloid neoplasms and acute leukemia. *Blood* **127**, 2391–405.

Baumann I, et al. (2012) Morphological differentiation of severe aplastic anaemia from hypocellular refractory cytopenia of childhood: reproducibility of histopathological diagnostic criteria. *Histopathology* **61**(1), 10–17.

Caye A, et al. (2015) Juvenile myelomonocytic leukemia displays mutations in components of the RAS pathway and the PRC2 network. *Nat Genet* **47**(11), 1334–40.

Chang TY1, et al. (2014) Bedside to bench in juvenile myelomonocytic leukemia: insights into leukemogenesis from a rare pediatric leukemia. *Blood* **124**(16), 2487–97.

Gohring G, et al. (2010) Complex karyotype newly defined: the strongest prognostic factor in advanced childhood myelodysplastic syndrome. *Blood* **116**, 3766–99.

Hasegawa D (2016) The current perspective of low-grade myelodysplastic syndrome in children. *Int J Hematol* **103**(4), 360.

Hasle H, Niemeyer CM (2011) Advances in the prognostication and management of advanced MDS in children. *Br J Haematol* **154**, 185–95.

Hasle H, et al. (2008) Myeloid leukemia in children 4 years or older with Down syndrome often lacks GATA1 mutation and cytogenetics and risk of relapse are more akin to sporadic AML. *Leukemia* **22**, 1428–30.

Klusmann JH, et al. (2008) Treatment and prognostic impact of transient leukemia in neonates with Down syndrome. *Blood* **111**(6), 2991–8.

Lipka DB, et al. (2017) RAS-pathway mutation patterns define epigenetic subclasses in juvenile myelomonocytic leukemia. *Nat Commun* **8**(1), 2126.

Locatelli F, Niemeyer CM (2015) How I treat juvenile myelomonocytic leukemia. *Blood* **125**(7), 1083–90.

Locatelli F, et al. (2005) Hematopoietic stem cell transplantation (HSCT) in children with juvenile myelomonocytic leukemia (JMML): results of the EWOG-MDS/EBMT trial. *Blood* **105**, 410–19.

Niemeyer CM, et al. (2015) Criteria for evaluating response and outcome in clinical trials for children with juvenile myelomonocytic leukemia. *Haematologica* **100**, 17–22.

Niemeyer CM, et al. (2010) Germline CBL mutations cause developmental abnormalities and predispose to juvenile myelomonocytic leukemia. *Nat Genet* **42**, 794–800.

Pastor V, et al. (2017) Mutational landscape in children with myelodysplastic syndromes is distinct from adults: specific somatic drivers and novel germline variants. *Leukemia* **31**, 759–62.

Roberts I, Izraeli S (2014) Haematopoietic development and leukaemia in Down syndrome. *Br J Haematol* **167**, 587–99.

Roberts I, et al. (2013) GATA1-mutant clones are frequent and often unsuspected in babies with Down syndrome: identification of a population at risk of leukemia. *Blood* **122**(24), 3908–17.

Sakaguchi H, et al. (2013) Exome sequencing identifies secondary mutations of SETBP1 and JAK3 in juvenile myelomonocytic leukemia. *Nat Genet* **45**(8), 937–41.

Stieglitz E, et al. (2015) Subclonal mutations in SETBP1 confer a poor prognosis in juvenile myelomonocytic leukemia. *Blood* **125**(3), 516–24.

Strahm B, et al. (2011) Hematopoietic stem cell transplantation for advanced myelodysplastic syndrome in children: results of the EWOG-MDS 98 study. *Leukemia* **25**(3), 455–62.

Taga T, et al. (2016) Preserved high probability of overall survival with significant reduction of chemotherapy for myeloid leukemia in Down Syndrome: a nationwide prospective study in Japan. *Pediatr Blood Cancer* **63**(2), 248–54.

Taub JW, et al. (1999) Expression of chromosome 21-localized genes in acute myeloid leukemia: differences between Down syndrome and non-Down syndrome blast cells and relationship to in vitro sensitivity to cytosine arabinoside and daunorubicin. *Blood* **94**(4), 1393–400.

Uffmann M, et al. (2017) Therapy reduction in patients with Down syndrome and myeloid leukemia: the international ML-DS 2006 trial. *Blood* **129**(25), 3314–21.

Wlodarski MW, et al. (2016) Prevalence, clinical characteristics and prognosis of GATA2-related MDS in children and adolescents. *Blood* **127**, 1387–97.

18

Non-Hodgkin Lymphomas in Children and Adolescents

Véronique Minard-Colin and Catherine Patte

Introduction

Non-Hodgkin's lymphoma (NHL) is a heterogeneous group of lymphoid malignancies. The histological classification of these diseases has changed many times over the years due to a better understanding of lymphomagenesis and to the development of new diagnostic tools. The World Health Organization (WHO) classification is now widely used, providing clinicians with a common language, and its revision in 2016 allowed identification of new/provisional entities in paediatric lymphomas.

NHL is the fourth most common malignancy in children (and the most common in sub-Saharan Africa) and can arise at any age. NHLs in children are rarer than in adults and exhibit significant differences in terms of the distribution of histological subtypes and clinical features, with virtually exclusively diffuse high-grade lymphomas and frequent extranodal involvement. Dramatic progress has been achieved in the treatment of NHL in children and adolescents, yielding an overall survival rate exceeding 80%. The progress in outcome is the consequence of a more accurate diagnostic process, of better risk-adapted chemotherapy approaches, and of the ability to prevent and control life-threatening treatment-related toxicities. Due to the rarity of each subtype, such progress could not have been achieved without international collaborations, especially through the European Intergroup for Childhood NHL (EICNHL) comprising most European countries, Japan, and Hong Kong, as well as collaborations between Europe and North America. Conversely, the outcome of patients with NHL treated in countries with limited resources is far worse, due to the unavailability of certain anti-cancer medicines and to the suboptimal diagnostic and therapeutic management of patients.

Increased knowledge in the field of biology of paediatric NHL will improve outcome through the use of more efficient multi-agent therapies and the introduction of novel agents, including targeted therapies. Nevertheless, conditions that allow the application of standard treatments on a global or international scale are needed, to provide a better chance of cure in less privileged areas of the world. These challenges will represent the new frontiers in paediatric NHL for the next decades.

Incidence and epidemiology

The overall incidence and frequency of the different histological subgroups varies according to age at diagnosis. Data from the American National Cancer Institute's Surveillance, Epidemiology, and End Results (SEER) programme show a steady increase in NHL with age. The annual incidence per million inhabitants ranges from 5.9 in children below five years of age to about 10 in children between the ages of five and fourteen, and to 15 in adolescents (and about 150 in adults). The increase in adolescents is essentially related to the higher incidence of large-cell lymphomas at that age. The vast majority of childhood NHL is high-grade lymphoma, mostly of B-cell origin. Burkitt lymphoma (BL) is by far the most frequent (50–60%, depending on the geographic region), followed by lymphoblastic lymphoma (LL) (20–25%), diffuse large B-cell lymphoma (DLBCL) (10–15%), and anaplastic large-cell lymphoma (ALCL) (10–12%) (**Table 18.1**). Other lymphomas, such as peripheral T-cell lymphoma, extranodal natural killer (NK)-cell/T-cell lymphoma, or paediatric follicular lymphomas may arise in children, but represent less than 5% of cases. Both the incidence and relative frequency of the different subtypes of NHL also vary considerably in different parts of the world; in equatorial Africa, lymphomas account for almost half of the childhood cancers, reflecting the very high incidence of Burkitt lymphoma but a relative paucity of LL in this region.

The aetiology of NHL is largely unknown. Immunodeficiency, whether inherited or acquired, is clearly related to the development of NHL. More recently described is the increased risk of NHL in the constitutional mismatch repair MMR deficiency syndrome, due to biallelic germline mutations of MMR genes and characterized by multiple cancers including NHL (mainly LL), brain tumours, and colorectal cancers in children with café au lait spots. The relationship between Epstein–Barr virus (EBV) and the pathogenesis of NHL began with the elegant investigations by Denis Burkitt in the late 1950s. Burkitt demonstrated that the disease was associated with climate and rainfall—in short, the regions where malaria is holoendemic. This observation led to a collaboration with Anthony Epstein and resulted in the discovery of a herpesvirus from cultures of endemic BL tissue, the first human tumour-associated virus.

Table 18.1 Immunophenotypical, cytogenetic, and molecular markers of paediatric non-Hodgkin lymphoma*

Histology (frequency)	BL (50–60%)	LBCL (10–15%)		LL (20–25%)		ALCL (10–12%)
Subtype		DLBCL	PMBL	B-LL	T-LL	
Immunohistochemistry						
MIB1	~100%	40–90%	30–90%	Not informative	Not informative	Not informative
CD10	+	+/−	−/+	+/−	+/−	−
CD19	+	+	+	+	−	−
CD20	+	+	+	+/−	−	−
CD79a	+	+	+	+	−	−
sIg	+	+/−	−	−	−	−
Bcl-6	+	+/−	+/−	−	−	+/−
MUM1	−	−/+	+	−	−	−
MAL	−	−/+	+	−	−	−
TdT	−	−	−	+	+	−
cCD3	−	−	−	−	+	−/+
CD4	−	−	−	−	+/−	−/+
CD8	−	−	−	−	+/−	−/+
CD7	−	−	−	−	+	−/+
CD5	−	−/+	−	−	+/−	+/−
CD30	−	§	+/−	−	−	+
ALK	−	£	−	−	−	+
Cytogenetic	t(8;14)(q24;q32) t(2;8)(p12;q24) t(8;22)(q24;q11)	R8q24 (~30%)	Few data	Few data	Translocations involving 14q11-13 Few other data	t(2;5)(p23;q35) >90% or variants involving 2p23
Molecular biology	*MYC/IGH* *IGK/MYC* *MYC/IGL*		NF-kappa B pathway dysregulation	*IGH/TCR* rearrangements	*IGH/TCR* rearrangements *NOTCH/FBXW7, PTEN*	*NPM/ALK* >90% or variants

BL, Burkitt lymphoma; LBCL, large B-cell lymphoma; DLBCL, diffuse large B-cell lymphoma; PMBL, primary mediastinal (thymic) large B-cell lymphoma; B-LL, B lymphoblastic lymphoma; T-LL, T lymphoblastic lymphoma; ALCL, anaplastic large-cell lymphoma, ALK-positive; +, >90% of cases; +/−, >50% of cases; −/+,<50% of cases; −, <10% of cases.

§, positive especially in the rare anaplastic variant; £, positive in the ALK-positive LBCL

* Other non-Hodgkin lymphomas, such as peripheral T-cell lymphoma, extranodal NK-/T-cell lymphoma, nasal type, and paediatric follicular lymphoma, represent <5% of paediatric NHL and are not indicated in the table.

Reproduced with permission from Minard-Colin, V. et al. 'Non-Hodgkin Lymphoma in Children and Adolescents: Progress Through Effective Collaboration, Current Knowledge, and Challenges Ahead.' *Journal of Clinical Oncology*, Volume 33, Issue 27, pp. 2963–74. Copyright © 2015 American Society of Clinical Oncology. doi:10.1200/JCO.2014.59.5827

Pathology and biology

Mature B-cell non-Hodgkin lymphomas

Burkitt lymphoma (BL) accounts for more than 80% of childhood B-cell NHL (Table 18.1). Morphologically, it is characterized by cells of intermediate size with nuclei containing prominent nucleoli and limited amount of basophilic cytoplasm in which vacuoles are almost invariably present. Tissue sections often show the 'starry-sky' morphology resulting from clear macrophages scattered among the rather intensely stained population of blasts. The current revised WHO classification of lymphoid malignancies also includes, under the term BL, the subtypes previously defined as Burkitt-like and atypical Burkitt lymphomas, since it is not possible to differentiate them based solely on morphology. Those tumours which present with features intermediate between BL and DLBCL are now placed into the category of unclassifiable B-cell lymphoma.

Immunophenotypical studies of BL demonstrate mature malignant B cells expressing CD19, CD20, CD22, CD10, CD79, and monoclonal surface immunoglobulin (sIg). Because BL is a very highly-proliferating human malignancy, with doubling time of less than 24 hours, analysis of proliferation markers such as Ki-67 or MIB-1 will show reactivity in more than 95% of the cells. BL cells harbour characteristic chromosomal translocations involving the MYC oncogene locus on chromosome 8q24. The most common translocation, t(8;14)(q24;q32), which involves the IgH gene locus, occurs in 80% of cases. The consequence of MYC rearrangements in BL is the deregulation of *MYC* expression, which promotes cell-cycle progression and cell transformation. The remaining 20% of BL cases have either a t(2;8)(p12;q24) or, less frequently, a t(8;22)(q24;q11) translocation involving MYC and either the kappa or lambda immunoglobulin light-chain gene loci, respectively, on chromosomes 2 or 22. While MYC is involved in both sporadic and endemic BL, the breakpoints within the MYC gene and in the IgH loci differ between the two BL subtypes. The most common translocation, t(8;14)(q24;q32), can be detected by long-distance polymerase chain reaction (LD-PCR) assay. Based on this approach, the MYC-IgH rearrangements can be used as markers to analyse minimal BM infiltration at diagnosis and its response to chemotherapy with a sensitivity of 10^{-4}.

One controversial issue, not fully resolved, is whether true BL without MYC translocations really exists. Some recent studies have identified a subset of lymphomas that resemble BL morphologically, to a large extent phenotypically, but which lack MYC rearrangements. Instead, they have a chromosome 11q alteration characterized by proximal gains and telomeric losses. Compared to BL, these lymphomas have more complex karyotypes, lower levels of MYC expression, a certain degree of cytological pleomorphism, occasionally a follicular pattern, and, frequently, a nodal presentation. The revised 2016 WHO classification considered this a new provisional entity designated as 'Burkitt-like lymphoma with 11q aberration'.

Recent findings with new biological tools—such as next-generation sequencing, microRNA and gene expression profiling, and single nucleotide polymorphism (SNP) array analysis—could also lead to novel and more effective therapies. In BL, genetic alterations other than the 8q24/*MYC* translocation participate in the deregulation of the *MYC* pathway and may be essential for disease initiation and progression. Recurrent mutations in the PI3K pathway suggest a cooperative role between MYC over-expression and deregulation of PI3K signalling. Other studies highlight the pathogenic and clinical relevance of mutations affecting the transcription factor *TCF3 (E2A)* or its negative regulator *ID3*, a novel tumour-suppressor gene, with *TCF3* or *ID3* mutations affecting nearly 70% of sporadic BL. Other mutations in genes including *CCND3, GNA13, TP53,* and *SMARCA4* have also been described.

Interestingly, a comparison between the frequency of mutations in BL and adult germinal centre B-cell (GCB) DLBCL revealed a stronger overlap, further supporting the notion that BL and GCB DLBCL both originate from germinal centre B cells. Altogether, these findings also support the development of drugs targeting the PI3K kinase pathway, antigen-independent B-cell receptor (BCR) signalling, and cyclin D3/CDK6 pathways in childhood B-NHL.

Similarly to BL, DLBCL is characterized by a mature B-cell phenotype, but cells display varying morphological and cytological appearances. Malignant cells are rather large in size and show more abundant cytoplasm compared to BL cells. Paediatric DLBCLs have a high proliferation rate (although lower than BL) as determined by Ki-67 or MIB-1 (i.e. less than 90%). They express cell sIg and a number of B-cell markers, including CD19, CD20, CD22, CD79, and PAX5. In contrast to adult DLBCL, paediatric cases are less frequently positive for BCL2, but can express high levels of the germinal centre markers CD10 and BCL6. No consistent cytogenetic abnormalities have been associated with DLBCL of children and adolescents, but more complex karyotypes than BL have been reported. Chromosomal translocations involving the MYC oncogene are more frequent in paediatric compared to adult DLBCL, whereas BCL2 translocations are rarely seen in paediatric cases. Recent gene-expression profile studies, together with specific immunostaining using markers of germinal centre, have demonstrated that more than 80% of the paediatric DLBCLs belong to the germinal centre B-cell-like subgroup, suggesting that DLBCLs of children and adolescents are biologically more similar to BL than to DLBCL seen in older patients.

Large B-cell lymphoma with IRF4 rearrangement is a new provisional entity in the WHO classification to distinguish from paediatric-type follicular lymphoma (FL) and other DLBCLs. It occurs most commonly in children and young adults, and typically develops in Waldeyer's ring and/or cervical lymph nodes and is low stage. Usually, strong IRF4/MUM1 expression is seen, with BCL6 and a high proliferative fraction. Most cases have IG/IRF4 rearrangements, sometimes together with BCL6 rearrangements, but they uniformly lack BCL2 rearrangements. This lymphoma is considered to be more aggressive than other paediatric-type FLs, but patients, at least when treated, have done very well.

A rare (1–2% of all paediatric NHL) and clinically distinct entity among large B-cell lymphomas is primary mediastinal large B-cell lymphoma (PMBL). It originates from thymic B cells and is characterized by diffuse proliferation of large cells and evident sclerosis. Due to both the almost exclusive mediastinal localization and the morphological appearance, PMBL may be difficult to distinguish from Hodgkin lymphoma. Cell surface markers in PMBL are similar to those seen in DLBCL and include CD19, CD20, CD22, CD79, and PAX5, but, very often, only cytoplasmic Ig and not SIg are present. CD30 is commonly expressed. Studies of gene expression show overlap of gene-expression profiles between PMBL and HL suggesting that, biologically, PMBL is more similar to HL than to DLBCL.

Lymphoblastic lymphoma

Lymphoblastic lymphoma (LL) accounts for 1520% of paediatric NHL (**Table 18.1**). Conventionally, LL is distinguished from acute lymphoblastic leukaemia (ALL) based on the extent of bone-marrow (BM) involvement (ALL is defined when BM blasts are more than 25%), but gene expression and genetic studies would suggest that they may differ biologically. LL includes both precursor T (T-LL) and B (pB-LL) NHL. Unlike ALL, with predominant pB-cell diseases, most LLs are of T-cell origin (80–90% versus 10–20%).

Morphologically, the malignant cells of LL appear indistinguishable from ALL, being of small or intermediate size, with high nuclear/cytoplasm ratio and finely dispersed chromatin. Nucleoli may be evident and, occasionally, blasts may have cytoplasmic vacuoles morphologically resembling L3 blasts (a feature that is not exclusive of BL). LL blasts in the lymph nodes show a high mitotic rate and cause diffuse absence of nodal architecture, with occasionally spared reactive follicles.

Immunophenotypically, LL blasts do not express sIg but, characteristically, are positive for terminal deoxynucleotidyl transferase (TdT) in more than 95% of cases and often for CD99, independently of their T- or B-cell lineage. TdT expression is the best immunohistochemical marker for determining the precursor origin of the proliferation. This is very useful for differentiating pB-LL from mature B-cell NHL, since they can express other similar markers (CD79a, CD10, CD19, +/-CD20) (**Table 18.1**). T-LLs express, in different combinations, T-cell markers typical of middle to late stages of thymocyte differentiation, including CD1a, CD2, CD5, CD7, CD4, and/or CD8. T-cell receptor antigens are frequently not expressed and CD3 is more often detected in the cytoplasm than on the cell surface. pB-LLs usually express CD19 and CD10, and have variable expression of HLA-DR and CD20, but not sIg.

Although specific data on LL are scarce, chromosomal translocations described in ALL have been reported also in LL. Translocations often involve rearrangements of T-cell receptor (TCR) or Ig gene rearrangements with proto-oncogenes, resulting in the juxtaposition of promoter and enhancer elements of TCR or Ig genes, and transcription factor genes including HOX11, TAL1, and LYL1. T-LL displays early TCR gene rearrangements that can be detected by molecular assays, whereas B-cell precursor LL usually shows Ig gene rearrangements. They represent a unique marker that can be exploited through the use of molecular assays to determine clonality, thus assisting in the differential diagnosis between LL and atypical or reactive lymphadenopathy. Unlike ALL, the prognostic value of minimal disseminated disease (MDD) and minimal residual disease (MRD) using either polymerase chain reaction (PCR)-based methods, molecular techniques, or flow cytometry, has not yet been proven in LL (unlike ALL).

Several biological characteristics considered of prognostic relevance in T-LL have been described: in the Berlin–Frankfurt–Munster (BFM) series, loss of heterozygosity (LOH) on chromosome 6q, found in 12% of the patients, was significantly associated with a poorer outcome (event-free survival (EFS): 27%±9% versus 86%±3% if no LOH6q16), while the presence of NOTCH1 mutations (60% of patients) was associated with a favourable outcome (EFS 84%±5% versus 66%±7%). NOTCH1 mutations and LOH6q16 were almost mutually exclusive. In a French series studying *FLASH* deletion on chromosome 6q, *TCR* rearrangements and NOTCH1/FBXW7 mutations (the last events found in 55% of cases) were the only prognostic factors in a multivariate analysis, with an EFS rate of 96%±0.04% versus 45%±0.13% ($p<0.01$). Finally, the prognostic value of an RAS/PTEN alteration and of the absence of biallelic TCR gamma deletion also warrants evaluation in T-LL.

Anaplastic large-cell lymphoma

Anaplastic large-cell lymphoma (ALCL) accounts for 10–15% of childhood/adolescent NHL (**Table 18.1**). More than 90% of systemic ALCLs in children carry a translocation resulting in the fusion of the anaplastic lymphoma kinase (ALK) gene to one of several partners. The most common ALK fusion protein is nucleophosmin (NPM)-ALK resulting from the t(2;5) translocation. The fusion protein can be detected using fluorescent in situ hybridization (FISH), reverse transcription-polymerase chain reaction (RT-PCR), or immunohistochemistry. Detection of the NPM-ALK transcript is increasingly applied in the diagnosis of ALCL but, most importantly, is exploited in the assessment of MDD that has been shown to be one of the most relevant prognostic parameters in ALK-positive ALCL of childhood. Indeed, less than 15% of patients exhibit cytologically detectable BM disease, whereas RT-PCR for NPM-ALK can detect MDD in blood or BM in around 50% of patients at diagnosis. A number of variant partners of ALK have been reported in the ALK gene rearrangements and they are often characterized by a specific pattern of cellular ALK expression, as detected by anti-ALK antibodies.

Characteristically, ALCL cells are large, pleomorphic, multinucleated, or horse-shoe-shaped cells (hallmark cells). They are present in differing proportions in the various morphological subtypes of ALCL. The most frequent morphological subtype (more than 70% of cases) is the 'common type' in which typical anaplastic and hallmark cells predominate. The lymphohistiocytic and small-cell variants account for about 20% of cases and appear to be clinically more aggressive. ALCL express CD30 and, in most cases, EMA and cytotoxic molecules like TIA1, granzyme B, or perforin. Most cases express at least one T-cell antigen and exhibit clonal rearrangement of the T-cell receptor.

Accumulating evidence indicates that the immune system plays a major role in both the pathogenesis and final control of ALK-positive ALCL. Antibodies against ALK and cytotoxic T-cell (CTL) and CD4 T-helper responses to ALK have been detected in patients with ALK-positive ALCL, both at diagnosis and during remission, with a significant inverse correlation between ALK-antibody titres and the incidence of relapses. The presence of germline monoallelic mutations of the perforin gene has been demonstrated in patients with ALCL, suggesting that impairment of the cytotoxic machinery may predispose to ALCL.

Rare non-Hodgkin lymphomas in paediatrics

Paediatric FL has become a definite entity in the WHO 2016 classification but is already known as paediatric-type FL because similar lymphomas may occur in adults. It is a nodal disease characterized by large, expansile, highly-proliferative follicles that often have prominent blastoid follicular centre cells, rather than classic centroblasts (or centrocytes). Some have reported a moderate number of cases as grade 1–2 (of 3). BCL2 rearrangements must not be present, but there may be some BCL2 protein expression. They also lack BCL6 and MYC rearrangements, with ongoing investigations of their genetic/molecular landscape. Nearly all cases are localized and may not require treatment other than excision. The criteria for paediatric-type FL, however, must be strictly applied to avoid underdiagnosing conventional grade 3 FL, with particular caution required before making this diagnosis in an adult. This category also excludes cases with diffuse areas (i.e. foci of DLBCL).

Some studies have raised the possibility that paediatric-type FL might be a 'benign clonal proliferation with low malignant potential'. Recently, genome analysis of paediatric-type FL revealed unique molecular features (i.e. low genetic complexity, recurrent alterations of *TNFRSF14* gene, and high prevalence of MAPK pathway mutations) that define it as a biologically and clinically distinct indolent **lymphoma** of children and adults.

Other rare B-cell lymphomas are nodal and extranodal (mucosa-associated) marginal-zone lymphomas (MZLs). These entities histologically overlap with the adult lymphomas and may be difficult to differentiate from reactive lymphocytic proliferations. Another rare group of paediatric NHL is represented by the peripheral T-cell lymphomas (PTCLs). Except for ALCL, the not otherwise specified (NOS) category of PTCL is the most common. Morphologically, they have variable appearances with medium- to large-size neoplastic cells, with irregular nuclei and basophilic cytoplasm, infiltrating the lymph node. Cells show aberrant expression of T-cell markers (CD2, CD3, CD5, or CD7) and may co-express or lack both CD4 and CD8. TCR rearrangements are almost invariably detectable.

Staging

The Ann Arbor classification is not adapted to childhood NHL because of predominantly extranodal primary sites. The usual staging classification is the St Jude's classification in which mediastinal and extensive abdominal lesions are classified as stage III, and stage IV is restricted to bone marrow (BM) and central nervous system (CNS) involvement regardless of involvement of other visceral sites. The International Prognostic Index (IPI) is not used in childhood NHL due to a difference in staging and because the performance status index does not reflect quality-of-life deterioration but, rather, the rapidity of growth and the tumour volume.

The role of fluorodeoxyglucose (FDG)-positron emission tomography (PET)/computed tomography (CT) in the management of childhood NHL has not been assessed as yet. FDG-PET may be more accurate than conventional imaging to assess disease extension since high FDG uptake has been shown in most subtypes, but the impact on therapeutic stratification has not been evaluated. The role of FDG-PET for the assessment of remission has only been investigated in small series and most reports indicate high rates of false positive results requiring histological examination of all residual masses before any changes in treatment.

Several groups are working on the prognostic impact of MDD in the blood, BM, and/or CNS, identified by molecular techniques or flow cytometry. Recently, a group of paediatricians worked on a proposal for a Revised International Paediatric NHL Staging System Classification (IPNHLSS), to add these results to the final staging of childhood NHL (Box 18.1).

Box 18.1 International paediatric non-Hodgkin lymphoma staging system

Stage I

- Single tumour with exclusion of mediastinum and abdomen (N; EN; B or S: EN-B, EN-S)

Stage II

- Single EN tumour with regional node involvement
- Two N areas on same side of diaphragm
- Primary GI tract tumour (usually in ileocecal area), involvement of associated mesenteric nodes, completely resectable (if malignant ascites or extension of tumour to adjacent organs, it should be regarded as stage III)

Stage III

- Two EN tumours (including EN-B or EN-S) above and/or below diaphragm
- Two N areas above and below diaphragm
- Any intrathoracic tumour (mediastinal, hilar, pulmonary, pleural, or thymic)
- Intra-abdominal and retroperitoneal disease, including liver, spleen, kidney, and/or ovary localizations, regardless of degree of resection (except primary GI tract tumour (usually in ileocecal region) with involvement of associated mesenteric nodes that is completely resectable)
- Any paraspinal or epidural tumour, regardless of whether other sites are involved
- Single B lesion with concomitant involvement of EN and/or non-regional N sites

Stage IV

- Any of the above findings with initial involvement of CNS (stage IV CNS), BM (stage IV BM), or both (stage IV combined) based on conventional methods

Note: For each stage, type of examination and degree of BM and CNS involvement should be specified.

B, bone; BM, bone marrow; EN, extranodal; N, nodal; S, skin.

Reproduced with permission from Rosolen A, et al. 'Revised International Pediatric Non-Hodgkin Lymphoma Staging System'. *Journal of Clinical Oncology*, Volume 33, Issue 18, pp. 2112–2118. Copyright © 2015, American Society of Clinical Oncology. Doi: 10.1200/JCO.2014.59.7203

Clinical presentation and treatment

Mature B-cell non-Hodgkin lymphomas

BL generally arises in the abdomen and head and neck region, and presents as advanced stage disease, with BM and CNS involvement in about 20–25% of cases. However, the predominant sites of involvement and patterns of spread are different in patients with sporadic compared to endemic BL. Jaw involvement is the most common site of disease in endemic BL. In endemic cases of BL, lesions in multiple quadrants of the jaw or orbital tumours (with or without maxillary disease) are observed in the majority of children, especially those younger than five years. Abdominal disease is also very common. In contrast to sporadic BL, BM infiltration at diagnosis and at relapse is uncommon, but CNS disease occurs in almost one third of patients. CNS disease may present as headache and increased intracranial pressure from meningeal infiltration, cranial nerve palsies, or an isolated epidural tumour and paraplegia. The most common site of disease in sporadic cases of BL is the abdomen. Abdominal disease may present with pain or distention, nausea and vomiting, gastrointestinal bleeding, or, rarely, intestinal perforation. Approximately 25–30% of children present with a right lower quadrant mass or acute abdominal pain caused by an ileocecal intussusception, which is often confused with acute appendicitis. The majority of patients with abdominal BL have massive disease involving the mesentery, retroperitoneum, kidneys, ovaries, and peritoneal surfaces (often associated with malignant ascites). Therefore, surgical debulking is neither feasible nor appropriate in these patients.

The head and neck region is the second most common site of disease in sporadic BL, but in contrast to patients with endemic BL, jaw involvement is observed in fewer than 10% of cases of sporadic disease. BM involvement occurs in approximately 20% of cases of sporadic BL. Almost 20% of patients present without lymphomatous masses but with fever, pallor, and/or bleeding secondary to pancytopenia from extensive marrow replacement by tumour cells. These children may also have peripheral lymphadenopathy and hepatosplenomegaly; however, mediastinal primaries are more rarely seen than in other paediatric NHL. BL can involve almost any organ including testes, breasts, thyroid gland, skin, epidural space, bone, or pancreas.

Children with DLBCL have a more heterogeneous range of clinical presentations compared to patients with BL. In contrast to BL, the BM and CNS are unusual sites of disease. DLBCL usually presents with nodal disease, though bone involvement (single or multiple sites) is relatively common. In immunocompromised individuals, extranodal disease is common, and primary DLBCL of the brain is not uncommon. Primary mediastinal B-cell lymphoma is a distinct entity. It is typically diagnosed in young adult females in the third to fourth decades of life. The tumour is locally invasive (e.g. pericardial and lung extension) andoften associated with superior vena cava (SVC) syndrome. Additionally, there is often extrathoracic involvement of the kidney.

Outcomes of paediatric BL have improved dramatically due to the implementation of the results of several prospective national and multinational studies (**Table 18.2**). Clinical prognostic factors are already known in B-cell NHL: stage, lactate dehydrogenase (LDH) level, CNS involvement (especially the presence of blasts in the cerebrospinal fluid (CSF) and treatment-related factors such as early response), initial dose intensity, and complete response (CR). Biological characteristics could also have a prognostic value: the presence of abnormalities on 13q, the presence of MYC rearrangement in DLBCL, and a high level of MDD and MRD in BL. However, these findings should still be confirmed in larger and prospective studies.

Treatment of BL is based on two to six months of intensive pulse polychemotherapy. Relapses occur early, within the first year. The French (Lymphomes Malins B) (LMB) studies and the international FABLMB96 trial demonstrated that:

1. high-dose (HD) methotrexate (MTX) was a very effective drug for CNS prophylaxis,
2. patients with leukaemic presentation (mature B-cell acute leukaemia, B-AL) and CNS-positive disease benefitted from a higher dose of HDMTX and the introduction of HD cytarabine (Ara-C) (CYVE courses),
3. treatment intensity should not only be adapted to the stage and resection, but also to response to chemotherapy (at D7 and after three courses),
4. early dose intensity is essential: in the FABLMB96 trial, EFS in the intermediate-risk group was 10% lower when the second induction course started later than 21 days after the first one,
5. the total dose of cyclophosphamide and doxorubicin could be reduced to 3.3 g/m^2 and 120 mg/m^2 respectively for more than 70% of the patients, allowing clinicians to anticipate fertility preservation and the absence of long-term cardiac toxicity.

The German BFM studies showed that treatment intensity can also be adapted to the LDH level and that HDMTX is a very effective systemic drug, and more prolonged drug exposure is required for more advanced disease. They also confirmed that HDAra-C is important in advanced diseases. Although stratification and the weight of therapy are not exactly comparable in both strategies, the results are very similar. CNS prophylaxis should comprise HDMTX +/– HDAra-C and intrathecal (IT) injections of MTX +/–Ara-C, but no cranial irradiation. With all these current strategies in Western countries, EFS of BL attains 80–90%, but immediate treatment-related toxicities require adequate supportive care and protocol management experience.

BL frequently occurs in countries with fewer resources, especially in sub-Saharan countries (where Burkitt first described the disease). Treatment should be adapted to find a compromise between sufficient effectiveness and tolerable toxicity. Several groups have published interesting results showing cure in about half of the children with adapted protocols. These cure rates will improve with experience, better resources, and less family abandonment of treatment.

DLBCL accounts for 10–20% of B-cell lymphoma in children and occurs more frequently in adolescents. Outcomes are similar in children and adolescents to that of BL, with the same protocols, except that relapses can occur up to three years later. The subgroup of primary mediastinal large B-cell lymphoma (PMBL) has to be separated from other DLBCLs. In paediatric protocols, treatment outcome is lower, with EFS around 70%, but is similar to that obtained with adult protocols. Its biology is similar in both age groups (but grey-zone lymphomas are not seen in children) indicating that rituximab should improve outcomes, as seen in adults.

The anti-CD20 chimeric monoclonal antibody rituximab (Mabthera®, Rituxan®) improves survival of adult B-cell malignancies. In childhood B-NHL, pilot studies have yielded responses for single-drug rituximab use in newly diagnosed BL and immediate good tolerance when combined with induction chemotherapy. However, considering the very high cure rates obtained in children and adolescents with no/minimal long-term toxicity, the benefit of adding rituximab to conventional chemotherapy in BL should be evaluated. The international 'Inter-B NHL ritux 2010' trial, with the participation of several countries in Europe and of the Children's Oncology Group (COG) of North America, combined a phase III study testing the impact of adding rituximab to the LMB regimen for advanced-stage B-cell lymphoma (excepting PMBL, for which this trial includes a phase II study of the DA-EPOCH-R regimen (http://clinicaltrials.gov/ct2/show/record/NCT01760226)). The randomized phase III trial compared the standard LMB chemotherapy to the same chemotherapy with rituximab in patients less than 18 years of age with high-risk B-NHL (stage III with LDH level more than 2N, stage IV) and mature B leukaemia. Rituximab was given (375 mg/m^2) on days minus two and one during the first two chemotherapy courses, and on day one of the two following courses (in total, six infusions). The first interim analysis was based on 27 events (37.5% of information) occurring in 310 patients (155/arm) (85% BL). With a median follow-up of 11.5 months, patients on the rituximab arm achieved better EFS than those on the control arm: one-year EFS (95%CI) was 94.2% (88.5–97.2%) versus 81.5% (73.0–87.8%). The hazard ratio (HR) was 0.33 (90%CI: 0.16–0.69), one-sided p-value = 0.006. This p-value was higher than the nominal alpha (0.0014) of this first interim analysis. However, the conditional power analysis demonstrated high likelihood of getting a positive study in later interim/final analyses (from 100% to 87% for HR = 0.33 to 0.75).

Thus, rituximab, in addition to standard LMB therapy, improves EFS of children/adolescents with high-risk B-NHL and mature B leukaemia. However, the use of rituximab in addition to current chemotherapy backbone in standard-risk B-NHL is still questionable. Indeed, survival in standard-risk B-NHL (stages I/II and III LDH $\leq$ 2N) is very high, about 97–98%, with chemotherapy only. This chemotherapy is associated with acute toxicity but exceptional toxic deaths and no expected long-term sequelae. In this risk group, the use of rituximab is questionable, and more data are needed on its long-term safety when used in addition to chemotherapy in children before introducing it (and reducing chemotherapy intensity) in standard-risk B-NHL.

Relapses in mature B-cell NHL are rare, but their outcome is dismal, with a cure rate below 30%. The first step is to obtain a second CR. CYVE or ifosfamide, carboplatin, and etoposide (ICE) regimens are effective salvage chemotherapy. Consolidation with HD chemotherapy and haematopoietic support is needed after a second CR. An allograft does not afford more benefit than an autograft but could be considered to maintain dose intensity and/or in case of leukaemic involvement. Adverse prognostic factors at relapse are early relapse (within six months), but also multiple sites of recurrence (versus one site), BL histology (versus DLBCL), and initial high-risk features (e.g.

Table 18.2 Characteristics and results of main studies in childhood (less than 18 years of age) B-cell lymphoma

Protocol	Study groups	Ran domi za tion	Criteria for stratification and risk groups		No. patients	3-yr or 5-yr EFS	No. courses	CNS prophylaxis MTX g/m² (infusion duration)	TD Cyclo g/m² (Ifo g/m²)	TD Doxo mg/m²	TD VP16 g/m²
LMB89 Patte C, et al. (2001)	SFOP	No	Stage, resection, CNS, response at D7		561	91%					
			A	Stage 1 & 2 resected	52 (9%)	98%	2	No	3	120	0
			B	Not A, not C	386 (69%)	92%	5	5 HDMTX=3 g/m²(3h) 10 DIT	5.3	180	0
			C	CNS+ and/or BM >70%	123 (22%)	84% CNS 90% CNS+79%	8	5 HDMTX=8 g/m²(4h) 2 HDAra-C (CYVE) 10 TIT	6.8	240	2.5
FAB **LMB96** Gerrard M, et al. (2008) Patte C, et al. (2008) Cairo MS, et al. (2007)	SFOP UKCCSG CCG	Yes	Idem LMB89		1111	88%					
			A	Idem LMB89	132 (12%)	99%	2	No	3	120	0
		Yes	B	Not A, not C	744 (67%)	89%	4	Idem LMB89	3.3*	120*	0
		Yes	C	CNS+, BM >25%	235 (21%)	79%	8	Idem LMB89	6.8*	240*	2.5
BFM90 Reiter A, et al. (1999)	BFM	No	Resection, site, LDH (500), BM, CNS		413	88%					
			R1	Complete resection	71 (17%)	100%	2	2 MTX 0.5 g/m² (24h) 3 TIT	2 (4)	50	0.2
			R2	Extra abdominal only or abdominal & LDH <500	167 (40%)	96%	4	4 HDMTX 5 g/m²(24h) 5 TIT	3 (8)	100	0.4
			R3	Abdominal & LDH >500 and/or CNS+, and/or BM+, and/or multifocal bone	175 (43%)	79% CNS+ 65%	6	6 HDMTX 5 g/m²(24h) 7 TIT	4 (12)	150	0.6
BFM95 Woessmann W, et al. (2005)	BFM	Yes	Resection, stage, CNS LDH (<500,500–1000, >1000) Random: HDMTX 4h vs 24h		505	89%					
		Yes	R1	Stage 1 & 2 resected	48 (10%)	94%	2	2 HDMTX 1 g/m² (4h)* 3 TIT	2 (4)	50	0.2
		Yes	R2	Stage 1 & 2 non-resected Stage 3 & LDH <500	233 (46%)	94%	4	4 HDMTX 1 g/m² (4h)* 5 TIT	2.4 (8)	100	0.4
		Yes	R3	Stage 3 & LDH <1000 Stage 4/B-AL & LDH <1000	82 (16%)	85%	5	4 HDMTX 5 g/m² (24h) 1 HDAra-C (CC) 6 TIT	2.4 (8)	100	0.9
		Yes	R4	LDH > 1000 CNS+	142 (28%)	81% CNS+ 69%	6	4 HDMTX 5 g/m² (24h) 2 HDAra-C 7 TIT	2.4 (8)	100	1.4

B-NHL03 Tsurusawa M, et al. (2014)	JPLSG	No	Stage, resection, BM, CNS		321	87%					
			G1	Stage 1 & 2 resected	17	94%	2	2 DIT	1.5	120^	0
			G2	Stage 1 & 2 non-resected	103	99%	4	2 TIT, 2 DIT 2 HDMTX 3 g/m² (24h) 2 MTX 0.5 g/m² (6h)	1.5	120^	0
			G3	Stage 3 & 4 CNS-	111	84%	6	4 TIT, 2 DIT 4 HDMTX 3 g/m² (24h) 2 MTX 0.5 g/m² (6h)	3	240^	0.6
			G4	Stage 4 CNS+ & B-AL	90	78%	6	6 TIT, 2 DIT 4 HDMTX 5 (24h) 2 HDAra-C	5.5	240^	0.9
Inter-B-NHL ritux 2010	Part of EICNHL & COG	Yes	Stage, LDH /x2N, CNS, CSF Randomization: with or without rituximab (R)		600 pts planned	First interim analysis (n=310 pts)[57]: 1-year EFS (95%CI) Pts on the R is 94.2% (88.5–97.2) vs. 81.5% (73.0–87.8) on the control arm. HR=0.33.					
		Yes	B high	Stage 3 & 4 and LDH >Nx2			4	5 HDMTX=3 g/m²(3h) 10 DIT	3.3	120	0
		Yes	C1	Stage 4 CNS- & B-AL and CSF-			6	3–4 HDMTX=8 g/m²(4h) 2 HDAra-C (CYVE) 10–12 TIT	5.8	180	1.6
		Yes	C3	CSF+			6	4 HDMTX=8 g/m²(24h) 2 HDAra-C (CYVE) 12 TIT	5.8	180	1.6
		No	PMBL	PMBL CNS- DA-EPOCH-R regimen	40 pts planned	Ended 2016. Analysis in progress	6		>6	>240	>1.2

SFOP: Société Francaise d'Oncologie Pédiatrique; UKCCSG: United Kingdom Children's Cancer Study Group; CCG: Cancer Children Group (USA); JPLSG: Japanese Pediatric Leukemia/Lymphoma Study Group; COG: Children Oncology Group (North America, Australia, New Zealand); LMB: Lymphoma Malin B; FAB Franco-American-British; BFM: Berlin-Frankfurt-Munster; EICNHL: European Intergroup for Childhood NHL; Inter-B-NHLritux2010: clinical trial.gov identifier: NCT01760226; B-AL: mature B-cell acute leukaemia; PMBL: primary mediastinal B-cell lymphoma; TD: total (cumulative) dose; HDMTX: high dose methotrexate (with folinic rescue); DIT: double intrathecal injection (two drugs injected, either MTX or cytarabine with corticosteroid); TIT: triple intrathecal injection (corticosteroids, methotrexate, cytarabine); HDAra-C: high-dose cytarabine; CYVE course: combination of cytarabine in continuous infusion and HDAra-C with VP16; CC course: combination of HDAra-C with VP16, vindesine; CNS+: central nervous system involvement; CNS-: without central nervous system involvement; BM >70%: bone-marrow involvement with more than 70% blasts; LDH > 2N: LDH level more than twice the institutional normal value; DA-EPOCH-R: dose adjusted of VP16, prednisone, vincristine, cyclophosphamide, doxorubicin with rituximab.

* As results of the randomizations, these are the doses and the MTX infusion durations which are the standards in the current protocols.

^ p rarubicin instead of doxorubicin.

elevated LDH and advanced-stage disease versus a low LDH and stage I and II disease).

Innovative therapies are difficult to explore in childhood B-NHL due to the small numbers of cases of refractory/relapsed disease (in France, for example, there are about five relapses per year of BL and DLBCL). The most promising therapies include new antibody therapies, along with immunomodulatory agents that improve antibody-coated tumour-cell-killing, cytotoxic T cells genetically engineered to express a chimeric antigen receptor (CAR) recognizing CD19 expressed by B cells, and BTK inhibitors. Additionally, for some lymphomas, it has been demonstrated that PDL1 expression is driven by constitutive oncogenic signalling pathways in the tumour cell ('intrinsic' immune resistance). In PMBL, as in Hodgkin lymphoma, chromosome 9p24.1/PDL1/PDL2 alterations are frequent and anti-PD1 pembrolizumab has been recently reported to have promising activity in heavily pre-treated PMBL (overall response rate 41% and, with a median follow-up of 11.3 months, the median duration of response was not reached).

Lymphoblastic lymphoma

T-LLs generally present as mediastinal masses with advanced-stage disease ($\geq$III in more than 90% of cases), may involve the BM at diagnosis (around 30%), but less often the CNS (around 5%). Symptoms often include cough, wheezing, shortness of breath, orthopnoea; though swelling of the neck, face, and upper extremities from SVC obstruction can occur. Haemodynamic compromise due to pericardial effusions may also occur. Subdiaphragmatic disease is often present and may include hepatosplenomegaly, kidney infiltration, and retroperitoneal nodal disease. In contrast to the clinical features associated with precursor T-cell LL, children and adolescents with pB-LL tend to have limited disease in sites including skin, soft tissue, bone, testes, and peripheral lymph nodes. The cutaneous lesions are typically in the scalp and appear as enlarging, discoloured masses. Morphologically detectable BM involvement is uncommon at presentation.

The best treatment approaches for childhood advanced LL are ALL-based therapeutic regimens (e.g. LSA2L2 and the BFM regimens) (**Table 18.3**). These protocols were modified by adding HDMTX to the original LSA2L2 protocol to improve CNS prophylaxis, and by gradually excluding local and CNS radiotherapy. They are based on semi-continuous intensive polychemotherapy followed by maintenance therapy for a total duration of two years. Numerous drugs are given including corticosteroids, vincristine, anthracyclines, cyclophosphamide, cytarabine, asparaginase, and methotrexate. The major role of asparaginase was shown in several studies in which outcome was correlated with the dose intensity of the drug. CNS prophylaxis is generally based on HDMTX and intrathecal injections.

However, outcomes have not changed significantly since the 1980s, with EFS around 75–85% in most clinical trials in children and adolescents (**Table 18.2**). The only exception was the BFM90 study, with EFS attaining 90%, but this result was not reproduced in the following BFM95 study. Despite minimal differences between the two protocols, the divergent results obtained may be explained by a different dose and type of asparaginase. To date, except in the case of localized versus advanced stages, no clinical prognostic factors have been identified. A trend towards a better prognosis was shown in patients with a very good response after the seven-day pre-phase of corticosteroids. The international Euro-LB02 trial was designed by the EICHNL group to compare dexamethasone (known to better penetrate the CNS) to prednisone in the induction phase, and to evaluate the possibility of **decreasing** the duration of treatment from 24 to 18 months (second randomization). The reference arm was the NHL-BFM90 regimen without cranial irradiation, and only T-LLs were randomized. The study had to be closed prematurely because of excess toxic deaths. Final analysis showed an EFS rate of 821%±2% for the 319 eligible patients (75% T-LL), with a median follow-up of 6.8 years. Although no CNS relapses occurred in the dexamethasone arm, there was no trend towards better survival in this arm.

With intensive frontline treatment such as the BFM regimen, refractory disease/relapses are rare and have a dismal outcome, with a cure rate generally below 30%. In LL, there is a clear indication for an allograft if a second CR is achieved. However, the difficulty of obtaining a second CR emphasizes the need for new treatments. So far, the more recent drugs for T-LL such as nelarabine or clofarabine have proved disappointing. Blinatumumab, a bispecific CD19/CD3 antibody, may be promising for pB-LL.

Anaplastic large-cell lymphoma

Two forms of ALCL have been described: systemic ALCL and cutaneous ALCL. Primary cutaneous ALCLs usually lack ALK translocations and belong to the spectrum of primary cutaneous CD30-positive lymphoproliferations, a group that also comprises lymphomatoid papulosis. They remain confined to the skin and usually have an excellent prognosis after surgical resection without systemic therapy.

The clinical presenting features of systemic ALCL in children are quite variable but often include constitutional symptoms of fever and weight loss. About two thirds of cases present with disseminated disease. The most frequent sites of involvement in systemic ALCL are peripheral nodes, mediastinal adenopathy, and extranodal sites including skin, soft tissue, and bone. Skin involvement is much more frequent than in other childhood lymphomas and is a most common site of extranodal disease in ALCL. Spontaneous regression or waxing and waning of skin disease has been observed in systemic ALCL, albeit less frequently than in primary cutaneous ALCL. Bone disease is also common and it is multifocal in as many as 10% of patients. The CNS and BM are occasionally involved, and in several cases a leukaemic presentation has been described. Diagnosis of marrow involvement may be difficult and require immunostaining with CD30 and/or ALK or molecular analysis to identify rare tumour cells.

In recent trials with very diverse first-line chemotherapy regimens (in terms of the duration of treatment, and the number and cumulative doses of drugs), similar EFS rates of about 65–75% have been achieved in children and adolescents (**Table 18.4**). In the largest multinational trial, ALCL99, comprising more than 400 children, a 73% five-year EFS rate was achieved using NHL-BFM-B chemotherapy as the reference arm. This trial showed that the methotrexate schedule of the BFM protocol, including IT therapy, can be safely replaced by a less toxic schedule of methotrexate 3 g/m^2 in a three-hour infusion without IT therapy, and that adding vinblastine to each course and as maintenance for a total treatment duration of 12 months significantly delayed the occurrence of relapses, but did not reduce the absolute risk. Similarly, the COG group ANHL0131

Table 18.3 Characteristics and results of main series of paediatric lymphoblastic lymphoma*

Protocol	Study group (period of the study)	Study patients	Treatment strategy	Treatment duration in months	RTH	CNS Prophy laxis	Number patients with LL	3-5y EFS	3-5y OS
CCG-551 (COMP vs LSA2L2) Anderson, J. R. et al.1993	CCG (1977–82)	NHL	LSA2L2	18	local	IT	124 st 3&4	64%	67%
LSA2L2 Mora, J. et al. 2003	NY (1971–90)	LL all stages	LSA2L2	24-36	local	IT	95 (80%T)	75%	79%
LMT81 Patte, C. et al.*1992*	IGR (1981–89)	LL all stages	LSA2L2 +HDMTX	24	cranial if CNS+	HDMTX IT	84	75%	76%
CCG 502 (LSA2L2 vs ADCOMP) Tubergen, D. G. et al.1995	CCG (1983–90)	LL	LSA2L2	24	local craniospinal if CNS+	IT	143	74%	77%
POG 9404 (HDMTX vs no) Asselin, B. L. et al. 2011	POG (1996–2000)	T-ALL & T-LL	Dana Farber backbone	24	cranial	IT +/- HDMTX cranial RTX	137	85%	NA
COG 5941 Abromowitch, M. et al. 2008	COG (1994–97)	LL advanced stages	"condensed"	12	cranial if CNS+	IT HDMTX	85 (91%T)	78%	85%
BFM86 Reiter, A. et al. 1995	BFM (1986–1990)	LL all stages	NHL-BFM-nonB	24	cranial	IT HDMTX cranial RTX (st III/IV)	63 (91%T)	84%	88%
BFM90 Reiter, A. et al.*2000*	BFM (1990–95)	LL all stages	NHL-BFM-nonB	24	cranial	IT HDMTX cranial RTX (st III/IV)	136 (81%T)	90%	92%
BFM95 Burkhardt, B. et al. 2006	BFM (1995–2001)	LL all stages	NHL-BFM-nonB	24	cranial if CNS+	IT HDMTX	198 (73%T)	80%	86%
CLG 58881 Uyttebroeck, A. et al. 2008	EORTC (1989–98)	T-LL	NHL-BFM-nonB	24	no	IT HDMTX	119	77.5%	86%
LMT96 Bergeron, C. et al. 2015	SFOP (1997–2003)	T-LL	Modified BFM	18-24	cranial if CNS+	IT HDMTX	79	85%	89%
AIEOP92 Pillon, M. et al. 2009	AEIOP (1992–97)	LL all stages	LSA2L2	24	cranial if CNS+	IT HDMTX	55 (85%T)	69%	74%
COG A5971 1/ "CCG/ALL" vs NHL/BFM95 2/ Intensification: yes vs no Termuhlen, A. M. et al. 2013	COG (2000–05)	LL advanced stages	Modified BFM	24	cranial if CNS+	IT +/- HDMTX	266 (86%T)	82%	85%
EuroLb02 dexamethasone vs prednisone Landmann et al. 2017	EICNHL (2003–08)	LL all stages	NHL-BFM90	24 vs 18	cranial if CNS+	IT HDMTX	319 (73%T)	82±2%	87±2%

* Series of localized diseases or B-LL are not presented

See Table 18.2 for CCG, COG, SFOP, BFM, EICNHL, HDMTX, IT, CNS+

RTH: radiation therapy; ref: reference; NA: not available; LMT: lymphomes malins T; POG: Pediatric Oncology Group (USA); EORTC: European Organization for Research and Treatment of Cancer; AEIOP: Italian Association of Pediatric Hematology and Oncology; NY: New York Memorial Sloan-Kettering Cancer Center; IGR: Institut Gustave Roussy, France

Table 18.4 Results of the main series of paediatric anaplastic large-cell lymphoma

Protocol	Study group (period of the study)	Treatment strategy	Treatment duration	No. of patients	3-5-yr EFS	3-5-yr OS
HM89-91 Brugières L, et al. (1998)	SFOP (1989–97)	B-cell regimen (COPADM + maintenance)	7–8 m	82	66%	83%
NHL-BFM90 Seidemann K, et al. (2001)	BFM (1990–95)	B-cell regimen (BFM-B)	2–5 m	89	76%	-
NHL 9000 & 9602 Williams DM, et al. (2002)	UKCCSG (1990–98)	B-cell regimen (LMB)	4–5 m	72	59%	65%
LNH92 Rosolen A, et al. (2005)	AIEOP (1993–97)	T-cell regimen	24 m	34	65%	85%
POG9315 Laver JH, et al. (2005)	POG (1994–2000)	APO + randomization of HDMTX & HDAra-C	12 m	86	72%	88%
CCSG5941 Lowe EJ, et al. (2009)	CCSG (1996–2001)	Compressed T-cell regimen	11 m	86	68%	80%
ALCL99 Brugières L, et al. (2009)	EICNHL (1999–2006)	B-cell regimen (BFM-B) + randomization of vinblastine	4–12 m	352	73%	92%
ANHL0131 Alexander S, et al. (2014)	COG (2004–08)	APO + randomization of vinblastine	12 m	125	74%	84%

See abbreviations of Box 18.1 and Table 18.2 for the study groups
APO: doxorubicin, prednisone, vincristine.

trial showed that replacing vincristine by weekly vinblastine, as part of multi-agent maintenance therapy from the adriamycin, prednisone, and vincristine (APO) regimen, did not improve EFS or overall survival (OS).

One of the unique features of ALCL compared to other paediatric NHLs is its sensitivity to chemotherapy after recurrence, leading to a survival rate of more than 90% in the recent ALCL99 study. Several strategies, including re-induction chemotherapy followed by autologous or allogeneic haematopoietic stem-cell transplantation (SCT) or weekly vinblastine, can be successful. The efficacy of vinblastine, initially shown in a small series of patients with multiple relapses, was confirmed in the European ALCL relapse study. An interim analysis in August 2011 confirmed the efficacy of vinblastine, showing an 87% two-year EFS rate in a small series of patients with a late relapse (median follow-up 34 months).

Interestingly, vinblastine is one of the most potent drugs capable of enhancing the anti-cancer immune response by stimulating dendritic cell (DC) function. *In vitro*, vinblastine was found to induce the production of IL-1α, IL-6, and IL-12, increase surface expression of CD40, CD80, CD86, and MHC class II, and to enhance T-cell stimulatory capacity of DCs. One of the mechanisms of DC maturation induced by vinblastine is thought to be the release of the high mobility group box 1 protein (HMGB1), a major molecule involved in DC stimulation and immunogenic cell death.

Prognostic factors associated with an increased risk of failure have been identified in ALCL: the presence of mediastinal or visceral involvement and skin lesions, and histological lymphohistiocytic and small-cell variant subtypes. More recently, new parameters such as the detection of MDD in BM and/or blood, the persistence of positive MRD after four weeks of treatment, and low production of anti-ALK titres were also identified. Using MDD and antibody titre results in a series of 128 patients allowed them to be classified into three biological risk groups, each with a different prognosis: high risk: MDD-positive and low antibody titre (20% of patients with five-year progression-free survival (PFS) of 28%); low risk (MDD-negative and high antibody titre (31% of patients with five-year EFS of 93%); and intermediate risk: all the remaining patients (48% with five-year PFS of 68%).

Several new drugs have recently been implemented in the treatment of ALCL. Brentuximab vedotin (BV) is an anti-CD30 monoclonal antibody conjugated to the antimicrotubule cytotoxic monomethyl auristatin-E (MMAE). A study on 58 patients with relapsed/refractory ALCL (16 ALK-positive) treated with BV reported an objective response rate of 86%, with a median duration of 12.6 months. Following these results, BV was approved by the Federal Drug Agency (FDA) and European Medical Agency (EMA) for the treatment of systemic ALCL after failure of at least one chemotherapy regimen in adults.

ALK inhibitors such as crizotinib, an ALK/MET inhibitor, are also promising drugs. Crizotinib is now approved by the FDA and EMA for the treatment of ALK-dependent lung cancers. The results in ALCL are also promising with seven out of nine CRs in patients with relapsed/refractory ALCL included in a paediatric phase I trial of crizotinib. The same results were obtained, with a response rate of 91%, in 11 patients with ALK+ resistant/refractory adult lymphoma. Following these results, the COG is currently investigating the feasibility of BV or crizotinib combined with ALCL99 chemotherapy in children with newly diagnosed stage II–IV ALCL (http://clinicaltrials.gov/ct2/show/record/NCT01979536/). The EICNHL, however, is planning a randomized trial with risk stratification, based on MDD and the antibody level, aimed at evaluating the efficacy of adding crizotinib to ALCL99 in frontline therapy for intermediate- and high-risk ALCL, and comparing weekly vinblastine to ALCL99 in low- and intermediate-risk disease.

NPM-ALK has also been shown to promote immune evasion by inducing the expression of the immunosuppressive cell-surface protein, programmed death ligand 1 (PD-L1), through the activation of the *STAT3* pathway. Remarkably, ALK+ ALCL cell lines express PD-L1 (both mRNA and protein). Furthermore, all patient tissue samples reported to date have exhibited strong PD-L1 immunostaining. Indeed, two refractory ALK+ ALCL patients demonstrated durable response with anti-PD1 therapy after failure to chemotherapy and ALK inhibitors (in one patient, also after allogeneic haematopoietic stem-cell transplantation). Thus, the development of PD-1 inhibitors in refractory/relapsed ALCL, either in case of progression after targeted therapies or as consolidative immunotherapy in patients in CR after ALK inhibitors or brentuximab vedotin, may be promising.

Conclusion

Thanks to better recognition of the diseases, and to national and international collaborations, dramatic improvements of cure rates have been obtained in childhood/adolescent NHL, with chemotherapy adapted to subtypes and to disease extension. Most of these treatments trigger immediate toxicities, commonly aplasia and mucositis, which not only hamper quality of life during treatment but can also be life-threatening. However, most of the current treatments have few expected long-term toxicities. Furthermore, the therapeutic strategy and treatment intensity vary considerably between paediatric and adult approaches for similar subtypes. The lack of uniform criteria for staging and the limited data concerning age-related biological characteristics of each subtype prevent us from knowing the impact of these differences on patient outcomes. The use of excellent chemotherapy combination has gradually reduced the role of radiotherapy. However, radiotherapy can still be useful as a form of urgent treatment in children with large mediastinal masses compromising respiration, in selected relapse cases, or as palliation.

Defining new prognostic factors will help better develop risk-adapted strategies. Major progress is expected, with new treatments including antibodies and/or targeted therapies. It is improbable that they will cure NHL on their own, but their subtle combinations with chemotherapy may allay some of the chemotherapy-related toxicities. Except for high-risk patients who require further therapeutic improvements, the challenge over the coming years will not be to increase already high cure rates but, rather, to strike a balance between immediate toxicity and no long-term toxicity versus potentially decreased immediate toxicity but unknown long-term toxicity. This requires further paediatric international collaboration along with partnerships with adult lymphoma groups.

FURTHER READING

Abromowitch M, et al. (2008) Shortened intensified multi-agent chemotherapy and non-cross resistant maintenance therapy for advanced lymphoblastic lymphoma in children and adolescents: report from the Children's Oncology Group. *Br J Haematol* **143**, 261–7.

Ait-Tahar K, et al. (2006) B and CTL responses to the ALK protein in patients with ALK-positive ALCL. *Int J Cancer* **118**, 688–95.

Ait-Tahar K, et al. (2010) Correlation of the autoantibody response to the ALK oncoantigen in pediatric anaplastic lymphoma kinase-positive anaplastic large cell lymphoma with tumor dissemination and relapse risk. *Blood* **115**, 3314–19.

Alexander S, et al. (2014) Advanced stage anaplastic large cell lymphoma in children and adolescents: results of ANHL0131, a randomized phase III trial of APO versus a modified regimen with vinblastine. A report from the Children's Oncology Group. *Pediatr Blood Cancer* **61**(12), 2236–42. doi:10.1002/pbc.25187

Anderson JR, et al. (1993) Long-term follow-up of patients treated with COMP or LSA2L2 therapy for childhood non-Hodgkin's lymphoma: a report of CCG-551 from the Children's Cancer Group. *J Clin Oncol* **11**, 1024–32.

Anoop P, et al. (2012) Outcome of childhood relapsed or refractory mature B-cell non-Hodgkin lymphoma and acute lymphoblastic leukemia. *Leuk. Lymphoma* **53**, 1882–8.

Asselin BL, et al. (2011) Effectiveness of high-dose methotrexate in T-cell lymphoblastic leukemia and advanced-stage lymphoblastic lymphoma: a randomized study by the Children's Oncology Group (POG 9404). *Blood* **118**, 874–83.

Bergeron C, et al. (2015) Treatment of childhood T-cell lymphoblastic lymphoma—long-term results of the SFOP LMT96 trial. *Pediatr Blood Cancer* **62**, 2150–6.

Bhojwani D, et al. (2015) The role of FDG-PET/CT in the evaluation of residual disease in paediatric non-Hodgkin lymphoma. *Br J Haematol* **168**, 845–53.

Bienemann K, et al. (2011) Promising therapy results for lymphoid malignancies in children with chromosomal breakage syndromes (Ataxia teleangiectasia or Nijmegen-breakage syndrome): a retrospective survey. *Br J Haematol* **155**, 468–76.

Bonn BR, et al. (2013) Incidence and prognostic relevance of genetic variations in T-cell lymphoblastic lymphoma in childhood and adolescence. *Blood* **121**, 3153–60.

Bouda GC, Traore F, Couitchere L, et al. (2019) Advanced Burkitt Lymphoma in Sub-Saharan Africa Pediatric Units: Results of the Third Prospective Multicenter Study of the Groupe Franco-Africain d'Oncologie Pediatrique. *J Global Oncol* in press.

Brugières L, et al. (1998) CD30(+) anaplastic large-cell lymphoma in children: analysis of 82 patients enrolled in two consecutive studies of the French Society of Pediatric Oncology. *Blood* **92**, 3591–8.

Brugières L, et al. (2000) Relapses of childhood anaplastic large-cell lymphoma: treatment results in a series of 41 children—a report from the French Society of Pediatric Oncology. *Ann Oncol ESMO* **11**, 53–8.

Brugières L, et al. (2009) Impact of the methotrexate administration dose on the need for intrathecal treatment in children and adolescents with anaplastic large-cell lymphoma: results of a randomized trial of the EICNHL Group. *J Clin Oncol* **27**(6), 897–903.

Burkhardt B, et al. (2005) The impact of age and gender on biology, clinical features and treatment outcome of non-Hodgkin lymphoma in childhood and adolescence. *Br J Haematol* **131**, 39–49.

Burkhardt B, et al. (2006) Impact of cranial radiotherapy on central nervous system prophylaxis in children and adolescents with central nervous system-negative stage III or IV lymphoblastic lymphoma. *J Clin Oncol* **24**, 491–9.

Burkhardt B, et al. (2009) Poor outcome for children and adolescents with progressive disease or relapse of lymphoblastic lymphoma: a report from the Berlin-Frankfurt-Muenster group. *J Clin Oncol* **27**, 3363–9.

Burkhardt B (2010) Paediatric lymphoblastic T-cell leukaemia and lymphoma: one or two diseases? *Br J Haematol* **149**, 653–68.

Burkitt D (1962) Determining the climatic limitations of a children's cancer common in Africa. *BMJ* **2**, 1019–23.

Cairo MS, et al. (2007) Results of a randomized international study of high-risk central nervous system B non-Hodgkin lymphoma and B acute lymphoblastic leukemia in children and adolescents. *Blood* **109**, 2736–43.

Cairo MS, et al. (2012) Advanced stage, increased lactate dehydrogenase, and primary site, but not adolescent age (≥ 15 years), are associated with an increased risk of treatment failure in children and adolescents with mature B-cell non-Hodgkin's lymphoma: results of the FAB LMB 96 study. *J Clin Oncol* **30**, 387–93.

Callens C, et al. (2012) Clinical impact of NOTCH1 and/or FBXW7 mutations, FLASH deletion, and TCR status in pediatric T-cell lymphoblastic lymphoma. *J Clin Oncol* **30**, 1966–73.

Ciambotti B, et al. (2014) Monoallelic mutations of the perforin gene may represent a predisposing factor to childhood anaplastic large cell lymphoma. *J Pediatr Hematol Oncol* **36**, e359–65.

Coustan-Smith E, et al. (2009) Minimal disseminated disease in childhood T-cell lymphoblastic lymphoma: a report from the Children's Oncology Group. *J Clin Oncol* **27**, 3533–9.

Damm-Welk C, et al. (2007) Prognostic significance of circulating tumor cells in bone marrow or peripheral blood as detected by qualitative and quantitative PCR in pediatric NPM-ALK-positive anaplastic large-cell lymphoma. *Blood* **110**, 670–7.

Ducassou S, et al. (2011) Clinical presentation, evolution, and prognosis of precursor B-cell lymphoblastic lymphoma in trials LMT96, EORTC 58881, and EORTC 58951. *Br J Haematol* **152**, 441–51.

Epstein MA, et al. (1964) Virus particles in cultured lymphoblasts from Burkitt's lymphoma. *Lancet* **1**, 702–3.

Gambacorti Passerini C, et al. (2014) Crizotinib in advanced, chemoresistant anaplastic lymphoma kinase-positive lymphoma patients. *J Natl Cancer Inst* **106**, djt378.

Gerrard M, et al. (2008) Excellent survival following two courses of COPAD chemotherapy in children and adolescents with resected localized B-cell non-Hodgkin's lymphoma: results of the FAB/LMB 96 international study. *Br J Haematol* **141**, 840–7.

Gerrard M, et al. (2013) Outcome and pathologic classification of children and adolescents with mediastinal large B-cell lymphoma treated with FAB/LMB96 mature B-NHL therapy. *Blood* **121**, 278–85.

Greenough A, Dave SS (2014) New clues to the molecular pathogenesis of Burkitt lymphoma revealed through next-generation sequencing. *Curr Opin Hematol* **21**, 326–32.

Goldman S, et al. (2014) Rituximab with chemotherapy in children and adolescents with central nervous system and/or bone marrow-positive Burkitt lymphoma/leukaemia: a Children's Oncology Group report. *Br J Haematol* **167**(3), 394–401. doi:10.1111/bjh.13040

Goldman S, et al. (2013) Rituximab and FAB/LMB 96 chemotherapy in children with stage III/IV B-cell non-Hodgkin lymphoma: a Children's Oncology Group report. *Leukemia* **27**, 1174–7.

Gross TG, et al. (2010) Hematopoietic stem cell transplantation for refractory or recurrent non-Hodgkin lymphoma in children and adolescents. *Biol Blood Marrow Transplant* **16**, 223–30.

Haddy TB, et al. (1991) CNS involvement in small noncleaved-cell lymphoma: is CNS disease per se a poor prognostic sign? *J Clin Oncol* **9**, 1973–82.

Hebart H, et al. (2016) Nivolumab for refractory anaplastic large cell lymphoma: a case report. *Ann Intern Med* **165**, 607–8.

Hesseling P, et al. (2013) Practical recommendations for the management of children with endemic Burkitt lymphoma (BL) in a resource limited setting. *Pediatr Blood Cancer* **60**, 357–62.

Jourdain A, et al. (2015) Outcome and prognostic factors of relapse in children and adolescents with mature B-cell lymphoma and leukemia treated in three consecutive prospective LMB protocols. Study by the SFOP/SFCE (Société Française d'Oncologie Pédiatrique/Société Française des Cancers de l'Enfant). *Haematologica* **100**(6), 810–17.

Lamant L, et al. (2011) Prognostic impact of morphologic and phenotypic features of childhood ALK-positive anaplastic large-cell lymphoma: results of the ALCL99 study. *J Clin Oncol* **29**, 4669–76.

Landmann E, Burkhardt B, Zimmermann M, et al. (2017) Results and conclusions of the European Intergroup EURO-LB02 trial in children and adolescents with lymphoblastic lymphoma. *Haematologica* **102**, 2086–96. doi:10.3324/haematol.2015.139162

Lavoine N, et al. (2015) Constitutional mismatch repair deficiency syndrome: clinical description in a French cohort. *J Med Genet* **52**, 770–8.

Laver JH, et al. (2005) Advanced-stage large-cell lymphoma in children and adolescents: results of a randomized trial incorporating intermediate-dose methotrexate and high-dose cytarabine in the maintenance phase of the APO regimen: a Pediatric Oncology Group phase III trial. *J Clin Oncol* **23**, 541–7.

Le Deley MC, et al. (2008) Prognostic factors in childhood anaplastic large cell lymphoma: results of a large European intergroup study. *Blood* **111**, 1560–6.

Le Deley MC, et al. (2010) Vinblastine in children and adolescents with high-risk anaplastic large-cell lymphoma: results of the randomized ALCL99-vinblastine trial. *J Clin Oncol* **28**, 3987–93.

Louissaint A, et al. (2012) Pediatric-type nodal follicular lymphoma: an indolent clonal proliferation in children and adults with high proliferation index and no BCL2 rearrangement. *Blood* **120**, 2395–404.

Louissaint A, et al. (2016) Pediatric-type nodal follicular lymphoma: a biologically distinct lymphoma with frequent MAPK pathway mutations. *Blood* **128**, 1093–100.

Love C, et al. (2012) The genetic landscape of mutations in Burkitt lymphoma. *Nat Genet* **44**, 1321–5.

Lowe EJ, et al. (2009) Intensive chemotherapy for systemic anaplastic large cell lymphoma in children and adolescents: final results of Children's Cancer Group Study 5941. *Pediatr Blood Cancer* **52**, 335–9.

Magrath IT (1991) African Burkitt's lymphoma. History, biology, clinical features, and treatment. *Am J Pediatr Hematol Oncol* **13**, 222–46.

Marzec M, et al. (2008) Oncogenic kinase NPM/ALK induces through STAT3 expression of immunosuppressive protein CD274 (PD-L1, B7-H1). *Proc Natl Acad Sci USA* **105**, 20852–7.

Meinhardt A, et al. (2010) Phase II window study on rituximab in newly diagnosed pediatric mature B-cell non-Hodgkin's lymphoma and Burkitt leukemia. *J Clin Oncol* **28**, 3115–21.

Miles RR, et al. (2008) Pediatric diffuse large B-cell lymphoma demonstrates a high proliferation index, frequent c-Myc protein expression, and a high incidence of germinal center subtype: report of the French–American–British (FAB) international study group. *Pediatr Blood Cancer* **51**, 369–74.

Minard-Colin V, et al. (2015) Non-Hodgkin lymphoma in children and adolescents: progress through effective collaboration, current knowledge, and challenges ahead. *J Clin Oncol* **33**, 2963–74.

Minard-Colin V, et al. (2016) Results of the randomized intergroup trial Inter-B-NHL Ritux 2010 for children and adolescents with high-risk B-cell non-Hodgkin lymphoma (B-NHL) and mature acute leukemia (B-AL): evaluation of rituximab (R) efficacy in addition to standard LMB chemotherapy (CT) regimen. *J Clin Oncol* **34**(15), suppl 10507.

Mora J, et al. (2003) Lymphoblastic lymphoma of childhood and the LSA2-L2 protocol: the 30-year experience at Memorial–Sloan–Kettering Cancer Center. *Cancer* **98**, 1283–91.

Mossé YP, et al. (2013) Safety and activity of crizotinib for paediatric patients with refractory solid tumours or anaplastic large-cell lymphoma: a Children's Oncology Group phase 1 consortium study. *Lancet Oncol* **14**, 472–80.

Murphy SB (1980) Classification, staging and end results of treatment of childhood non-Hodgkin's lymphomas: dissimilarities from lymphomas in adults. *Semin Oncol* **7**, 332–9.

Mussolin L, et al. (2003) Prospective analysis of minimal bone marrow infiltration in pediatric Burkitt's lymphomas by long-distance polymerase chain reaction for t(8;14)(q24;q32). Leukemia **17**, 585–9.

Mussolin L, et al. (2011) Minimal disseminated disease in high-risk Burkitt's lymphoma identifies patients with different prognosis. *J Clin Oncol* **29**, 1779–84.

Mussolin L, et al. (2013) Use of minimal disseminated disease and immunity to NPM-ALK antigen to stratify ALK-positive ALCL patients with different prognosis. *Leukemia* **27**, 416–22.

Neth O, et al. (2000) Precursor B-cell lymphoblastic lymphoma in childhood and adolescence: clinical features, treatment, and results in trials NHL-BFM 86 and 90. *Med Pediatr Oncol* **35**, 20–7.

Oschlies I, et al. (2006) Diffuse large B-cell lymphoma in pediatric patients belongs predominantly to the germinal-center type B-cell lymphomas: a clinicopathologic analysis of cases included in the German BFM (Berlin–Frankfurt–Munster) multicenter trial. *Blood* **107**, 4047–52.

Oschlies I, et al. (2011) Clinical, pathological and genetic features of primary mediastinal large B-cell lymphomas and mediastinal gray zone lymphomas in children. *Haematologica* **96**, 262–8.

Patte C, et al. (1991) High survival rate in advanced-stage B-cell lymphomas and leukemias without CNS involvement with a short intensive polychemotherapy: results from the French Pediatric Oncology Society of a randomized trial of 216 children. *J Clin Oncol* **9**, 123–32.

Patte C, et al. (1992) Results of the LMT81 protocol, a modified LSA2L2 protocol with high dose methotrexate, on 84 children with non-B-cell (lymphoblastic) lymphoma. *Med Pediatr Oncol* **20**, 105–13.

Patte C, et al. (2001) The Société Française d'Oncologie Pédiatrique LMB89 protocol: highly effective multiagent chemotherapy tailored to the tumor burden and initial response in 561 unselected children with B-cell lymphomas and L3 leukemia. *Blood* **97**, 3370–9.

Patte C, et al. (2007) Results of the randomized international FAB/LMB96 trial for intermediate risk B-cell non-Hodgkin lymphoma in children and adolescents: it is possible to reduce treatment for the early responding patients. *Blood* **109**, 2773–80.

Pelicci PG, et al. (1986) Chromosomal breakpoints and structural alterations of the c-myc locus differ in endemic and sporadic forms of Burkitt lymphoma. *Proc Natl Acad Sci USA* **83**, 2984–8.

Percy C, et al. (1999) Lymphomas and reticuloendothelial neoplasms. In: L. Ries, et al. (eds) *Cancer Incidence and Survival Among Children and Adolescents: United States SEER Program 1975–1995*, pp. 35–50. Bethesda, MD: National Cancer Institute.

Pillon M, et al. (2009) Long-term results of AIEOP LNH-92 protocol for the treatment of pediatric lymphoblastic lymphoma: a report of the Italian Association of Pediatric Hematology and Oncology. *Pediatr Blood Cancer* **53**, 953–9.

Poirel HA, et al. (2009) Specific cytogenetic abnormalities are associated with a significantly inferior outcome in children and adolescents with mature B-cell non-Hodgkin's lymphoma: results of the FAB/LMB 96 international study. *Leukemia* **23**, 323–31.

Pro B, et al. (2012) Brentuximab vedotin (SGN-35) in patients with relapsed or refractory systemic anaplastic large-cell lymphoma: results of a phase II study. *J Clin Oncol* **30**, 2190–6.

Reiter A, Klapper, W (2008) Recent advances in the understanding and management of diffuse large B-cell lymphoma in children. *Br J Haematol* **142**, 329–47.

Reiter A, et al. (1995) Non-Hodgkin's lymphomas of childhood and adolescence: results of a treatment stratified for biologic subtypes and stage—a report of the Berlin–Frankfurt–Münster Group. *J Clin Oncol* **13**, 359–72.

Reiter, A, et al. (1999) Improved treatment results in childhood B-cell neoplasms with tailored intensification of therapy: a report of the Berlin–Frankfurt–Münster Group Trial NHL-BFM 90. *Blood* **94**, 3294–306.

Reiter A, et al. (2000) Intensive ALL-type therapy without local radiotherapy provides a 90% event-free survival for children with T-cell lymphoblastic lymphoma: a BFM group report. *Blood* **95**, 416–21.

Rigaud C (2018) Efficacy of nivolumab in a patient with systemic refractory ALK+ anaplastic large-cell lymphoma. *Pediatr Blood Cancer*, **65**(4). doi: 10.1002/pbc.26902

Rohde M, et al. (2017) Relevance of ID3-TCF3-CCND3 pathway mutations in pediatric aggressive B-cell lymphoma treated according to the non-Hodgkin lymphoma Berlin–Frankfurt–Münster protocols. *Haematologica* **102**, 1091–8.

Rosenwald A, et al. (2003) Molecular diagnosis of primary mediastinal B cell lymphoma identifies a clinically favorable subgroup of diffuse large B cell lymphoma related to Hodgkin lymphoma. *J Exp Med* **198**, 851–62.

Rosolen A,et al. (2005) Anaplastic large cell lymphoma treated with a leukemia-like therapy: report of the Italian Association of Pediatric Hematology and Oncology (AIEOP) LNH-92 protocol. *Cancer* **104**, 2133–40.

Rosolen A, et al. (2015) A revised international pediatric non-Hodgkin lymphoma (NHL) staging system classification (IPNHLSS): a report from the Fourth International Childhood, Adolescent and Young Adult NHL Symposium. *J Clin Oncol* **20**, 33(18), 2112–18.

Salaverria I, et al. (2011) Translocations activating IRF4 identify a subtype of germinal center-derived B-cell lymphoma affecting predominantly children and young adults. *Blood* **118**, 139–47.

Salaverria I, et al. (2014) A recurrent 11q aberration pattern characterizes a subset of MYC-negative high-grade B-cell lymphomas resembling Burkitt lymphoma. *Blood* **123**, 1187–98.

Sander S, et al. (2012) Synergy between PI3K signaling and MYC in Burkitt lymphomagenesis. *Cancer Cell* **22**, 167–79.

Sandlund JT, et al. (1994) Clinical features and treatment outcome for children with CD30+ large-cell non-Hodgkin's lymphoma. *J Clin Oncol* **12**, 895–8.

Sandlund JT, et al. (2014) Pilot study of modified LMB-based therapy for children with ataxia-telangiectasia and advanced stage high-grade mature B-cell malignancies. *Pediatr Blood Cancer* **61**, 360–2.

Schmidt J, et al. (2016) Genome-wide analysis of pediatric-type follicular lymphoma reveals low genetic complexity and recurrent alterations of TNFRSF14 gene. *Blood* **128**, 1101–11.

Seidemann K, et al. (2001) Short-pulse B-non-Hodgkin lymphoma-type chemotherapy is efficacious treatment for pediatric anaplastic large cell lymphoma: a report of the Berlin–Frankfurt–Münster Group Trial NHL-BFM 90. *Blood* **97**, 3699–706.

Swerdlow SH, et al. (2016) The 2016 revision of the World Health Organization classification of lymphoid neoplasms. *Blood* **127**, 2375–90.

Tanaka H, et al. (2009) Dual therapeutic efficacy of vinblastine as a unique chemotherapeutic agent capable of inducing dendritic cell maturation. *Cancer Res* **69**, 6987–94.

Termuhlen AM, et al. (2013) Disseminated lymphoblastic lymphoma in children and adolescents: results of the COG A5971 trial—a report from the Children's Oncology Group. *Br J Haematol* **162**, 792–801.

Tsurusawa M, et al. (2014) Improved treatment results of children with B-cell non-Hodgkin lymphoma: a report from the Japanese Pediatric Leukemia/Lymphoma Study Group B-NHL03 study. *Pediatr Blood Cancer* **61**, 1215–21.

Tubergen DG, et al. (1995) Comparison of treatment regimens for pediatric lymphoblastic non-Hodgkin's lymphoma: a Children's Cancer Group study. *J Clin Oncol* **13**, 1368–76.

Uyttebroeck A, et al. (2008) Treatment of childhood T-cell lymphoblastic lymphoma according to the strategy for acute lymphoblastic leukaemia, without radiotherapy: long-term results of the EORTC CLG 58881 trial. *Eur J Cancer* **44**, 840–6.

Williams DM, et al. (2002) Anaplastic large cell lymphoma in childhood: analysis of 72 patients treated on the United Kingdom Children's Cancer Study Group chemotherapy regimens. *Br J Haematol* **117**, 812–20.

Wimmer K, et al. (2014) Diagnostic criteria for constitutional mismatch repair deficiency syndrome: suggestions of the European consortium 'Care for CMMRD' (C4CMMRD). *J Med Genet* **51**, 355–65.

Woessmann W, et al. (2005) The impact of the methotrexate administration schedule and dose in the treatment of children and adolescents with B-cell neoplasms: a report of the BFM Group Study NHL-BFM95. *Blood* **105**, 948–58.

Woessmann W, et al. (2011) Relapsed or refractory anaplastic large-cell lymphoma in children and adolescents after Berlin–Frankfurt–Muenster (BFM)-type first-line therapy: a BFM group study. *J Clin Oncol* **29**, 3065–71.

Woessmann W, et al. (2012) Risk-adapted therapy for patients with relapsed or refractory ALCL—interim results of the prospective EICNHL-trial ALCL-relapse. *Br J Haematol* **159**(S1), 41.

Zinzani PL, et al. (2017) Safety and tolerability of pembrolizumab in patients with relapsed/refractory primary mediastinal large B-cell lymphoma. *Blood* **130**, 267–70.

19

Hodgkin Lymphoma

Modern Management of Children and Young Adults

Judith Landman-Parker and Françoise Montravers

Introduction

In three decades, Hodgkin lymphoma (HL) has become a highly curable lymphoid malignancy with an expected survival rate at ten years of over 90%. The number of patients cured of their disease is estimated at 100,000 in Europe, and long-term management of treatment-related subsequent morbidity is now a relevant health question. Moreover, new drugs have recently emerged targeted at Hodgkin/Reed–Sternberg (H/RS) cells and their environment, leading to new therapeutic opportunities in patients with relapsed or refractory disease

Epidemiology

Exceptional before five years of age, HL is the most common cancer in adolescence. In the European Union, the crude incidence of HL is 2.3–3 cases per 100,000 people per year. Sex ratio varies with age, with a higher incidence in boys when HL is diagnosed below 12 years. HL displays a bimodal distribution in adults, with an initial peak in young adults and a later peak among patients over 55 years. Childhood and adolescent HL represents around 10% of the cases. Patterns of incidence are variable worldwide: lower in Asia and higher in the Middle East and Mediterranean area. In economically less developed regions, the initial HL peak is earlier among children and teenagers.

Pathology

HL is characterized by the presence of multinucleated giant H/RS cells or large mononuclear cell variants (lymphocytic and histiocytic cells) accounting for 1% of the cells surrounded by polymorphic inflammatory tissue reaction with lymphoid cells, macrophages, eosinophilia, and fibrosis.

World Health Organization classification

Since 2001, the World Health Organization (WHO) classification has defined the classical variant of Hodgkin lymphoma (cHL): 90% of cases characterized histologically by HRS cells and a rare and distinct nodular lymphocyte predominant Hodgkin lymphoma (NLPHL) subtype with unique clinico-pathological features and detection of histiocytic 'pop corn' cells. cLH is subdivided into four subtypes: nodular sclerosis, 70–80%; mixed cellularity, 20–30%; lymphocyte-rich, 2–5%; and lymphocyte depletion, less than 1%. Immunostaining of HRS is typically CD30+, CD15+, PAX5+, ALK-, CD45-, and CD 20+/-.

Biology

Recent insights into the biology of H/RS cells are beginning to provide a better understanding of HL pathogenesis. H/RS cells are clonal, arise from germinal centre B-cell lymphocytes in virtually all cases, and present crippling mutations of immunoglobulin genes. Their failure to express a normal B-lymphocyte phenotype is related to multiple molecular and epigenetic mechanisms leading to survival and proliferation of H/RS cells. Most H/RS cells constitutively express the anti-apoptotic NF-kB pathway as a result of somatic mutation or amplification of REL, TNFα-induced protein3, and NFKBIA genes and upregulate the JAK-Stat pathway by somatic mutations in 40% of cases.

Moreover, H/RS cells suppress anti-tumour immunity through expression of CD30, CD40, CD80, and PD1. They secrete numerous cytokines, such as TARC (CCL17), CCL5, CCL22, and interleukin-7, attracting T-helper 2 and regulatory T (Treg) cells to the tumour microenvironment. In 2016, a report by Roemer et al., combining fluorescent *in situ* hybridization (FISH), single nucleotide polymorphism (SNP) arrays, and immunohistochemical analysis in 108 biopsy specimens from patients with newly diagnosed cHL, identified rearrangements of the PDL1/PDL2 genes locus in 97% of cases and, therefore, confirmed a potential major role of this mechanism in cLH development.

Hodgkin lymphoma and Epstein-Barr virus

Epstein–Barr virus (EBV) is associated with cHL development in 30–50% of cases in children and adolescents, depending on age, socioeconomic context, and histopathology. In these cases, HR/S cells express latency type II EBV genes: LMP1, LMP2, EBNA1, and BamH1A. Transfection of viral genes in lymphocytes reproduces the HR/S phenotype. High levels of antibodies against EBV are associated with HL, and a population-based study has confirmed a four-times higher risk to develop EBV-associated HL up to five years after a mononucleosis infection.

Predisposition to Hodgkin lymphoma: a link with immune system control?

Familial Hodgkin lymphoma

Familial HL has been described since the 1970s. There is an estimated seven-fold risk to develop HL in siblings and first-degree relatives. GWAS (genome-wide association) analysis and more classical candidates' gene approaches have reported a possible locus of interest in HLA and DNA repair genes.

Paediatric immune deficiencies

Paediatric immune deficiencies are associated with HL development. Although rare, reports concern common variable immunoglobulin deficiency, X-LP, Ataxia telangiectasia, Wiskott–Aldrich syndrome, CD27/CD70 deficiency, DNA repair disorders, and other exceptional entities. In oncology practice, any familial history or unusual clinical or histopathological presentation such as very young age, consanguinity, Ig-deficiency, or interfollicular subtype has to lead to immunological investigations. Reports of HL cases in the context of defined acquired immune deficiency such as HIV, organ transplantation, or immunosuppressive treatment are important as providing clinical information about risk and outcome. However, few of these concern children and adolescents. In those cases, HL is mostly EBV-associated and in an advanced stage.

Autoimmune disease and Hodgkin lymphoma predisposition

Such as acute autoimmune cytopenias, glomerulopathy with nephrotic syndrome, and neurological inflammatory disease have been reported concomitant with, before, or after HL. GWAS analysis, as well as epidemiological studies, have described common polymorphisms in autoimmune disease and cHL. From a practical point of view, treatment of HL in these patients should follow the actual guidelines as much as possible, except in case of organ failures that require therapeutic modifications.

Clinical management and work-up in classical variant of Hodgkin lymphoma

Initial peripheral node enlargement is described in 85% of patients with cHL. Indolent progression of the disease leads frequently to delayed diagnosis (median six months between first reported symptoms and diagnosis). Systemic symptoms such as unexplained fever, drenching night sweats, or weight loss have to be collected, as well as detailed clinical node involvement and splenic or hepatic enlargement. Usual blood tests such as erythrocyte sedimentation rate (ESR), haemogram, white blood cell (WBC) count, immunoglobulin dosage, human immunodeficiency virus (HIV) serology, and renal and hepatic tests, as well electrocardiogram (ECG) and echocardiography, have to be performed before treatment.

Imaging in Hodgkin lymphoma

Initial work-up comprises X-ray chest with measure of the mediastinal diameter, cervico–thoracic–abdominal pelvis contrast-enhanced computed tomography (CT) or magnetic resonance imaging (MRI), and abdominal ultrasonography. Diagnostic CT and MRI reliably detect enlarged lymph nodes; intravenous (IV) contrast is mandatory to distinguish lymphadenopathy from other structures in the mediastinum and abdomen. Diagnostic CT allows detailed evaluation of pulmonary parenchyma, pleura, and pericardium. MRI is superior to contrast CT for evaluation of bone marrow, liver, soft tissue, and central nervous system, and is currently performed as a complement to other imaging examinations.

[^{18}F] fluorodeoxyglucose-positron emission tomography/computed tomography in Hodgkin lymphoma

Metabolic scintigraphy by [^{18}F] fluorodeoxyglucose-positron emission tomography/computed tomography (FDG-PET/CT) is indicated in cHL and highly recommended before any treatment as part of initial staging. In 97–100% of HL, FDG-PET/CT is positive (at least one [^{18}F]FDG-avid HL site). Low-dose CT, usually performed with PET, is more accurate than PET alone. However, contrast-enhanced CT or MRI with thoracic CT remain mandatory, at least at diagnosis, and can be performed either simultaneously with PET or separately.

[^{18}F]FDG-PET detects nodal and extranodal disease sites that are missed by CT/MRI staging methods, and improves the characterization of lesions (e.g. bone/bone marrow disease) that are equivocal on other types of imaging. Bone marrow biopsy indicated previously in stage III or above HL can now be replaced by [^{18}F]FDG-PET. In contrast, [^{18}F]FDG-PET/CT can under-stage disease, especially in lung localizations and because some lesions, even large, may not be [^{18}F]FDG-avid. Therefore, careful comparison of [^{18}F]FDG-positive lesions and morphological imaging is essential for accurate staging, according to the Ann Arbor revised Cotswolds classification. In children, [^{18}F]FDG-PET modified the stage in 10–23% of patients as a consequence. Patient stage distribution in the Euronet paediatric Hodgkin trial is stage I–II, 55%; stage III, 20%, and stage IV, 25%, if FDG-PET/CT is integrated in the staging modalities.

Imaging during treatment and response-adapted strategy

Initial [^{18}F]FDG-PET/CT provides a reference for subsequent treatment evaluation in cHL. Since the first reports on inferior outcome of patients with [^{18}F]FDG-PET positivity during treatment after two ABVD (doxorubicin, bleomycin, vinblastine, dacarbazine) cycles or escalated BEACOPP (bleomycin, etoposide, doxorubicin, cyclophosphamide, vincristine, prednisone, procarbazine), consensus about standard definition of [^{18}F]FDG-PET positivity in HL has been reported and the five-point Deauville scale is used to define criteria for treatment intensification or reduction (Box 19.1); a Deauville score of three or less is considered as metabolic complete remission (Figure 19.1).

Box 19.1 Semi-quantitative Deauville five-point scale

1 no residual positivity
2 fixation < mediastinum blood pool
3 fixation > mediastinum < liver
4 fixation moderately > liver
5 fixation higher > foie

Adapted with permission from Meignan M., et al. 'Report on the First International Workshop on interim-PET scan in lymphoma'. *Leukemia & Lymphoma*, Volume 50, Issue 8, pp. 1257–1260. Copyright © 2009 Informa UK Limited. DOI: 10.1080/10428190903040048

Treatment

Stratification

Worldwide, treatment groups based on previous trial results and prognostic factors are not identical between adult and paediatric collaborative groups, and a harmonization process is ongoing to specify the definition of bulky disease, E-lesion (organ and parietal involvement), as well as biological criteria of inflammatory HL. Based on previous studies, the Euronet Paediatric Hodgkin Lymphoma Group currently defines localized disease as:

- stage I/IIA—ESR less than 30 and no bulky mass more than 200 ml
- intermediate disease: stage I/IIA—ESR more than or equal to 30 or bulky disease more than or equal to 200 ml; stage IIB—no E-lesion
- advanced disease: stages IIIA, IIIB, and IV—stage IIB with E-lesion

Treatment strategy

With an actuarial survival of over 95% at ten years in children and adolescents with cHL, major efforts are undertaken to provide treatment with a low rate of adverse long-term events such as secondary malignancies (notably breast cancer), fertility impairment, cardiac and pulmonary toxicity, thyroid dysfunction, musculoskeletal abnormalities, and fatigue. These events are largely related to radiation therapy, cumulative doses of alkylating agents and anthracyclines, and steroid treatment.

Led by the EuroNet Paediatric Hodgkin Lymphoma Group, a large study was conducted in Europe, between 2007 and 2013, recruiting 2,111 patients with a median age of 14.8 years. Objectives of the EuroNet PHL-C1 trial (Box 19.2) were to limit the indication for radiotherapy (RT) to patients with an inadequate response defined at

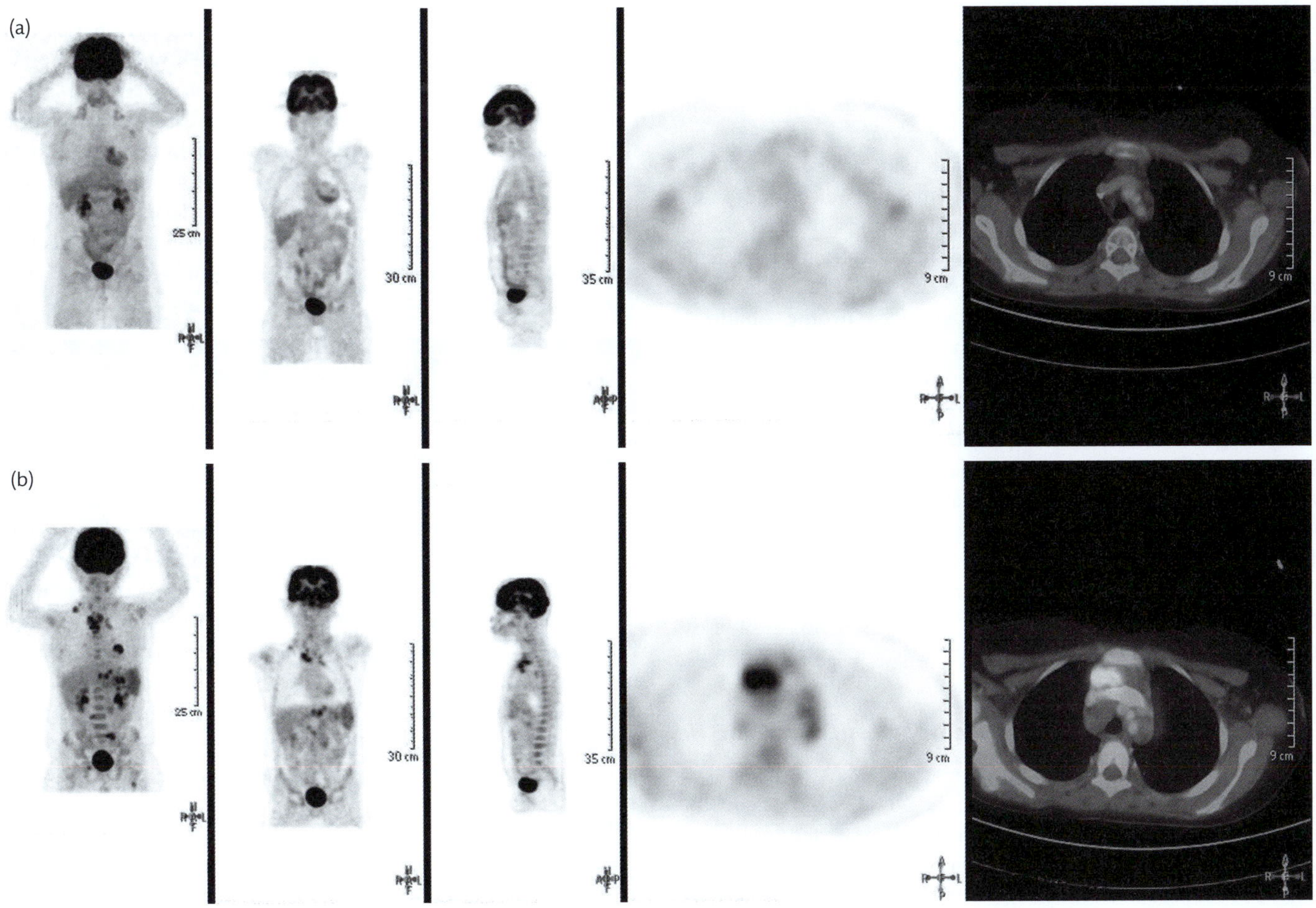

Figure 19.1 cLH stade IV. (a) Diagnostic; (b) Complete metabolic response after 2 OEPA.
Reproduced courtesy of Françoise Montravers, Hôpital Tenon APHP, Paris, France.

Box 19.2 Chemotherapy in classical variant of Hodgkin lymphoma: Euronet paediatric Hodgkin lymphoma C1 trial

Two OEPA cycles every 28 days

- Prednisone: 60 mg/m²; days 1–15
- Vincristine: 1.5 mg/m²; days 1, 8, and 15
- Adriamycine: 40 mg/m²; days 1 and 15
- VP-16: 125 mg/m²; days 1–5

COPDAC cycles every 21 days

- Prednisone: 40 mg/m²; days 1–15
- Dacarbazine: 250 mg/m²; days 1, 2, and 3
- Vincristine: 1.5 mg/m²; days 1 and 8
- Endoxan: 500 mg/m²; days 1 and 8

an intermediate [^{18}F]FDG-PET and CT evaluation after two OEPA (vincristine, etoposide, prednisone, adriamycin) cycles, and to replace procarbazine by dacarbazine in order to limit the impact on fertility. At the latest interim analysis, 48-month overall survival (OS) and event-free survival (EFS) were 98% and 88%, respectively. The EFS in patients with or without RT was 88% and 87%. EFS did not differ between the COPP (vincristine, cyclophosphamide, procarbazine, prednisone) and the COPDAC (vincristine, cyclophosphamide, dacarbazine, prednisone) arm. In this trial, RT could be avoided in about 50% of patients without impairing treatment results, and COPDAC is now considered as standard consolidation. The EuroNet PHL-C2 trial will further focus on reducing RT indication by proposing a moderate increase of chemotherapy in a randomized fashion.

Meanwhile, the current standard of care in Europe is induction treatment by two OEPA cycles in all patients, followed by one to four cycles of COPDAC in localized, intermediate, and advanced disease groups; 20 Gy radiotherapy to involved sites is restricted to patients with inadequate response after two cycles of OEPA. Alternative chemotherapy strategies are being developed by the Children's Oncology Group (COG), mainly with an ABV-PC and DBVE-PC regimen and restricted use of RT in advanced stages, based on response after two or three cycles.

In young adults with cHL, the ABVD regimen followed by 20–30 Gy RT to involved sites is the standard of care in localized disease. In intermediate and advanced stages, ABVD and escalated BEACOPP provide excellent results, but cumulative doses of alkylating agents or anthracyclines, with or without RT, are not considered adaptable to children or adolescents. Nevertheless, studies are ongoing, with response-adapted strategies leading to reduction of cumulative chemotherapy dose and restriction in indications for RT.

Treatment in relapsed and refractory classical variant of Hodgkin lymphoma

Cumulative relapse rates in cHL are around 10–15%. More than 90% arise within three years of diagnosis. In reports restricted to children and adolescents, the only prognostic factor associated with adverse outome in relapsed and refractory (RR) cHL is a time lag of less than 12 months from the end of primary treatment. This has nevertheless to be tempered by initial stage and initial treatment, as well as stage at relapse. Recently, several publications have demonstrated [^{18}F]FDG-PET response before intensification as an independent prognostic factor in RR cHL, leading to subsequent adapted strategies in this context. Commonly used salvage regimens include ifosfamide, carboplatin, and etoposide (ICE), the combination of dexamethasone, high-dose cytarabine, and cisplatin (DHAP), and other gemcitabine-based combination regimens, including gemcitabine, prednisone, ifosfamide, and vinorelbine (IGEV). As many drug regimens are efficient in RR cHL, and in absence of randomized studies, the choice depends on age, first-line treatment, and response. There is consensus for high-dose chemotherapy (BEAM) with haematopoietic stem-cell support in most cases of relapse occurring within one year after first treatment.

Recently, two new drugs have been registered for RR cHL: brentuximab vedotin, an anti-CD30 coupled with monomethyl auristatin-E (MMAE), and nivolumab, an anti-PDL1 monoclonal antibody showing promising results in RR cHL, with complete remission (CR) rates in monotherapy and overall response rates of 15–20% and 60–80%, respectively. Their place in RR strategy, alone or in combination with chemotherapy, is currently being explored in numerous trials, along with other immunotargeted compounds and antibodies.

Clinical management and work-up in nodular lymphocyte predominant Hodgkin lymphoma

NLPHL is a rare form of HL accounting for 5–10% of HL cases. Clinical characteristics of patients with NLPHL are different, with a vast majority of boys, localized disease with peripheral lymph nodes, and rarity of clinical or biological inflammatory symptoms. Histopathology and immunophenotype shows typical CD20-positive 'popcorn' cells. A strategy based on limited treatment associated to monoclonal anti-CD20 antibodies in rare advanced cases, or 'watch and wait' after initial lymph node resection in stage I limited disease, is currently proposed. Long-term follow-up is recommended as subsequent high-grade lymphomas have been described in adult cohorts of patients with previous NLPHL.

Long-term outcome and follow-up after Hodgkin lymphoma during childhood and adolescence

Secondary malignancies

The risk of secondary RT-induced cancers is well documented in cHL and has led to consensus guidelines for follow-up and screening. Breast cancer is the most frequent secondary cancer and needs screening from a median time of 8–13 years after RT for cHL. Other cancers are mainly gastric cancer and lung carcinoma. The cumulative incidence of secondary cancers increases with time and reaches 25–30% at 25-year follow-up. Leukaemia after cHL is reported mainly during the five first years following treatment. Leukaemia has an incidence of less than 1% and is associated with alkylating agents or inhibitors of topoisomerase.

Cardiovascular events

Cardiovascular events are the second major cause of significant long-term morbidity and premature deaths. Information to patients and recommendations about lifestyle, including avoiding smoking and other risk factors of cardiovascular morbidity, is essential. Echocardiography every three years, to detect valvular dysfunction and impaired cardiac function, is recommended a fortiori in cases of mediastinal RT in association with anthracycline treatment. Significant premature coronary disease in young adults after RT on the heart is possible, but there is no consensus for systematic screening yet.

Impaired fertility

Impaired fertility in boys is related to cumulative doses of procarbazine and cyclofosphamide. In adolescents and young adults, sperm cryopreservation has to be proposed before treatment. In girls and young women, fertility damage is mainly linked to premature menopause or pelvic RT. Cryopreservation of oocytes before or after treatment should be discussed, particularly in cases of advanced stage or relapse.

Thyroid dysfunction

Thyroid dysfunction occurs in 5–10% of cases after five years and can be detected by annual thyroid-stimulating hormone (TSH) dosage. Thyroid echography is recommended every three to five years for screening of thyroid carcinoma.

Late effects

Late-effect clinics are currently under development in some American and European countries. Major challenges are to provide accurate patient information and promote adherence to recommendations. Social and psychological distress and fatigue after cancer in childhood and adolescence is better documented, with published results from long-term cohorts of patients treated for HL. Improvements in the care and management of these adverse effects are necessary.

FURTHER READING

Ansell SM, et al. (2015) PD-1 blockade with nivolumab in relapsed or refractory Hodgkin'slymphoma. *N Engl J Med*, **372**, 311–19.

Bhatia S, et al. (2003) High risk of subsequent neoplasms continues with extended follow-up of childhood Hodgkin's lymphoma: report from the Late Effects Study Group. *J Clin Oncol* **21**, 4386–94.

Bhakta N, et al. (2016) Cumulative burden of cardiovascular morbidity in paediatric, adolescent, and young adult survivors of Hodgkin's lymphoma: an analysis from the St Jude Lifetime Cohort Study. *Lancet Oncol* **17**, 1325–34.

Cerhan JR, Slager SL (2015) Familial predisposition and genetic risk factors for lymphoma. *Blood* **126**, 2265–73.

Chen R, et al. (2017) Phase II study of the efficacy and safety of pembrolizumab in relapsed/refractory Hodgkin lymphoma *J Clin Oncol* **35**, 2125–32.

Daw S, et al. (2011) Management of relapsed and refractory classical Hodgkin's lymphoma in children and adolescents. *Br J Haematol* **152**, 249–60.

Friedman DL, et al. (2014) Dose-intensive response-based chemotherapy and radiation therapy for children and adolescents with newly diagnosed intermediate-risk Hodgkin lymphoma: a report from the Children's Oncology Group Study AHOD0031. *J Clin Oncol* **32**, 3651–58.

Furth C, et al. (2009) Early and late therapy response assessment with [18F]fluorodeoxyglucose positron emission tomography in pediatric Hodgkin's lymphoma: analysis of a prospective multicenter trial. *J Clin Oncol* **27**, 4385–91.

Gallamini A, et al. (2014) The predictive role of interim positron emission tomography for Hodgkin lymphoma treatment outcome is confirmed using the interpretation criteria of the Deauville five-point scale. *Haematologica* **99**, 1107–13.

Gorde-Grosjean S, et al. (2012) Outcome of children and adolescents with recurrent/refractory classical Hodgkin lymphoma, a study from the Société Française de Lutte contre le Cancer des Enfants et des Adolescents (SFCE). *Br J Haematol* **158**, 649–56.

Jaffe ES, et al. (2008) *WHO Classification of Tumors: Pathology and Genetics of Tumors of Haematopoietic and Lymphoid Tissues*. Lyon: IARC Press.

Hjalgrim H, et al. (2003) Characteristics of Hodgkin's lymphoma after infectious mononucleosis. *N Engl J Med* **349**, 1324–32.

Kharazmi E, et al. (2015) Risk of familial classical Hodgkin lymphoma by relationship, histology, age, and sex: a joint study from five Nordic countries. *Blood* **126**, 1990–5.

Küppers R (2009) Molecular biology of Hodgkin lymphoma. *Hematology Am Soc Hematol Educ Program* 491–6. doi: 10.1182/asheducation-2009

Küppers R (2012) New insights in the biology of Hodgkin lymphoma. *Hematology Am Soc Hematol Educ Program* 328–34. doi: 10.1182/asheducation-2012.1.328

Lee AI, LaCasce AS (2009) Nodular lymphocyte predominant Hodgkin lymphoma. *Oncologist* **14**, 739–51.

Mauz-Körholz C, et al. (2007) Resection alone in 58 children with limited stage, lymphocyte-predominant Hodgkin lymphoma—experience from the European network group on pediatric Hodgkin lymphoma. *Cancer* **110**, 179–85.

Mauz-Körholz C, et al. (2015) Pediatric Hodgkin lymphoma. *J Clin Oncol* **33**, 2975–85.

Moskowitz CH, et al. (2015) Brentuximab vedotin as consolidation therapy after autologous stem-cell transplantation in patients with Hodgkin's lymphoma at risk of relapse or progression (AETHERA): a randomised, double-blind, placebo-controlled, phase 3 trial. *Lancet* **385**, 1853–62.

Nachman JB, et al. (2002) Children's Cancer Group: randomized comparison of low-dose involved-field radiotherapy and no radiotherapy for children with Hodgkin's disease who achieve a complete response to chemotherapy. *J Clin Oncol* **20**, 3765–71.

Ng AK, Mauch PM (2009) Late effects of Hodgkin's disease and its treatment. *Cancer J* **15**, 164–8.

Pellegrino B, et al. (2003) Lymphocyte-predominant Hodgkin's lymphoma in children: therapeutic abstention after initial lymph node resection—a study of the French Society of Pediatric Oncology. *J Clin Oncol* **21**, 2948–52.

Purz S1, et al. (2011) [18F]fluorodeoxyglucose positron emission tomography for detection of bone marrow involvement in children and adolescents with Hodgkin's lymphoma. *J Clin Oncol* **29**, 3523–8.

Roemer MG, et al. (2016) PD-L1 and PD-L2 genetic alterations define classical Hodgkin lymphoma and predict outcome. *J Clin Oncol* **34**, 2690–7.

Shankar A, et al. (2012) Treatment outcome after low intensity chemotherapy [CVP] in children and adolescents with early stage nodular lymphocyte predominant Hodgkin's lymphoma—an Anglo-French collaborative report (2012). *Eur J Cancer* **48**, 1700–6.

Sklar C, et al. (2000) Abnormalities of the thyroid in survivors of Hodgkin's disease: data from the Childhood Cancer Survivor Study. *J Clin Endocrinol Metab* **85**, 3227–32.

Steliarova-Foucher E, et al. (2017) International incidence of childhood cancer, 2001–10: a population-based registry study. *Lancet Oncol* **18**, 719–31.

Thorley-Lawson DA, Gross A (2004) Persistence of the Epstein–Barr virus and the origins of associated lymphomas. *N Engl J Med* **350**, 1328–37.

Wallace WH, et al. (2005) Fertility preservation for young people with cancer: who is at risk and what can be offered? *Lancet Oncol* **6**, 209–18.

Younes A, et al. (2010) Brentuximab vedotin (SGN-35) for relapsed CD30-positive lymphomas. *N Engl J Med* **363**, 1812–21.

20

Childhood Histiocytoses

Maurizio Aricò, Cor van den Bos, and Sheila Weitzman

Langerhans cell histiocytosis

Langerhans cell histiocytosis (LCH) is a rare clonal inflammatory myeloid neoplasm with a reported incidence in children of between two and eight per million per year. In the recently revised classification of the histiocytoses, it is placed in the L-group, together with Erdheim–Chester disease and indeterminate cell histiocytosis. The diagnosis is based on pathological findings in the correct clinical setting. Lesions are characterized by infiltration by cells originating from the myelomonocytic lineage—the LCH cells. Morphologically, LCH cells are mononuclear, express CD1a and/or CD207 (Langerin), have coffee-bean-shaped or kidney-shaped nuclei, and are often accompanied by abundant eosinophils and multinucleated giant cells. It is a disorder with a striking clinical heterogeneity, ranging from spontaneously healing single-system bone and skin lesions to a life-threatening multisystem disease.

Recently, considerable progress has been made in the understanding of LCH biology. In 2010, the constitutive activation of the RAS–RAF–MEK–ERK pathway in LCH was first described. It was shown that, in approximately half the cases, the *BRAF-V600E* mutation is present. Other mutations in *BRAF* (including small in-frame deletions) and in other pathway genes such as *ARAF, MAP2K*,as well as *FAM73A-BRAF* fusions have subsequently been described. On the basis of further studies in patients and murine models, a model has been postulated whereby somatic mutations in an early myeloid progenitor cell lead to multisystem LCH, while mutations in more differentiated cells lead to localized, single-system LCH.

Clinical manifestations of Langerhans cell histiocytosis

LCH can manifest itself in many tissues and organs. Bone is most frequently affected, being observed in 80–100% of cases in large series, most commonly presenting as painful swellings. The skull, long bones, and then flat bones are most frequently involved. In the spine, typical vertebra plana may be observed. In the case of isolated vertebra plana without a soft-tissue component, the risk of biopsy may outweigh the need for tissue diagnosis, but the patient should be closely followed to exclude malignancy. Clinical features and possible complications of osseous lesions depend on the bone involved.

Skin involvement is observed in over one third of children with LCH. Most frequently affected sites are scalp and nappy areas, but any area may be affected, including the nails. Cutaneous LCH can present with a wide range of clinical manifestations, from reddish papules and nodules to blisters, tumour-like lesions, and scaling or purpuric macules.

Hepatomegaly is common in patients with disseminated disease. Evidence of altered liver function (e.g. hypoalbuminaemia) is less commonly observed. A common complication of liver LCH is the development of sclerosing cholangitis (SC), which may be present at diagnosis. In patients with SC, the progression of liver damage may become independent of LCH activity, and progression to end-stage liver failure can occur. Spleen involvement presents as splenomegaly.

Anaemia, leukocytopenia, and thrombocytopenia are manifestations of 'bone-marrow involvement'. These cytopenias most often occur in the absence of morphological bone-marrow infiltration. Pathological confirmation of LCH in bone marrow is unnecessary if bi- or tri-lineage cytopenia is present that is not explained by another cause. Haemophagocytosis can be observed in severe forms of LCH, reflecting the hyperinflammatory state of the patient.

In children, pulmonary LCH is usually part of multisystem disease, although in adolescents, isolated lung LCH is sometimes observed. Clinically, lung involvement leads to respiratory distress with tachypnoea, retractions, and persistent cough. Rupture of superficial cysts may lead to pneumothorax. As in the liver, progression of lung fibrosis may become independent of LCH activity.

Diabetes insipidus (DI) is the most commonly observed endocrine complication in LCH, involving up to 35% of children with LCH. DI may present as the first manifestation of LCH, or it may occur later, months or even many years after diagnosis. Patients with DI may progress to multiple anterior pituitary hormone deficiencies, the first usually being growth hormone deficiency.

In the central nervous system, LCH can manifest as cerebral mass lesions. In a minority of patients, most often with preceding DI, a progressive neurodegeneration (ND) can develop with ataxia, as well as cranial nerve palsies and neuropsychological defects. Biopsies of LCH ND lesions do not show CD1a positive cells, but more recent biopsies have demonstrated presence of the *BRAF-V600E* mutation suggesting that inhibitor therapy might be effective.

Involvement of the gastrointestinal tract can manifest as intestinal malabsorption, (bloody) diarrhoea, or protein-losing enteropathy. Lymphadenopathy is seen in a minority of patients.

Table 20.1 Clinical classification of Langerhans cell histiocytosis

Main category	Subcategories	Definition
Single-system LCH (SS LCH)	Unifocal bone	One bone involved
	Multifocal bone	More than one bone involved
	Skin	
	Lymph node	
	Central nervous system	
	Isolated lung	
	Other organs	
Multisystem LCH (MS LCH)	MS LCH RO negative (RO–)	Two or more organs/systems involved without liver, spleen, or bone marrow
	MS LCH RO positive (RO+)	Two or more organs/systems involved with liver and/or spleen and/or bone marrow

Source: data from 'LCH-IV, International Collaborative Treatment Protocol for Children and Adolescents with Langerhans Cell Histiocytosis', NIH US Library of Medicine, https://clinicaltrials.gov/show/NCT02205762

Clinical classification and evaluation of Langerhans cell histiocytosis

The diagnosis of LCH is made pathologically, together with the clinical picture. LCH can present as single-system (SS) disease, at one site (unifocal), or at multiple sites (multifocal). In multisystem (MS) LCH, the disease involves multiple tissues or organs. MS LCH is subdivided into 'risk-organ positive (RO+)' and 'risk-organ negative (RO–)'. MS-RO+ LCH is defined by involvement of 'risk' organs—liver, spleen, and haematopoetic system. Involvement of risk organs is associated with the risk of mortality (Table 20.1).

Thorough clinical evaluation at diagnosis is obligatory to determine disease extent and treatment. For bony lesions, plain radiography remains the first-line approach for detection. In the current LCH-IV protocol of the Histiocyte Society, only the bone lesions detected by plain radiography are considered for stratification. Lesions detected by alternative imaging, like Tc-bone scan or fluorodeoxyglucose-positron emission tomography/computed tomography (FDG-PET/CT), will be documented but, according to the LCH-IV protocol 'are not considered for stratification unless proven by plain radiography or MRI or pathology'. Total-body magnetic resonance imaging (MRI), as well as FDG-PET/CT, have been shown to detect lesions not otherwise visualized, but their clinical relevance is unproven. Nonetheless, some studies have upstaged patients based on these results. Results of the LCH-IV study might allow insight into the clinical relevance of these total-body imaging techniques. Only a well-designed prospective study, however, will yield definitive results. An MRI of the spine is indicated in the case of vertebra plana to exclude spinal cord compression from an associated soft-tissue mass.

Abdominal ultrasound and physical examination are used to detect hepatosplenomegaly. Liver function is evaluated by standard laboratory tests, including albumin levels and coagulation parameters. A chest X-ray is routine at diagnosis. In case of suspected pulmonary involvement, a CT scan of the lungs is mandatory. If age appropriate, lung function studies should be performed.

Table 20.2 Response evaluation in paediatric Langerhans cell histiocytosis

Main category	Subcategories	Definition
Non-active disease (NAD)		Resolution of all signs/symptoms (no evidence of disease)
Active disease (AD) Better	Regressive disease	Regression of signs/symptoms, no new lesions
Active disease (AD) Stable	Stable disease	Persistence of signs or symptoms, no new lesions

Source: data from 'LCH-IV, International Collaborative Treatment Protocol for Children and Adolescents with Langerhans Cell Histiocytosis', NIH US Library of Medicine, https://clinicaltrials.gov/show/NCT02205762

DI is confirmed by a water deprivation test and imaging of the pituitary stalk. MRI may show absence of the posterior bright spot on T2-weighted imaging and thickening of the pituitary stalk.

Evaluation of the efficacy of treatment is not always easy. Criteria have been developed by the Histiocyte Society (Table 20.2), but the determination of disease activity in the most common lesions (i.e. bone lesions) can be especially problematic. For patients with MS LCH, a disease activity score has been developed that includes both clinical and laboratory parameters such as albumin levels. The recent studies reporting measures of levels of circulating mutated DNA (circulating tumour DNA; ctDNA) need further confirmation to allow determination of clinical relevance.

Progression of skeletal lesions is defined as unequivocal enlargement of the size of existing lesions and/or appearance of new lesions

Treatment of paediatric Langerhans cell histiocytosis

Treatment of paediatric LCH should be directed by the extent and quality of disease involvement. While for patients with involvement of vital organs (liver, spleen, haematopoietic system)—which bears a risk of mortality—systemic therapy is warranted, for single-bone lesions and isolated skin LCH, a 'wait and see' policy is often sufficient.

Single-system skin Langerhans cell histiocytosis

The only indication for therapy in skin-only LCH is bleeding, ulceration, or pain. However, skin-only LCH in very young infants can progress within weeks to months to high-risk MS LCH, and these infants should be closely watched. For patients who deserve therapy for skin LCH, numerous approaches have been published: topical corticosteroids, nitrogen mustard, or tacrolimus; narrow band UVB or PUVA. If systemic therapy is required, low-dose methotrexate, alone or with the addition of 6 mercaptopurine, can be tried first before going onto the more standard chemotherapy approaches described below. Oral etoposide or azathioprine, which have been shown to be useful therapy in adults, are rarely used in paediatrics.

Single-system bone Langerhans cell histiocytosis

For unifocal disease, curettage alone allows for pathological diagnosis and is often followed by spontaneous healing. If necessary, intralesional methylprednisolone can be safely used but, to date, no study has ever shown a clear superiority of intralesional steroids over observation only. The exception to observation alone for unifocal bone disease includes a vertebral body lesion with a soft-tissue mass, with risk to the spinal cord. Craniofacial bone lesions have been reported to be associated with increased risk of developing DI and LCH-associated ND ('CNS-risk lesions'), thus deserving systemic chemotherapy. However, this 'CNS-risk lesion' is still a matter of debate. Multifocal bone disease is usually an indication for systemic treatment.

Multisystem Langerhans cell histiocytosis

Multisystem LCH is always treated systemically. The backbones most broadly used are either vinblastine–prednisone (the mainstay of the four consecutive LCH I–IV trials), or the combination of vincristine–cytarabine–prednisone. Recently, single-agent cytarabine has been suggested but remains to be proven, particularly in high-risk young infants. Over the years, clinical studies performed by different study groups have led to the following conclusions:

- In patients with MS-RO+ LCH, early response is an important predictor of survival, necessitating a timely switch to intensified therapy in non-responders.
- In partial responders or non-responders without risk organ, a second induction treatment has been shown to increase the NAD rate.
- Prolongation of treatment to 12 months decreases the reactivation rate in high- and low-risk MS LCH patients from 50% to around 30%.

To date, none of the treatment backbones has been shown to be clearly superior, and the optimal treatment duration for both multifocal bone LCH and MS LCH is still being studied (e.g. in the current Histiocyte Society LCH-IV protocol, 12-month versus 24-month duration). There is also an ongoing need for better understanding of the disease, since it is impossible to distinguish, at diagnosis or early in treatment, the MS LCH patients who will benefit from long maintenance from those for whom treatment prolongation is unnecessary.

For non-responding MS-RO+ LCH patients, the combination of high-dose cytarabine and cladribine has been shown to be an effective but toxic salvage therapy, as has allogeneic stem-cell transplantation. More recently, inhibitors to mutated *BRAF* have been shown to lead to a quick response in those patients, but after cessation of short-term treatment, reactivation of the disease has been observed. Based on the present knowledge, the use of targeted therapy with inhibitors appears very useful to speed up initial disease control, but the combination with standard LCH-directed chemotherapy appears still warranted. Future cooperative studies addressing the combination of inhibitors (such as *BRAF* and *MEK* inhibitors) and the use of limited chemotherapy appear justified.

Permanent consequences of Langerhans cell histiocytosis

There is a long list of potential permanent consequences of LCH, but the commonest and most important relate to the endocrine system and the CNS.

The commonest late effect, DI, can be managed with oral or intranasal desmopressin. Other hormonal deficiencies such as growth-hormone deficiency or secondary hypothyroidism require substitution therapy.

Management of ND remains a major problem and represent a really unmet need for patients with LCH. On MRI, the characteristic pattern of usually bilateral and symmetrical demyelination starting from the cerebellum is seen. Not all patients with MRI signs of ND will develop clinical ND, and neurophysiological tests such as basal evoked potentials, as well as cerebrospinal fluid (CSF) cytokine patterns or continued *BRAF* mutation positivity in blood, are being studied for their ability to identify patients in need of treatment. A major obstacle is the absence of a clearly effective therapy. Intravenous immunoglobulin (IVIG), cytarabine, and retinoic acid have been used. The efficacy of those treatments appears to depend on early diagnosis and therapy, which generally results in prevention of progression at best. Based on the finding of positive immunostaining for the *BRAF-V600E* mutation in ND LCH lesions, targeted therapy has been given to a limited number of patients. Results of these early-phase studies and the development of specific trials are eagerly awaited. The neuropsychological consequences of ND LCH may be severe.

Haemophagocytic lymphohistiocytosis

Haemophagocytic lymphohistiocytosis (HLH) is a disorder characterized by a hyperinflammatory syndrome with fever, hepatosplenomegaly, cytopenia, liver dysfunction, and sometimes CNS involvement, which may lead to multi-organ failure and death. The disease may be inherited (so-called 'primary') or apparently sporadic, and in these cases is usually triggered by malignancies, rheumatological disorders, or infections (so-called 'secondary'). The familial form of the disease (FHL) is genetically heterogeneous, involving genes important to the normal function of cytotoxic T cells and natural killer (NK) cells. The recent discovery of sporadic HLH patients with monoallelic mutations or polymorphisms in typical FHL-associated genes, as well as non-cytotoxicity-related genes, has led to the blurring of the distinction between "primary" and "secondary" HLH. Nonetheless, it remains true that patients with familial disease (FHL) have an earlier onset, a more aggressive clinical course, and need allogeneic transplantation for cure. Otherwise, patients who lack biallelic mutations in FHL-related genes usually have a later onset, a less aggressive clinical course, and do not require haematopoietic stem-cell transplantation for cure.

The disease manifestations are due to excessive inflammatory response caused by hypersecretion of pro-inflammatory cytokines such as interferon-γ, tumour necrosis factor-α, interleukin(IL)-6, and macrophage-colony-stimulating factor (M-CSF). These mediators are secreted by activated T lymphocytes and macrophages that infiltrate all tissues, and lead to tissue necrosis and organ failure.

Differential diagnosis of HLH may be difficult and diagnostic guidelines for HLH have been established by the Histiocyte Society (**Box 20.1**).

There are ongoing efforts among specialists to replace these criteria with others more specific for the diagnosis. The clinical relevance of items such as hypertriglyceridaemia, hypofibrinogenaemia, haemophagocytosis, and NK activity testing is questionable, and for different reasons, including low sensitivity or limited access. Bone-marrow haemophagocytosis, for example, is neither specific nor sensitive for HLH and, contrary to common belief, is not by itself a useful criterion.

The combination of fever, splenomegaly, thrombocytopenia, and hyperferritinaemia (and/or high levels of sCD25) may positively identify the population deserving an immediate genetic and immunological work-up such as the granule release assay (see below). This is only useful in centres where these tests are readily available, however.

Additional laboratory tests that are not 'diagnostic criteria' but that may help in diagnosis and in evaluation of therapeutic response, include measurement of transaminases and bilirubin,

Box 20.1 Clinical and laboratory criteria for haemophagocytic lymphohistiocytosis*

- Fever
- Splenomegaly
- Cytopenia affecting at least two of three lineages in the peripheral blood:
  - Haemoglobin <9 g/dl (below 4 weeks <12 g/dl)
  - Neutrophils <1 × 10^3/mm^3
  - Platelets <100 × 10^3/mm^3
- Hypertriglyceridaemia (fasting, ≥265 mg/dl) and/or hypofibrinogenaemia (<150 mg/dl)
- Ferritin ≥500 μg/l
- Soluble CD25 (that is, soluble IL-2 receptor) ≥2400 U/ml
- Decreased or absent NK-cell activity

In patients with familial disease or known genetic defect (i.e. biallelic pathogenic mutations in genes related to the autosomal recessive form of the disease or single mutations in males with the X-linked forms of disease), the diagnosis can be established even with incomplete criteria.

* Five of the criteria are considered diagnostic

Adapted with permission from Henter JI et al. 'HLH-2004: Diagnostic and Therapeutic Guidelines for Hemophagocytic Lymphohistiocytosis'. *Pediatric Blood and Cancer*, Volume 48, Issue 2, pp. 124–131. Copyright © 2006, John Wiley and Sons. DOI: https://doi.org/10.1002/pbc.21039

lactate dehydrogenase (LDH), and D-dimers (even when INR, PTT, and fibrinogen are normal), and CSF pleocytosis. Hyponatraemia and hypoalbuminaemia may also be present. The utility of requiring multiple clinical and laboratory abnormalities, none of which are specific for diagnosis, is that they reflect the uncontrolled hyper-immune status which is damaging the body—a criterion which has been called 'immunopathology' by some investigators.

Pathogenesis of haemophagocytic lymphohistiocytosis

The pathogenic mechanisms of FHL are based on insufficient control of target antigens by cellular cytotoxicity. As a result, excessive cytokine production induces lymphocyte overstimulation. In this vicious loop, the patient is unable to get rid of the target, often a common viral pathogen such as Epstein–Barr virus (EBV) or cytomegalovirus (CMV). Failure to terminate the immune response (defect in immune homeostasis) is also believed to be important.

Within the cytoplasm of NK cells and cytotoxic lymphocytes (CTLs) are cytolytic granules containing perforin and granzyme. Upon contact between the effector killer cells and their target, an immunological synapse is formed and cytolytic granules traffic to the contact site, dock, and fuse with the plasma membrane and release their contents into the synapse. Perforin, a pore-forming protein, produces a channel in the target-cell membrane allowing entry of granzymes, activation of caspases, and apoptosis of target cells. Most known defects in FHL seem to be involved in this process, although there remains a very small minority of patients with unassigned defects. An increasing number of other congenital immunodeficiencies, such as X-linked SCID and X-line hypogammaglobulinaemia, have been described as being associated with HLH.

Genetic forms of haemophagocytic lymphohistiocytosis

The identification of the causative gene(s) of FHL has been a long process. In 1999, the first defect in the perforin gene (*PRF1*) was described (FHL2). Patients with FHL2 have different ethnic origins, with cases documented from all continents. Age at disease onset is usually very young, median three months, but with a wide range reaching the third decade. Mutations of *UNC13D* have been associated with FHL3. It encodes the Munc13–4 protein, which results in defective cellular cytotoxicity and a clinical picture very similar to FHL2. Genotype/phenotype correlations do not identify ethnic-specific mutations; CNS involvement is more frequent and age at diagnosis is significantly higher than FHL2. FHL4 is due to deficiency of syntaxin 11, a protein that contributes to cytotoxic cell degranulation; most patients are of Turkish/Kurdish descent. FHL5 is due to mutations in the *Munc18–2* gene encoding syntaxin-binding protein-2.

A few additional genetic conditions may have a clinical picture overlapping HLH. Chédiak–Higashi syndrome (CHS), Griscelli syndrome type II (GSII), and X-linked lymphoproliferative syndrome (XLP) types 1 and 2 are immune deficiencies with distinctive clinical features in which the development of HLH is sporadic, though frequent. HLH is often the presenting symptom, but may also occur later in the disease. Patients with CHS and GSII show partial albinism as melanin granules move by the pathway described earlier. XLP1 is mainly characterized by a defect of specific effective immune responses to EBV. Following exposure to EBV, these subjects are prone to develop HLH; if they survive, they may develop lymphoma or dysgammaglobulinaemia. Similarly, patients with XLP2 may develop HLH as part of their clinically heterogenous phenotype.

Prompt identification of FHL in the absence of a positive family history is an ongoing challenge, even in young children. The approach to this problem has changed over the years. Initially, the diagnosis was based on the identification of HLH in very young patients with recurrence of disease after cessation of therapy and/or a positive family history. Identification of the genetic defects has allowed investigation of novel tools for rapid screening of FHL. For example, perforin protein can be measured by flow cytometry, providing a reliable and rapid identification of FHL-2 patients. Other proteins measurable by flow cytometry include UNCD (*MUNC13.4*) and SAP (XLP1). In addition, flow cytometry has been shown to be a useful screening tool for absence of degranulation of the PRF/granzyme-containing granules. CD107a (LAMP-1) lines the cytotoxic granule to protect the host cell from damage by granule content and is expressed on the surface of the NK/T cell after granule exocytosis. Lack of surface CD107a expression represents a rapid tool for identification of patients with FHL and degranulation defects, in contrast to healthy control subjects or perforin-deficient NK cells where degranulation is normal but perforin is absent. Thus, this assay rapidly became the standard for identification of patients with degranulation defects who need formal genetic sequencing studies.

New methodologies, such as next-generation sequencing (NGS), are now available for genetic testing, allowing all HLH-associated genes to be evaluated at significantly lower cost.

The aforementioned tools are extremely useful in the diagnostic approach to a child with HLH, allowing discrimination of those patients with a genetic defect who require aggressive therapy followed by haematopoietic stem-cell transplantation (HSCT), from those in whom HLH may develop as a temporary complication of another underlying condition, who nonetheless require anti-HLH therapy but who do not generally require HSCT.

Therapy of haemophagocytic lymphohistiocytosis

In most cases, the natural course of FHL is rapidly fatal within a few weeks, unless appropriate treatment, including corticosteroids, etoposide, or anti-thymocyte globuline can obtain transient disease control. Therapy duration for good responders is usually around eight weeks.

In FHL, disease reactivation is inevitable, leading to a rapidly fatal outcome unless the immune system cells with a defective gene are replaced by allogeneic HSCT. The very high transplant-related mortality associated with HSCT, for both LCH and HLH, has led to current trials of reduced-intensity conditioning for these diseases.

For patients with reactivated FHL as well as patients with insufficient response to standard front-line therapy, recent introduction of a novel anti-gamma interferon agent (emapalumab) may represent a novel therapeutic opportunity, which deserves prospective randomized evaluation versus standard therapeutic approach.

Gene replacement therapy, although very appealing as in other monogenic diseases, and shown to be effective in mouse models, is unlikely to be a reality soon for most patients, although human trials are starting in several countries.

Macrophage activation syndrome

The term 'macrophage activation syndrome' (MAS) has been used to describe patients with rheumatological diseases, most commonly sJIA, who develop a clinical syndrome similar to HLH. Many patients with sJIA-associated MAS have been shown to have monoallelic defects in the FHL genes. Different and less stringent diagnostic criteria have been established for sJIA MAS, and the patients tend to respond to less aggressive therapy such as corticosteroids and IVIG. Anti-cytokine therapy, such as the inhibition of the IL1 receptor by anakinra and others, is being investigated in these patients.

Malignancy-associated haemophagocytic lymphohistiocytosis

HLH can be triggered by malignancy, seen most often in mature T-cell malignancies including anaplastic large-cell lymphoma, but also described in B-cell disease including Hodgkin lymphoma and diffuse large B-cell lymphoma. Therapy consists of treatment of the underlying malignancy, but specific HLH therapy may also be required. HLH in cancer patients may also occur later, in patients in remission, and is thought to be due to infection and chemotherapy-induced immunosuppression. Treatment of this latter form includes therapy of the underlying infection and possibly delay in chemotherapy until recovery, but corticosteroid and/or etoposide therapy may be required to control the HLH until regular chemotherapy can be restarted.

Uncommon histiocytic disorders

Uncommon histiocytic (UCH) disorders are a diverse group of disorders that do not meet diagnostic criteria for LCH or HLH. The commonest UCH disorders in childhood are juvenile xanthogranuloma (JXG) and sinus histiocytosis with massive lymphadenopathy (Rosai–Dorfman disease).

The juvenile xanthogranuloma family

The JXG family comprises a number of the UCH disorders with an identical immunophenotype, with lesional cells positive for vimentin, factor XIIIa, CD68, CD163, fascin, CD68, and CD14, and negative for CD1a, S100, and langerin. Pathologically, they show well-circumscribed nodules with a dense infiltrate of histiocytes. Touton giant cells, seen in 85% of cases of JXG, but not limited to JXG, are characterized by a wreath of nuclei around a homogenous eosinophilic cytoplasmic centre, while the periphery shows prominent xanthomatization. Mutations in *BRAF* have been shown in a minority of JXG patients.

The commonest members of the JXG family in childhood are benign cephalic histiocytosis (BCH) and JXG. BCH presents with multiple cutaneous lesions confined to the head and neck area in a young child. These lesions either spontaneously disappear or progress to JXG clinically or pathologically. No therapy is necessary. Cutaneous JXG is a benign proliferative disorder that usually resolves spontaneously within one to five years but may leave residual scarring. Long-term sequelae of JXG are rarely reported. Diagnosis is made on biopsy and immunohistochemistry. Extensive work-up should be reserved for those with clinical suspicion of systemic involvement.

Median age of onset of JXG is two years, but lesions may be present at birth. Most JXG presents with solitary lesions which vary in size. Infants less than six months old tend to present with multiple lesions, with a predisposition for the head and neck. The male preponderance is much higher (12:1) in young infants with multiple skin lesions. JXG is associated with other diseases including the triad of JXG, neurofibromatosis type 1 (NF1), and juvenile myelomonocytic leukaemia (JMML).

Extracutaneous involvement (systemic JXG) occurs in around 4% of children and 30% overall, with half of the patients having no skin involvement. Median age at presentation is 0.3 years. The commonest extracutaneous site is a solitary mass in the subcutis and/or deeper soft tissues, followed by the liver, spleen, CNS, and lungs. Like cutaneous JXG, most systemic lesions undergo spontaneous involution, but ocular and CNS involvement may cause significant problems and fatality. CNS involvement may result in seizures, ataxia, increased intracranial pressure, subdural effusions, developmental delay, DI, and other neurological deficits. In one series, two out of thirty-six children died of progressive CNS disease, while in another, two neonates died of hepatic failure.

Ocular JXG occurs in the very young child (92% are less than two years of age), and may be without skin involvement. When skin lesions coexist, they are always multiple. Eye involvement is usually unilateral and commonly presents with an asymptomatic iris tumour, a red eye with signs of uveitis, unilateral glaucoma, spontaneous hyphaema, or heterochromia iridis. Less commonly, other areas of the eye may be involved. Early diagnosis and treatment determine the final visual outcome. Ophthalmological surveillance is recommended for high-risk patients less than two years of age, who should undergo screening every three to six months until the age of three.

Therapy

The management of JXG depends upon the site(s) of involvement. Patients with JXG isolated to skin should be treated only for pain or ulceration, and not for cosmetic appearance. Single and accessible lesions may be amenable to surgical excision. For systemic JXG, there is currently no established standard chemotherapeutic regimen. A variety of regimens have been tried with variable results. LCH-like therapy, with corticosteroids alone or with vinblastine or vincristine, appear to have the highest response rate, but chemotherapy response is less predictable than in LCH. Patients responding to cladribine and cytosine arabinoside, alone and in combination, have been reported, and clofarabine has been reported to have activity in a small number of heavily pretreated, refractory patients. Other published therapies include methotrexate, etoposide, cyclosporine, interferon, and radiation therapy. A trial of different agents may be needed in individual patients.

For ocular JXG, therapy includes topical, intralesional, and subconjunctival corticosteroids; surgery may be required to treat complications such as hyphaema and glaucoma; and systemic corticosteroids, chemotherapy, or low-dose 'non-cataractogenic' radiation therapy (300–400 cGy) may be required for non-responders. CNS involvement has been successfully treated with cladribine, but the disease does not always respond. Thalidomide has been tried successfully in a few cases.

As in LCH, when *BRAF* mutations are found in JXG, inhibitor therapy may be a useful therapy option.

Rosai-Dorfman disease

Sinus histiocytosis with massive lymphadenopathy (SHML), or Rosai-Dorfman disease (RDD), is a non-neoplastic, polyclonal, usually self-limited disease due to accumulation of S100+, CD1a−, CD68++, CD163++ histiocytes. Pathologically, lymph nodes show massive sinus infiltration of large histiocytes admixed with lymphocytes and plasma cells. Intact erythrocytes, lymphocytes, and plasma cells may be engulfed by histiocytes—a process known as emperipolesis. Emperipolesis in histiocytes expressing S100 in the appropriate clinico-pathological setting is considered diagnostic of SHML. The mean age of onset is 20.6 years, with a wide age distribution. A familial form of RDD with mutations in *SLC29A3* has recently been described. The aetiology of SHML is unknown. An increased incidence of autoimmune disorders, such as autoimmune haemolytic anaemia, and various rheumatological disorders have been reported. Evaluation of pathology specimens for *BRAF-V600E* mutations in SHML have shown no mutations except in a few adult patients presenting with simultaneous SHML and Erdheim–Chester disease.

Clinical presentation

The commonest presentation is with bilateral painless cervical adenopathy associated with fever, night sweats, malaise, weight loss, and polyclonal hypergammaglobulinaemia. Other nodal groups may be involved, and involvement of extranodal tissue such as skin, soft tissue, upper respiratory tract, bone, eye, retro-orbital tissue, and other sites occurs in 43% of cases as the sole initial manifestation or with lymphadenopathy. Involvement of the CNS, seen in 4% (8 out of 200) of RDD cases in an early series, poses a significant diagnostic and therapeutic challenge, usually occurring without extracranial lymphadenopathy and clinically and radiologically resembling meningioma due to the propensity of all of the intracranial UCH disorders to be dural-based. Patients presenting with isolated intracranial disease tend to be older (mean age 37.5 years). Pulmonary RDD is uncommon but carries a significantly worse prognosis. While skin involvement occurs commonly, disease limited to skin is uncommon.

The clinical course of SHML is unpredictable, with episodes of exacerbation and remission which may extend over many years. The outcome is usually good and disease is often self-limiting; nonetheless, about 5% of patients die from disease.

Therapy

Patients with RDD isolated to nodes should be observed without therapy. Surgery may be indicated when localized nodal obstruction of a vital organ is present. First-line systemic therapy, utilized for patients with vital organ compression or dysfunction, is usually corticosteroids, which are often effective, but off-therapy relapses are common. Chemotherapy, including vinblastine (alone or in combination with corticosteroids), cytosine arabinoside, methotrexate, and other agents, produces variable to poor responses. Cladribine, alone and in combination, has been successful in some patients, as has clofarabine. Imatinib, targeting platelet-derived growth factor receptor and KIT-positive tumours, has resulted in good responses in some patients but not others. Rituximab therapy induced remission in a child with long-standing refractory disease. Other innovative therapies (including interferon-alfa, thalidomide, and retinoids) have been reported, and therapies that target cytokines such as TNF-alfa and IL6 have been used successfully in some patients. Recurrence of SHML after cessation of therapy (including after rituximab, interferon, and thalidomide) may occur, but retreatment with the same agents may induce a second response.

Treatment options for CNS and orbital RDD include surgery for diagnosis, relief of compression or excision if possible, stereotactic fractionated radiotherapy or radiosurgery, or chemotherapy (as outlined earlier). As with JXG, different therapies may have to be tried with an individual patient until a response is obtained.

FURTHER READING

Abla O, Janka G (eds) (2018) *Histiocytic Disorders*. Switzerland: Springer International Publishing.

Abla O, Weitzman S (2015) Treatment of Langerhans cell histiocytosis: role of BRAF/MAPK inhibition. *Hematology Am Soc Hematol Educ Program* 565–70. doi: 10.1182/asheducation-2015.1.565

Allen CE, et al. (2015) How I treat Langerhans cell histiocytosis. *Blood* **126**, 26–35.

Aricò M, et al. (2001) Pathogenesis of haemophagocytic lymphohistiocytosis. *Br J Haematol* **114**, 761–9.

Aricò M (2016) Langerhans cell histiocytosis in children: from the bench to bedside for an updated therapy. *Br J Haematol* **173**, 663–70.

Badalian-Very G, et al. (2013) Pathogenesis of Langerhans cell histiocytosis. *Ann Rev Pathol* **8**, 1–20.

Berres ML, et al. (2014) BRAF-V600E expression in precursor versus differentiated dendritic cells defines clinically distinct LCH risk groups. *J Exp Med* **211**, 669–83.

Brisse E, et al. (2016) Advances in the pathogenesis of primary and secondary hemophagocytic lymphohistiocytosis: differences and similarities. *Br J Haematol* **174**, 203–17.

Brown NA, et al. (2014) High prevalence of somatic MAP2K1 mutations in BRAF V600E-negative Langerhans cell histiocytosis. *Blood* **124**, 1655–8.

Bryceson YT, et al. (2012) A prospective evaluation of degranulation assays in the rapid diagnosis of familial hemophagocytic syndromes. *Blood* **119**, 2754–63.

Cetica V, et al. (2016) Genetic predisposition to hemophagocytic lymphohistiocytosis: report on 500 patients from the Italian registry. *J Allergy Clin Immunol* **137**, 188–96.

Delprat C, Aricò M (2014) Blood spotlight on Langerhans cell histiocytosis. *Blood* **124**, 867–72.

Donadieu J, et al. (2015) Cladribine and cytarabine in refractory multisystem Langerhans cell histiocytosis: results of an international phase 2 study. *Blood* **126**, 1415–23.

Donadieu J, et al. (2019) Vemurafenib for refractory multisystem Langerhans Cell Histiocytosis in children: An international observational study. *J Clin Oncol* **37**, 2857–65.

Eckstein OS, et al. (2019) Clinical responses and persistent BRAF V600E+ blood cells in children with LCH treated with MAPK pathway inhibition. *Blood* **133**, 1691–94.

Gadner H, et al. (2013) Therapy prolongation improves outcome in multisystem Langerhans cell histiocytosis. *Blood* **121**, 5006–14.

Hackmann Y, et al. (2013) Syntaxin binding mechanism and disease-causing mutations in Munc18-2. *Proc Natl Acad Sci USA* **110**, E4482–91.

Haroche J, et al. (2012) High prevalence of BRAF V600E mutations in Erdheim–Chester disease but not in other non-Langerhans cell histiocytoses. *Blood* **120**(13), 2700–3.

Haroche J, et al. (2015) Reproducible and sustained efficacy of targeted therapy with vemurafenib in patients with BRAFV600E-mutated Erdheim–Chester disease. *J Clin Oncol* **33**, 411–18.

Haroche J, et al. (2017) Histiocytoses: emerging neoplasia behind inflammation. *Lancet Oncol* **18**, e113–25.

Henter JI, et al. (2007) HLH-2004: diagnostic and therapeutic guidelines for hemophagocytic lymphohistiocytosis. *Pediatr Blood Cancer* **48**, 124–1.

Hutter C, Minkov M. (2016) Insight into the pathogenesis of Langerhans cell histiocytosis: the development of targeted therapies. *Immunotargets Ther* **5**, 81–91.

Jordan MA, et al. (2011) How I treat hemophagocytic lymphohistiocytosis. *Blood* **118**, 4041–52.

Lehmberg K, et al. (2015) Malignancy-associated haemophagocytic lymphohistiocytosis in children and adolescents. *Br J Haematol* **170**, 539–49.

Maghnie M, et al. (2000) Central diabetes insipidus in children and young adults. *N Engl J Med* **343**, 998–1007.

Marcenaro S, et al. (2006) Analysis of natural killer-cell function in familial hemophagocytic lymphohistiocytosis (FHL): defective CD107a surface expression heralds Munc13-4 defect and discriminates between genetic subtypes of the disease. Blood 108, 2316–23.

Meazza R, et al. (2016) Diagnosing XLP1 in patients with hemophagocytic lymphohistiocytosis. *J Allergy Clin Immunol* **134**, 1381–7.

Picarsic J, et al. (2019) BRAF V600E mutation in Juvenile Xanthogranuloma family neoplasms of the central nervous system (CNS-JXG): a revised diagnostic algorithm to include pediatric Erdheim-Chester disease. *Acta Neuropathol Commun* **7**(1), 168. doi:10.1186/s40478-019-0811-6.

Ravelli A, et al. (2016) Classification criteria for macrophage activation syndrome complicating systemic juvenile idiopathic arthritis: a European League Against Rheumatism/American College of Rheumatology/Paediatric Rheumatology International Trials Organisation Collaborative Initiative. *Ann Rheum Dis* **75**(3), 481–9.

Rollins BJ (2015) Genomic alterations in Langerhans cell histiocytosis. *Hematol Oncol Clin North Am* **29**, 839–51.

Sieni E, et al. (2015) Early diagnosis and monitoring of neurodegenerative Langerhans cell histiocytosis. *PLoS One* **10**(7), e0131635.

Sieni E, et al. (2014) Familial hemophagocytic lymphohistiocytosis: when rare diseases shed light on immune system functioning. *Front Immunol* **5**, 167.

Simko SJ, et al. (2014) Clofarabine salvage therapy in refractory multifocal histiocytic disorders, including Langerhans cell histiocytosis, juvenile xanthogranuloma and Rosai-Dorfman disease. *Pediatr Blood Cancer* **61**, 479–8.

Tran TH, et al. Cutaneous histiocytoses. In: C. Griffiths, et al. (eds) *Rooks Textbook of Dermatology* (9th edn), Chapter 136. Oxford: Wiley-Blackwell.

Trottestam H, et al. (2011) Chemoimmunotherapy for hemophagocytic lymphohistiocytosis: long-term results of the HLH-94 treatment protocol. *Blood* **118**(17), 4577–84.

Veys PA, et al. (2015) Haematopoietic stem cell transplantation for refractory Langerhans cell histiocytosis: outcome by intensity of conditioning. *Br J Haematol* **169**(5), 711–18.

21

Symptoms and Emergencies in Children with Brain and Spinal Tumours

Michel Zerah, David Walker, and Shaarna Whitton

Introduction

Childhood central nervous system (CNS) tumours are the most common solid tumour in childhood, accounting for a quarter of all childhood cancers. Despite being the commonest cancer cause of death, the time from symptom onset to diagnosis, known as the total diagnostic interval (TDI), is one of the longest for all childhood cancers. The international median TDI for brain tumours is reported as 8.5 weeks (range) and 5.6 months (range) for spinal tumours. Five-year survival rates for brain tumours have improved to over 80% across Europe; however, two-thirds of survivors are left with a life-changing disability.

As oncologists, we receive children who have been given a new diagnosis of a brain or spinal cord tumour. The start of symptoms indicates the start of brain/spinal injury and accelerating diagnosis is increasingly recognized as a crucial step in order to reduce long-term brain injury for all. Childhood CNS tumours pose a particular diagnostic challenge for all clinicians, but especially for family and hospital clinicians who meet these children at the start of their journey to diagnosis; the signs and symptoms that precede diagnosis are non-specific, fluctuate in severity, and can mimic other common illnesses. The aim of highlighting this issue is to understand these difficulties and raise awareness amongst colleagues to seek ways to accelerate diagnosis so as to minimize neurological injury.

Delays in diagnosis

Along this pathway of initial symptom onset to diagnosis, symptom progression linked to tumour growth inevitably occurs. In the early stages, due to the rarity of the disease, conventional approaches in primary care, using positive predictive values of red-flag symptoms, are recognized as insufficiently sensitive. In the later stages, the accumulation of signs and symptoms becomes increasingly helpful in localizing the problem within the nervous system, at which point the neurological outcome is poorer. A prolonged TDI in childhood brain tumours is associated with an increased risk of life-threatening neurological complications at presentation and a worse cognitive outcome in survivors. It has also been associated with a reduced likelihood of achieving complete tumour resection, which is an important prognostic indicator in some tumour types.

The reasons for prolonged TDIs are multi-factorial. Firstly, the rarity of brain tumours means health professionals do not routinely consider this as a diagnosis when presented with non-specific symptoms. The presenting symptoms of brain tumours include headache, vomiting, and lethargy, which are commonly misdiagnosed as gastroenteritis, migraine, or behavioural problems. Furthermore, the majority of children who present with a brain tumour have a completely normal neurological examination, contrary to the beliefs of many health professionals. Reluctance to consider brain imaging in children also contributes to the delay; it is an alarming investigation for the child and family, often requires general anaesthesia or sedation, and is mistakenly considered costly. All too frequently, the diagnosis is suggested by the parents who have noticed an abnormal behaviour or insidious onset of symptoms and have asked, for many weeks, for access to imaging for their child.

A very specific situation is represented by the antenatal diagnosis of a brain tumour. The diagnosis is made predominantly during the third trimester due to observation of macrocrania, disorganization of the brain, and hydramnios. In most of the cases, they are very malignant tumours, that lead to a termination of pregnancy or to a prenatal or neonatal death. Occasionally, prenatally diagnosed choroid plexus papillomas or craniopharyngiomas can be treated postnatally with good results.

In order to diagnose brain tumours effectively, we need to have knowledge of the risk of the disease in children and young people, and be aware of the signs and symptoms of brain tumours at all ages.

Predisposing factors

There are a number of predisposing factors which are associated with an increased risk of childhood CNS tumours. These include important familial genetic syndromes such as neurofibromatosis types 1 and 2 (see Table 21.1), as well as a personal or family history of a brain tumour, leukaemia, sarcoma or early-onset breast cancer,

Table 21.1 Central nervous system tumours and their genetic association

Syndrome (gene)	Associated CNS tumours
Ataxia-telangiectasia (ATM)	• Medulloblastoma
Constitutional mismatch repair deficiency syndrome (MSH2, MSH6 MLH1, PMS2)	• Astrocytoma • Glioblastoma • CNS embryonic tumour • Medulloblastoma
Familial adenomatous polyposis (APC)	• Astrocytoma • Medulloblastoma • Ependymoma • Pineoblastoma
Carney complex (PRKAR1A)	• Schwannoma (psammomatous melanotic)
Cowden syndrome (PTEN)	• Dysplastic gangliocytoma of cerebellum • Meningioma
DICER1 syndrome (DICER1)	• CNS embryonic tumour (specifically medulloepithelioma) • Pineoblastoma • Pituitary blastoma
Fanconi anaemia (FANCD1/ BRCA2, FANC-N, or PALB2)	• CNS embryonic tumour • Medulloblastoma
Hereditary retinoblastoma (RB1)	• Pineoblastoma
Li-Fraumeni syndrome (TP53)	• Astrocytoma • High-grade glioma (diffuse astrocytoma, anaplastic astrocytoma, glioblastoma) • Choroid plexus tumour • CNS embryonic tumour • Medulloblastoma
Neurofibromatosis type 1 (NF1)	• Pilocytic astrocytoma/optic pathway/ brainstem, neuraxial glioma • Diffuse astrocytoma • High-grade glioma • Malignant peripheral nerve sheath tumour • Neurofibroma
Neurofibromatosis type 2 (NF2)	• Astrocytoma • Ependymoma • Meningioma • Neurofibroma • Schwannoma • Vestibular schwannoma
Nevoid basal-cell carcinoma syndrome (PTCH/SUFU)	• Astrocytoma • Craniopharyngioma • Medulloblastoma (desmoplastic subtype) • Meningioma • Oligodendroglioma
Rhabdoid tumour predisposition syndrome (SMARCB1)	• Atypical teratoid/rhabdoid tumour • Malignant peripheral nerve sheath tumour
Rubinstein-Taybi syndrome (CREBBP)	• Medulloblastoma
Schwannomatosis (SMARCB1)	• Schwannoma
Tuberous sclerosis complex (TSC)	• Subependymal giant-cell astrocytoma
Von Hippel-Lindau (VHL)	• Haemangioblastoma (intracranial, spinal)

Source: data from de Kock L, et al. (2014); Dubuc AM, et al. (2010); Foulkes W, et al. (2011); Hasselblatt M, et al. (2014); Hottinger AF, Khakoo Y (2007); Kimmelman A, Liang BC (2001); Kirschner L, et al. (2000); Louis D, et al. (2007); Ohgaki H, et al. (2010); Stefanaki K, et al. (2012); Tabori U, et al. (2015); Taylor M, et al. (2001); and Villani A, et al. (2012)

and prior therapeutic CNS irradiation. Recognition of predisposing factors would not only lower the threshold for investigation but also affect treatment options and prognosis. Table 21.1 outlines a comprehensive list of the genetic associations. The more common presentations are discussed below.

Neurofibromatosis type 1

Neurofibromatosis type 1 (NF1) is associated with visual pathway gliomas and other tumours of the CNS. Approximately 20% of NF1 cases are associated with low-grade gliomas which are almost always pilocytic astrocytomas. They can occur anywhere in the CNS, with the commonest locations being the visual pathways, cerebellum, and brainstem. They classically affect the visual pathways in early childhood, which justifies visual screening during early childhood.

Neurofibromatosis type 2

Neurofibromatosis type 2 (NF2) is characterized by the presence of acoustic neuromas or auditory nerve sheath schwannomas, causing hearing difficulties. Other clinical features include skin nodules or plaque-like lesions, café au lait patches, mono- or polyneuropathies, and visual loss due to cataracts or post-lenticular opacities. In addition, there is a high risk of intracranial meningioma affecting 18–58% of patients, and astrocytomas and ependymomas in about 3% of patients. When present in the adolescent age group, they may represent the more aggressive version of the disease called the 'Wiseheart' type, which is progressive and has a reduced life expectancy.

Tuberous sclerosis complex

Tuberous sclerosis complex (TSC) phenomena can affect any organ; however, they affect the brain and skin in up to 80%. Other organ phenomena manifest at different times in life. Thus, cardiac rhabdomyomas occur in infancy, grow, and then involute within the first year. Subependymal giant-cell astrocytomas (SEGAs) present symptomatically or on brain imaging as part of diagnostic screening during childhood, and grow during adolescence. Recently published guidelines recommend surveillance imaging to diagnose the development of SEGAs and other TSC phenomena earlier during childhood. Worsening epilepsy and raised intracranial pressure due to obstruction of the lateral/third ventricles are common presenting symptoms; occasionally, massive spontaneous haemorrhage can occur.

Brain tumours

Symptomatology

Symptoms of CNS tumours can be non-specific and can occur singularly or in combination. Symptoms frequently fluctuate in severity; resolution and then recurrence does not exclude a CNS tumour. It is important to note that presentation depends on the age of the child, as well as tumour location and biology.

Wilne and colleagues provided data on the most common presenting signs and symptoms. Ranking of symptoms based on location is outlined in Figure 21.1 and highlights the variability of presentation depending on location. For example, brainstem tumours present most commonly with abnormal gait and cranial

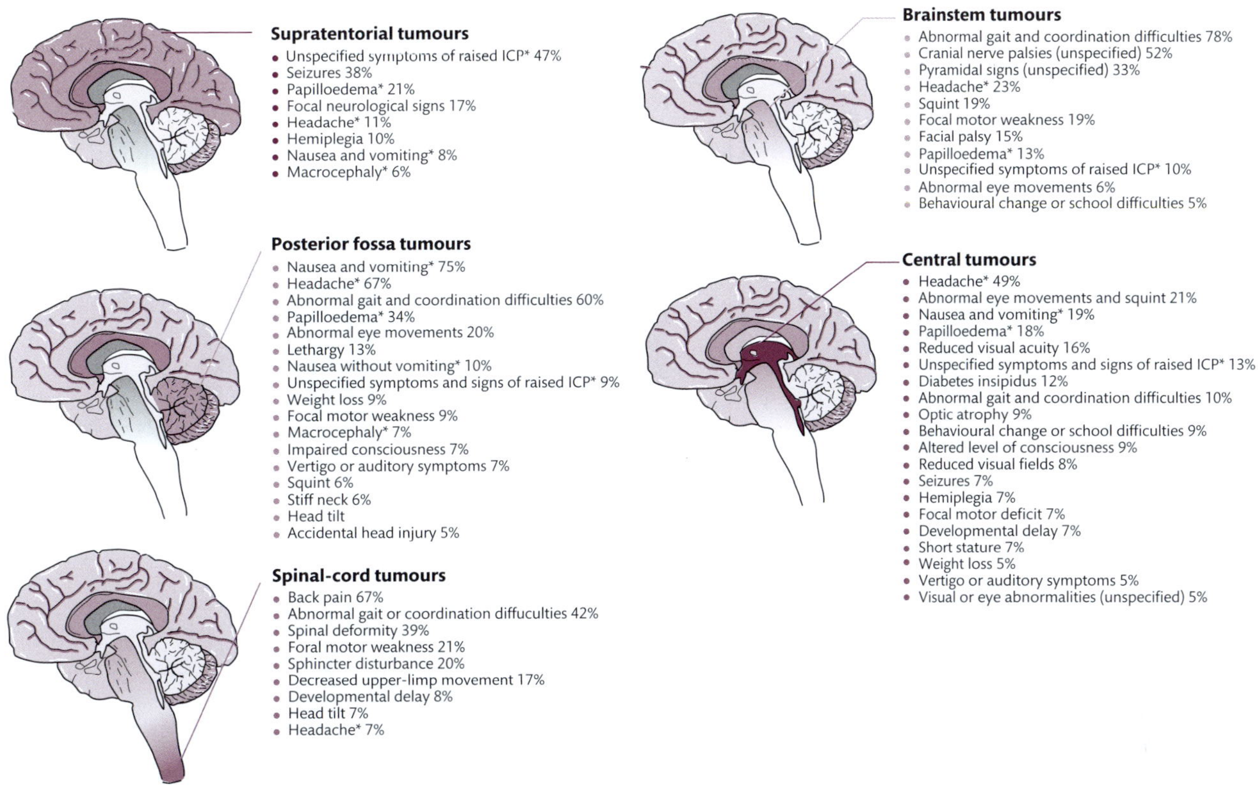

Figure 21.1 Presenting symptoms of central nervous system tumours ranked according to location, based on a systematic meta-analysis.
Reproduced with permission from Wilne S, et al. 'Presentation of childhood CNS tumours: a systematic review and meta-analysis', *Lancet Oncology*, Volume 8, Issue 8, pp. 685–95. Copyright © 2007 Elsevier Ltd. All rights reserved. DOI: https://doi.org/10.1016/S1470-2045(07)70207-3

nerve palsies, whereas posterior fossa tumours present with nausea and/or vomiting and headaches.

A UK-based cohort study highlighted that the symptom profile also changes over time from symptom onset to diagnosis. Visual and motor symptoms increase the most, by 53% and 45% respectively, from symptom onset to diagnosis. This is important to consider when reassessing patient symptoms over time; looking at the progression of visual, motor, or behaviour symptoms over multiple consultations should alert clinicians to a possible diagnosis of brain tumour.

It is also recognized that the non-specificity of symptoms can result in numerous consultations with different subspecialties in order to find a cause. Subspecialty clinicians need to be aware of a brain tumour as a potential diagnosis in order to accelerate diagnosis, thereby limiting brain injury (Figure 21.2).

'HeadSmart: Early Diagnosis of Brain Tumour' campaign

In the UK, a national public and professional awareness campaign named 'HeadSmart: Early Diagnosis of Brain Tumour' was launched to amplify the national evidence-based clinical professional guidance in order to promote earlier diagnosis (www.headsmart.org.uk). As a quality-improvement project, the driver for change was chosen as the TDI, which was collected nationally across 18 UK Children's CNS tumour treatment centres. Following the launch of the guideline and two years after the subsequent awareness campaign, the median TDI had reduced from 14 weeks (mean 35.4 weeks) to 6.7 weeks (mean 22.3 weeks). The campaign did enhance awareness of signs and symptoms amongst paediatricians nationally. About 20% of the UK public also became aware of the campaign.

Further analysis of the TDI data showed that the tumour subtypes with the greatest proportion of prolonged TDI were mid-line supratentoral tumours including craniopharyngiomas, intracranial germ-cell tumours, low-grade gliomas, and optic pathway gliomas, with median TDIs of 15.1, 5.6, 11.9, and 10.4 weeks respectively. Moreover, the 12–18 age group were found to have the longest delay, with a median of 12.1 weeks, compared to six weeks for the 0–5 age group and eight weeks for the 5-11 age group.

The next phase of the campaign involves strategies targeting the adolescent age group, as well as those tumour subtypes with longest delays; the website and media campaign has been designed to appeal to the adolescent age group, with symbols to represent the symptoms, a website designed for mobile devices, and the use of musical content to attract attention. In the UK, the campaign was relaunched by the Royal College of General Practitioners in conjunction with the Royal College of Paediatrics and Child Health, to emphasize the priority across the primary–secondary care interface. The overall success of this programme, using public-awareness techniques, is worthy of consideration.

Emergency presentations

Sudden coma

Sudden coma due to brain tumour is diagnosed in the emergency room, necessitating admission to an intensive-care unit (ICU),

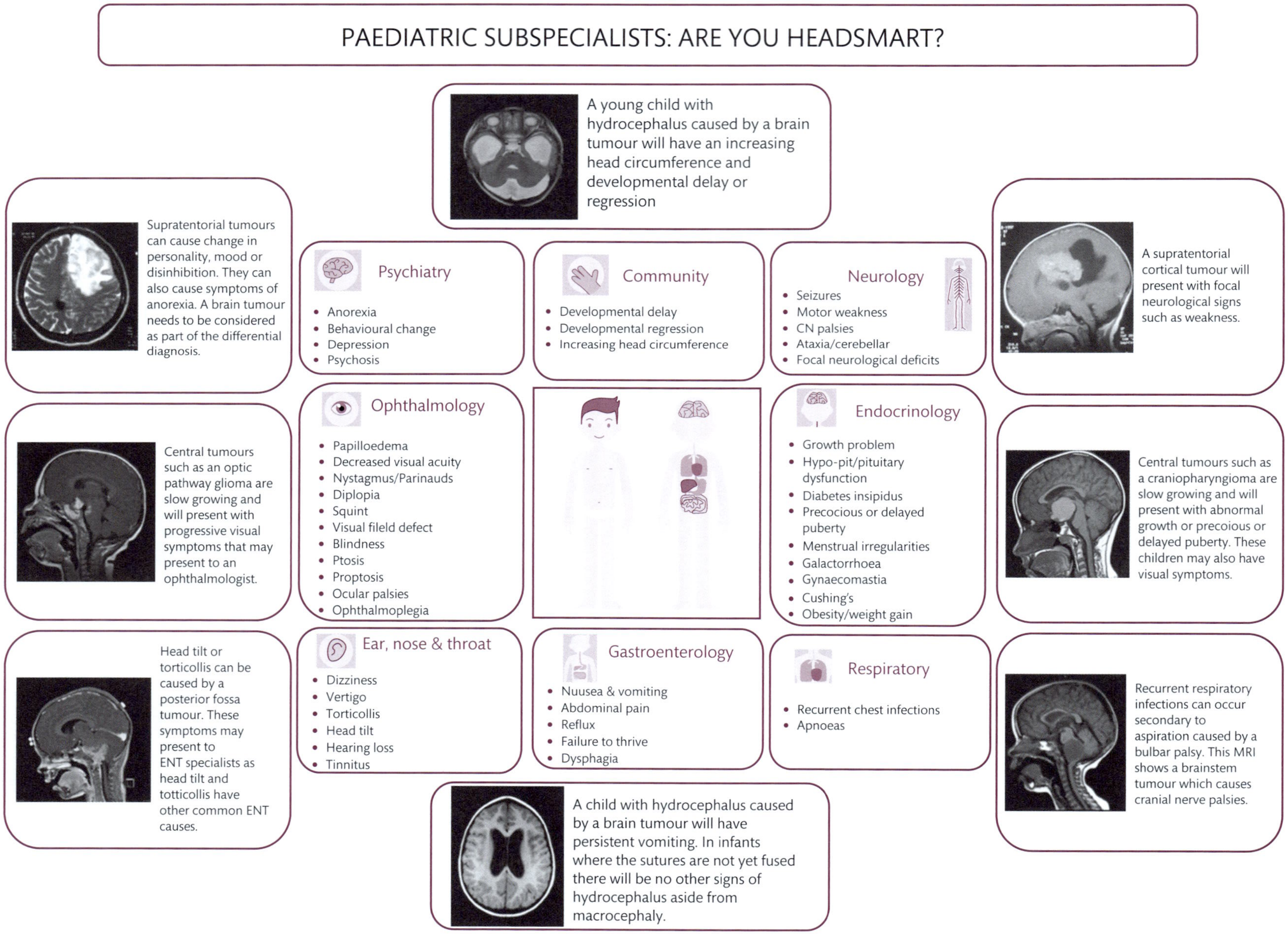

Figure 21.2 Subspecialty involvement in central nervous system tumour diagnosis.

intubation, and emergency computed tomography (CT) (magnetic resonance imaging (MRI) is often difficult to achieve in such emergencies). The sudden deterioration is frequently due to intra-tumoural haemorrhage in hemispheric tumours, or acute hydrocephalus in pineal or posterior fossa tumours. Mannitol or hyperosmotic saline must be given, and emergency surgery is mandatory to debulk the tumour, control the bleeding, and/or treat the hydrocephalus.

Hydrocephalus

If recognized and diagnosed, hydrocephalus is not life-threatening, but it does need urgent treatment. If a pineal tumour is the cause, then endoscopic third ventriculostomy (ETV) with sampling of cerebrospinal fluid (CSF) markers and, if it is safely possible, tumour biopsy, is recommended. In posterior fossa tumours, the approach is more controversial as surgical approaches include four options:

- direct approach of the tumour,
- external ventricular drainage,
- ventriculo-peritoneal shunt, or
- ETV.

ETV remains the best option as it allows the surgeon to operate on the tumour when the patient is in a better clinical condition, and also allows the surgeon time to discuss alternative therapeutic strategies, especially in very young children, children with metastatic disease, and those with the possibility of desmoplastic histology.

Vision or visual-field loss

Acute visual impairment can be the first noticed symptom. The most frequent situation is a cystic craniopharyngioma with neglected endocrinological symptoms or ignored diabetes insipidus. There is a high risk of irreversible blindness associated with immediate tumour surgery, and most neurosurgical teams favour stereotactic or endoscopic tapping of cysts with the positioning of an intracystic reservoir for further tapping or local treatment. Similarly, optic pathway gliomas, whether associated with NF1 or not, can present with visual impairment. Sustained raised intracranial pressure causing papilloedema and subsequent optic atrophy can cause lifelong visual impairment. Together, about 6% of children are registered blind within two years of diagnosis, and historical follow-up studies identify visual impairment in up to 20% of survivors.

A diagnostic emergency

In some situations, the emergency is not to treat but to have access to a diagnosis to initiate non-surgical approaches to treatment. Many such situations have been described here: CSF and CSF markers or endoscopic biopsy for pineal tumours, for example. More and more often, as stereotactic biopsy is the first diagnostic step for diffuse intrinsic pontine gliomas (DIPGs), it is also a requirement in new therapeutic trial protocols.

Spinal-cord tumours

Spinal-cord tumours in childhood account for about 5–10% of all CNS tumours. There is a wide range of tumour types which can present in this way, ranging from benign slow-growing tumours of spinal nerve roots through to tumours of the spinal cord itself or tumours of spinal coverings, vertebrae, or tissues of the paraspinal regions (Figure 21.3).

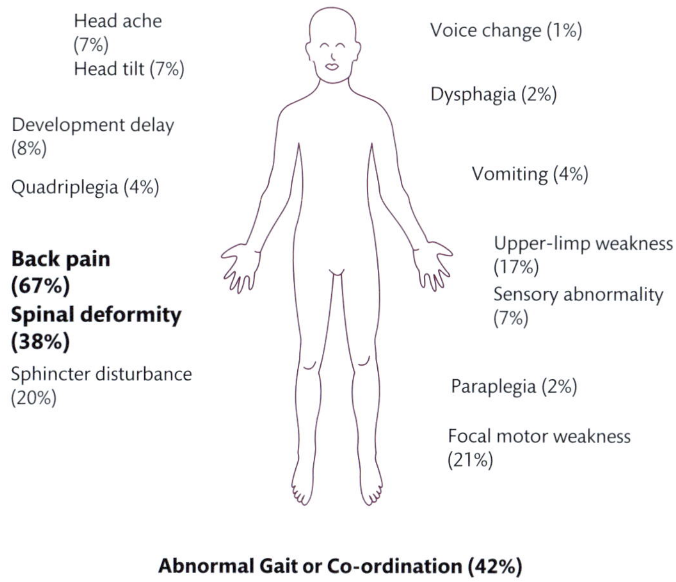

Figure 21.3 Presenting symptoms and signs of spinal tumours in childhood and young people.

Reproduced with permission from Wilne S, Walker D 'Spine and spinal cord tumours in children: a diagnostic and therapeutic challenge to healthcare systems', *British Medical Journal*, Volume 95, Issue 2, pp. 47–54. Copyright © BMJ Publishing Group Ltd. DOI: http://dx.doi.org/10.1136/adc.2008.143214

Risks of delays in diagnosis

Initial signs are often relatively subtle and their initial symptoms may easily be disregarded as trivial complaints. Delays are common due to multiple consultations where the significance of symptoms of spinal origin are not appreciated at first. A review of the diagnostic and therapeutic challenges that these initial symptoms pose is provided by Wilne and Walker (see 'Further reading').

A study of 134 cases from Italy provides information on delay between clinical presentation and diagnosis, age incidence, clinical presentation, and outcome. This large, single-centre experience identified that delay in diagnosis was frequent, with a median symptom interval before diagnosis of 5.3 months (range one day to two years). There was a bimodal age distribution, with a peak in the first 12–18 months followed by a second peak in adolescence. Symptoms reported at presentation were, in order of frequency, pain, palpable mass, paraparesis, torticollis, spinal deformity, sphincteric problems, dyspnoea, weight loss, headache, hemiparesis, and vomiting. From this analysis, the most progressive problems at the time of diagnosis were pain, paraparesis, spinal deformity, sphincter problems, and hemiparesis. The tumours predominantly involved the upper spinal cord in cervical and thoracic regions, but all regions were represented. Intramedullary tumours accounted for 34.3%, intradural extramedullary tumours, 18.7%, and extradural tumours, 39.5%, of which 60% involved the vertebrae, 39% did not, and 7.5% were classified as paravertebral. The range of histologies extended to 29 subtypes of benign and malignant tumours.

A second population-based study of children aged less than three years is reported, where gait disorder affected over 70%, followed by developmental delay, abnormal eye movements, seizures, head tilt, vomiting, and failure to thrive. The range of tumour types was much more restricted, involving low-grade astrocytoma (70%), CNS embryonic tumour (15%), and rhabdoid tumour (15%). Outcomes were significantly different between benign and malignant tumours, the malignant tumours doing significantly worse.

A third institutional report focused upon presentation, imaging, and pathological characteristics in addition to clinical features and outcomes. Mean symptom delay was 7.8 months (0.25–60 months). A notable presenting feature was early handedness in under three year olds. Radiographically, homogenous gadolinium enhancement on MRI correlated with low-grade histology. The degree of resection was strongly predictive of survival.

From these reports, we can conclude that tumours can arise anywhere along the spinal cord, and that delays in diagnosis are frequent and longer for low-grade tumours. The distribution between extradural and intradural tumours is similar. The range of histological subtypes is extremely wide, especially when the whole childhood age range is studied. Children less than three years of age present with a narrower range of tumour types. Surgical management is important for obtaining histology in this extremely diverse range of tumour types but, more importantly, complete resection, where it is achieved, contributes to significant functional and survival advantage.

Clinical description

The clinical features of spinal-cord compression include three groups of symptoms and signs:

- back pain and rigidity,
- signs of segmental spinal involvement, and
- signs resulting from interruption of long tracts within the spinal cord.

The importance of back pain and, especially, of spinal rigidity as an early symptom of tumour of the cord has long been known. Pain may have a radicular distribution but is more often diffuse and is usually predominantly nocturnal. Rigidity is frequently associated with scoliosis. It must be re-emphasized that a painful or rigid scoliosis is a completely abnormal situation and must lead in any case to MRI. Segmental weakness, hyporeflexia, sensory disturbances, and amyotrophy can result from involvement of the central grey matter or nerve roots. Segmental myoclonus is a rare presentation. Spasticity evolving into paraplegia, sphincter disturbances, and sensory deficits results from long-tract involvement. Disturbances of walking, with claudication and stiffness, may be present long before other symptoms. The presence of a definable sensory level, which may be difficult to demonstrate in young children, indicates the upper level of compression. Bilateral pyramidal tract signs are present with Babinski and Rossolimo signs. Initial bladder symptoms are increased urgency followed by retention or incontinence. Sphincter disturbances, especially urinary retention, indicate an urgent need for decompression.

The main clinical problem with these tumours is functional disturbance (gait, sensory, sphincters, pain, spinal deformity, and pulmonary restriction). McCormick's widely used classification divides these spinal-cord tumour patients into four groups (see Box 21.1).

Box 21.1 Classification of spinal-cord tumours

Grade one
- Is neurologically normal.
- The mild focal deficit does not significantly affect the function of the involved limb.
- There is mild spasticity or reflex abnormality.
- Patient's gait is normal.

Grade two
- Sensorimotor deficit affects the function of the involved limb.
- Severe pain or dysaesthetic syndrome present which impairs the patient's quality of life.
- Patient has mild to moderate gait difficulty.
- Patient can still function and ambulate independently.

Grade three
- The neurological deficit is more severe.
- Patient requires a cane or brace for ambulation, or there is significant bilateral upper-extremity impairment.
- Patient may or may not be able to function independently.

Grade four
- The neurological deficit is severe.
- Patient requires a wheelchair or a cane/brace, and there is bilateral upper-extremity impairment.
- Patient is usually not independent.

Source: data from McCormick, P. et al. 'Intramedullary ependymoma of the spinal cord'. *Journal of Neurosurgery*. Volume 72, Issue 4. pp. 523–32. Copyright © 1990, American Association of Neurological Surgeons

Diagnosis

The diagnosis of a spinal-cord tumour should be quickly confirmed by MRI since the risk of sudden aggravation, with complete paraplegia due to compromised circulation in the anterior cerebral artery and its branches, although very rare, may occur at any time. One should be exceedingly suspicious of recurrent back pain and, in some patients, of recurrent abdominal pain. Atypical presentations with paroxysmal attacks of arm pain or isolated abdominal discomfort simulating an irritable bowel syndrome may delay recognition of a tumour.

Plain X-rays of the spine may be diagnostic by showing bone destruction, erosion of the spinal pedicles or of the posterior vertebral bodies, and widening of both the anteroposterior and transverse diameters of the spinal canal. MRI is the imaging technique of choice. CT scanning involves relatively high doses of radiation for young children; it does show bony structures but is less precise at showing neural tissue. MRI clearly shows both intra- and extramedullary lesions and associated cystic formation, thus permitting separation of intramedullary tumours with associated cysts from syringomyelia. However, distinguishing a tumour from an area of increased signal due to oedema, haemorrhage, or inflammation can be difficult. Gadolinium enhancement, when homogenous, selects low-grade lesions, and diffusion-weighted MRI may be useful in some cases. CSF protein, where obtained, is usually increased below the level of the block. However, there is a serious risk of damage to the cord by lumbar puncture at the site of compression, possibly due to slight downward displacement of the cord (Figure 21.4).

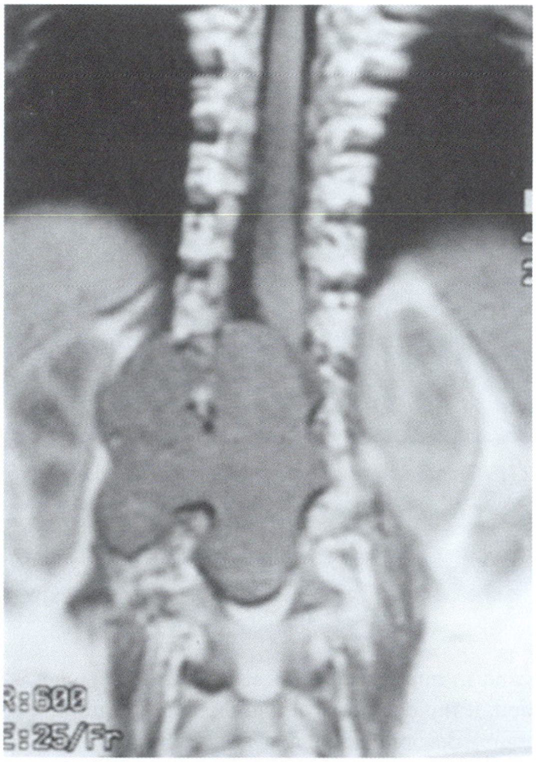

Figure 21.4 Paraspinal neuroblastoma entering the spinal canal through the intervertebral foramen, displacing and compressing the lower spinal cord roots.

Emergency presentation

The emergency context of clinical presentation is worthy of specific comment. If a spinal tumour is diagnosed, then the rate of progression of neurological signs must be kept under regular review. The nature of many children's tumours is that they can progress rapidly. Extramedullary tumours in particular (e.g. neuroblastoma, lymphoma, Ewing's tumour) can grow across the spinal canal in a few days to a week or two. Clinical priority for referral, diagnostic biopsy, and possible medical or surgical decompression needs to be classified as urgent, imaging and referral actions being completed in emergency. Where spinal-cord compression is identified, the use of immediate steroid medication such as dexamethasone in high dose (up to 10 mg/m^2/day), in preparation for surgical decompression, can be critical to saving neurological function. In parallel, achieving a histological diagnosis remains a strong priority. Lymphomas can melt away under the influence of steroids and the possibility of a tissue diagnosis can be lost as a consequence. Close collaboration with the neuro-oncology team can help minimize these risks. Individualized management is critical as the use of steroids in a lymphoma can also precipitate tumour lysis syndrome with the risk of acute renal failure.

Intramedullary spinal-cord tumours

Intramedullary tumours are mainly represented by astrocytomas, ependymomas and gangliogliomas/cavernomas, and haemangio-blastomas. They are frequently associated with cystic cavitation of the central cord, which may be difficult to differentiate from purely cystic intramedullary lesions. Their presentations are often subacute or diagnosed in patients under investigation for spinal surgery or associated with inherited predisposition states (NF2, NF1, and von Hippel–Lindau). They can produce symmetrical weakness of the limbs and are often unassociated with pain. They often do not produce a clear-cut sensory level and some of them may be surprisingly well tolerated for long periods, despite considerable anatomical extension.

Some spinal astrocytomas may present with the clinical manifestations of raised intracranial pressure (ICP) without local signs. Cinalli and colleagues reported eight cases in which hydrocephalus was the initial manifestation and reviewed 38 cases from the literature. Intracranial hypertension may result from metastatic disease, meningeal fibrosis due to haemorrhage from the tumour, or decreased resorption of CSF because of its high protein content 'clogging' the arachnoid granulations.

Diagnosis and management

The diagnosis of intramedullary tumours is dependent upon MRI clearly delineating the extent, the gross tumour morphology, and neuronal involvement. Astrocytomas may extend over considerable lengths of cord. Yet their removal, specifically in the paediatric population, has been made possible in most (more than 90% of the ependymomas and 80% of the astrocytomas) cases by modern neurosurgical techniques. Obtaining a tissue biopsy is the prime reason for operating and surgical resectability is discovered at operation. This, however, is not always possible, and so selected cases may be offered a trial of chemotherapy to see if tumour shrinkage and symptom relief can be achieved after histological diagnosis.

Spinal ependymomas that complicate NF2 are often multiple and are progressive during adolescence and adulthood. When not associated with NF2, they are uncommon and not infrequently present in conus medullaris where they often demonstrate myxo-papillary histology and are reported to metastasize throughout the CNS. The role of chemotherapy versus radiotherapy has not been studied in low-grade astrocytomas. Primary chemotherapy, particularly in younger children, with vincristine and carboplatin (or other drug combinations), is being investigated in clinical trials and in selected spinal-cord cases. Non-progression rates of 70% and response rates of 50% can be expected with all drug regimens. As in all CNS tumours, treatment selection by the neuro-oncology multidisciplinary team is the recommended approach.

Other rare spinal tumour types, such as gangliogliomas and haemangioblastomas, may be a part of the von Hippel–Lindau complex. These tumours are often cystic and commonly extend over considerable lengths in the cervico-dorsal part of the cord. Some of them also involve the lower brainstem. Surgery is the only option in symptomatic haemangioblastomas. It is very complex and dangerous surgery which can be helped by pre-surgical embolization (Figure 21.5).

Treatment of intramedullary tumours raises special problems. If removal proves impossible, decompression of surrounding bony structures, chemotherapy, or irradiation may afford fairly long symptomatic relief in 30–50% of cases. Astrocytomas, even when incompletely resected and treated with adjuvant chemotherapy, can remain static for sustained periods. One study found that the overall long-term survival was only of the order of 50%, but such figures

(a) (b)

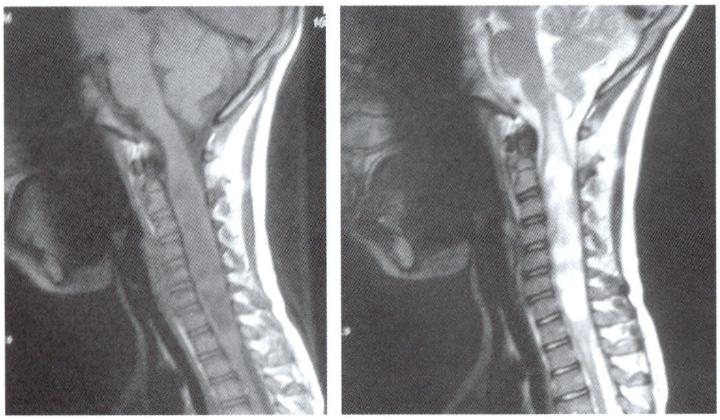

Figure 21.5 Intramedullary astrocytoma of the spinal cord: (a) T1-weighted MRI showing enlarged cervical cord with multiple low-signal areas; and (b) T2-weighted MRI showing high signal in the same areas.

(a) (b)

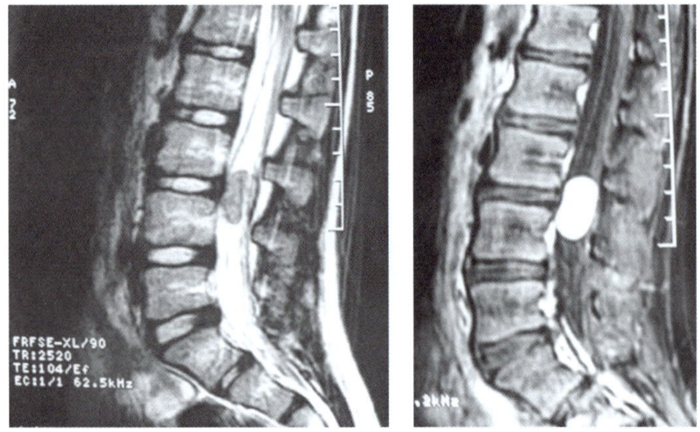

Figure 21.6 Spinal schwannoma (neurinoma) of cauda equine: (a) T1-weighted MRI; (b) T2-weighted high-signal image.

require interpretation with specific histologies. Patients with malignant tumours such as glioblastomas do poorly.

Intradural tumours account for approximately 25% of cases, and meningiomas are the most common histological type, followed by schwannomas. Metastases from intracranial tumours, especially ependymomas and medulloblastomas, are usually multiple.

Extramedullary tumours

Approximately two thirds of extramedullary tumours are extradural in origin, spreading from nearby bone or through intervertebral foramina. About a quarter are intradural. Neuroblastoma is the most frequent cause but other tumours are of osseous or soft-tissue origin such as rhabdomyosarcoma, Ewing sarcoma, aneurysmal bone cysts, metastases, lymphomas, or bony deposits of Langerhans cell histiocytosis (LCH).

Extramedullary tumours tend to manifest initially with unilateral pain in segmental distribution, often in association with paraesthesiae and weakness. Brown–Séquard syndrome is observed in a small proportion of children with extramedullary tumours. More commonly, there is only predominant weakness, spasticity, and deep sensory loss on the side of the tumour, with more marked contralateral loss of pain and temperature sensation. Schwannomas (neurinomas) are more common than meningiomas (Figure 21.6).

Acute spinal-cord compression

There is some controversy regarding the role of surgical decompression in tumour-related presentations. On the one hand, acute neurological deterioration is reversible with early decompressive surgery; it offers the opportunity to obtain tissue for histological diagnosis without attempting to access retroperitoneal tissues in the thorax or abdomen. The risk of subsequent spinal deformity linked to delamination is thought to be limited by the use of osteoplastic laminotomy and replacement of lamina post surgery, subsequent surgical instability affecting only a minority (mainly the youngest patients and in tumours of cervical or junctional regions). On the other hand, if the neurological injury is long-standing (more than 24–48 hours), decompression may not be effective in saving spinal-cord function, although remarkable late recoveries can occur in children, when not expected in adults.

Selection of the tissue site for biopsy is critical, especially if it can offer decompression to prevent further progression of spinal injury associated with delayed tumour response to chemotherapy. The significant differences between the treatment programmes justifies the need for tissue for histology and biology, as well as for research purposes. In acute presentations, where spinal-nerve injury is progressive, chemotherapy may be used as empirical treatment pending histological classification, if steroids alone are not holding neurological deterioration or a full histological/molecular diagnosis will be delayed.

Spinal-cord tumours can arise throughout childhood, are frequently delayed in diagnosis, and, when presenting acutely, are associated with risk of serious spinal injury justifying timely intervention. Histological diagnosis is crucial for treatment planning and prognostication. Successful surgical intervention is central to a successful outcome in most cases.

There are two completely different situations for emergency presentations of spinal-cord tumours:

1. **Intramedullary tumours**
   True emergency situations are exceptional, requiring mostly speedy surgery in the case of intractable pain or rapidly progressive symptoms.
2. **Extramedullary tumours**
   On the other hand, emergency presentation is frequent in extramedullary tumours. The decision making depends on the age, the topography, the supposed diagnosis, the clinical condition, the evolution, and the MR images. However, acute surgery is very often mandatory. Laminectomy, which was once the only option, has been progressively in competition with different or combined approaches and the use of instrumentation, even in

emergency surgery. These types of approaches need well-trained neurosurgical and orthopaedic paediatric teams with significant experience of these complex spinal-surgery techniques. Two specific situations where this surgery must be discussed are:

- **Neuroblastoma**: There is no surgical indication in case of antenatal or neonatal neuroblastoma. The possibility of recovery is nil and the effect on the spine growing is catastrophic. Surgery is not indicated as a first option except to do a biopsy, if impossible by another approach (exceptional), or in case of clinical impairment after one or two courses of chemotherapy.
- **Ewing sarcoma**: Spinal Ewing sarcomas are very often diagnosed in emergency, in the face of very severe clinical deterioration. The role of the surgery is to do a biopsy and to protect the spinal cord by a reasonable decompression. Sparing of the spinal capital and the planning process for the next surgery must always be taken into account, and a frozen section can be helpful to challenge the diagnosis and stop the surgery.

Conclusion

Clinical presentations of brain and spinal tumours include slow, gradually progressive symptomatology which can mimic a wide variety of clinical conditions, leading to avoidable delays. Acute presentations, on the other hand, can constitute emergencies threatening life due to raised ICP or sudden onset of paralysis due to spinal cord compression, the risk of acute intra-tumoural haemorrhage can complicate avoidable delays in diagnosis. Any neurological symptoms of the brain can constitute the beginning of brain injury, which is likely to be lifelong. Accelerating diagnosis is therefore emerging as a top priority for reducing the late neurological consequences for survivors. Emergencies associated with brain and spinal tumours need to be recognized as such by health systems to offer the optimal response.

FURTHER READING

Albanese V, Platania N (2002) Spinal intradural extramedullary tumors. Personal experience. *J Neurosurg Sci* **46**, 18–24.

Allen J, et al. (1998) Treatment of high-grade spinal cord astrocytoma of childhood with '8-in-1' chemotherapy and radiotherapy: a pilot study of CCG-945. *J Neurosurg* **88**, 215–20.

Celli P, et al. (2005) Spinal extradural schwannorna. *J Neurosurg* **2**, 447–56.

Cinalli G, et al. (1995) Hydrocephalus associated with intramedullary low-grade glioma—illustrative cases and review of the literature. *J Neurosurg* **83**, 480–5.

Costello F, et al. (2002) Papilledema as the presenting manifestation of spinal schwannoma. *J Neuro-ophthalmol* **22**, 199–203.

Crawford J, et al. (2009) Primary spinal tumors of childhood: effects of clinical presentation, radiographic features, and pathology on survival. *J Neuro-oncology* **95**(2), 259–69.

Daley M, et al. (2003) Primary epidural Burkitt lymphoma in a child: case presentation and literature review. *Pediatr Hematol Oncol* **20**, 333–8.

de Kock L, et al. (2014) Germ-line and somatic DICER1 mutations in pineoblastoma. *Acta Neuropathol* **128**(4), 583–95.

de Kock L, et al. (2014) Pituitary blastoma: a pathognomonic feature of germ-line CICER1 mutations. *Acta Neuropathol* **128**(1), 111–22.

Di Rocco C, et al. (1994) Spinal epidural meningiomas in childhood: a case report. *J Neurosurg Sci* **38**, 251–4.

Dixon-Woods M, et al. (2001) Parents' accounts of obtaining a diagnosis of childhood cancer. *Lancet* **357**, 670e4.

Dubuc AM, et al. (2010) The genetics of pediatric brain tumors. *Curr Neurol Neurosci Rep* **10**(3), 215–23.

Epstein F, Wisoff J (1987) Intra-axial tumors of the cervicomedullary junction. *J Neurosurg* **67**, 483–7.

Flores LE, et al. (1986) Delay in the diagnosis of paediatric brain tumors. *Am J Dis Child* **140**, 684e6.

Foulkes W, et al. (2011) Extending the phenotypes associated with DICER1 mutations. *Hum Mutat* **32**(12), 1381–4.

Gelabert M, et al. (1990) Hydrocephalus and intraspinal tumor in childhood. *Child Nerv Syst* **6**, 110–12.

Hasselblatt M, et al. (2014) SMARCA4-mutated atypical teratoid/rhabdoid tumors are associated with inherited germline alterations and poor prognosis. *Acta Neuropathol* **128**(3), 453–6.

HeadSmart website: www.headsmart.org.uk

Hottinger AF, Khakoo Y (2007) Update on the management of familial central nervous system tumor syndromes. *Curr Neurol Neurosci Rep* **7**(3), 200–7.

Houten J, Weiner H (2000) Pediatric intramedullary spinal cord tumors: special considerations. *J Neuro-oncol* **47**, 225–30.

Jallo GI, et al. (2004) Spinal cord gangliogliomas: a review of 56 patients. *J Neuro-Oncol* **68**, 71–7.

Kimmelman A, Liang BC (2001) Familial neurogenic tumor syndromes. *Hematol Oncol Clin North Am* **15**(6), 1073–84.

Kirschner L, et al. (2000) Mutations of the gene encoding the protein kinase A type I-α regulatory subunit in patients with the Carney complex. Nat Genet **26**(1), 89–92.

Louis D, et al. (2007) The 2007 WHO classification of tumours of the central nervous system. *Acta Neuropathol* **114**(5), 97–109.

McCormick P, et al. (1990) Intramedullary ependymoma of the spinal cord. *J Neurosurg* **72**, 523–32.

Mora J, et al. (2007) Successful treatment of childhood intramedullary spinal cord astrocytomas with irinotecan and cisplatin. *Neuro Oncol* **9**(1), 39–46.

Nagib M, O'Fallon M (1997) Myxopapillary ependymoma of the Conus medullaris and filum terminale in the pediatric age group. *Pediatr Neurosurg* **26**, 2–7.

Ohgaki H, et al. (2010) Nervous system tumors associated with familial tumor syndromes. *Curr Opin Neurol* **23**(6), 583–91.

Orbach D, et al. (2013) Neonatal cancer. *Lancet Oncol* **14**, e609–20.

Pascual-Castraviejo I (ed.) (1990) *Spinal Tumors in Children and Adolescents*. New York: Raven Press.

Phan T, et al. (2000) Recurrent lumbar ependymoma presenting as headache and communicating hydrocephalus. *Mayo Clin Proc* 75, 850–2.

Pui M, et al. (2005) Diffusion-weighted magnetic resonance imaging of spinal infection and malignancy. *J Neuroimaging* **15**, 164–70.

Renault F, et al. (1995) Segmental myoclonus in a child with spinal cord tumour. *Dev Med Child Neurol* **37**, 354–61.

Rifkinson-Mann S, et al. (1990) The association of hydrocephalus with intramedullary spinal cord tumors: a series of 25 patients. *Neurosurgery* **27**, 749–54.

Robertson P, et al. (1994) Cervicomedullary tumors in children: a distinct subset of brainstem gliomas. *Neurology* **44**, 1798–803.

Roig M, et al. (1988) Congenital spinal cord haemangioblastoma: another cause of spinal cord section syndrome in the newborn. *J Neurol Neurosurg Psychiatry* **51**, 1091–103.

Royal College of Paediatric and Child Health (RCPCH) (2008) *The Brain Pathways Guideline: A Guideline to Assist Healthcare*

Professionals in the Assessment of Children Who May Have a Brain Tumour. London: RCPCH.

Spacca B, et al. (2015) Spinal tumors in children: long term retrospective evaluation of a series of 134 cases treated in a single unit of pediatric neurosurgery. *Spinal J* **15**, 1949–55.

Stefanaki K, et al. (2012) Tumors of central and peripheral nervous system associated with inherited genetic syndromes. *Pediatr Neurosurg* **48**, 271–85.

Tabori U, et al. (2015) Cancer predisposition in children with brain tumors. In: K Scheinemann, E Bouffet E (eds) *Pediatric Neuro-Oncology*, pp. 69–89. New York: Springer.

Taylor M, et al. (2001) Medulloblastoma in a child with Rubenstein–Taybi syndrome: case report and review of the literature. *Pediatr Neurosurg* **35**(5), 235–8.

Uesaka T, et al. (2003) Intradural, extramedullary spinal Ewing's sarcoma in childhood. *J Clin Neurosci* **10**, 112–25.

Villani A, et al. (2012) Syndromes predisposing to pediatric central nervous system tumors: lessons learned and new promises. *Curr Neurol Neurosci Rep* **12**(2), 153–64.

Walker D, et al. (2013) A multi-disciplinary consensus statement concerning surgical approaches to low-grade, high-grade astrocytomas and diffuse intrinsic pontine gliomas in childhood (CPN Paris 2011) using the Delphi method. *Neuro Oncol* 15(4), 462–8.

Williams A, et al. (1987) Differentiation of intramedullary neoplasms and cysts by MR. *Am J Roentgenol* **149**, 159–64.

Wilne S, et al. (2012) Progression from first symptom to diagnosis in childhood brain tumours. *Eur J Pediatr* **171**(1), 87–93.

Wilne S, et al. (2007) Presentation of childhood CNS tumours: a systematic review and meta-analysis. *Lancet Oncol* **8**(8), 685–95.

Wilne S, et al. (2010) The diagnosis of brain tumors in children: a guideline to assist healthcare professionals in the assessment of children who may have a brain tumour. *Arch Dis Child* **95**, 534e9.

Wilne S, Walker D (2010) Spine and spinal cord tumours in children: a diagnostic and therapeutic challenge to healthcare systems. *Arch Dis Child Educ Pract Ed* **95**, 47–54.

Zelcer S, et al. (2011) Spinal cord tumors in children under the age of 3 years: a retrospective Canadian review. *Child Nerv Syst* **27**, 1089–94.

22

Glial Central Nervous System Tumours of Childhood

Dannis van Vuurden, Darren Hargrave, Dominik Sturm, and David T.W. Jones

Low-grade gliomas

Classification and pathology

Low-grade gliomas (LGGs) are the most common primary central nervous system (CNS) tumours in children and adolescents (more than 30%) and consist of a variety of histopathological entities classified as grade I or grade II (relatively benign, slow-growing lesions) by the World Health Organization (WHO) classification of tumours of the CNS. The largest proportion of these tumours presents as WHO grade I pilocytic astrocytoma (PA), accounting for approximately 20% of brain tumours in patients under the age of 20 years, with an average age-adjusted annual incidence rate of 0.84 cases per 100,000. Other frequent histopathological entities classified as paediatric LGG include subependymal giant-cell astrocytoma (SEGA), pleomorphic xanthoastrocytoma (PXA), paediatric-type diffuse astrocytoma, and mixed low-grade glial-neuronal tumours (LGGNTs) such as dysembryoplastic neuroepithelial tumours (DNTs), ganglioglioma (GG), and desmoplastic infantile astrocytoma/ganglioglioma (DIA/DIG), as well as other, less frequent diagnoses. The majority of paediatric LGGs harbour a variety of genetic abnormalities frequently causing aberrant intracellular signalling via the Ras mitogen-activated protein kinase (MAPK) pathway (see the section 'Biology').

Paediatric PAs (WHO grade I) can occur throughout the neuraxis, but arise predominantly in infratentorial regions. Commonly affected sites include (but are not restricted to) the cerebellum, optic nerve/chiasm, hypothalamus, thalamus, and cerebral hemispheres. PAs appear circumscribed upon imaging, with little (or no) oedema, and display variable proportions of cyst-like areas intermixed with contrast-enhancing solid components. Optic-pathway tumours can be sporadic but are a hallmark of neurofibromatosis type 1 (NF1), an autosomal dominant tumour predisposition syndrome caused by germline mutations affecting the *neurofibromin 1* gene; about 20% of NF1 patients develop a PA. Upon microscopy, they are characterized by a biphasic pattern with compacted bipolar cells, with Rosenthal fibres alongside loose-textured multipolar cells with microcysts. A histological variant, with tumour cells in a prominent myxoid background, is termed pilomyxoid astrocytoma. By far the most frequent (more than 70%) genetic MAPK pathway alteration is a tandem duplication involving the *BRAF* gene, resulting in an oncogenic *KIAA1549-BRAF* fusion.

Subependymal giant-cell astrocytomas (WHO grade I) typically present as solid, partially calcified masses in the wall of the lateral ventricles adjacent to the foramen of Monro. They are composed of large ganglionic astroyctes arranged in sweeping fascicles, sheets, and nests. Up to 15% of patients with tuberous sclerosis syndrome (TSC), an autosomal dominant genetic disease (caused by inactivating germline mutations in *TSC1/2*) predisposing to benign tumour growth, develop SEGAs during childhood or adolescence. It is uncertain whether SEGAs occur outside a TSC setting.

PXAs (WHO grade II) account for about 0.3 cases per 100,000 population, typically developing in children and adolescents. They arise almost exclusively in supratentorial regions, often involving the leptomeninges and cerebrum. Neuroimaging shows a tumour mass with frequently cystic portions, moderate contrast enhancement, and no pronounced oedema. The histological appearance of the tumour is very variable, containing large pleomorphic and frequently multinucleated cells, spindle and lipidized cells, a dense pericellular reticulin network, and numerous eosinophilic granular bodies. An often present diffusely infiltrating component may render paediatric-type diffuse astrocytoma (WHO grade II) a differential diagnosis, especially in the absence of a typical pleomorphic pattern. The majority of PXAs harbour point mutations in the *BRAF* gene (V600E; 50–80%), and concomitant homozygous 9p21.3 deletions targeting the *CDKN2A/CDKN2B* loci are common. If five or more mitoses per ten high-power fields are present, tumours are diagnosed as anaplastic PXAs (WHO grade III), which are associated with comparably worse overall survival.

Among the group of mixed glial-neuronal tumours are DNTs (WHO grade I), which typically occur in children (or young adults) with early-onset epilepsy and account for more than 20% of long-term epilepsy-associated tumours. They predominantly arise in cortical regions of the temporal lobe and, in contrast to diffuse gliomas, show little mass effect and no significant perifocal oedema upon imaging. Specific glioneuronal elements, characterized by columns made up of bundles of axons orientated perpendicularly to the cortical surface, are a histological hallmark of DNTs.

Gangliogliomas (WHO grade I) most frequently occur in the temporal lobe (more than 70%) of children and young adults. Imaging usually demonstrates a circumscribed solid or mixed solid and cystic mass with variable contrast enhancement and occasional tumour calcification. Gangliogliomas are well-differentiated glioneuronal neoplasms composed of dysplastic ganglion cells in combination with neoplastic glial cells. *BRAF V600E* point mutations are present in up to 50% of gangliogliomas . The presence of an anaplastic glial component with elevated mitotic activity corresponds to a diagnosis of anaplastic ganglioglioma (WHO grade III).

DIAs/DIGs (WHO grade I) are rare neoplasms of early childhood, accounting for about 15% of infant tumours. Tumour location is always supratentorial, frequently involving more than one lobe. Neuroimaging usually demonstrates a solid, superficial, enhancing portion extending to the leptomeninges, and a cystic portion reaching into the cerebrum. Tumours are characterized by a prominent desmoplastic stroma with a neoplastic glial component (DIAs) or neoplastic glioneuronal component (DIGs).

Biology

Genetic aberrations targeting the MAPK signalling pathway are a hallmark molecular feature of paediatric LGGs as well as some LGGNTs. As the most prominent example, a variety of single-hit MAPK abnormalities, including gene fusions and point mutations, can be found in essentially all PAs, which therefore has been hypothesized to represent a prototypical single-pathway disease.

The most frequent genetic event are *KIAA1549:BRAF* fusion genes detectable in 70–80% of PAs, with a number of less frequent *BRAF* fusion gene partners representing variants of a common molecular mechanism of MAPK activation (i.e. loss of the autoinhibitory N′-terminal region of *BRAF* while retaining its active kinase domain). Similar rearrangements involving upstream receptor tyrosine kinase genes *NRTK2* or *NTRK3* (previously observed in infant high-grade gliomas) have recently been identified across various histological subtypes of LGG, as well as fusion events involving *FGFR1* or *FGFR3*, previously observed in adult high-grade gliomas and resulting in constitutive *FGFR* signalling. Duplications of the whole kinase domain (internal tandem duplication, ITD) have been described as a frequent alternative mechanism of *FGFR1* activation in DNT and some PAs. The occurrence of *NTRK* and *FGFR* gene-family rearrangements in both low- and high-grade gliomas suggests some overlap in their molecular genetic make-up in some instances.

The most common point mutations in LGG and LGGNT also target the *BRAF* gene, typically resulting in a hotspot *V600E* alteration, and occur with high incidence in GG and PXA as well as supratentorial PA. Hotspot mutations were also shown to occur in *FGFR1* (at p.N546 or p.K656) in some tumours, highlighting the growing evidence for *FGFR1* alterations as a molecular driver in LGG.

In line with location-specific differences in DNA methylation and gene-expression patterns of LGG and LGGNT, the aforementioned aberrations in the canonical MAPK pathway differ in their anatomical distribution, with *BRAF* fusions predominating in cerebellar tumours, *BRAF V600E* and *NTRK* gene-family fusions more commonly found in hemispheric supratentorial tumours, and *FGFR1* alterations typically occurring in midline tumours.

Outside of the MAPK pathway, and enriched in paediatric-type diffuse astrocytomas and angiocentric gliomas (AGs—epilepsy-associated, slow-growing cerebral tumours histologically characterized by an angiocentric growth pattern), are alterations in the *MYB* and *MYBL1* oncogenes. In contrast to the typical kinase fusions, *MYB* and *MYBL1* rearrangements result in loss of their C′-terminal portion (encoding a negative regulatory domain) but retention of the transactivating N′-terminus. The most commonly identified variant is a *MYB:QKI* fusion gene, acting through a tripartite mechanism of *MYB* activation by truncation, enhancer translocation driving aberrant *MYB-QKI* expression, and hemizygous loss of the tumour suppressive functions of *QKI* at the same time.

Low-grade tumours arising in children with NF1 represent a distinct molecular subset of LGG, characterized by biallelic inactivation of the *NF1* gene accompanied by increased MAPK signalling.

While certain histologies are enriched for recurrent molecular alterations (e.g. *BRAF* in PA/ganglioglioma, *FGFR1* in DNT, *MYB* in AG), it is becoming increasingly evident that classification schemes based purely on histological criteria fail to recapitulate the substantial heterogeneity of molecular LGG/LGGNT subgroups. Some of these represent very rare but distinct biological entities, reflecting the complex interplay among cellular origins, anatomical tumour location, and susceptibility to particular oncogenic insults. Future molecularly guided classification approaches may therefore distinguish between *BRAF* fusion-positive, *BRAF V600E*-positive, and *BRAF* wildtype LGG/LGGNT, and paediatric-type diffuse gliomas driven by *MYB/MYBL1*, *FGFR*, and *NRTK* abnormalities, while still acknowledging histopathological variants in each of these categories.

However, the diagnostic, prognostic, or predictive value of the aforementioned molecular genetic markers remains to be determined. Their integration into a new standard of an integrated, multi-layered, histopathologic-molecular diagnosis is therefore crucial for their prospective evaluation in not only improving diagnostic accuracy, but also identifying patients that may potentially benefit from targeted therapeutic strategies such as BRAF V600E or MEK inhibitors.

Current treatment strategies

Paediatric low-grade gliomas (pLGGs) are the most common brain tumours in children, and the majority of patients will survive, but often with significant long-term deficits either from the tumour itself or secondary to treatment. These tumours can return multiple times over many years and follow a chronic disease course, with a cumulative treatment burden. This makes the choice and sequencing of therapy complex, with a need to balance durable tumour control with protecting neurological function.

Surgery is the treatment of choice for some hemispheric and cerebellar LGGs when total resection can be accomplished with little morbidity. The six-year progression-free survival (PFS) of a gross total resection alone is 70% to 100%. However, owing to their proximity to vital brain structures (e.g. the hypothalamus, pituitary, optic pathways), many pLGGs can only undergo partial resection to facilitate mechanical decompression or biopsy, and have a significantly higher rate of progression post surgery. Asymptomatic pLGGs (e.g. optic-pathway gliomas in NF1 patients, tectal-plate tumours post CSF diversion) may not require immediate or even any treatment, whereas those that progress or present with symptoms often require non-surgical treatment. Poor prognostic factors include young age (under one year old), grade II histology, and dissemination.

The selection of adjuvant therapy varies according to age, location, and the presence of NF1. Children with NF1 and optic-pathway gliomas often have an indolent course and, in many patients, careful observation may safely be undertaken, as up to 50% of tumours will not progress. Radiotherapy has been considered a definitive treatment of pLGGs, with overall survival (OS) in excess of 90% and PFS of 60–85%. However, it is associated with late effects which depend on location, dose, volume, and age of the child. The most frequent reported deficits are in neurocognition and neuroendocrine function, but vasculopathy and second malignancy have also been documented, especially for NF1 patients, where irradiation is usually avoided. Advances in radiotherapy have led to increasingly conformal focal approaches to reduce treatment volumes, and to try and reduce side effects. Proton beam radiotherapy is one such technique which can decrease the dose to normal brain by the possible lower entrance dose and elimination of the exit dose, compared with conventional photon beams. Reports from pLGG show good disease control with 83% PFS and 100% OS rates, respectively, at eight years. Even with proton beams, significant neurocognitive decline has been seen in younger patients (under seven years), but for older patients and with sparing of the left temporal lobe, hippocampus, and hypothalamic-pituitary good clinical outcomes have been reported.

To avoid or delay radiotherapy, those young patients (typically under seven to eight years of age) and patients with NF1 requiring treatment usually receive chemotherapy. The combination of vincristine and carboplatin is currently regarded as the standard regimen, and several studies report five-year PFS rates of 35–45% for sporadic pLGG and higher in those with NF1 (60–65%). Disease control tends to plateau in many NF1 patients over the first five years, but in sporadic patients this tends to fall over the first five to ten years. This means that patients will often require several rounds of treatment and may have to discontinue initial therapy due to treatment-related effects (e.g. carboplatin allergy). This has resulted in many alternative chemotherapy regimens being explored, either to try and improve PFS by intensification (e.g. multi-agent regimens such as TPCV (thioguanine, procarbazine, CCNU, vincristine) or to reduce toxicity and maintain PFS (e.g. single-agent carboplatin, vinblastine, vinorelbine).

With increasing knowledge of the underlying biology of pLGG and the desire to improve function whilst decreasing treatment burden, targeted therapy is now being explored. One example has been SEGA in TSC, where mTOR inhibition has been used when surgical resection is difficult. Whether mTOR inhibitors have a role in PA remains unclear. The anti-angiogenic agent bevacizumab has been combined with chemotherapy and shown good short-term response rates with functional improvement (e.g. vision recovery) in some patients, and optimization of this agent with standard chemotherapy is now being investigated.

Most recently, the main focus has been on agents targeting the MAPK pathway, which has been shown to be activated in the majority of pLGGs. The first attempt at targeting this pathway in pLGG used the agent sorafenib as a BRAF inhibitor, but this resulted in rapid disease progression in patients with tumours with *KIAA1549:BRAF* fusions. This occurred as the *KIAA1549:BRAF* protein functions as a homodimer, which results in resistance to first-generation BRAF inhibitors due to paradoxical MAPK activation. Targeting more downstream targets with a MEK inhibitor is thought to overcome this problem, and several of these inhibitors are being studied in progressive/relapsed pLGG with preliminary results reported in a phase I study of the MEK inhibitor selumetinib. In this study, selumetinib demonstrated encouraging preliminary activity, with 20% sustaining partial responses and a two-year PFS for those treated at the recommended phase II dose of 69%. The phase 2 study has been published and confirms this preliminary activity: NF1-associated pLGG had a 40% objective response rate and 96% two-year PFS, and sporadic pLGG (either BRAF fusion- or BRAF V600E-positive) had a 36% objective response rate and 70% two-year PFS. The toxicity profile was similar to that seen in adults, with rash and mucositis, asymptomatic CPK elevation, and no retinal toxicity, all of which will need monitoring in subsequent late phase trials.

Confirmatory data, including response rates according to underlying biology (e.g. NF1, BRAF fusion, BRAF V600E) and duration of tumour control off treatment, are eagerly awaited from studies of selumetinib, trametinib, cobimetinib, and MEK-162 in pLGG. For BRAF V600E-mutated pLGG, selective BRAF inhibitors represent an attractive option and the first results using dabrafenib have been reported in abstract form. The drug was well tolerated, with the most common side effects related to skin rash being similar to those observed in adults. Promising response rates were reported for all but three out of the 32 enrolled, demonstrating tumour control with a high objective response rate. Such responses have also been reported with other BRAF inhibitors in pLGG.

Future outlook

It is likely that future clinical trials and treatment strategies will concentrate on the dual aim of durable tumour control and improving the quality of survival. This will be achieved by focusing on protecting or improving neurological function and decreasing the overall treatment burden, with an emphasis on using biology to optimize patient selection and risk stratification. The use of molecular analysis as a prognostic and predictive tool will lead to more patients being biopsied and considered for targeted therapies. Over the next few years, studies will assess the impact of MAPK inhibitors as single agents and in combinations, and explore agents such as bevacizumab which may play a role not just in tumour control but also in protecting against or reversing neurological deficits.

High-grade gliomas

Classification and pathology

High-grade gliomas (HGGs) in children and adolescents comprise a group of diffusely infiltrating, malignant CNS tumours, that are situated supratentorially, as well as in midline structures of the brain and (more rarely) the spinal cord. These tumours occur in any age group, ranging from neonates to young adults, with a peak incidence in the second decade of life, and display a relatively equal sex distribution.

Apart from specific genetic tumour-predisposition syndromes such as DNA mismatch repair, Li–Fraumeni syndrome (LFS), and neurofibromatosis type I, aetiology is largely unknown.

On magnetic resonance imaging (MRI), supratentorial HGGs usually present as poorly defined tumour masses. Irregular-shaped contrast enhancement around a dark central core of necrosis, which may have a haemorrhagic component, is a typical radiological feature of glioblastomas. Surrounding oedema is frequent and often contains infiltration by neoplastic cells. Where possible, tumour resection or biopsy, followed by histopathological and molecular work-up, establish an integrated diagnosis for clinical management.

On pathology, paediatric HGGs have a varying histological appearance. Most display morphological and immunohistochemical features of anaplastic astrocytoma (i.e. atypia, anaplasia, and mitotic activity) or glioblastoma (with additional microvascular proliferation and/or pseudopalisading necrosis). The vast majority of *supratentorial* paediatric HGGs are classified as 'anaplastic astrocytoma, isocitrate dehydrogenase (IDH)-wildtype' (WHO grade III) or 'glioblastoma, IDH-wildtype' (WHO grade IV) according to the revised 2016 fourth edition of the WHO classification of tumours of the CNS. In contrast to adult HGG, *IDH1/2* mutations in this age group are very rare (see the section 'Biology').

Of specific interest, the 2016 WHO classification has introduced a new category of HGGs situated in the *midline* of the brain, called 'diffuse midline glioma, H3 K27M-mutant' (WHO grade IV), referring to infiltrative midline HGGs with predominantly astrocytic differentiation that primarily affect children, harbouring highly specific mutations in histone genes (see the section 'Biology'). On morphology/immunohistochemistry, these tumours can show low- to high-grade histology with equally poor outcomes, clearly discerning them from non-histone-mutated LGGs. This new pathological entity not only relates to tumours that have been termed 'diffuse intrinsic pontine glioma' (DIPG), but also to diffuse gliomas in non-pontine midline structures such as the thalamus, medulla oblongata, or spinal cord. Initially thought to only occur in paediatric high-grade astrocytic tumours, the histological spectrum of CNS tumours with H3 K27M mutations has recently been expanded to lower-grade lesions and rare instances of posterior fossa ependymomas.

Although paediatric HGGs are rare compared to their adult counterparts, they altogether add up to be one of the most common malignant childhood CNS tumours, with an age-adjusted incidence of 0.26 per 100,000. This might also be an underestimation, as tumours classified as H3 K27-mutant diffuse midline gliomas might have previously been classified as low-grade malignant/diffuse astrocytomas (or not have been biopsied at all), and another fraction might previously have been classified as CNS-primitive neuroectodermal tumours, a term describing a heterogeneous group of CNS neoplasms and no longer used in the WHO classification.

Due to their critical anatomical location precluding surgical resection, the diagnosis of DIPG has historically been based on the combination of characteristic clinical symptoms (signs of brainstem dysfunction and/or CSF obstruction, developing over a short period of time) and radiological parameters (large, expansile, often asymmetrical brainstem mass occupying more than two thirds of the pons). Reintroducing safe stereotactic biopsies in these pontine tumours has led to the identification of pathognomonic DNA mutations (H3 K27M; see the section 'Biology') that also occur across other midline locations, and that now serve as robust molecular markers for pathological diagnosis with additional prognostic value.

Both anaplastic astrocytomas and glioblastomas, as well as diffuse midline gliomas, may manifest at initial clinical presentation with a 'gliomatosis cerebri pattern'—an extremely diffuse phenotype, with the affected area ranging from most of one cerebral hemisphere (three lobes or more) to both cerebral hemispheres with additional involvement of the brainstem, cerebellum, and spinal cord. Since gliomatosis cerebri is lacking a unique underlying molecular biology, it is considered a more invasive phenotype of HGG (rather than a distinct nosological entity). The mechanisms by which these tumours display this extensively diffuse phenotype are yet unknown.

Biology

Recent collaborative efforts directed at the underlying molecular biology of paediatric HGG have unravelled fundamental differences compared to other CNS neoplasms arising in both adults and children, highlighted by the discovery of somatic histone mutations in up to 50% of these tumours, affecting key residues for post-translational histone tail modification.

The majority of diffuse midline gliomas in the brainstem (more than 85%), thalamus (about 50%), and spinal cord (about 60%) harbour mutations at position 27 (K27M; lysine replaced by methionine) in genes coding for histone variants H3.3 (*H3F3A*; about 75%) and H3.1 (*HIST1H3B/C*; about 25%), or rare variations. Independent of which histone 3 variant is affected, the K27M-mutant protein inhibits polycomb repressive complex 2 (PRC2) activity—via sequestration of its catalytic subunit EZH2—resulting in a global decrease of H3 K27 trimethylation (which can serve as a molecular surrogate marker). The exact downstream processes driving the evolution of H3 K27M-mutated gliomas remain to be elucidated, but likely involve other non-recurrent mutations targeting the epigenetic machinery such as members of the lysine-specific methyltransferase (KMT), lysine-specific demethylase (KDM), and chromodomain helicase DNA-binding protein (CHD) families. Additional mutations in canonical cancer pathways target the receptor tyrosine kinase/RAS/PI3K pathway (e.g. mutations in *PDGFRA, PIK3CA, PIK3R1*, or *PTEN*; occurring in about 50% of tumours), the p53 pathway (e.g. mutations in *TP53, PPM1D, CHEK2*, or *ATM*; occurring in about 70% of tumours), and the retinoblastoma protein pathway. Structural variations across diffuse midline gliomas include focal gene amplifications of *PDGFRA, MYC/MYCN, CDK4/6, CCND1–3, ID2*, or *MET*.

Location-specific patterns of genetic alterations and clinical characteristics suggest biological diversity within diffuse midline K27M-mutated gliomas. Tumours harbouring H3.3 mutations develop across midline structures (co-occurring with *FGFR1* mutations in some thalamic gliomas), typically affect children aged seven to ten years, and are associated with very poor outcome. In contrast, H3.1 mutations are largely restricted to diffuse pontine gliomas with earlier onset (four to six years), have been associated with distinct clinicopathological and radiological features as well as a slightly better prognosis, and frequently co-occur with mutations in *ACVR1*.

Up to one third of non-midline paediatric HGGs carry mutations at position 34 (G34R/V; glycine replaced by arginine/valine) in the *H3F3A* gene (encoding histone 3.3), the exact molecular consequences of which are not yet fully understood. However, associations with mutations in *ATRX* and/or *DAXX* and subtelomeric DNA hypomethylation point towards a role for telomerase-independent telomere maintenance mechanisms (i.e. alternative lengthening of telomeres; ALT) in this subset of tumours, in which mutations in *TP53* and *MGMT* promoter methylation are also commonly observed. Restricted to hemispheric locations, H3.3 G34R/V-mutated gliomas manifest during adolescence or young adulthood

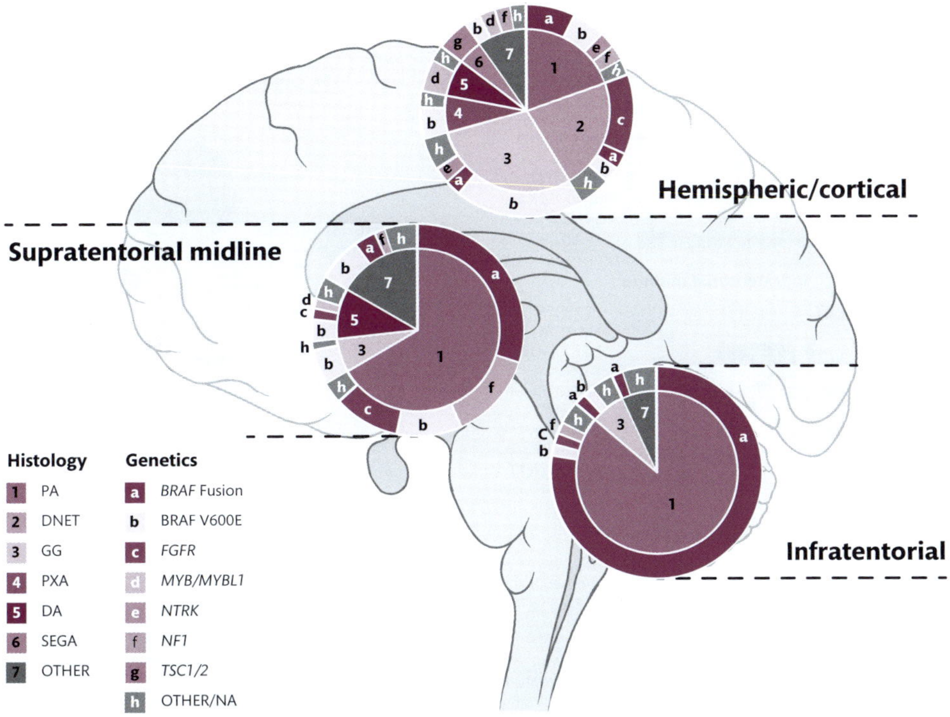

Figure 22.1 Distribution of paediatric low-grade glioma histologies and molecular genetic alterations by anatomical tumour location. Inner pie charts represent relative frequencies of the most common paediatric low-grade glioma histological entities, indicated by different shading. Outer rings represent the most common molecular genetic alterations associated with each histological entity in a given location.

DA, diffuse astrocytoma; DNET, dysembryoplastic neuroepithelial tumour; GG, ganglioglioma; PA, pilocytic astrocytoma; PXA, pleomorphic xanthoastrocytoma; SEGA, subependymal giant-cell astrocytoma.

Adapted with permission from Sturm D, et al. 'Pediatric Gliomas: Current Concepts on Diagnosis, Biology, and Clinical Management'. *Journal of Clinical Oncology*, Volume 35, Issue 21, pp. 2370–2377. DOI: 10.1200/JCO.2017.73.0242

(10–25 years) and are associated with prolonged overall survival compared with other HGGs.

A minor fraction (less than 5%) of hemispheric HGGs in older adolescents display hotspot mutations in *IDH1/2* genes—a *quasi*-defining hallmark of secondary glioblastomas and lower-grade diffuse gliomas from which they develop—and therefore represent the lower-age spectrum of gliomas in young adults (40–50 years) that are enriched in the frontal lobe and share the overall best prognosis.

The associations of hotspot mutations in histone (H3.3/H3.1) and *IDH1/2* genes with anatomical location, patient age, and outcome have led to our understanding of distinct biological variants of (paediatric) HGG (Figure 22.2). Each of these variants displays a unique DNA methylation pattern thought to be an imprint of different cell-of-origin populations during neurodevelopment, and shaped by mutations rewiring their epigenome.

The remaining proportion of non-H3/non-IDH-mutated HGGs (less than 50%) is likely to include further biological subtypes, some of which might be driven by *MYC(N)* amplifications, receptor tyrosine kinase amplifications, *BRAF* mutations, or fusion events involving, for example, *NTRK* or *FGFR* genes. However, there are a substantial number of paediatric malignant gliomas with relatively stable genomic profiles for which the molecular mechanisms underlying gliomagenesis are yet to be elucidated.

Current treatment strategies

The treatment of paediatric HGG patients is challenging. For patients suffering from DIPG and other WHO grade IV diffuse midline gliomas, resection is not an option. Radiotherapy is considered to be the standard, albeit palliative care modality in these patients, improving PFS and OS by some months and positively influencing quality of life. Although not investigated in randomized studies and distilled from retrospective data, chemotherapy in addition to radiotherapy seems to convey a minor benefit in PFS and OS. Very rarely, long-term survival is reported in these diseases.

For supratentorial HGG, standard therapy consists of multimodal treatment combining maximal resection, post-operative conformal (chemo-) radiotherapy, and adjuvant chemotherapy. Neurosurgical resection of supratentorial and spinal paediatric HGG is an important part of therapy, as the extent of tumour resection is positively correlated with long-term survival. As HGGs invade brain tissue beyond the tumour margins visible on MRI, maximal surgery alone is not considered curative, necessitating adjuvant radio- and chemotherapy. Since the 1960s, radiation therapy (RT) adjuvant to surgery has been the mainstay of therapy, improving survival, although not proven in a randomized fashion. Focal radiation of 54 Gy is usually employed in fractions of 1.8–2 Gy, with boosts up to 59.4 Gy to residual tumour. Intensification of radiotherapy by hyperfractionation to a total dose of 72 Gy has failed to improve outcome. New radiotherapy techniques, such as intensity-modulated radiation therapy (IMRT) and proton-beam radiotherapy, have been developed to allow for more precise delivery to the tumour bed while sparing normal brain tissue, but the efficacy in the context of diffusely infiltrating gliomas needs to be ascertained.

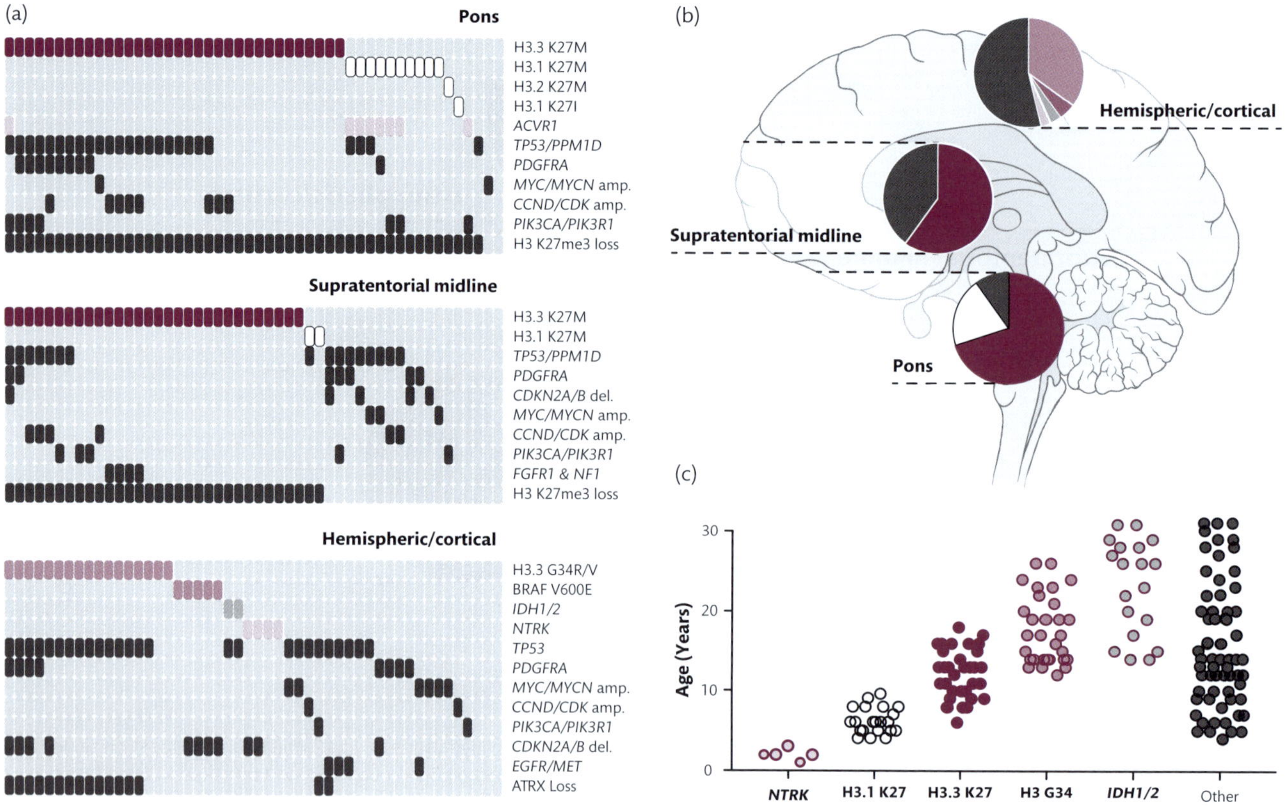

Figure 22.2 Molecular patterns and clinical features of paediatric high-grade glioma subgroups. (A) Oncoprints schematically depicting selected common molecular alterations in paediatric high-grade gliomas by anatomical location. Shaded boxes indicate alterations being present. (B) Pie charts representing relative frequencies of common paediatric high-grade glioma molecular alterations represented by shading corresponding to (A) and (C). (C) Age distribution of common paediatric high-grade glioma molecular alterations in children and young adults (age younger than 30 years).

amp, amplification; del, deletion

Adapted with permission from Sturm D, et al. 'Pediatric Gliomas: Current Concepts on Diagnosis, Biology, and Clinical Management'. *Journal of Clinical Oncology*, Volume 35, Issue 21, pp. 2370–2377. Copyright © 2017 American Society of Clinical Oncology. All rights reserved. DOI: 10.1200/JCO.2017.73.0242

Because of its detrimental neurological long-term sequelae, especially in tumours situated supratentorially, radiotherapy is usually either omitted or postponed in children under four years of age, and replaced by high-dose chemotherapy regimens. Although profound evidence of efficacy is lacking, most children suffering from HGGs are nowadays treated with chemotherapy concomitant and adjuvant to radiotherapy, based on experiences in adult HGG. In the late 1980s, the Children's Cancer Group (CCG) showed improved survival in a first randomized study (CCG-943) for paediatric patients with non-brainstem anaplastic astrocytoma and glioblastoma treated with radiotherapy with concomitant and maintenance prednisone, CCNU (procarbazine, 6-thioguanine, dibromodulcitol, and lomustine) and vincristine (pCV), compared to radiotherapy alone. Glioblastoma multiforme (GBM) patients seemed to particularly benefit from the addition of chemotherapy. A later study of central neuropathological review of cases treated in the CCG-943 study indicated that a large proportion of patients randomized could actually be reclassified to LGGs, possibly influencing the reported survival. The subsequent randomized CCG-945 study—two cycles of post-operative pre-radiotherapy multi-drug chemotherapy (vincristine, hydroxyurea, procarbazine, CCNU, cisplatin, cytarabine, methylprednisolone, and cyclophosphamide or dacarbazine)—failed to show a benefit over the CCG-943 pCV scheme.

With significant improvement in survival reported in adults with GBM treated with temozolomide (TMZ) added to radiation and maintenance therapy, the non-randomized single-arm ACNS0126 study investigated the use of TMZ in paediatric HGG, showing equal survival rates to the more toxic CCG-943 and CCG-945 trials. Based on this study, radiochemotherapy with TMZ has been more or less considered a backbone for HGG therapy. More recently, results from the non-randomized, single-arm ACNS0423 study indicate that the reintroduction of CCNU to the backbone of TMZ-RT has a survival benefit over TMZ-RT, most notably in GBM, although survival is still poor, with a three-year PFS of 22%. Anti-angiogenesis strategies to the TMZ-RT backbone, in analogy to adult GBM studies, are currently being investigated.

In younger children in whom radiotherapy is postponed or omitted, high-dose chemotherapy with stem-cell support regimens has yielded promising results, albeit these are studies with small numbers of patients with potentially different tumour biology and/or blood–brain barrier dynamics.

Future outlook

Future studies need to be focused on analysis of retrospective and prospective paediatric HGG patient data from multiple trials, correlating clinical, radiological, pathological, and molecular biology data to treatment and outcome data. As it is more and more evident that these diffusely infiltrative diseases show large intratumoural heterogeneity, both of the tumour cells and the micro-environment, including the blood–brain barrier, research needs to be addressed at combinational (targeted) treatment strategies. Novel drug targeting and delivery systems, such as convection-enhanced, interstitial delivery of drugs and oncolytic viruses, and focused ultrasound-assisted (nanocarrier-mediated) drug delivery, as well as immunotherapies, are of particular interest in this respect.

FURTHER READING

Adamski J, et al. (2014) Advances in the management of paediatric high-grade glioma. *Curr Oncol Rep* **16**, 414.

Ater JL, et al. (2016) Nonrandomized comparison of neurofibromatosis type 1 and non-neurofibromatosis type 1 children who received carboplatin and vincristine for progressive low-grade glioma: a report from the Children's Oncology Group. *Cancer* **122**, 1928–36.

Ater JL, et al. (2012) Randomized study of two chemotherapy regimens for treatment of low-grade glioma in young children: a report from the Children's Oncology Group. *J Clin Oncol* **30**, 2641–7.

Bandopadhayay P, et al. (2014) Long-term outcome of 4,040 children diagnosed with pediatric low-grade gliomas: an analysis of the Surveillance Epidemiology and End Results (SEER) database. *Pediatr Blood Cancer* **61**, 1173–9.

Bandopadhayay P, et al. (2016) MYB-QKI rearrangements in angiocentric glioma drive tumorigenicity through a tripartite mechanism. *Nat Genet* **48**, 273–82.

Banerjee A, et al. (2017) A phase I trial of the MEK inhibitor selumetinib (AZD6244) in pediatric patients with recurrent or refractory low-grade glioma: a Pediatric Brain Tumor Consortium (PBTC) study. *Neuro Oncol* **19**(8), 1135–44.

Blumcke I, et al. (2014) A neuropathology-based approach to epilepsy surgery in brain tumors and proposal for a new terminology use for long-term epilepsy-associated brain tumors. *Acta Neuropathol* **128**, 39–54.

Brada M, Haylock B (2014) Is current technology improving outcomes with radiation therapy for gliomas? *Am Soc Clin Oncol Educ Book* e89–94. doi: 10.14694/EdBook_AM.2014.34.e89

Broniscer A, Gajjar A (2004) Supratentorial high-grade astrocytoma and diffuse brainstem glioma: two challenges for the pediatric oncologist. *Oncologist* **9**, 197–206.

Broniscer A, et al. (2016) Gliomatosis cerebri in children shares molecular characteristics with other pediatric gliomas. *Acta Neuropathol* **131**, 299–307.

Cappellano AM, et al. (2015) Single agent vinorelbine in pediatric patients with progressive optic pathway glioma. *J Neurooncol* **121**, 405–12.

Castel D, et al. (2015) Histone H3F3A and HIST1H3B K27M mutations define two subgroups of diffuse intrinsic pontine gliomas with different prognosis and phenotypes. *Acta Neuropathol* **130**, 815–27.

Chamdine O, et al. (2016) Metastatic low-grade gliomas in children: 20 years' experience at St Jude Children's Research Hospital. *Pediatr Blood Cancer* **63**, 62–70.

Chappe C, et al. (2013) Dysembryoplastic neuroepithelial tumors share with pleomorphic xanthoastrocytomas and gangliogliomas BRAF(V600E) mutation and expression. *Brain Pathol* **23**, 574–83.

Chintagumpala M, et al. (2015) A pilot study using carboplatin, vincristine, and temozolomide in children with progressive/symptomatic low-grade glioma: a Children's Oncology Group study dagger. *Neuro Oncol* **17**, 1132–8.

Cohen KJ, et al. (2011) Temozolomide in the treatment of high-grade gliomas in children: a report from the Children's Oncology Group. *Neuro Oncol* **13**, 317–23.

Dodgshun AJ, et al. (2016) Single agent carboplatin for pediatric low-grade glioma: a retrospective analysis shows equivalent efficacy to multiagent chemotherapy. *Int J Cancer* **138**, 481–8.

Dohrmann GJ, et al. (1976) Glioblastoma multiforme in children. *J Neurosurg* **44**, 442–8.

Dougherty MJ, et al. (2010) Activating mutations in BRAF characterize a spectrum of pediatric low-grade gliomas. *Neuro Oncol* **12**, 621–30.

Fangusaro J (2012) Pediatric high grade glioma: a review and update on tumor clinical characteristics and biology. *Front Oncol* **2**, 105.

Fangusaro J, et al. (2019) Selumetinib in paediatric patients with BRAF-aberrant or neurofibromatosis type 1-associated recurrent, refractory, or progressive low-grade glioma: a multicentre, phase 2 trial. *Lancet Oncol* **20**(7), 1011–22. doi: 10.1016/S1470-2045(19)30277-3.

Fisher PG, et al. (2008) Outcome analysis of childhood low-grade astrocytomas. *Pediatr Blood Cancer* **51**, 245–50.

Fouladi M, et al. (2003) Outcome of children with centrally reviewed low-grade gliomas treated with chemotherapy with or without radiotherapy on Children's Cancer Group high-grade glioma study CCG-945. *Cancer* **98**, 1243–52.

Franz DN, et al. (2013) Efficacy and safety of everolimus for subependymal giant cell astrocytomas associated with tuberous sclerosis complex (EXIST-1): a multicentre, randomised, placebo-controlled phase 3 trial. *Lancet* **381**, 125–32.

Fulton DS, et al. (1992) Increasing radiation dose intensity using hyperfractionation in patients with malignant glioma. Final report of a prospective phase I-II dose response study. *J Neurooncol* **14**, 63–72.

Gessi M, et al. (2016) Evidence of H3 K27M mutations in posterior fossa ependymomas. *Acta Neuropathol* **132**, 635–7.

Gnekow AK, et al. (2012) Long-term follow-up of the multicenter, multidisciplinary treatment study HIT-LGG-1996 for low-grade glioma in children and adolescents of the German Speaking Society of Pediatric Oncology and Hematology. *Neuro-Oncology*, **14**, 1265–84.

Gnekow AK, et al. (2004) Low grade chiasmatic-hypothalamic glioma-carboplatin and vincristin chemotherapy effectively defers radiotherapy within a comprehensive treatment strategy—report from the multicenter treatment study for children and adolescents with a low grade glioma—HIT-LGG 1996—of the Society of Pediatric Oncology and Hematology (GPOH). *Klin Padiatr* **216**, 331–42.

Greenberger BA, et al. (2014) Clinical outcomes and late endocrine, neurocognitive, and visual profiles of proton radiation for pediatric low-grade gliomas. *Int J Radiat Oncol Biol Phys* **89**, 1060–8.

Grill J, et al. (1999) Radiation-induced cerebral vasculopathy in children with neurofibromatosis and optic pathway glioma. *Ann Neurol* **45**, 393–6.

Gururangan S, et al. (2014) Efficacy of bevacizumab plus irinotecan in children with recurrent low-grade gliomas—a Pediatric Brain Tumor Consortium study. *Neuro Oncol* **16**, 310–17.

Gururangan S, et al. (2007) Temozolomide in children with progressive low-grade glioma. *Neuro Oncol* **9**, 161–8.

Hargrave D, et al. (2006) Diffuse brainstem glioma in children: critical review of clinical trials. *Lancet Oncol* **7**, 241–8.

Hersh DS, et al. (2016) Emerging applications of therapeutic ultrasound in neuro-oncology: moving beyond tumor ablation. *Neurosurgery* **79**, 643–54.

Hutt-Cabezas M, et al. (2013) Activation of mTORC1/mTORC2 signaling in pediatric low-grade glioma and pilocytic astrocytoma reveals mTOR as a therapeutic target. *Neuro Oncol* **15**, 1604–14.

Jakacki RI, et al. (2011) A phase 1 study of vinblastine in combination with carboplatin for children with low-grade gliomas: a Children's Oncology Group phase 1 consortium study. *Neuro Oncol* **13**, 910–15.

Jakacki RI, et al. (2016) Phase 2 study of concurrent radiotherapy and temozolomide followed by temozolomide and lomustine in the treatment of children with high-grade glioma: a report of the Children's Oncology Group ACNS0423 study. *Neuro Oncol* **18**, 1442–50.

Jansen MH, et al. (2012) Diffuse intrinsic pontine gliomas: a systematic update on clinical trials and biology. *Cancer Treat Rev* **38**, 27–35.

Jansen MH, et al. (2015) Survival prediction model of children with diffuse intrinsic pontine glioma based on clinical and radiological criteria. *Neuro Oncol* **17**, 160–6.

Jaspan T, et al. (2016) Response assessment in pediatric neuro-oncology: implementation and expansion of the RANO criteria in a randomized phase II trial of pediatric patients with newly diagnosed high-grade gliomas. *Am J Neuroradiol* **37**, 1581–7.

Johansson G, et al. (2016) Recent developments in brain tumor predisposing syndromes. *Acta Oncol* **55**, 401–11.

Jones C, Baker SJ (2014) Unique genetic and epigenetic mechanisms driving paediatric diffuse high-grade glioma. *Nat Rev Cancer* **14**(10). doi: 10.1038/nrc3811

Jones DT, et al. (2013) Recurrent somatic alterations of FGFR1 and NTRK2 in pilocytic astrocytoma. *Nat Genet* **45**, 927–32.

Jones DT, et al. (2008) Tandem duplication producing a novel oncogenic BRAF fusion gene defines the majority of pilocytic astrocytomas. *Cancer Res* **68**, 8673–7.

Kalra M, et al. (2015) Confirmation of bevacizumab activity, and maintenance of efficacy in retreatment after subsequent relapse, in pediatric low-grade glioma. *J Pediatr Hematol Oncol* **37**, e341–46.

Karajannis MA, et al. (2014) Phase II study of sorafenib in children with recurrent or progressive low-grade astrocytomas. *Neuro Oncol* **16**, 1408–16.

Karim R, et al. (2016) Nanocarriers for the treatment of glioblastoma multiforme: current state-of-the-art. *J Control Release* **227**, 23–37.

Kieran MW, et al. (2016) The first study of dabrafenib in pediatric patients with BRAF V600—mutant relapsed or refractory low-grade gliomas. *Ann Oncol* **27**(Suppl 6), LBA19_PR. *of Oncology*, Volume 27, Issue suppl_6, 1 October 2016, LBA19_PR. doi.org/10.1093/annonc/mdw435.09

Krueger DA, et al. (2010) Everolimus for subependymal giant-cell astrocytomas in tuberous sclerosis. *N Engl J Med* **363**, 1801–11.

Lassaletta A, et al. (2016) Profound clinical and radiological response to BRAF inhibition in a 2-month-old diencephalic child with hypothalamic/chiasmatic glioma. *Pediatr Blood Cancer* **63**, 2038–41.

Lassaletta A, et al. (2016) Phase II weekly vinblastine for chemotherapy-naive children with progressive low-grade glioma: a Canadian Pediatric Brain Tumor Consortium Study. *J Clin Oncol* **34**(29), 3537–43.

Lassaletta A, et al. (2016) An integrative molecular and genomic analysis of pediatric hemispheric low-grade gliomas: an update. *Childs Nerv Syst* **32**, 1789–97.

Lewis PW, et al. (2013) Inhibition of PRC2 activity by a gain-of-function H3 mutation found in pediatric glioblastoma. *Science* **340**, 857–61.

Listernick R, et al. (1999) Intracranial gliomas in neurofibromatosis type 1. *Am J Med Genet* **89**, 38–44.

Louis DN, et al. (2016) *WHO Classification of Tumours of the Central Nervous System*. Switzerland: WHO Press.

Massimino M, et al. (2010) Is there a role for myeloablative chemotherapy with autologous hematopoietic cell rescue in the management of childhood high-grade astrocytomas? *Pediatr Blood Cancer* **54**, 641–3.

Merchant TE, et al. (2009) Late effects of conformal radiation therapy for pediatric patients with low-grade glioma: prospective evaluation of cognitive, endocrine, and hearing deficits. *J Clin Oncol* **27**, 3691–7.

Miller C, et al. (2017) Report of effective trametinib therapy in 2 children with progressive hypothalamic optic pathway pilocytic astrocytoma: documentation of volumetric response. *J Neurosurg Pediatr* **19**, 319–24.

Northrup H, et al. (2013) Tuberous sclerosis complex diagnostic criteria update: recommendations of the 2012 International Tuberous Sclerosis Complex Consensus Conference. *Pediatr Neurol* **49**, 243–54.

Olow A, et al. (2016) BRAF status in personalizing treatment approaches for pediatric gliomas. *Clin Cancer Res* **22**, 5312–21.

Ostrom QT, et al. (2016) CBTRUS statistical report: primary brain and other central nervous system tumors diagnosed in the United States in 2009–2013. *Neuro-Oncology*, **18**, v1–75.

Packer RJ, et al. (1997) Carboplatin and vincristine chemotherapy for children with newly diagnosed progressive low-grade gliomas. *J Neurosurg* **86**, 747–54.

Packer RJ, et al. (2009) Objective response of multiple recurrent low-grade gliomas to bevacizumab and irinotecan. *Pediatr Blood Cancer* **52**, 791–5.

Qaddoumi I, et al. (2016) Genetic alterations in uncommon low-grade neuroepithelial tumors: BRAF, FGFR1, and MYB mutations occur at high frequency and align with morphology. *Acta Neuropathol* **131**, 833–45.

Ramkissoon LA, et al. (2013) Genomic analysis of diffuse pediatric low-grade gliomas identifies recurrent oncogenic truncating rearrangements in the transcription factor MYBL1. *Proc Natl Acad Sci USA* **110**, 8188–93.

Sanders RP, et al. (2007) High-grade astrocytoma in very young children. *Pediatr Blood Cancer* **49**, 888–93.

Schindler G, et al. (2011) Analysis of BRAF V600E mutation in 1,320 nervous system tumors reveals high mutation frequencies in pleomorphic xanthoastrocytoma, ganglioglioma and extra-cerebellar pilocytic astrocytoma. *Acta Neuropathol* **121**, 397–405.

Schwartzentruber J, et al. (2012) Driver mutations in histone H3.3 and chromatin remodelling genes in paediatric glioblastoma. *Nature* **482**, 226–31.

Sievert AJ, et al. (2013) Paradoxical activation and RAF inhibitor resistance of BRAF protein kinase fusions characterizing pediatric astrocytomas. *Proc Natl Acad Sci USA* **110**, 5957–62.

Skrypek M, et al. (2014) Pilomyxoid astrocytoma treated successfully with vemurafenib. *Pediatr Blood Cancer* **61**, 2099–100.

Stokland T, et al. (2010) A multivariate analysis of factors determining tumor progression in childhood low-grade glioma: a population-based cohort study (CCLG CNS9702). *Neuro Oncol* **12**, 1257–68.

Stupp R, et al. (2005) Radiotherapy plus concomitant and adjuvant temozolomide for glioblastoma. *N Engl J Med* **352**, 987–96.

Sturm D, et al. (2014) Paediatric and adult glioblastoma: multiform (epi)genomic culprits emerge. *Nat Rev Cancer* **14**, 92–107.

Sturm D, et al. (2016) New brain tumor entities emerge from molecular classification of CNS-PNETs. *Cell* **164**, 1060–72.

Sturm D, et al. (2017) Pediatric gliomas: current concepts on diagnosis, biology, and clinical management. *J Clin Oncol* **35**(21), 2370–7.

Sturm D, et al. (2012) Hotspot mutations in H3F3A and IDH1 define distinct epigenetic and biological subgroups of glioblastoma. *Cancer Cell* **22**, 425–37.

Tatevossian RG, et al. (2010) MYB upregulation and genetic aberrations in a subset of pediatric low-grade gliomas. *Acta Neuropathol* **120**, 731–43.

Vanan MI, Eisenstat DD (2014) Management of high-grade gliomas in the pediatric patient: Past, present, and future. *Neuro-Oncol Pract* **1**, 145–57.

Vogelbaum MA, Aghi MK (2015) Convection-enhanced delivery for the treatment of glioblastoma. *Neuro Oncol* **17**(Suppl 2), ii3–ii8.

Weber RG, et al. (2007) Frequent loss of chromosome 9, homozygous CDKN2A/p14(ARF)/CDKN2B deletion and low TSC1 mRNA expression in pleomorphic xanthoastrocytomas. *Oncogene* **26**, 1088–97.

Willard VW, et al. (2015) Prospective longitudinal evaluation of emotional and behavioral functioning in pediatric patients with low-grade glioma treated with conformal radiation therapy. *J Neuro-oncol* **122**, 161–8.

Wisoff JH, et al. (2011) Primary neurosurgery for pediatric low-grade gliomas: a prospective multi-institutional study from the Children's Oncology Group. *Neurosurgery* **68**, 1548–54.

Wu G, et al. (2012) Somatic histone H3 alterations in pediatric diffuse intrinsic pontine gliomas and non-brainstem glioblastomas. *Nat Genet* **44**, 251–3.

Wu G, et al. (2014) The genomic landscape of diffuse intrinsic pontine glioma and pediatric non-brainstem high-grade glioma. *Nat Genet* **46**, 444–50.

Zhang J, et al. (2013) Whole-genome sequencing identifies genetic alterations in pediatric low-grade gliomas. *Nat Genet* **45**, 602–12.

Zhang X, et al. (2016) Targeting immune checkpoints in malignant glioma. *Oncotarget* **8**(4), 7157–74.

Zuccaro G, et al. (1986) Intracranial neoplasms during the first year of life. *Surg Neurol* **26**, 29–36.

23 Embryonal Tumours

Maura Massimino, Eric Bouffet, and Vijay Ramaswamy

Introduction and epidemiology

Among the various tumours of the central nervous system (CNS) occurring in childhood, 20% are medulloblastomas (MB). The disease has an annual incidence of 5–6.8 per million children (aged 0–14 years) in the USA and Europe. Higher rates are observed in Southern and Central Europe. The disease has a higher incidence in boys. Embryonal tumours represented 23.2% of all cases seen at the Children's Cancer Hospital in Egypt between 2007 and 2013, similar to Europe and North America. Some genetic disorders that predispose patients to cancer, including Turcot (APC mutation), Li–Fraumeni (TP53 mutations), and Rubinstein–Taybi (CREB/BP mutation) syndromes, mismatch repair deficiency (PMS2, MLH1, MSH2, or MSH6 mutations), and abnormalities in the 'sonic hedgehog' (SHH) pathway (Gorlin syndrome with PTCH1 mutation, SUFU mutations), are associated with an increased risk of MB.

The one-, three-, and five-year survival rates among European children with MB diagnosed from 2000 to 2007 were 81%, 63%, and 56%, respectively. Survival rates remained much the same during the period between 1999 and 2007, having improved before the end of the 1990s. Very recent data from the American National Cancer Data Base indicate that five-year overall survival (OS) is around 82% for children with no metastases who are treated with post-operative radiotherapy.

The incidence and epidemiology of non-MB and non-atypical teratoid rhabdoid (ATR) CNS embryonal tumours, known as 'other CNS embryonal tumours' (and previously as primitive neuroectodermal tumours (PNETs)) is extraordinarily difficult to discern. Best estimates suggest they represent approximately 2–3% of all paediatric brain tumours. Due to their heterogeneity and diagnostic uncertainty, their incidence is unclear, varying significantly by study. This has led to the removal of 'other CNS embryonal tumours' from the 2016 revised World Health Organization (WHO) classification of CNS tumours. Moreover, entities comprising CNS embryonal tumours vary tremendously in outcome, with ETMRs (embryonal tumours with multilayered rosettes) having a dismal prognosis, while survival in other CNS embryonal tumours ranges from 17–60%.

The incidence and epidemiology of atypical teratoid rhabdoid tumours (ATRTs) is also difficult to discern. In the USA, the best estimate is 0.12 per 100,000 children, accounting for 2–3% of all paediatric brain tumours, but is predominantly diagnosed in children under the age of three. An additional difficulty in discerning the incidence of ATRTs is that prior to the late 1990s, they were commonly diagnosed as MBs or CNS-PNETs, as *SMARCB1* loss as its defining feature had not been well established. ATRTs can be familial in up to 25% due to germline inactivating lesions in *SMARCB1*. Until recently, there have been no dedicated data pertaining to either demographics or survival of ATRTs. The most recent issue of the Central Brain Tumour Registry of the United States (CBTRUS) estimates five-year survival to be 12.1% in those under one year of age and 33.9% in those over one year of age.

Diagnosis

The differential diagnoses of posterior fossa tumours include MB, cerebellar astrocytoma, ependymoma, brainstem glioma, and ATRT. Computed tomography (CT) is often the first choice for neuroimaging because of its availability in an emergency setting. A typical picture of MB on CT is a midline, homogeneous, contrast-enhancing cerebellar vermian mass. Follow-on magnetic resonance imaging (MRI) is needed before any surgery, and typically shows a heterogeneous hypointense mass on T1-weighted images. Contrast enhancement is usually heterogeneous. Up to 40% of patients have spinal metastases, best seen on post-contrast images, making spinal MRI essential before any adjuvant treatment.

It has been suggested recently that MRI features can distinguish between different histological subtypes and molecular subgroups of MB: WNT tumours occur frequently in the cerebellar peduncle and cerebellar-pontine angle, while SHH tumours arise in the cerebellar hemispheres; and Group 3 and 4 tumours predominate within the midline fourth ventricle. Midline Group 4 tumours also show little or no enhancement.

On neuroimaging, the appearance of CNS-PNET is highly variable, although usually displaying restricted diffusion (Figure 23.1). Controversy has always existed as to whether CNS-PNET truly represents one entity, and the key to diagnosis is to exclude other morphological mimics. A study by the Children's Oncology Group (COG) suggests that up to 50% of institutionally diagnosed CNS-PNETs are high-grade gliomas on centralized review, and an integrated genomic study suggests that by using a combined molecular

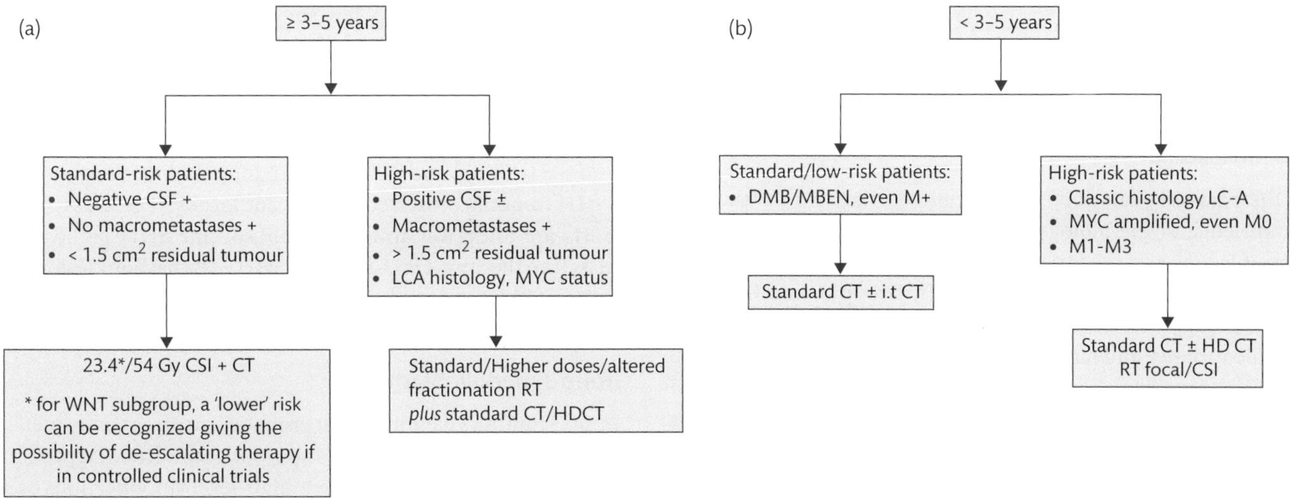

Figure 23.1 Current clinical-risk stratification employed by both European and North American Cooperative Groups. (A) Patients over the age of three to five are classified as standard risk if they have no evidence of residual disease either in the tumour bed or along the leptomeninges, and classified as high risk if they have residual disease. In some studies, large-cell/anaplastic histology and MYC amplification are also considered higher-risk features. (B) Proposed risk stratification for children under the age of three to five in the upcoming International Society of Paediatric Oncology infant medulloblastoma study. Children with desmoplastic histology and/or SHH-driven tumours are considered standard risk, and receive lower doses of chemotherapy. Children with non-desmoplastic histology and/or non-SHH-driven tumours are classified as higher risk, and proceed to either high-dose chemotherapy with autologous stem-cell support and/or external beam irradiation.

Reproduced courtesy of Maura Massimino, IRCCS National Cancer Institute Foundation, Milan, Italy

approach, up to 70% of CNS-PNETs can be reclassified as a multitude of different entities.

ATRTs can occur anywhere within the nervous system, and on neuroimaging can mimic other embryonal tumours and high-grade gliomas. Thus, as such, INI1 immunoreactivity should be determined in all malignant infant brain tumours. The diagnosis of ATRT should include renal ultrasounds to exclude extracranial rhabdoid tumours, and genetic counselling to determine germline SMARCB1 status. In rare instances, INI1 immunoreactivity is retained with either functional loss of INI1 or mutations in SMARCA4.

Pathology

The recent WHO classification of CNS tumours acknowledges both the histological classification and the biological subtypes of MB. There are four histological variants: classic, desmoplastic/nodular, MB with extensive nodularity (MBEN), and large-cell/anaplastic (LC/A) (**Figure 23.2**).

The combined LC/A form accounts for 10–22%, while nodular/desmoplastic MB and MBEN represent approximately 7% and 3% of cases, respectively. Classic tumours make up the remainder. Clinical data firmly support a favourable prognosis for nodular/desmoplastic MB in some age and risk groups, and especially in young children. The prognosis of the LC/A variant is significantly worse. However, the high interobserver variability of these histological subtypes significantly impairs global interpretation and clinical applicability. Currently, the biological subtypes are divided into WNT-activated, SHH-activated TP53 wild-type, SHH-activated TP53 mutant, and non-WNT/SHH with Group 3 and Group 4 listed as provisional entities. There is overlap between the histological and biological classifications, where desmoplastic and MBEN tumours are almost exclusively SHH-activated MBs, while the LC/A variant is enriched for very high-risk biological groups, specifically high-risk Group 3 and TP53-mutated SHH. The prognostic of LC/A in WNT and Group 4 is unclear.

The revised 2016 WHO classification has removed CNS-PNET as a distinct entity and replaced it with CNS neuroblastoma, CNS ganglioneuroblastoma, and CNS embryonal tumour not otherwise specified (NOS). ETMR is now accepted as a distinct entity defined by an amplification of a microRNA cluster on chromosome 19. ATRT is described as mixed small blue-cell tumour and rhabdoid cells, characterized by loss of INI1/BAF47 immunoreactivity. A small proportion of ATRTs have retained INI1/BAF47 immunoreactivity,

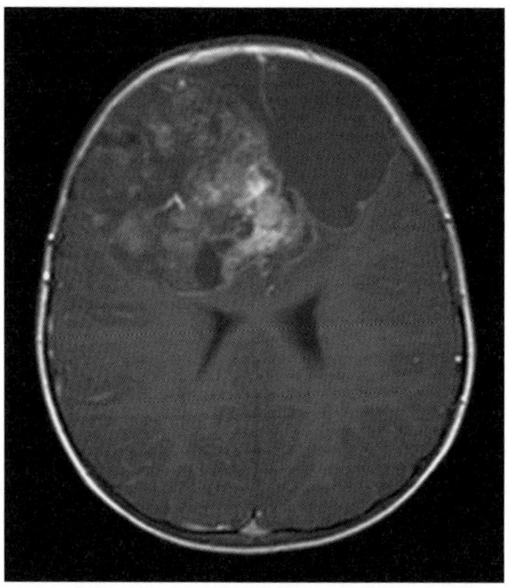

Figure 23.2 MRI of CNS embryonal tumour: axial T1-enhanced image of the entity (formerly termed CNS-PNET) showing a heterogeneously enhancing mass in the left frontal lobe with associated cyst.

Reproduced courtesy of Maura Massimino, IRCCS National Cancer Institute Foundation, Milan, Italy

with functional loss of the *SMARCB1* gene or mutations in the *SMARCA4* gene.

Biology

Medulloblastoma

Over the past ten years there have been considerable advances in our knowledge of the biology of MB. Historically considered one disease, it is now accepted that MB actually comprises four distinct molecular subgroups termed WNT, SHH, Group 3, and Group 4. These subgroups have distinct demographics, cytogenetics, somatic nucleotide variants, and outcomes, and are now included in the 2016 revised WHO classification of CNS tumours. The clinical utility of molecular subgrouping is apparent when applying risk-stratification schemes, which are significantly more robust than standard-risk stratification when incorporating subgrouping, and will form the basis of future clinical trials.

WNT medulloblastoma

WNT tumours are unique in that they have an excellent prognosis across many studies, where survival consistently approaches 95% in patients under the age of 16. Biologically, they are characterized by activation of the WNT pathway, resulting in nuclear translocation of beta-catenin. WNT tumours have a relatively quiet genome with mutations in exon 3 of the gene coding for b-catenin (CTNNB1) being the most frequent aberration, followed by monosomy 6. Less frequently, TP53 and DDX3X mutations are observed. WNT tumours can be diagnosed using a variety of methods including direct sequencing of exon 3 of CTNNB1, methylation profiling, or gene-expression profiling. Immunohistochemistry showing nuclear beta-catenin immunoreactivity is a hallmark of WNT tumours. However, it should be used with caution and in isolation, due to false positive results. Similarly, identification of monosomy 6, while highly enriched in WNT tumours, should be used with caution.

Demographically, WNT tumours present in older children and a minority of adults. An international consensus suggests that childhood WNT tumours are now considered very low-risk tumours. They seem to have a worse prognosis in patients over the age of 16. Histologically, most WNT tumours are classic histology, although a small proportion can have LC/A histology, which is of dubious clinical significance.

SHH medulloblastoma

SHH tumours are characterized by lesions within the SHH pathway, and are thought to arise from the external granular layer, hence their cerebellar location. They are observed across all ages, and are the predominant subgroup in infants and adults. The most common aberrations are inactivating mutations of PTCH1, SMO, and SUFU and amplifications of GLI2 and MYCN. TP53 mutations (usually germline mutations) are found in children aged 3–16, and these patients have a near universally fatal prognosis, succumbing to local recurrence or, less frequently, secondary malignancies. TP53-mutated SHH usually occurs with significant genomic instability and high-level amplifications of GLI2 and MYCN.

All SHH MBs in non-infants warrant urgent testing for germline TP53 mutations in the context of Li–Fraumeni syndrome. Non-TP53-mutated SHH MBs in older children confer an excellent prognosis. Infant SHH MBs frequently harbour mutations in PTCH1 and SUFU, and display desmoplastic or MBEN histology, and integrated clustering has suggested two distinct infant SHH groups, SHH1 and SHH2, with significant differences in outcome. PTCH1 and SUFU mutations can be germline, and all infants should undergo genetic counselling for potential Gorlin syndrome. Adults with SHH medulloblastomas frequently harbour somatic mutations in PTCH1, TERT, and SMO, with an intermediate prognosis.

SHH tumours most frequently recur locally, regardless of therapy. Efforts are underway to incorporate specific SHH-pathway antagonists into therapy. TP53-mutated SHH MBs harbour lesions downstream of SMO and are unlikely to respond to the current generation of SHH inhibitors.

Group 3 medulloblastoma

Group 3 tumours have the worst prognosis, are frequently metastatic, and occur mainly in infants and young children. Approximately 20% of Group 3 tumours harbour high-level amplifications of MYC, are frequently metastatic, and comprise a very high-risk group. Histologically, Group 3 are frequently LCA/anaplastic and are likely associated with MYC amplifications. Other aberrations in Group 3 include OTX2 amplifications, isochromosome 17q, gains of ACVR1/2, and activation of GFI1/GFI1b through enhancer hijacking. Infant Group 3 patients pose a particularly difficult challenge. However, recent studies have suggested that survival for non-metastatic Group 3 can approach 40–50% using high-dose chemotherapy (HDCT) with autologous stem-cell transplantation (ASCT), such as the CCG99703 protocol. Metastatic Group 3 have a dismal prognosis, particularly in infants.

Recent drug screening has suggested pemetrexed and gemcitabine as rationale therapies for Group 3 patients—a combination currently being evaluated in the SJMB12 study. Panobinostat has also been proposed as a Group 3 specific therapy. Irradiated Group 3 patients almost exclusively recur with metastatic dissemination, usually with a tumour bed devoid of disease, suggesting that future therapies need to be tailored to the metastatic compartment.

Group 4 medulloblastoma

Group 4 tumours comprise over 40% of all patients, and are primarily observed between the ages of three and seventeen. They are usually of classic histology, although it is unclear what the significance of anaplasia is in this group. Group 4 are frequently metastatic, portending to a worse prognosis, although non-metastatic Group 4 patients with loss of chromosome 11 have an excellent prognosis and are now considered very low-risk patients. Nearly 80% of Group 4 tumours harbour isochromosome 17q, with less frequent aberrations being amplifications of CDK6, MYCN, chromosome 7q gain, and chromosome 8p loss. KDM6A mutations are the most common recurrent SNV, occurring in 10% of patients, and tandem duplications of SNCAIP are found in 20% of Group 4 patients. Unlike SHH, the presence of MYCN amplifications in Group 4 confers no prognostic significance. Infant and adult Group 4, while rare, appear to have a poor prognosis, and similar to Group 3, irradiated Group 4 patients recur almost exclusively with metastatic dissemination.

Other embryonal tumours

The first suggestion that PNET was not a single entity was a gene-expression study of medulloblastoma, ATRT, and PNET, in which PNETs did not form a clear cluster on their own. Further work suggested that a proportion of PNETs harbour high-level amplifications of a microRNA cluster on chromosome 19, and should be considered a distinct entity known as ETMR/ETANTR (embryonal tumour with abundant neuropil and true rosettes). ETMRs arise in very young children and have a dismal prognosis. An integrated genomic study of PNET showed that it comprises three groups, with one group harbouring the C19MC amplicon. Further work has shown that up to 70% of institutionally diagnosed PNET can be reclassified as another entity after careful molecular analysis. As such, the diagnosis of PNET should include evaluation for RELA fusion for ependymoma, SMARCB1 alterations for ATRT, G34V and K27M mutations for high-grade glioma, and C19MC amplicon for ETMR. Genome-wide methylation profiling is emerging as a powerful tool in the evaluation of CNS embryonal tumours. Pineoblastoma represents a distinct entity, although little is known regarding its genomic landscape. Germline DICER1 mutations are found in a small proportion of patients and warrant genetic testing for all patients.

The small proportion of PNETs/other embryonal tumours, which could not be reclassified, harbour unique rearrangements comprising four distinct groups. Alterations of FOXR2, CIC, MN1, and BCOR comprise these new molecular entities provisionally designated 'CNS neuroblastoma with FOXR2 activation (CNS NB-FOXR2)', 'CNS Ewing sarcoma family tumour with CIC alteration (CNS EFT-CIC)', 'CNS high-grade neuroepithelial tumour with MN1 alteration (CNS HGNET-MN1)', and 'CNS high-grade neuroepithelial tumour with BCOR alteration (CNS HGNET-BCOR)'. The clinical significance of these alterations is still unknown and requires large multicentre collaboration.

Atypical teratoid rhabdoid tumour

ATRTs are almost universally defined by a genetic lesion in SMARCB1, either broad events resulting in deletions or point mutations, with a small proportion harbouring lesions in SMARCA4. Recent integrated genomic studies have shown that ATRT comprises three distinct molecular variants. These groups are termed Group 1/ATRT-SHH, Group 2A/ATRT-TYR, and Group 2B/ATRT-MYC, defined by distinct gene expression and DNA-methylation patterns. Group 1/ATRT-SHH are more frequently supratentorial with focal alterations in SMARCB1, with a trend towards a more favourable prognosis. This group have a more closed chromatin pattern and activation of NOTCH and SHH pathways. Group 2A/ATRT-TYR are more frequently infratentorial, with a mix of broad and focal alterations in SMARCB1, and a trend towards a poorer prognosis. This group have activation of PDGFRB and overactivation of multiple receptor tyrosine kinases. Spinal tumours are enriched in group 2B/ATRT-MYC, with broad alterations in SMARCB1 and a globally hypomethylated DNA-methylation landscape. The clinical implications of these subgroups are still being discerned, although clear trends are emerging from retrospective data.

Staging

MB, other embryonal tumour, and ATRT staging and risk stratification are crucial for management. Staging is based on MRI of the brain and spine, with and without gadolinium, and on cytology of cerebrospinal fluid (CSF) drawn from the lumbar region two weeks after surgery (to avoid false positive findings).

Table 23.1 Chang's classification for metastases

Stage	Description
M0	No gross nodular or laminar subarachnoid or haematogenous metastasis
M1	Microscopic tumour cells found in CSF
M2	Gross nodular or laminar seeding in the cerebellum, cerebral subarachnoid space, or third or fourth ventricles
M3	Gross nodular or laminar seeding in the spinal subarachnoid space
M4	Extra-neuraxial metastasis

Adapted with permission from Chang C, et al. 'An operative staging system and a megavoltage radiotherapeutic technic for cerebellar medulloblastomas'. *Radiology*, Volume 93, Issue 6, pp.1351–9. Copyright © 1969 Radiological Society of North America. DOI: https://doi.org/10.1148/93.6.1351

MB patients are stratified as standard- or high-risk for treatment purposes, depending on the clinical presentation, metastatic status (M1–M4), and/or residual disease of more than 1.5 cm^2 on early post-operative MRI (within 24–72 hours). The risk grouping of MB patients is based on Chang's classification for metastases (Table 23.1). Historically, patients with other embryonal tumours and ATRTs have been treated on MB protocols and, due to their poorer survival, as high-risk patients, although dedicated ATRT studies have become more prevalent.

Patients have generally been risk stratified by age, extent of residual disease, spread, LC/A-MB in some protocols, and (more recently) by biological features such as MYC and WNT status (Figure 23.3).

The standard-risk group applies to 60–70% of patients over three years old. High-risk patients are those with disseminated disease and/or less than a gross or near-total resection (arbitrarily defined as 1.5 cm^2 or more residue). Histologically, LC/A MB is considered high-risk. The value of staging in the context of molecular subgrouping is unclear, particularly for WNT and Group 4 patients. In forthcoming trials, staging will be done by combining histological and biological variables. CNS embryonal tumour patients over the age of three receive similar staging to medulloblastoma patients; however, the value of biological markers is currently unclear.

Prognosis

With modern treatment protocols combining surgery with craniospinal irradiation (CSI) and CT, five-year OS for MB is now higher than 80% for standard-risk patients. Until a few years ago, the outcome for metastatic MB was poor, with five-year OS around 30–40%. Intensified CT regimens and high-dose RT schedules (including hyperfractionated accelerated radiotherapy—HART) have considerably improved outcomes, achieving five-year survival rates around 70%.

Younger children (up to five years of age, depending on group policies) have traditionally been treated with prolonged CT schedules in an effort to contain late sequelae, especially of RT. More recently, using systemic CT combined with intraventricular methotrexate or HDCT, five-year progression-free survival (PFS) has risen to more than 70%, showing that a tailored use of CT can make RT unnecessary, in some patient subgroups at least.

Other embryonal tumours have a variable prognosis. ETMR and CNS embryonal tumours harbouring C19MC amplicons are near

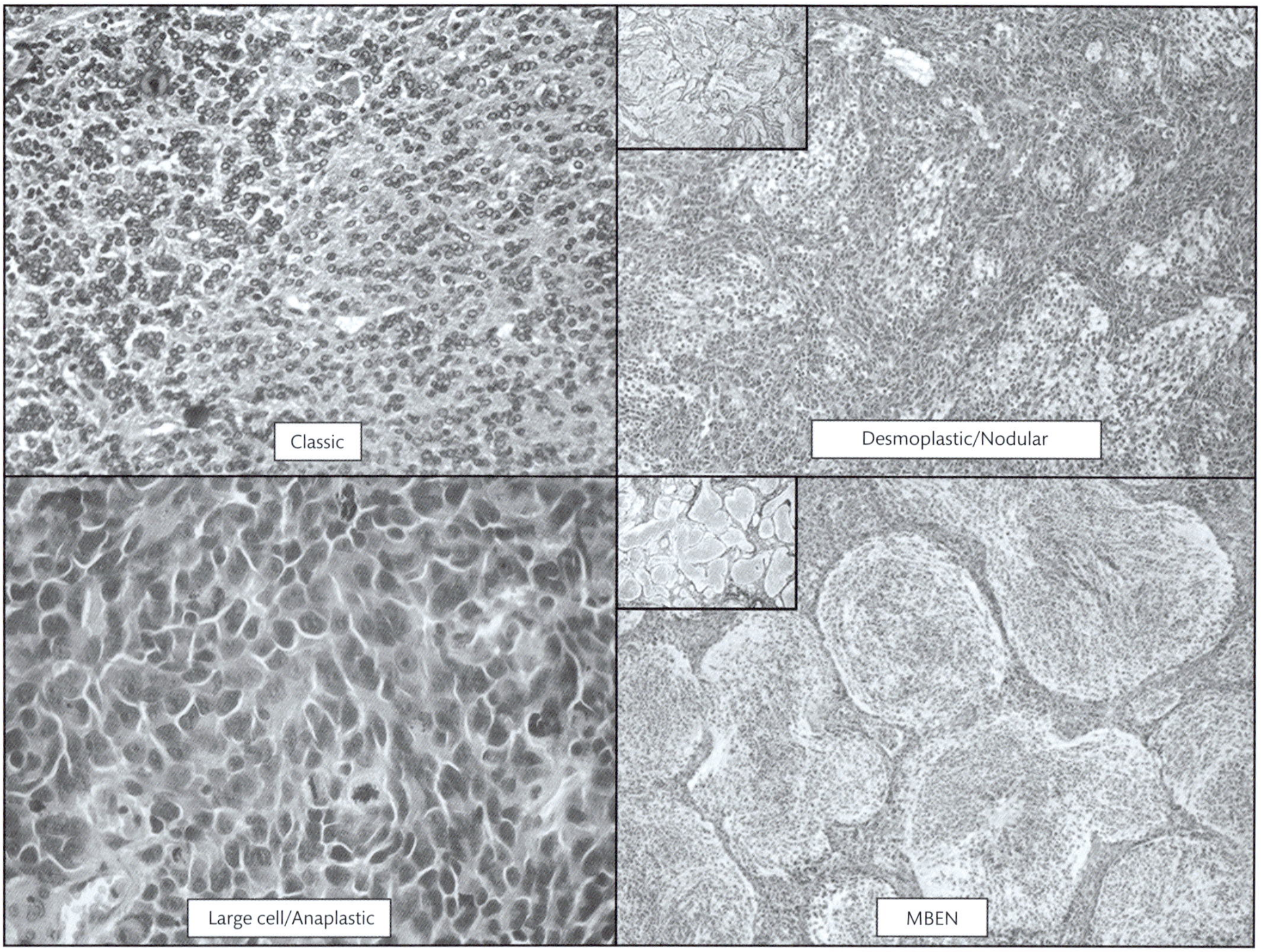

Figure 23.3 Histological classification of medulloblastoma: microscopic haematoxylin and eosin-stained sections of medulloblastoma depicting the four histological variants in the WHO classification.

Reproduced with permission from Maura Massimino, et al. 'Childhood medulloblastoma', *Critical Reviews in Oncology/Hematology*, Volume 105, pp. 35–51. DOI: https://doi.org/10.1016/j.critrevonc.2016.05.012

universally fatal. A major factor in the interpretation of studies of other embryonal tumours is the inclusion of small-cell high-grade gliomas which have a worse outcome. However, a pineal location portends to a better outcome, with three- to five-year event-free survival (EFS) between 38% and 69%. Currently, there is a paucity of studies enrolling other embryonal tumours, making it difficult to provide accurate risk stratification and prognosis.

Treatment

The aim of ongoing and future clinical trials is to improve the prognosis for MBs and CNS embryonal tumours, and to contain the sequelae of treatments by:

1. Testing the feasibility of reducing the dose of CSI and the volume of the posterior fossa boost in standard-risk patients in the light of the recently-identified biological stratification factors;
2. Establishing whether intensifying CT or RT can improve outcome in high-risk MB patients;
3. Introducing any available targeted therapies in suitable constellations;
4. Considering other radiation techniques, such as proton therapy, with a view to limiting late sequelae. This is particularly of interest in younger children who are at high risk to suffer long-term side effects of cranial radiation.

Surgery

Surgical resection is fundamental to the treatment of MB. Though there is a substantial risk of morbidity, expert paediatric neurosurgeons can usually achieve gross total resection without causing major damage. Recent studies have shown that the value of extent of surgery in MB is less pronounced when accounting for molecular subgroups. A permanent CSF diversion will be necessary for about 20–30% of patients due to scarring of the CSF pathways. In addition to the risk of infections and mechanical complications (fluid leak, pseudomeningocele), surgery can lead to posterior fossa mutism syndrome developing 48–72 hours after the surgical procedure. In around one third of cases, this condition is associated with severe cerebellar impairments, including dysmetria, hypotonia, paresis, and depressed mood, which may persist for months.

Surgical resection is also fundamental in the treatment of other embryonal tumours. Although historically, a gross total resection is thought to confer a better prognosis, it fails to reach significance, likely due to small patient numbers. The prognostic role of surgical resection in ATRTs is not clear. A pooled retrospective data analysis failed to show a clear benefit to gross total resection when correcting for HDCT and radiation; however, this has not been confirmed in a prospective study.

Early post-operative brain MRI (within 48 hours after the procedure) should be obtained to assess the extent of the resection. In the event of residue, patients whose tumour can be reduced by means of a second surgical resection to no more than 1.5 cm^2 are eligible for standard-risk protocols—providing this approach is undertaken in good time (generally within two weeks after the first surgical procedure).

Non-surgical treatment

Standard-risk medulloblastoma

After surgical resection, the mainstay for patients aged three to five years or more is 'reduced-dose' CSI, with a total dose of 23.4 Gy, plus a boost to the tumour bed up to a total dose of 54–55.8 Gy. Historically, whole posterior fossa boosts were considered the standard; however, reduced-volume tumour-bed boost spares a significant proportion of the occipital lobes from exposure to radiation without a reduction in survival. This is often combined with weekly vincristine, and is then followed by a multi-drug platinum-based regimen. With this approach, the five-year EFS rate is over 80%.

The clinical target volume (CTV) for CSI includes the whole brain and spinal cord with the meninges, down to the thecal sac on level L5 or S3. Modern protocols include frontline central review of RT planning to assure the best possible quality control. An 18 Gy CSI dose has been investigated in the randomized COG trial ACNS0331, and showed a higher rate of relapse in the reduced-dose CSI arm. Still, reduced-dose CSI is being tried in a subset of standard-risk patients under 16 years old with WNT-MB in the SIOP-PNET5, ACNS1422, and SJMB12 trials.

Another solution that might reduce the late sequelae of RT lies in proton therapy, but the follow-up is very short in the experiences published to date, and only carefully selected cases have been treated so far. Obviously, proton therapy may only spare normal brain during the boost phase of the treatment, not during the CSI phase. However, during the CSI phase, proton therapy may spare other normal tissues like the oesophagus and intestine, which often receive a higher dose with photon therapy.

High-risk patients

Intensified cyclophosphamide-based regimens, including HDCT with ASCT and high-dose RT schedules, seem to have improved the prognosis for high-risk patients, whose five-year survival rates have risen from under 40% to 70%. The COG is currently assessing a randomized treatment with concurrent carboplatin and vincristine plus RT (versus vincristine and RT), followed by maintenance CT with or without 13-cis retinoic acid, for newly diagnosed high-risk MB (unpublished data). The 13-cis retinoic-acid arm was closed early due to lack of efficacy in an interim analysis.

None of the studies conducted to date have demonstrated that combinations of high-dose CSI (be it hyperfractionated/accelerated or not) with HDCT can improve disease control. Wider, phase 3 trials may soon begin to seek more evidence, but any effort to improve the prognosis by intensifying treatments should meet accurate quality assurance and feasibility criteria to avoid undue toxicities.

Infant medulloblastoma

Infants have either SHH tumours with a better prognosis, or Group 3 tumours with a higher incidence of metastatic disease and a worse prognosis.

Some studies have tried intensifying systemic CT, while others have added intraventricular CT or HDCT in an effort to avoid the unacceptably severe sequelae seen in long-term survivors treated with CSI at a young age. High response rates have been reported after sequential HDCT, particularly in the CCG99703 protocol with three tandem cycles of myeloablative carboplatin and thiotepa, which is being investigated in second-generation studies. A French group has also reported that smaller volumes of RT after HDCT contributed to long-term survival. Further research should ascertain whether these regimens can also increase the proportion of patients curable without RT in the M0/T0 group, particularly when accounting for molecular subgrouping.

Whether the subset of infants cured in each study had particular biological features that favoured survival remains to be seen. The HIT (Hirntumoren Säuglinge und Kleinkinder—the German group for brain tumour study in children) SKK 1992 study reported a higher frequency of desmoplastic MBs (40%), which carry a significantly better prognosis than the classic variant. A meta-analysis of infant studies conducted in Europe and North America, between 1987 and 2004, included 270 children under five years old and confirmed a significantly better EFS and OS for infants with nodular/desmoplastic MB and patients with completely resected localized disease (M0R0). This histological subtype is mainly associated with SHH activation and emerges as a major positive prognostic factor in young children, whatever therapy they receive, whereas HDCT seems to be needed for higher-risk histotypes and clinical presentations. Every attempt should be made to avoid RT for infants with associated Gorlin syndrome or at risk of developing secondary tumours later in life. In conclusion, the last 10-15 years have seen improvements in the treatment for infant MB, tending towards less RT and more CT. Recent evidence suggests that age per se is no longer an adverse prognostic factor. The SIOPE is considering an international phase III trial for young children with MB, to compare survival rates and neurocognitive outcomes achievable with different treatment strategies based on recognized prognostic factors (**Figure 23.2**).

Treatment of other embryonal tumours

Post-surgical treatment for other embryonal tumours has historically followed that of MB. Results of these protocols have consistently shown inferior survival rates.

Results in infants

Infants have classically been treated with a CT-only approach. However, the results of early trials should be interpreted with caution, as they certainly included a number of patients with ATRTs and high-grade gliomas. Duffner reported the result of the first large, infant, brain-tumour collaborative study that included 17 patients with supraPNETs/supratentorial CNS embryonal tumours and 11 with pineoblastomas. Patients were treated with a four-drug combination (vincristine–cyclophosphamide/cisplatin–etoposide) until the age of three, and then received CSI. The five-year EFS rate was 27% for patients with sPNETs and 0% for those with pineoblastomas. Similar results were reported by the French and UK groups and the Children's Cancer Group (CCG). A subsequent study conducted by the CCG used a more intensive CT approach without adjuvant radiation, and reported 8% five-year PFS.

The best results were reported by Fangusaro and colleagues, using consolidation with HDCT and ASCT. In this experience, EFS and OS were 39% and 49%, with a better survival rate for non-pineal sPNETs (57% versus 23%). Twelve patients did not receive any radiation. However, these results should be taken with caution, as there was no central pathology review in this trial. The HIT-SKK group analysed its experience of CT only followed by delayed radiation in 29 young children. They reported a dismal EFS and OS of 14.9% and 17.2%, respectively. Based on their findings, they recommended limiting any delay of RT to a maximum of six months.

Overall, the management of young children with CNS embryonal tumours remains a challenge. A benefit of HDCT has been suggested in some series, and this approach has become standard in many places. In CT-only protocols, there is a lack of agreement regarding the role of focal irradiation following completion of therapy in patients with no evidence of disease.

Results in older children

Children over the age of three to five are treated with CSI, with a boost to the primary tumour bed. Due to their relatively poor outcome, sPNET/supratentorial CNS embryonal tumour patients have traditionally been treated as high-risk patients with 36 Gy of CSI, even in the absence of metastatic dissemination. Currently, accrual for sPNET patients in the COG ACNS0332 was discontinued in 2013 and there are no open North American or European studies. However, the CCG99701 study suggested PFS of almost 50% for sPNETs treated with 36 Gy of CSI with a focal boost and concurrent carboplatin as a radiosensitizer, followed by six cycles of cisplatin, cyclophosphamide, and vincristine. A limited series has shown encouraging survival rates using CSI followed by four cycles of HDCT and ASCT. Interestingly, in this protocol, children with average-risk features were treated with reduced-dose CSI. Massimino reported the result of a pilot study using HDCT and HART in 15 sPNET patients. Three-year EFS and OS were 51% and 61%, respectively.

Currently, there is no clear consensus, particularly in the context of recent advances in biology. However, the standard of care in most centres remains CSI with a tumour-bed boost, followed by cisplatin-based maintenance CT. By contrast with the results observed in younger children, outcomes of pineoblastoma patients treated with CSI are constantly better than those observed in other sPNETs, with five-year survival rates in the range of 60–70% in patients without metastatic disease.

Atypical teratoid rhabdoid tumour

There are still a number of uncertainties concerning optimal management of ATRT patients. Early reports stated that ATRTs rarely respond to CT, with an overall response rate of less than 20% and median survival of six months in an early report. In 1995, Olson and colleagues described patients who showed sustained response using multidisciplinary management, with an approach similar to that used to treat rhabdomyosarcomas. The possibility to successfully manage ATRT patients was further confirmed by Hilden and colleagues in a report on 42 patients enrolled into the ATRT registry. Although 14 patients were alive in this report, the heterogeneity of treatments administered precluded any conclusions regarding the respective role of surgery, CT, and radiation. However, a simultaneous publication from the St Jude group described a high survival rate in older children treated with CSI and chemotherapy, and emphasized the role of early radiation. This approach was used by Chi and colleagues, who reported two-year PFS and OS rates of 53% and 70%, respectively, in a prospective multi-institutional trial of 20 evaluable patients treated with a chemotherapy backbone of the sarcoma IRS-III regimen.

The results of the recently closed COG ACNS0333 protocol are awaited. This protocol used an intensive induction, followed by focal irradiation and HDCT with ASCT. Although RT is advocated by many, its role continues to be controversial, and some series report successful outcomes with a radiation-sparing approach. There are similar controversies regarding the respective role of anthracyclines, high-dose methotrexate, HDCT, and intrathecal therapy. Whether these questions should be addressed in future protocols, or whether the focus should be on tailored management of ATRTs based on their molecular subgroups, is a challenge for the years to come. The efficacy of molecularly targeted agents, such as alisertib, suggests that future protocols should not be limited to addressing chemotherapy questions but, rather, should look for new drug opportunities.

Follow-up

Patients enrolled in study protocols undergo scheduled imaging, but after they have completed their treatment, the timing of their MRI scans becomes more arbitrary. Imaging of the brain and spine generally occurs every three months for the first two years; then brain MRI is every four months in the third year, six-monthly up until the fifth year, and yearly thereafter. Further imaging of the spine is usually only warranted for suspect clinical signs. Late medulloblastoma relapses in previously irradiated patients should be approached with caution; a significant proportion are radiation-induced secondary malignancies, particularly in locally relapsing Group 4 patients. Guidelines for patients with other embryonal tumours and ATRTs follow the same rules. However, overall, patients with previously irradiated embryonal tumours are extremely challenging, with dismal survival rates.

The follow-up should include all the appropriate clinical, radiological, and biochemical assessments, and tests tailored to a patient's neurofunctional capabilities (see the chapter 'Late Effects of Therapy and Survivorship Issues').

Treatment at relapse

MB relapses occur within two years of diagnosis in nearly 75% of paediatric patients, and more than half of them have disseminated disease. Several factors influence how patients with relapsing MB are treated. The initial treatment, and specifically whether the patient was treated with radiation, is crucial when considering treatment for relapse. Infants who were treated with a radiation-sparing approach comprise a distinct group where salvage is possible with CSI. This principle guided the initial studies of deferred radiation; however, more recent studies attempted to avoid radiation altogether. CSI at relapse, in this context, can result in survival approaching 60%, although the optimal dose of CSI remains unknown.

Older children who relapse after CSI cannot be cured by salvage therapy, with some very rare exceptions (less than 5%). Further surgery, followed by focal (re-)irradiation with or without CT, might be an option for solitary recurrences, but should be considered case by case, and only after complete staging to ascertain the extent of dissemination.

Many phase II trials have reported a poor response in nearly all recurrent MB patients. Several groups are investigating low-dose CT regimens called 'metronomic' therapy. It has proven feasible for treating paediatric brain tumours in case series, though it raises concerns about haematological toxicities and the risk of secondary malignancies. Furthermore, Group 4 patients relapse later and have significantly longer survival post recurrence, and, as such, should be taken into account when interpreting Phase II trials which suggest activity based on a small proportion of short-term survivors.

There are 'druggable' mutations and copy number variations in the genomic landscape of MB, but the only targeted therapy to have been examined so far in the clinical setting involved the use of smoothened (SMO) inhibitors. These inhibitors are only effective in the case of PTCH or SMO mutations (more common in adult MB), while they are useless when mutations downstream, including SUFU, GLI2, or MYCN, are responsible for SHH-pathway activation (as in childhood tumours), and any response to SMO inhibitors is transient due to downstream pathway activation. In addition to their limited efficacy, their use in children has to be balanced against the risk of their long-term toxicity.

The pattern of relapse in MB is highly subgroup-dependent, with SHH patients recurring most frequently locally, and Group 3 and 4 patients (particularly those who were irradiated) recurring almost exclusively with metastatic dissemination. As such, future therapies for Group 3 and 4 MB will undoubtedly need to include new therapies directed at the metastatic compartment. Moreover, it has been recently shown that the relapse sample is highly divergent from the diagnostic sample, and biopsy at the time of relapse should be considered if targeted therapies are to be employed.

There is no consensus on the treatment of other embryonal tumours or ATRTs at relapse, except for infants who were not irradiated, who may benefit from salvage radiation. The recent identification of novel groups of embryonal brain tumours and ATRTs with distinct molecular alterations may soon provide potential salvage options for these patients.

Future directions

The advent of integrated genomics has significantly changed our approach to MB, and has the potential to influence future therapies for ATRTs and other embryonal tumours. The current generation of MB studies are more molecularly informed, and the next generation of trials in MB will incorporate more robust molecular risk stratification and introduce novel agents for very high-risk subsets of patients. Moreover, the current and next generation of MB studies will consider therapy de-escalation for low-risk patients such as those with WNT MB and low-risk Group 4 tumours with chromosome 11 loss. As preclinical models of MB mature, new therapies are likely to emerge for high-risk patients which can be rapidly incorporated into clinical trials.

Although still in the conceptual stages, the next generation of ATRT studies will also likely be molecularly informed. More importantly, the discovery of discrete biological subsets of ATRT may help inform novel therapies. Unfortunately, other embryonal tumours are a group of rare tumours that have no open clinical trials. As such, there is a paucity of existing and ongoing prospective clinical data, which will make the design of any future clinical trial exceedingly difficult. International collaborations and pooled analyses will be required to determine the optimal therapy for the subsets of other embryonal tumours, to plan any future molecularly informed studies.

FURTHER READING

Bakst RL, et al. (2011) Reirradiation for recurrent medulloblastoma. *Cancer* **117**, 4977–82.

Bergthold G, et al. (2014) High-dose busulfan-thiotepa with autologous stem cell transplantation followed by posterior fossa irradiation in young children with classical or incompletely resected medulloblastoma. *Pediatr Blood Cancer* **61**, 907–12.

Biegel JA, et al. (1999) Germ-line and acquired mutations of INI1 in atypical teratoid and rhabdoid tumours. *Cancer Res* **59**, 74–9.

Broniscer A, et al. (2004) High-dose chemotherapy with autologous stem-cell rescue in the treatment of patients with recurrent non-cerebellar primitive neuroectodermal tumours. *Pediatr Blood Cancer* **42**, 261–7.

Chi SN, et al. (2009) Intensive multimodality treatment for children with newly diagnosed CNS atypical teratoid rhabdoid tumour. *J Clin Oncol* **27**, 385–9.

Chintagumpala M, et al. (2009) A pilot study of risk-adapted radiotherapy and chemotherapy in patients with supratentorial PNET. *Neuro Oncol* **11**, 33–40.

Clifford SC, et al. (2015) Biomarker-driven stratification of disease-risk in non-metastatic medulloblastoma: results from the multi-center HIT-SIOP-PNET4 clinical trial. *Oncotarget* **6**(36), 38827–39.

Cohen BH, et al. (2015) Pilot study of intensive chemotherapy with peripheral hematopoietic cell support for children less than 3 years of age with malignant brain tumours, the CCG-99703 phase I/II study. A report from the Children's Oncology Group. *Pediatr Neurol* **53**, 31–46.

Cohen BH, et al. (1995) Prognostic factors and treatment results for supratentorial primitive neuroectodermal tumours in children using radiation and chemotherapy: a Children's Cancer Group randomized trial. *J Clin Oncol* **13**, 1687–96.

de Kock L, et al. (2014) Germ-line and somatic DICER1 mutations in pineoblastoma. *Acta Neuropathol* **128**, 583–95.

Duffner PK, et al. (1993) Postoperative chemotherapy and delayed radiation in children less than three years of age with malignant brain tumours. *N Engl J Med* **328**, 1725–31.

Dufour C, et al. (2014) Tandem high-dose chemotherapy and autologous stem cell rescue in children with newly diagnosed high-risk medulloblastoma or supratentorial primitive neuro-ectodermic tumours. *Pediatr Blood Cancer* **61**, 1398–402.

Eberhart CG, Burger PC (2003) Anaplasia and grading in medulloblastomas. *Brain Pathol* **13**, 376–85.

Ezzat S, et al. (2016) Pediatric brain tumours in a low/middle income country: does it differ from that in developed world? *J Neurooncol* **126**, 371–6.

Fangusaro J, et al. (2008) Intensive chemotherapy followed by consolidative myeloablative chemotherapy with autologous hematopoietic cell rescue (AuHCR) in young children with newly diagnosed supratentorial primitive neuroectodermal tumours (sPNETs): report of the Head Start I and II experience. *Pediatr Blood Cancer* **50**, 312–18.

Friedrich C, et al. (2013) Treatment of young children with CNS-primitive neuroectodermal tumours/pineoblastomas in the prospective multicenter trial HIT 2000 using different chemotherapy regimens and radiotherapy. *Neuro Oncol* **15**, 224–34.

Gajjar A, et al. (2006) Risk-adapted craniospinal radiotherapy followed by high-dose chemotherapy and stem-cell rescue in children with newly diagnosed medulloblastoma (St Jude Medulloblastoma-96): long-term results from a prospective, multicentre trial. *Lancet Oncol* **7**, 813–20.

Gandola L, et al. (2008) Hyperfractionated accelerated radiotherapy in the Milan strategy for metastatic medulloblastoma. *J Clin Oncol* **27**, 566–71.

Garre ML, et al. (2009) Medulloblastoma variants: age-dependent occurrence and relation to Gorlin syndrome—a new clinical perspective. *Clin Cancer Res* **15**, 2463–71.

Gatta G, et al. (2014) Childhood cancer survival in Europe 1999–2007: results of EUROCARE-5—a population-based study. *Lancet Oncol* **15**, 35–47.

Gerber NU, et al. (2014) Treatment of children with central nervous system primitive neuroectodermal tumours/pinealoblastomas in the prospective multicentric trial HIT 2000 using hyperfractionated radiation therapy followed by maintenance chemotherapy. *Int J Radiat Oncol Biol Phys* **89**, 863–71.

Geyer JR, et al. (2005) Multiagent chemotherapy and deferred radiotherapy in infants with malignant brain tumours: a report from the Children's Cancer Group. *J Clin Oncol* **23**, 7621–31.

Grill J, et al. (2005) Treatment of medulloblastoma with postoperative chemotherapy alone: an SFOP prospective trial in young children. *Lancet Oncol* **6**, 573–80.

Grundy RG, et al. (2010) Primary postoperative chemotherapy without radiotherapy for treatment of brain tumours other than ependymoma in children under 3 years: results of the first UKCCSG/SIOP CNS 9204 trial. *Eur J Cancer* **46**, 120–33.

Hasselblatt M, et al. (2014) SMARCA4-mutated atypical teratoid/rhabdoid tumours are associated with inherited germline alterations and poor prognosis. *Acta Neuropathol* **128**, 453–6.

Hilden JM, et al. (2004) Central nervous system atypical teratoid/rhabdoid tumour: results of therapy in children enrolled in a registry. *J Clin Oncol* **22**, 2877–84.

Jakacki RI, et al. (2015) Outcome and prognostic factors for children with supratentorial primitive neuroectodermal tumours treated with carboplatin during radiotherapy: a report from the Children's Oncology Group. *Pediatr Blood Cancer* **62**, 776–83.

Jakacki RI, et al. (2012) Outcome of children with metastatic medulloblastoma treated with carboplatin during craniospinal radiotherapy: a Children's Oncology Group phase I/II study. *J Clin Oncol* **30**, 2648–53.

Johann PD, et al. (2016) Atypical teratoid/rhabdoid tumours are comprised of three epigenetic subgroups with distinct enhancer landscapes. *Cancer Cell* **29**, 379–93.

Kann BH, et al. (2016) Postoperative radiotherapy patterns of care and survival implications for medulloblastoma in young children. *JAMA Oncol* **2**, 1574–81.

Kool M, et al. (2014) Genome sequencing of SHH medulloblastoma predicts genotype-related response to smoothened inhibition. *Cancer Cell* **25**, 393–405.

Korshunov A, et al. (2014) Embryonal tumour with abundant neuropil and true rosettes (ETANTR), ependymoblastoma, and medulloepithelioma share molecular similarity and comprise a single clinicopathological entity. *Acta Neuropathol* **128**, 279–89.

Lafay-Cousin L, et al. (2016) Clinical, pathological, and molecular characterization of infant medulloblastomas treated with sequential high-dose chemotherapy. *Pediatr Blood Cancer* **63**(9), 1527–34.

Louis DN, et al. (2016) The 2016 World Health Organization classification of tumours of the central nervous system: a summary. *Acta Neuropathol* **131**, 803–20.

Marec-Berard P, et al. (2002) Supratentorial embryonal tumours in children under 5 years of age: an SFOP study of treatment with postoperative chemotherapy alone. *Med Pediatr Oncol* **38**, 83–90.

Massimino M, et al. (2009) No salvage using high-dose chemotherapy plus/minus reirradiation for relapsing previously irradiated medulloblastoma. *Radiat Oncol Biol* **73**, 1358–63.

Massimino M, et al. (2006) Supratentorial primitive neuroectodermal tumours (S-PNET) in children: a prospective experience with adjuvant intensive chemotherapy and hyperfractionated accelerated radiotherapy. *Int J Radiat Oncol Biol Phys* **64**, 1031–7.

Morrissy AS, et al. (2016) Divergent clonal selection dominates medulloblastoma at recurrence. *Nature* **529**, 351–7.

Muller K, et al. (2014) Postponed is not canceled: role of craniospinal radiation therapy in the management of recurrent infant medulloblastoma—an experience from the HIT-REZ 1997 & 2005 studies. *Int J Radiat Oncol Biol Phys* **88**, 1019–24.

Northcott PA, et al. (2012) Medulloblastomics: the end of the beginning. *Nat Rev Cancer* **12**, 818–34.

Northcott PA, et al. (2014) Enhancer hijacking activates GFI1 family oncogenes in medulloblastoma. *Nature* **511**, 428–34.

Olson TA, et al. (1995) Successful treatment of disseminated central nervous system malignant rhabdoid tumour. *J Pediatr Hematol Oncol* **17**, 71–5.

Ostrom QT, et al. (2015) Alex's Lemonade Stand Foundation Infant and Childhood Primary Brain and Central Nervous System Tumours Diagnosed in the United States in 2007–2011. *Neuro Oncol* **16** (Suppl 10), x1–x36.

Packer RJ, et al. (2006) Phase III study of craniospinal radiation therapy followed by adjuvant chemotherapy for newly diagnosed average-risk medulloblastoma. *J Clin Oncol* **24**, 4202–8.

Pei Y, et al. (2016) HDAC and PI3K antagonists cooperate to inhibit growth of MYC-driven medulloblastoma. *Cancer Cell* **29**, 311–23.

Peris-Bonet R, et al. (2006) Childhood central nervous system tumours—incidence and survival in Europe (1978–1997): report from Automated Childhood Cancer Information System project. *Eur J Cancer* **42**, 2064–80.

Perreault S, et al. (2014) MRI surrogates for molecular subgroups of medulloblastoma. *Am J Neuroradiol* **35**, 1263–9.

Picard D, et al. (2012) Markers of survival and metastatic potential in childhood CNS primitive neuro-ectodermal brain tumours: an integrative genomic analysis. *Lancet Oncol* **13**, 838–48.

Pietsch T, et al. (2014) Prognostic significance of clinical, histopathological, and molecular characteristics of medulloblastomas in the prospective HIT2000 multicenter clinical trial cohort. *Acta Neuropathol* **128**, 137–49.

Pizer B, et al. (2011) Treatment of recurrent central nervous system primitive neuroectodermal tumours in children and adolescents: results of a Children's Cancer and Leukaemia Group study. *Eur J Cancer* **47**, 1389–97.

Pomeroy SL, et al. (2002) Prediction of central nervous system embryonal tumour outcome based on gene expression. *Nature* **415**, 436–42.

Ramaswamy V, et al. (2011) FISH and chips: the recipe for improved prognostication and outcomes for children with medulloblastoma. *Cancer Genet* **204**, 577–88.

Ramaswamy V, et al. (2016) Medulloblastoma subgroup-specific outcomes in irradiated children: who are the true high-risk patients? *Neuro Oncol* **18**, 291–7.

Ramaswamy V, et al. (2016) Risk stratification of childhood medulloblastoma in the molecular era: the current consensus. *Acta Neuropathol* **131**, 821–31.

Ramaswamy V, et al. (2013) Recurrence patterns across medulloblastoma subgroups: an integrated clinical and molecular analysis. *Lancet Oncol* **14**, 1200–207.

Raybaud C, et al. (2015) Posterior fossa tumours in children: developmental anatomy and diagnostic imaging. *Childs Nerv Syst* **31**, 1661–76.

Remke M, et al. (2011) Adult medulloblastoma comprises three major molecular variants. *J Clin Oncol* **29**, 2717–23.

Remke M, et al. (2013) TERT promoter mutations are highly recurrent in SHH subgroup medulloblastoma. *Acta Neuropathol* **126**, 917–29.

Rorke LB, et al. (1996) Central nervous system atypical teratoid/rhabdoid tumours of infancy and childhood: definition of an entity. *J Neurosurg* **85**, 56–65.

Rudin CM, et al. (2009) Treatment of medulloblastoma with hedgehog pathway inhibitor GDC-0449. *N Engl J Med* **361**, 1173–8.

Rutkowski S, et al. (2005) Treatment of early childhood medulloblastoma by postoperative chemotherapy alone. *N Engl J Med* **352**, 978–86.

Rutkowski S, et al. (2010) Medulloblastoma in young children. *Pediatr Blood Cancer* **54**, 635–7.

Rutkowski S, et al. (2010) Survival and prognostic factors of early childhood medulloblastoma: an international meta-analysis. *J Clin Oncol* **28**, 4961–68.

Schrey D, et al. (2016) Multimodal therapy in children and adolescents with newly diagnosed atypical teratoid/rhabdoid tumour: individual pooled data analysis and review of the literature. *J Neuro-Oncol* **126**, 81–90.

Shih DJ, et al. (2014) Cytogenetic prognostication within medulloblastoma subgroups. *J Clin Oncol* **32**, 886–96.

Smith MJ, et al. (2014) Germline mutations in SUFU cause Gorlin syndrome-associated childhood medulloblastoma and redefine the risk associated with PTCH1 mutations. *J Clin Oncol* **32**, 4155–61.

Spence T, et al. (2014) A novel C19MC amplified cell line links Lin28/let-7 to mTOR signaling in embryonal tumour with multilayered rosettes. *Neuro Oncol* **16**, 62–71.

Sturm D, et al. (2016) New brain tumour entities emerge from molecular classification of CNS-PNETs. *Cell* **164**, 1060–72.

Taylor MD, et al. (2012) Molecular subgroups of medulloblastoma: the current consensus. *Acta Neuropathol* **123**, 465–72.

Tekautz TM, et al. (2005) Atypical teratoid/rhabdoid tumours (ATRT): improved survival in children 3 years of age and older with radiation therapy and high-dose alkylator-based chemotherapy. *J Clin Oncol* **23**, 1491–9.

Thompson EM, et al. (2016) Prognostic value of medulloblastoma extent of resection after accounting for molecular subgroup: a retrospective integrated clinical and molecular analysis. *Lancet Oncol* **17**(4), 484–95.

Timmermann B, et al. (2002) Role of radiotherapy in the treatment of supratentorial primitive neuroectodermal tumours in childhood: results of the prospective German brain tumour trials HIT 88/89 and 91. *J Clin Oncol* **20**, 842–9.

Torchia J, et al. (2016) Integrated (epi)-genomic analyses identify subgroup-specific therapeutic targets in CNS rhabdoid tumours. *Cancer Cell* **30**, 891–908.

Torchia J, et al. (2015) Molecular subgroups of atypical teratoid rhabdoid tumours in children: an integrated genomic and clinicopathological analysis. *Lancet Oncol* **16**, 569–82.

Villani A, et al. (2012) Syndromes predisposing to pediatric central nervous system tumours: lessons learned and new promises. *Curr Neurol Neurosci Rep* **12**, 153–64.

Wetmore C, et al. (2015) Alisertib is active as single agent in recurrent atypical teratoid rhabdoid tumours in 4 children. *Neuro Oncol* **17**, 882–8.

Wetmore C, et al. (2014) Reirradiation of recurrent medulloblastoma: does clinical benefit outweigh risk for toxicity? *Cancer* **120**, 3731–7.

Yock TI, et al. (2016) Long-term toxic effects of proton radiotherapy for paediatric medulloblastoma: a phase 2 single-arm study. *Lancet Oncol* **17**(3), 287–98.

24

Other Central Nervous System Tumours of Childhood

Cecile Faure Conter, Didier Frappaz, Kristian W. Pajtler, and Stefan M. Pfister

Germ-cell tumours

Diagnosis: radiology, (molecular) pathology

All germ-cell tumours (GCT), whether intra- or extracranial, derive from the primordial germ cell. During early embryogenesis, primordial germ cells migrate along the dorsal mesentery to populate the gonads. Aberrant migration may occur axially (i.e. suprasellar, pineal regions with 10% being bifocal). Intracranial GCT are pure or mixed tumours including undifferentiated (germinoma, embryonal carcinoma) and/or extraembryonic (choriocarcinoma, yolk sac) and/or somatic (teratomas) differentiating components.

In the pineal location, Parinaud's syndrome and/or raised intracranial pressure is recognized promptly. In the opposing suprasellar location, symptoms—diabetes insipidus, impairment of visual fields, or variation in onset of puberty—are often overlooked for long periods in adolescents due to the natural changes occurring within the body and mood. Basal ganglia germinomas usually develop in Asiatic patients following a longstanding history of focal deficit and/or mental deterioration.

Pathology is not always available. It may include one or several of the following components that may not all appear in a limited biopsy. Germinomas, which represent the most frequent histology, are composed of monotonous undifferentiated cells with some isolated syncitiotrophoblastic cells (explaining why germinomas may secrete ß-human chorionic gonadotropin (HCG)) intermixed with an inflammatory infiltrate. Immunohistochemistry (IHC) stains positive for placenta-like alkaline phosphatase (PLAP). The other components may show aberrant differentiation toward extraembryonic and/or somatic features: yolk sac tumours (YST) show a lace-like, papillary, or cord-like pattern of cuboidal/elongated cells; 50% of tumours have Schiller–Duval bodies; IHC is positive for alpha fetoprotein (AFP) and glypican 3; choriocarcinomas (CC) are composed of mononucleated (cytotrophoblastic) and multinucleated (syncitiotrophoblastic) cells that stain on IHC for HCG; and embryonal carcinomas (EC) are composed of primitive epithelial-type cells with minimal features of differentiation arranged as solid, pseudo glandular, alveolar, tubular, or papillary patterns with CD30 positivity on IHC. Teratomas are either mature, with the presence of mature structures derived from all three germ layers (e.g. hair, squamous and mucous epithelium, teeth, cartilage, bone, glial or thyroid tissue), or immature, with varying components of immature tissue that mostly resemble immature neural tissue with neurotubular structures. GCT are either pure or mixed. In the latter case, each component has its specific sensitivity to treatment, germinomas being exquisitely sensitive, teratomas resistant to radio-chemotherapy (indicating the need for surgical removal), and other components being somewhere in between.

Intracranial GCT have a distinctive age distribution: teratomas and pure YSTs develop during infancy and childhood and show imbalances at chromosome 1 (loss at 1p, gain at 1q), whereas all others have a peak incidence during adolescence and early adulthood and are characterized by isochromosome 12p or 12p amplification. There is a male predominance, especially for germinomas.

Pineal tumours may bulge in the third and/or fourth ventricle and invade the thalamic region. Suprasellar masses involve the pituitary stalk and third ventricle, and may compress or invade the optic chiasm. Primary tumours tend to propagate along the ventricular walls often causing endocrinological disorders even when they are not radiologically detectable. Disappearance of the spontaneously bright spot of the posterior pituitary on T1 is correlated to diabetes insipidus. Germinomas are iso- to hyperdense, sometimes calcified on computer tomography (CT) scan, iso- or hypointense on T1- and T2-weighted magnetic resonance imaging (MRI), with moderate to marked gadolinium enhancement without necrosis, a drop in apparent diffusion coefficient (ADC) values is classically observed. The diffusion-weighted imaging (DWI) is similar to that of Langerhans cell histiocytosis and lymphocytic hypophysitis, but differs from craniopharyngiomas and gliomas. Bifocal tumours (if pineal and suprasellar) are a specific entity, not a metastatic disease (**Figure 24.1**), and are typical of GCT, though not pathognomonic. Teratomas may be suggested when the three compartments (parenchymal, fat, and calcifications) are present. Basal ganglia germinoma MRI shows atrophy of the cerebral peduncle and/or basal ganglia and/or cerebral hemisphere. The contrast enhancement is inconstant and patchy. Spinal MRI without and with contrast will look

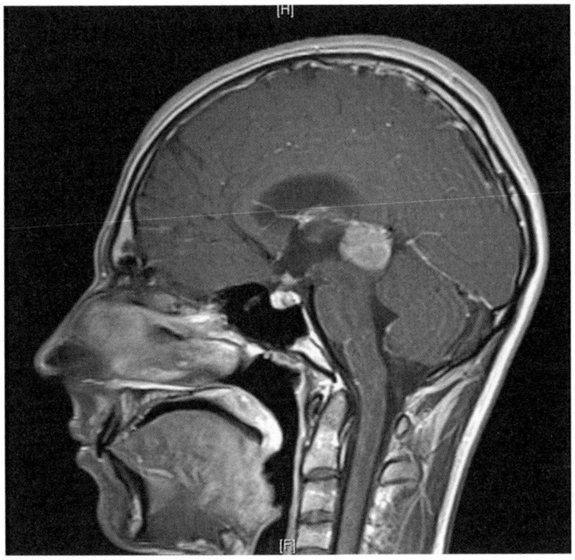

Figure 24.1 Bifocal germinoma on T1-weighted MRI showing gadolinium enhancement.

Reproduced courtesy of Cécile Faure-Conter, Institute of Hematology and Pediatric Oncology (iHOPe), Lyon, France

for nodules and/or linear enhancement. It should be performed preoperatively to avoid bloody artefacts. If not, and if doubtful, it should be repeated with both sagittal and axial sequences.

Biology

Certain markers are measurable in serum and cerebrospinal fluid (CSF) that can be used in diagnosis and monitoring: AFP is mainly produced by YST, though low levels may be detected from EC and immature teratomas. Its half-life is five to seven days. The high level at birth falls to adult limits at 12 months of age. During this period, an isolated measure should prompt further sampling at one-week intervals. Total HCG is produced by the placenta and is secreted by CC and at lower levels by germinomas and EC. Its half-life is two days. Total HCG measures both HCG and subunit β and is expressed as mUI/ml, while free-chain HCG only measures free subunit β. Positive cytology of CSF is found in 10% of cases.

Current treatment strategies

The initial strategy requires a multidisciplinary approach. The initial workflow includes craniospinal MRI and determination of markers (AFP and HCG) both in blood and CSF, and cytology of CSF. The incidence of relapses increased from 4% in fully staged to 24% in partially staged germinoma patients. Apart from the Japanese strategy (explained later), if markers (serum and CSF) are positive, histological confirmation is not required. Moreover, for non-secreting bifocal tumours (most likely germinomas) biopsy may be skipped. In the remaining cases, open surgery, stereotactic biopsy, or endoscopic third ventriculostomy may be used to obtain histological proof. The latter is often used to relieve hydrocephalus and allows inspection of the ventricles. In ongoing protocols, detection of ventricular nodules during this procedure does not qualify the patient as metastatic, provided they are not detectable on MRI, as it is considered that ventriculoscopy is a recent procedure that deserves prospective evaluation.

As all Japanese patients have histological documentation, the first Japanese study promoted a three-category strategy. Pure germinomas reached ten-year overall survival (OS) of 97% when treated with three courses of etoposide and carboplatin concomitant with whole ventricular irradiation (WVI) of 24 Gy. The intermediate group (HCG-secreting germinomas and mixed tumours composed of germinomas and immature teratomas) received similar treatment, with an increased dose to the ventricles (30 Gy) and a local boost (20 Gy); their ten-year OS was 89%. The high-risk group (non germinomatous tumours) received three courses of platinum–etoposide–ifosfamide concomitant with whole-brain irradiation (30 Gy) with a local boost (30 Gy) and spinal (24 Gy) radiotherapy; their ten-year OS was 58%. In the ongoing study, strategy for germinomas (including HCG-secreting tumours) remains the same. Those in the intermediate group receive similar chemotherapy with a decreased dose to the ventricles (23.4 Gy) and an increased boost to the tumour bed (27 Gy). Those in the high risk group receive a 30.6 Gy CSI plus 30.6 Gy additional boost to the tumour with concomitant and maintenance courses of platinum–etoposide–ifosfamide. Basal ganglia primaries with good or intermediate prognosis have a poor outcome and receive chemotherapy followed by a 27 Gy whole-brain irradiation. Those in the intermediate group receive similar chemotherapy but with a decreased dose to the ventricles (23 Gy) and an increased boost (30 Gy). Those in the high risk group received eight courses of platinum–etoposide–ifosfamide and a 30 Gy CSI with 30 Gy additional boost. Basal ganglia primaries with good or intermediate prognosis have a poor outcome and receive a 27 Gy whole-brain irradiation.

American and European groups do not advocate front-line biopsy in secreting tumours (i.e. non germinoma) and thus use a two-category strategy: germinomas and non-germinomas.

Localized germinomas were treated within the SIOP (International Society of Paediatric Oncology) GCT 96 protocol with either CSI of 24 Gy with a local boost of 16 Gy, or combined treatment with etoposide–carboplatin–ifosfamide (CarboPEI) followed by a 40-Gy focal boost. Due to potential neurotoxicity in the former, and excess of ventricular relapses in the latter, the current CGTII SIOP protocol explores the same induction chemotherapy followed by WVI of 24 Gy with a 16-Gy boost, delivered exclusively in patients who do not reach complete remission (CR) prior to radiation.The Children's Oncology Group (COG) launched ACNS 1123 that explores combined treatment by etoposide–carboplatin, followed by 18 Gy of WVI with a 12-Gy boost in patients reaching CR, or 24 Gy and 12 Gy respectively otherwise.

Localized non-germinomas were treated in the two successive SIOP trials (GCT96 and SIOPGCTII) with ifosfamide–etoposide–cisplatin (PEI) followed by a 54-Gy boost to the primary. The GCT96 cohort reported a poorer prognosis for patients with AFP more than 1,000 and/or with persisting viable tumour after chemotherapy. Hence, GCTII explores the role of high-dose therapy followed by stem-cell rescue, prior to radiation, in high-risk patients. ACNS 0122 delivered etoposide–carboplatin–ifosfamide with 36 Gy of CSI and a 18-Gy boost for patients in CR, and consolidation by high-dose etoposide thiotepa with stem-cell rescue followed by CSI otherwise. Five-year OS was 93%. The current ACNS 1123 for non-germinomas explores the feasibility of reducing the field to WVI. The overall prognosis for patients with recurrent germinomas remains excellent. Non-germinomatous GCT that recur may be salvaged, although the long-term outcome is worse.

Future outlook

Biology of intracranial (non-)germinomas is lagging behind due to the lack of availability of tumour tissue in most chemo-naive patients. Intracranial and extracranial tumours have similar mutations in KIT (26%: mostly exon 17), KRAS (15%), NRAS (5%; exclusive from KIT), mTor (8%), CBL (11%), with copy gain of AKT1 (19%). Potentially effective drugs in the future include sunitinib and mTor inhibitors. EC is CD30-positive and may benefit from brentuximab vedotin.

Liquid biopsy, especially in CSF, is an attractive surrogate for tissue sampling; miRNAs are potential candidates for the follow-up of tumour-mass response to therapy.

Craniopharyngiomas

Diagnosis: radiology, (molecular) pathology

Craniopharyngiomas are World Health Organization (WHO) grade I tumours of the intra/suprasellar region. Due to the proximity of the opto-chiamatic and hypothalamo-pituitary axis, the quality of life is often compromised in these children whose life expectancy is long (up to 95% at 20 years after diagnosis). With less than two cases per million persons per year, this orphan disease has a bimodal distribution: half before the end of adolescence (rarely prenatal or neonatal period), half during adulthood. No sex preference or predisposing factors are reported.

Adamantinomatous craniopharyngiomas (Figure 24.2) are composed of a solid portion formed by nests and trabeculae of epithelial tumour cells with calcifications, and a cystic component filled with a dark, oily fluid. They are most frequent in children, more locally aggressive with higher rate of recurrences than papillary tumours that occur primarily in adults, and have a well-differentiated squamous epithelium with picket-like palisades and wet keratin.

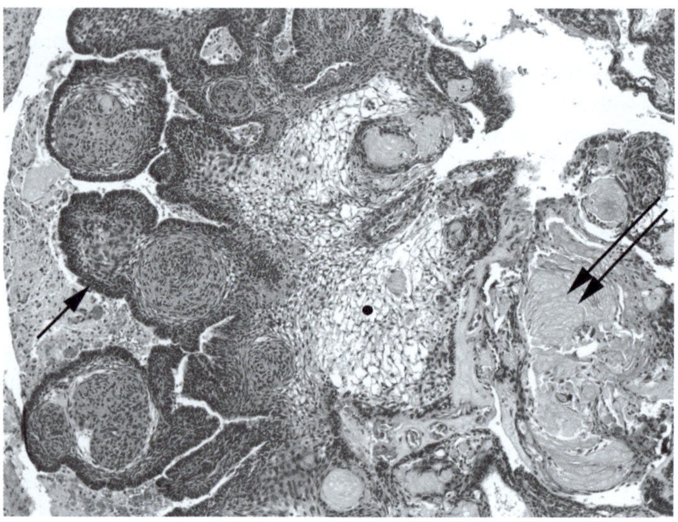

Figure 24.2 Adamantinomatous craniopharyngioma (hematoxylin-phloxine-saffron staining, original magnification × 100). Solid epithelial nests, that resemble the developing tooth, are bordered by basal cells (single arrow) and include loose areas called 'stellate reticulum' (black round) and a 'ghost' keratin called 'wet keratin' (double arrow).
Reproduced courtesy of Cécile Faure-Conter, Institute of Hematology and Pediatric Oncology (IHOPE), Lyon, France

The diagnosis is often overlooked for years, possibly due both to public and medical ignorance of the non-specific signs of intracranial pressure. Compression of optic nerves and/or chiasm induces loss of visual field and/or visual acuity in at least half of the cases. Most present with at least one hormonal deficit of growth hormone (GH: 75%), gonadotropins (40%), adrenocorticotropic hormone (ACTH: 25%), thyroid-stimulating hormone (TSH: 25%) secretions, or diabetes insipidus (30%). Significant weight gain, predictive of hypothalamic obesity, occurs shortly before diagnosis.

The majority of craniopharyngiomas (95%) have a suprasellar component (pure or with an intrasellar part), 5% are purely intrasellar. They combine solid, cystic, and calcified components. CT scan shows calcifications. On T1-weighted MRI, cyst-content intensity varies according to the protein content of fluid. They may extend intracranially and have an ectopic origin. The differential diagnoses include all tumours of the opto-chiasmato-hypothalamic region.

Current treatment strategies

In emergency, the management of raised intracranial pressure, visual compression, and rapid restoration or substitution of hormone deficits are crucial. According to the risk–benefit balance, first-line treatment—radical surgery and/or radiation therapy and/or cyst drainage—should be discussed in a multidisciplinary meeting.

Complete resection, preserving visual and hypothalamic function, is widely advised. No consensus exists when optic nerve and/or the hypothalamus are involved: complete resection versus planned limited resection followed by radiation therapy. In a report from Elowe Gruau, the rate of severe obesity decreased when extensive resective surgery was compared with hypothalamus-sparing surgical strategies tailored to an algorithm that took into account presurgical hypothalamic tumour involvement: 54% versus 28%. Merchant reported a 9.8 points IQ loss after complete resection versus 13.1 points after repeated surgery at relapse, versus 1.25 points after limited resection followed by radiation therapy. Treatment in large centres was less radical, and the rates of complete resection and hypothalamic surgical lesions were lower. A multinational prospective study is under way to adopt strategies tailored to risk factors for morbidity and quality of life.

Various surgical approaches have been described: pterional or subfrontal transcranial (for suprasellar tumours extending into the infundibulum); transventricular (for large tumours within the ventricle); and transsphenoidal (for infradiaphragmatic tumours with sellar enlargement). Tumour cysts can be opened for removal and decompression or insertion of catheters. Endoscopic procedures may treat occlusive hydrocephalus, and allow limited biopsies and catheter placement under optic control. Radiotherapy is very effective. The patient's age, site, and rate of progression dictate whether re-operation and/or radiotherapy should be performed at relapse. A prospective paediatric multinational trial (KRANIOPHARYNGEOM2007) randomizes between immediate radiotherapy versus radiotherapy at time of progression for patients older than five years of age with incomplete resection.

Craniopharyngiomas are not infiltrative and have sharp borders. They are ideally suited for using high-precision, three-dimensional conformational or intensity-modulated technology with a maximum

5-mm safety margin, delivering a conventionally fractionated target (total) volume dose of 54 Gy. The high-precision technique is sometimes also called fractionated stereotactic radiotherapy. Stereotactic radiosurgery requires sophisticated immobilization devices and is indicated in small, mainly solid tumours with more than 3 mm space between the tumour and critical structures. No treatment-related mortality has been reported.

Proton therapy is frequently considered to be the best option, when accessible, although no comparative study between proton-beam therapy and modern photon therapy is available. As reported by Fitzek, the combination of proton with photon irradiation for residual or recurrent disease provides a ten-year local control rate of 85% and OS of 72%, without treatment-related neurocognitive deficits, although newly diagnosed panhypopituitarism, cerebrovascular accident, and cyst enlargement have been described.

Multivariate analysis of a prospective programme reported by Muller showed that the risk for relapses after complete resection was 80% lower when compared to incomplete resection. The risk for progression was 88% lower in irradiated patients when compared with patients without or before irradiation. The tumour control rate was identical if radiation was offered after primary surgery or at the time of recurrence.

Local intracystic instillations—bleomycin or interferon-α—may be used in predominantly monocystic craniopharyngiomas. Emitting isotopes may be used for relapsing monocystic craniopharyngiomas after failure of surgery and external-beam irradiation.

Treatment-related morbidities are a major concern. Transient post-surgical diabetes insipidus occurs in almost all cases and persists in around 80%. Inappropriate antidiuretic hormone secretion and cerebral salt-wasting syndrome are usually transient. GH deficiency is found in most patients. Its therapy induces excellent linear growth, but has only a slight beneficial effect on body mass index (BMI) gain. A third of patients have neurological sequelae including both visual and neurological complications (e.g. epilepsy, motor or cranial nerve deficits), especially when the initial tumour volume was large. A series by Liu et al. described that one third of patients treated with irradiation develop some type of vasculopathy, half of them being symptomatic. However, treatment techniques dated back to the nineties and some patients received intracystic bleomycin.

Hypothalamic dysfunction is present in one third of patients preoperatively and manifests in behavioural changes, disturbed attention and impaired processing speed, obesity, perturbation of circadian rhythm and sleep, daytime sleepiness, imbalances in regulation of body temperature, thirst, heart rate, and/or blood pressure. Obesity and eating disorders result in increased risks of metabolic syndrome and cardiovascular disease, and increased premature mortality. Pharmacological interventions have little effect. Its incidence increases after radical surgery, especially when surgery reaches the mammillary bodies. A classification of presurgical involvement and post-surgical lesions of hypothalamic structures is now proposed to guide surgical decisions.

Future outlook

CTNNB1 mutations were exclusively detected in adamantinomatous craniopharyngiomas, whether adult or paediatric, whereas BRAF V600E mutations were solely found in the papillary subgroup. The methylome fingerprints perfectly matched with histology-based diagnosis. Gene-expression analysis confirmed over-activation of specific markers and important embryonic signalling pathways in adamantinomatous craniopharyngiomas: apart from significant upregulation of several direct targets of the WNT/β-catenin signalling pathway, important components of the hedgehog signalling pathway (e.g. GLI2, PTCH1, as well as SHH) were also over-expressed specifically. Gene-expression data showed increased expression of MAP2, tenascin C (TNC), and the stem-cell marker CD133 (PROM1). CD44 and claudin 1 (CLDN1) are significantly downregulated. All these alterations may be targeted by new compounds in the future and take an active part in the treatment of craniopharyngiomas.

Ependymomas

Ependymomas are the third most common paediatric tumour of the central nervous system (CNS), accounting for 10% of brain tumours in children. Ependymal tumours can arise along the entire neuraxis. In paediatric patients, more than 90% of ependymomas are located intracranially, with two thirds found in the infratentorial region. More than half of paediatric ependymomas occur in children younger than five years of age, with an overall male:female ratio of about 2:1. The aetiology of ependymal tumours is not yet known, and there are no reliable associations with environmental or infection-related factors. Ependymomas rarely occur in the context of cancer predisposition syndromes. Patients with neurofibromatosis type 2 may develop spinal ependymomas, while in both Turcot and Gorlin syndrome intracranial ependymomas may occur.

Progression-free survival (PFS) and OS rates of children with intracranial ependymomas vary significantly between different series, while all prior studies that evaluated the therapeutic value of interventions in these tumours have not accounted for molecular subgroup affiliation, and might therefore be confounded by clinical differences in response to therapy between these subgroups. Thus, clinical management of intracranial ependymomas (WHO Grade II/III) is challenging, and the optimal treatment strategy is contentious. Intracranial ependymomas, particularly before administration of any therapy, demonstrate predominantly locally invasive growth patterns and have only very low metastatic potential. However, late recurrence is frequent, especially in aggressive molecular subgroups (see Table 24.1).

Classic MRI appearance of ependymomas demonstrates a low T1-signal intensity, enhanced with gadolinium, and a heterogeneous T2 hyperintensity. Cystic components may be seen in supratentorial tumours. Posterior fossa ependymomas typically show an extension through the foramina of Luschka into the cerebellopontine angle and/or through the foramen of Magendie. This highly suggestive feature may help to distinguish ependymomas from medulloblastomas.

Histopathology, molecular classification, and risk stratification of ependymal tumours

Ependymomas from throughout the CNS are currently subdivided by three histology-based grades used to predict the natural course of the disease. WHO Grade I tumours include myxopapillary ependymomas, which typically occur in the spine, as well as subependymomas, which are usually intracranial and only rarely found in the spine. Grade I ependymomas are relatively easier to distinguish, occur predominantly in adults, and are usually associated

Table 24.1 Molecular subgroups of ependymal tumours

Molecular subgroup	Age group	Gender distribution	Prognosis	Genetics	Histopathology
SE	Adults	m>f	Good	Balanced	Subependymomo (WHO I)
EPN-YAP1	Children	m<f	Good	Focal aberrations Chrosome 11; YAP1-fusion	(Anaplastic) ependymoma (WHO I–III)
EPN-RELA	Children and adults	m>f	Poor	Aberrations Chrosome 11; chromothripsis; *RELA*-fusion	(Anaplastic) ependymoma (WHO I–III)
SE	Adults	m>f	Good	Balanced	Subependymoma (WHO I)
EPN-A	Children	m>f	Poor	Balanced	(Anaplastic) ependymoma (WHO I–II)
EPN-B	Children and adults	m<f	Good	CIN	(Anaplastic) ependymoma (WHO I–II)
SE	Adults	m=f	Good	6q deletion	Subependymoma (WHO I)
MPE	Predominantly adults	m=f	Good	CIN	Myxopapillary ependymoma (WHO I)
EPN	Predominantly adults	m>f	Good	CIN; *NF2* mutation	(Anaplastic) ependymoma (WHO I–II)

Adapted from Kristian W. Pajtler, et al. 'Molecular dissection of ependymomas,' *Oncoscience*, Volume 2, Number 10, pp. 827–828, 2015.

with favourable patient outcomes. The majority of ependymomas constitute WHO Grade II (classic) and WHO Grade III (anaplastic) tumours. While classic WHO Grade II ependymomas show a papillary, clear-cell, or tanycytic phenotype, anaplastic ependymomas exhibit additional features of elevated mitotic activity, microvascular proliferation, and tumour necrosis. Studies demonstrated a high variance in the utility of the Grade II versus Grade III distinction as a robust marker for clinical outcome, and conventional histological grading may be further confounded by anatomical compartment. Thus, the utility of histological grading of these tumours for risk stratification is controversial.

Recent advances in the biological characterization of ependymal tumours using genome-wide DNA methylation profiling have demonstrated the existence of nine clinically, demographically, and molecularly distinct entities, with three occurring in each anatomical compartment of the CNS—spine (SP), posterior fossa (PF), and supratentorial (ST) region. One of the molecular subgroups within each compartment was enriched with WHO Grade I subependymomas (SE)—named ST-SE, PF-SE, and SP-SE—occurring in adults only. The two other molecular subgroups within the spine predominantly matched the histopathology-based diagnoses myxopapillary ependymoma (SP-MPE) and WHO Grade II/III ependymoma (SP-EPN). The remaining two molecular types of ependymoma occurred in the posterior fossa, termed PF-EPN-A and PF-EPN-B (or, alternatively, posterior fossa Group A and B), and were independently identified in retrospective studies. PF-EPN-A tumours are predominantly diagnosed in infants and young children, and are associated with high recurrence rates and poor clinical outcome. In contrast, PF-EPN-B tumours are mainly found in adolescents and young adults, and are associated with a better prognosis. The majority of supratentorial ependymomas (more than 70%) are characterized by fusions between a gene with unknown function, *C11orf95*, and the NFkB effector, *RELA*, and are designated as ST-EPN-RELA tumours. ST-EPN-RELA tumours occur in both children and adults, while the remaining molecular subgroup of supratentorial ependymomas are characterized by recurrent fusions to the oncogene *YAP1*, and are mainly diagnosed in childhood.

Multivariate survival analyses demonstrated that molecular subgrouping is superior to histopathological grading of ependymal tumors, and the only other variables that endured as independent prognostic factors were extent of surgical resection and 1q gain. Molecular subclassification is expected to significantly simplify risk stratification processes in the near future. An interconnection of tissue-based information with more precise diagnostic aids gained from novel, unbiased, and observer-independent molecular analyses, as well as data from imaging methods including central pathology and radiological review, might finally converge at a refined diagnostic setting and improve treatment strategies for ependymoma. The updated fourth edition of the WHO classification of CNS tumours already recognizes the supratentorial molecular variant, ST-EPN-RELA, as a distinct pathological disease entity.

Surgery

Surgery is the mainstay for local tumour control and the extent of tumour resection has been demonstrated to be the most consistent independent prognostic factor in intracranial ependymomas. Treatment strategies increasingly comprise second-look surgeries, since there are marked outcome differences between patients with complete versus incomplete tumour resection. However, these concepts require experienced and comprehensive radiological assessment of the initial and residual disease status on which to base potential secondary neurosurgical intervention decisions.

In the context of molecular subgroups of ependymal tumours, it was recently demonstrated, in a huge retrospective study comprising four independent non-overlapping cohorts of PF ependymomas (n=820 cases), that patients with either PF-EPN-A or PF-EPN-B tumours benefit from gross total resection. However, survival rates are particularly poor for incomplete resected PF-EPN-A tumours, even after completion of radiation therapy. Notably, a subset of patients with gross totally resected PF-EPN-B tumours did not recur, even in the absence of radiotherapy. For ST ependymomas, series and collections of single cases markedly differ regarding age distribution, therapy modalities, and availability of molecular data. Thus, variations in outcome cannot be reliably linked to specific treatment approaches or molecular subgroups. Routine molecular analyses in the setting of prospective trials for ST ependymomas, as well as investigation of clinically well-annotated, large international retrospective cohorts with long-term follow-up, are expected to further clarify questions about the clinical outcome and adequate therapy regimens.

Radiotherapy and chemotherapy

In addition to surgery, post-operative involved-field radiotherapy dosed at 54–59.4 Gy is considered the standard of care for patients with non-disseminated ependymomas, to lower the risk of local recurrence. Safety margins around the target volume have decreased from 2.0 cm to 1.0 cm, or even 0.5 cm, without increased frequency of tumour recurrence. It is of note that extension of immediate post-operative high-dose conformal radiotherapy, even to children under the age of three years, led to seven-year PFS rates of 77%, albeit long-term follow-up for toxic effects on development is still pending. Since laterally located hindbrain ependymomas occur especially in young children, proton-beam therapy is under exploration to better spare eloquent neurological structures. There is also some evidence for reasonable treatment effects through re-irradiation in case of tumour recurrence, although this strategy was associated with a decline in intellectual function of affected patients.

In contrast to surgery and radiotherapy, the role of chemotherapy in the management of ependymoma remains unclear. Retrospective analyses of cohorts from paediatric patients, that investigated the role of chemotherapy, either failed to demonstrate a survival advantage or showed substantial variation between individual patients. Two ongoing international randomized trials in children—SIOP Ependymoma II (Europe) and ACNS0831 (USA)—are currently comparing post-irradiation chemotherapy to an observation-only strategy. In order to delay radiotherapy in infants, driven by concerns about long-term treatment toxicity, post-operative chemotherapy approaches in children under three years old were applied, with 42% being the highest rate of five-year PFS reached to date. Radiotherapy deferral strategies using chemotherapy in patients older than one year are, therefore, not frequently applied. Ongoing trials are currently exploring the role of neoadjuvant chemotherapy, since there is evidence for responses to chemotherapy after subtotal resection. To date, there is no chemotherapeutic regimen that can routinely be recommended, outside the context of a clinical trial, in paediatric patients with intracranial ependymoma.

Conclusion and outlook

Ependymal tumours from different compartments of the CNS are biologically distinct, and future therapy optimization trials, as well as testing of novel therapeutics, should accompany molecular classification in order to be useful to ependymoma patients. The differentiation between histologically defined WHO Grade II versus Grade III ependymomas is of limited utility for clinical decision making, and therefore should be used with great caution outside the setting of a clinical trial. For patients over the age of one year with PF-EPN-A ependymomas, the currently recommended standard of care is maximal safe neurosurgical resection complemented by local radiotherapy. There is no evidence to recommend routine use of chemotherapy outside of clinical trials. Randomized trial-based therapy de-escalation strategies should be explored in gross total resected PF-EPN-B ependymoma patients in order to test the possibility of avoiding radiotherapy.

There is an urgent need to clarify questions about the clinical outcome of the molecular variants of ST ependymoma, eventually allowing for explicit therapy recommendations of these subgroups. Further in-depth and comprehensive analyses of the molecular heterogeneity of ependymal tumours are expected to create new opportunities to identify promising therapeutic targets in these treatment-resistant tumours and facilitate risk stratification.

Choroid plexus tumours

Choroid plexus tumours (CPT) are rare intraventricular neoplasms derived from the choroid plexus epithelium and represent 0.2% of all CNS neoplasms. Within the first year of life, choroid plexus tumours even account for 10–20% of brain tumours. Paediatric CPT mainly occur in the lateral (80%) or third (15%) ventricles, whereas infratentorial tumours in the fourth ventricle or cerebellopontine angle are rare.

WHO classification of CNS tumours defines three histopathology-based entities. Choroid plexus papilloma (CPP, WHO Grade I) closely resembles normal choroid plexus tissue. Although malignant transformation of CPP to choroid plexus carcinoma (CPC) has been described, and even some cases with metastatic disease, CPP are considered as being of relatively low aggressiveness. Gross total resection of CPP is frequently achieved and is regarded as the therapeutic mainstay of these tumours. The five-year OS rates reach more than 90% with surgery alone. The defining feature of atypical choroid plexus papilloma (aCPP, WHO Grade II) is the presence of increased mitotic activity (two or more mitoses per ten high-power fields).

In infants, CPP and aCPP share molecular signatures and mostly show excellent outcome. However, in older children (above three years old) and adults, aCPPs are also associated with recurrent disease and intermediate outcome, and might also be difficult to distinguish from CPC by histology alone. It remains unclear which molecular mechanisms are driving these differences in aCPP between different age groups. CPC (WHO Grade III) is characterized by clear signs of malignancy including high mitotic activity, nuclear pleomorphism, high cellularity, blurring of the papillary growth pattern, and necrosis. CPCs exhibit a dismal prognosis, with long-term OS of about 30%. Despite aggressive treatment strategies, including surgical resection and combined radio-chemotherapy, the clinical behaviour of CPCs is variable and most of the few survivors exhibit long-term sequelae in cognitive functions and development.

To date, the optimal treatment regimen has not been defined, and only a few standardized trials have been performed. In an attempt to delay radiotherapy in very young children, a UKCCSG-SIOP trial applied post-operative chemotherapy only, but this resulted in dramatically low survival rates, with the primary tumour bed being the most frequent site of relapse. The previous study, CPT-SIOP-2000, established CPTs to be chemotherapy-responsive to combinations of etoposide, vincristine, and either carboplatin or cyclophosphamide, but which agent was superior could not be determined. The current

CPT-SIOP-2009 protocol randomizes CPCs, aCPP with residual disease or at relapse, and CPP in cases of metastases or unresectability to four different chemotherapy schedules. The majority of patients will not receive irradiation.

The indication for radiation, the treatment volume, and the dose is specified based upon the patient's age, tumour histology, staging, and response to the two first cycles of chemotherapy. Maximal radiation will be given to patients over three years of age with metastatic CPC not responsive to the first two cycles. These patients will also receive CSI. It is of note that over 50% of CPC harbour somatic *TP53* mutations, while germline *TP53* mutations are also frequently identified, since CPC is one of the hallmark cancers of the Li–Fraumeni syndrome. This cancer predisposition syndrome should be considered in the planning process for radiation therapy.

Recent classification approaches of CPT using DNA methylation profiling in a cohort across all age groups and CNS locations identified three distinct molecular clusters. These clusters are clinically relevant. Notably, some paediatric aCPP with favourable prognosis cluster together with CPP, thereby confirming previous studies that identified molecular similarities of CPP and aCPP in young children. However, a significant proportion of histologically diagnosed paediatric CPP and aCPP cluster together with CPC, and indeed have been associated with a higher risk of tumour progression. Further validation of these data in future prospective trials and in-depth molecular characterization of different CPT subgroups will inform risk stratification of affected patients and set the basis for future treatment intensification in high-risk patients and potentially de-escalation strategies in low-risk patients.

FURTHER READING

Amendola BE, et al. (2003) Role of radiosurgery in craniopharyngiomas: a preliminary report. *Med Pediatr Oncol* **41**(2), 123–7.

Aoyama H (2009) Radiation therapy for intracranial germ cell tumors. *Prog Neurolog Surg* **23**, 96–105.

Bahar M, et al. (2015) Radiation therapy for choroid plexus carcinoma patients with Li–Fraumeni syndrome: advantageous or detrimental? *Anticancer Res* **35**(5), 3013–17.

Beltran C, et al. (2012) On the benefits and risks of proton therapy in pediatric craniopharyngioma. *Int J RadiatOncol Biol Phys* **82**(2), e281–7.

Calaminus G, et al. (2013) SIOP CNS GCT 96: final report of outcome of a prospective, multinational nonrandomized trial for children and adults with intracranial germinoma, comparing craniospinal irradiation alone with chemotherapy followed by focal primary site irradiation for pat. *Neuro Oncol* **15**, 788–96.

Cavalheiro S, et al. (2010) Craniopharyngiomas: intratumoral chemotherapy with interferon-alpha: a multicenter preliminary study with 60 cases. *Neurosurg Foc* **28**(4), E12.

Chakrabarti I, et al. (2005) Long-term neurological, visual, and endocrine outcomes following transnasal resection of craniopharyngioma. *J Neurosurg* **102**(4), 650–7.

Derrey S, et al. (2008) Management of cystic craniopharyngiomas with stereotactic endocavitary irradiation using colloidal 186Re: a retrospective study of 48 consecutive patients. *Neurosurgery* **63**(6), 1045–52.

Dudley RW, et al. (2015) Pediatric choroid plexus tumors: epidemiology, treatments, and outcome analysis on 202 children from the SEER database. *J Neurooncol* **121**(1), 201–7. doi: 10.1007/s11060-014-1628-6

Elowe-Gruau E, et al. (2013) Childhood craniopharyngioma: hypothalamus-sparing surgery decreases the risk of obesity. *J Clin Endocrinol Metab* **98**(6), 2376–82.

Fitzek MM, et al. (2006) Combined proton and photon irradiation for craniopharyngioma: long-term results of the early cohort of patients treated at Harvard Cyclotron Laboratory and Massachusetts General Hospital. *Int J Radiat Oncol Biol Phys* **64**(5), 1348–54.

Flitsch J, et al. (2011) Surgical strategies in childhood craniopharyngioma. *Front Endocrinol* **2**, 96.

Geffner M, et al. (2004) Changes in height, weight, and body mass index in children with craniopharyngioma after three years of growth hormone therapy: analysis of KIGS (Pfizer International Growth Database). *J Clin Endocrinol Metab* **89**(11), 5435–40.

Goldman S, et al. (2015) Phase II trial assessing the ability of neoadjuvant chemotherapy with or without second-look surgery to eliminate measurable disease for nongerminomatous germ cell tumors: a Children's Oncology Group study. *J Clin Oncol* **33**(22), 2464–71.

González Briceño L, et al. (2014) Water and electrolyte disorders at long-term post-treatment follow-up in paediatric patients with suprasellar tumours include unexpected persistent cerebral salt-wasting syndrome. *Horm Res Pædiatr* **82**(6), 364–71.

Hardenbergh PH, et al. (1997) Intracranial germinoma: the case for lower dose radiation therapy. *Int J Radiat Oncol Biol Phys* **39**(2), 419–26.

Hölsken A, et al. (2016) Adamantinomatous and papillary craniopharyngiomas are characterized by distinct epigenomic as well as mutational and transcriptomic profiles. *Acta Neuropathol Comm* **4**(1), article 20.

Khatua S, et al. (2016) Current therapy and the evolving molecular landscape of paediatric ependymoma. *Eur J Cancer* **70**, 34–41. doi: 10.1016/j.ejca.2016.10.013

Laffond C, et al. (2012) Quality-of-life, mood and executive functioning after childhood craniopharyngioma treated with surgery and proton beam therapy. *Brain Inj* **26**(3), 270–81.

Liu AK, et al. (2009) Vascular abnormalities in pediatric craniopharyngioma patients treated with radiation therapy. *Pediatr Blood Cancer* **52**(2), 227–30.

Mason PW, et al. (2002) The use of dextroamphetamine to treat obesity and hyperphagia in children treated for craniopharyngioma. *Arch Pediatr Adol Med* **156**(9), 887–92.

Merchant TE (2017) Current clinical challenges in childhood ependymoma: a focused review. *J Clin Oncol* **35**(21), 2364–9. doi: 10.1200/JCO.2017.73.1265

Merchant TE, et al. (2002) Craniopharyngioma: the St Jude Children's Research Hospital experience 1984–2001. *Int J Radiat Oncol Biol Phys* **53**(3), 533–42.Merchant TE, et al. (2013) Disease control after reduced volume conformal and intensity modulated radiation therapy for childhood craniopharyngioma. *Int J Radiat Oncol Biol Phys* **85**(4), e187–92.

Merino DM, et al. (2015) Molecular characterization of choroid plexus tumors reveals novel clinically relevant subgroups. *Clin Cancer Res* **21**(1), 184–92. doi: 10.1158/1078-0432.CCR-14-1324

Modak S, et al. (2004) Thiotepa-based high-dose chemotherapy with autologous stem-cell rescue in patients with recurrent or progressive CNS germ cell tumors. *J Clin Oncol* **22**(10), 1934–43.

Mortini P, et al. (2011) Neurosurgical treatment of craniopharyngioma in adults and children: early and long-term results in a large case series. *J Neurosurg* **114**(5), 1350–9.

Mottolese C, et al. (2001) Intracystic chemotherapy with bleomycin in the treatment of craniopharyngiomas. *Childs Nerv Syst* **17**(12), 724–30.

Müller HL (2011) Diagnostics, treatment, and follow-up in craniopharyngioma. *Front Endocrinol* **2**, 70.

Müller HL (2014) Craniopharyngioma. *Endocr Rev* **35**(3), 513–43.

Müller HL, et al. (2004) Longitudinal study on growth and body mass index before and after diagnosis of childhood craniopharyngioma. *J Clin Endocrinol Metab* **89**(7), 3298–305.

Müller HL, et al. (2011) Post-operative hypothalamic lesions and obesity in childhood craniopharyngioma: results of the multinational prospective trial KRANIOPHARYNGEOM 2000 after 3-year follow-up. *Eur J Endocrinol* **165**(1), 17–24.

Murray MJ, et al. (2016) A pipeline to quantify serum and cerebrospinal fluid microRNAs for diagnosis and detection of relapse in paediatric malignant germ-cell tumours. *Br J Cancer* **114**(2), 151–62.

Özyurt J, et al. (2014) Neuropsychological outcome in patients with childhood craniopharyngioma and hypothalamic involvement. *J Pediatr* **164**(4), 876–81.Pajtler KW, et al. (2016) The current consensus on the clinical management of intracranial ependymoma and its distinct molecular variants. *Acta Neuropathol* **133**(1), 5–12.

Pajtler KW, et al. (2015) Molecular classification of ependymal tumors across all CNS compartments, histopathological grades, and age groups. *Cancer Cell* **27**(5), 728–43. doi: 10.1016/j.ccell.2015.04.002

Phi JH, et al. (2010) Germinomas in the basal ganglia: magnetic resonance imaging classification and the prognosis. *J Neuro-Oncol* **99**(2), 227–36.

Ramaswamy V, et al. (2016) Therapeutic impact of cytoreductive surgery and irradiation of posterior fossa ependymoma in the molecular era: a retrospective multicohort analysis. *J Clin Oncol* **34**(21), 2468–77. doi: 10.1200/JCO.2015.65.7825

Thomas C, et al. (2016) Methylation profiling of choroid plexus tumors reveals 3 clinically distinct subgroups. *Neuro Oncol* **18**(6), 790–6. doi: 10.1093/neuonc/nov322

Wang L, et al. (2014) Novel somatic and germline mutations in intracranial germ cell tumours. *Nature* **511**(7508), 241–5.

Winkfield KM, et al. (2009) Surveillance of craniopharyngioma cyst growth in children treated with proton radiotherapy. *Int J Radiat Oncol Biol Phys* **73**(3), 716–21.

25

Soft-Tissue Sarcomas

Gianni Bisogno and Hans Merks

Introduction

Soft-tissue sarcomas (STS) are a heterogeneous group of tumours derived from mesenchymal cells. As these cells normally mature into, for example, muscle, fibrous structures, and fat, the different histotypes of STS are designated according to the line of differentiation that may be recognized in the tumour.

STS comprise approximately 8% of all paediatric malignancies. They are conventionally divided into rhabdomyosarcoma (RMS), which account for 50–60% of the whole group, and non-rhabdomyosarcoma soft-tissue sarcoma (NRSTS) (**Figure 25.1**).

Rhabdomyosarcoma

Rhabdomyosarcoma (RMS) is an aggressive tumour that typically affects young children and can develop in almost any part of the body where mesenchymal tissue is present. Historically, until the 1960s, less than one third of children survived. In the 1970s, large co-operative national and international study groups started to adopt a systematic multidisciplinary approach, including multidrug chemotherapy coordinated with surgery and radiotherapy. This led to a progressive increase of survival (now above 70%) and to the identification of a number of prognostic factors that can be utilized to tailor the treatment. More recently, clinical protocols have been linked to pathology and biological studies that have added important insights into the nature of RMS and may provide new therapeutic opportunities in the near future.

Epidemiology and aetiology

RMS is a rare tumour with an annual incidence of 4.5 per million children under the age of 20. A male predominance is generally reported. In two thirds of cases, RMS arises before six years of age, but a second, smaller peak is evident in adolescence and the number of adults with RMS should not be neglected. The aetiology is not known. Genetic factors may play an important role, as demonstrated by an association between RMS and a familial cancer syndrome (Li–Fraumeni), congenital anomalies (involving the genitourinary and central nervous system), and other genetic conditions.

Pathology and biology

RMS is characterized by a variable degree of myogenic differentiation, a feature that results from the biological impact of aberrant transcription signals and the resultant production of myogenic proteins. Classically, RMS is histologically distinguished into two main subtypes: embryonal RMS (E-RMS), which accounts for approximately 70% of all RMS, and alveolar RMS (A-RMS) (20%). A third subtype, pleomorphic RMS, is described in adults but very rarely encountered in children; this entity is probably more closely related to adult pleomorphic STS than to other RMS subtypes.

E-RMS is characterized by a spindle and/or round cell tumour in a loose myxoid or dense collagenous stroma. Two variants have been described:

1. The **botryoid subtype**, found typically at vaginal or nasopharyngeal sites, where tumour grows into organ cavities. Histologically, it shows a characteristic condensed layer of tumour cells (cambium layer) under the overlying mucosa.
2. The **spindle-cell variant**, with either collagen-poor or collagen-rich leiomyomatous forms, with a storiform pattern, arising in paratesticular locations. Its distinction from other forms of STS relies on the presence of well-differentiated rhabdomyoblasts in the spindle-cell population.

Classical A-RMS displays well-defined alveolar-like spaces separated by thick collagenous bands and lined with round tumour cells showing variable myogenic features. A solid alveolar variant has been described and tumours exist with a mixed embryonal-alveolar appearance. Previously, it was generally accepted that the percentage of cells showing an alveolar pattern was unimportant and that even a focal presence was sufficient to justify the diagnosis of A-RMS. More recently, this concept has been challenged and the current histological definition of A-RMS requires that the majority of a tumour shows alveolar histology, or solid sheets of cells with monotonous round nuclei characteristic of A-RMS. Other variants have been proposed, such as pseudovascular sclerosing, rhabdoid, or anaplastic RMS, but the clinical significance of these entities is yet to be confirmed.

Desmin and muscle-specific actin are relatively sensitive immunohistochemical markers of RMS, but the most sensitive markers are the muscle transcription factors MyoD and myogenin.

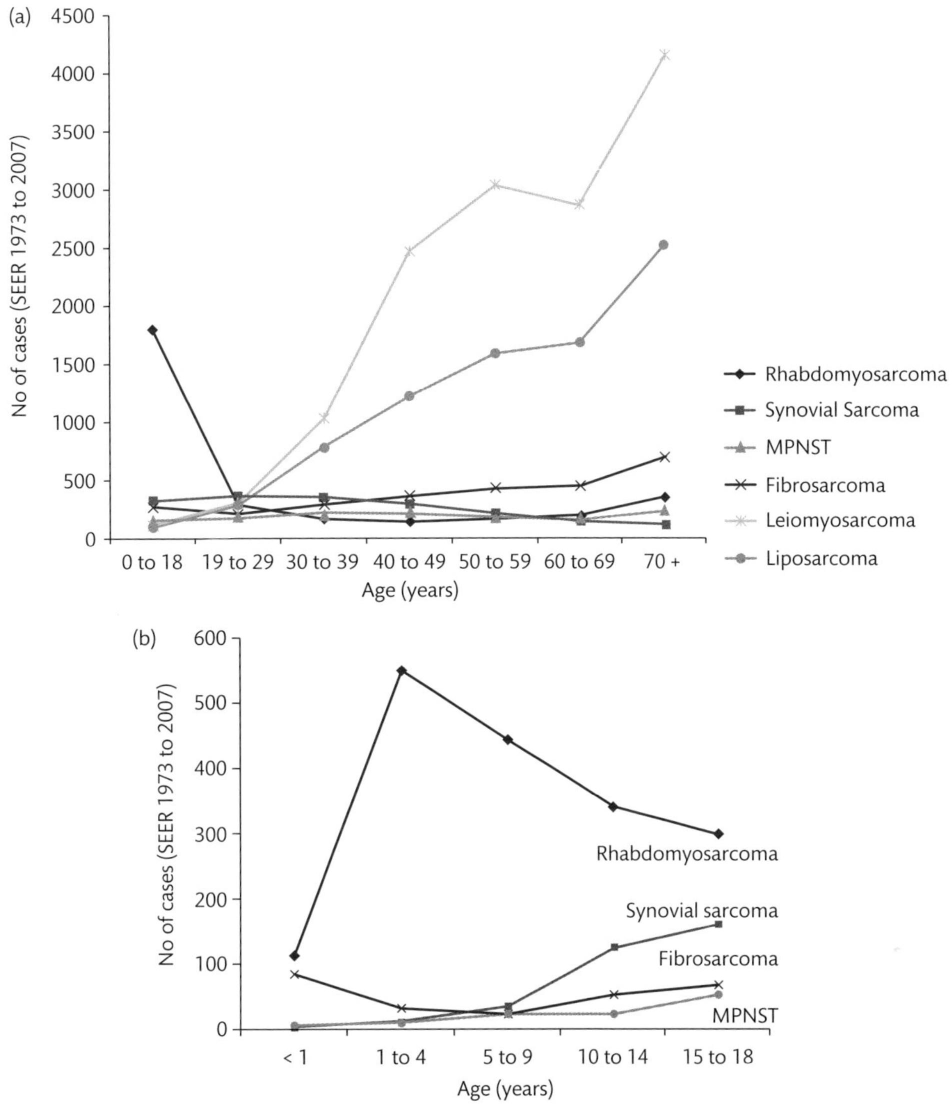

Figure 25.1 Frequency of soft-tissue sarcoma subtypes: (a) at all ages; and (b) for patients aged 0–18 years.
Source: data from the Survival Epidemiology and End result (SEER) public-access database (1973–2007) (www.seer.cancer.gov).

A high degree of nuclear staining of myogenin seems correlated with the alveolar subtype. Recently, gene-expression data have identified AP2Beta and P-cadherin as specific markers for A-RMS, and epidermal growth factor (EGF) receptor and fibrillin-2 as markers for E-RMS. The search for specific genetic alterations has identified two chromosomal translocations specifically associated with A-RMS, and the t(2;13)(q35;q14) and t(1;13)(p36;q14) translocations are found in more than 80% of cases. These abnormalities fuse the *FKHR* locus on chromosome 13 to either the *PAX3* gene on chromosome 2 (60%) or the *PAX7* gene on chromosome 1 (20%), producing the PAX3–FKHR and PAX7–FKHR chimeric proteins that are powerful transcription factors influencing cell growth, differentiation, and apoptosis. A minority of A-RMS do not show known translocations: this may be explained by the presence of rare alternative translocations such as t(2;2) and t(2;8). It seems, however, that most translocation-negative A-RMS are clinically and molecularly indistinguishable from embryonal cases and significantly different from fusion-positive A-RMS. As a consequence, in most current and future trials, fusion-gene status will be used in risk stratification of RMS irrespective of histology. No specific genetic alterations have been found in E-RMS but many of them exhibit a loss of heterozygosity at chromosome 11p15.5, although the biological implications of this are not yet understood.

The International Classification of Rhabdomyosarcoma identified three risk groups:

1. superior prognosis: botryoid and spindle-cell RMS
2. intermediate prognosis: E-RMS
3. poor prognosis: A-RMS

This classification was shown to be strongly predictive of survival, but it does not take into account the recent advances of molecular biology.

Clinical presentation and diagnosis

RMS is encountered at almost all anatomical sites, although head and neck (40%), genitourinary (20%), and extremities (15%) are the

(a)

(b)

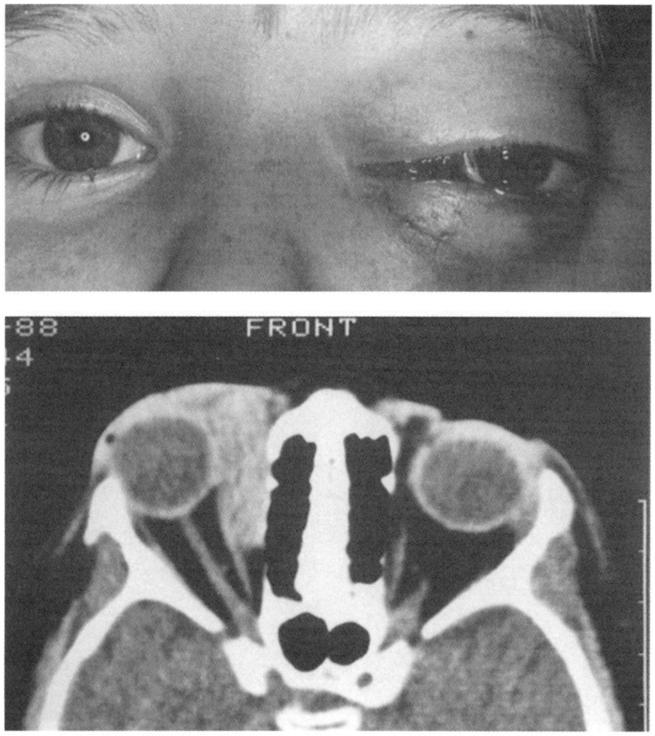

Figure 25.2 Orbital tumour: (a) clinical presentation with proptosis and deviation of globe; (b) CT scan shows large antero-medial soft-tissue mass without bone erosion.

most common locations. It tends to invade nearby organs and regional lymph nodes. Metastases at diagnosis are present in approximately 20% of cases, more frequently in the lungs, bone marrow, bones, and distant lymph nodes. Clinical presentation is strongly influenced by site; for example, tumours within the orbit tend to present early with obvious displacement of the ocular globe and are rarely associated with regional lymph node or distant metastatic spread (Figure 25.2), whilst tumours in the nasopharynx may result in a history of nasal discharge and obstruction and frequently involve local extension to the skull base, with the potential for associated cranial nerve palsies or visual loss. The definition of certain head–neck sites as 'parameningeal' relates to the risk of direct tumour extension into the meninges and beyond intracranially. Tumours within the genitourinary tract may present with urinary obstruction (in bladder and prostate sites), as a scrotal mass (paratesticular), or as a vaginal polyp or discharge (vaginal and uterine tumours).

Diagnostic and staging investigations

These must include adequate imaging of the primary site and regional lymph nodes by magnetic resonance imaging (MRI) scans, and accurate assessment of sites of potential metastatic spread by chest computed tomography (CT) scan, fluorodeoxyglucose (FDG)-positron emission tomography (PET)/CT scan, bone marrow biopsy, and aspirates. Cerebrospinal fluid should be sampled in the case of parameningeal/paraspinal tumours. The risk of involvement of regional lymph nodes depends on the primary site, and there is a general consensus to biopsy nodes when the RMS arises in the extremities (the use of sentinel lymph-node mapping techniques may be of help). Different strategies are adopted when RMS occurs in other sites; for example, systematic retroperitoneal lymph-node sampling is recommended in older children with paratesticular RMS in North American protocols, while radiological evaluation and selective biopsy is considered sufficient in Europe.

Diagnosis must be confirmed histologically and, although needle biopsy may be the simplest approach favoured by some clinicians, it has the disadvantage of limiting the tissue available for conventional histological examination, including immunohistochemistry, and may impede the need for fresh frozen tissue for cytogenetic and molecular genetic investigation. Open biopsy is therefore frequently preferred and should, when possible, be undertaken at the oncology centre where the initial surgical approach can be determined by the multidisciplinary team responsible for the child's subsequent treatment.

Treatment

The multidisciplinary risk-adapted management of RMS promotes chemotherapy as systemic treatment for both local and metastatic lesions, coordinated with local treatment that includes surgery and/or radiotherapy. Since the early 1970s, patients have been enrolled in large multi-institutional trials sequentially addressing crucial questions. Examples of successful models of clinical trials are the studies coordinated by the Intergroup Rhabdomyosarcoma Study (IRS) Group (now the Soft-Tissue Sarcoma Committee of the Children's Oncology Group (COG)) in the USA and those coordinated by the European paediatric Soft-Tissue Sarcoma Study Group (EpSSG) and the German Soft-Tissue Sarcoma Cooperative Group (CWS) in Europe.

Prognostic factors and staging

The presence of metastasis at diagnosis is the most powerful factor in determining an adverse outcome and groups of patients with localized or metastatic disease have often been investigated separately in the search for prognostic factors.

Localized disease

For non-metastatic RMS patients, several prognostic factors have emerged with the evolution of treatment. Table 25.1 describes the tumour and patient characteristics currently used to assign risk group and treatment strategy.

Histology

The IRS IV Study showed 88% relapse-free survival in E-RMS versus 66% in A-RMS. This prognostic distinction has been confirmed in most other studies and becomes more striking if only fusion-positive A-RMS is compared with E-RMS.

Fusion status

There is recent but increasing evidence that biological factors like the presence of the PAX3-FKHR or PAX7-FKHR gene fusions resulting from t(2;13) or t(1;13) translocations, typical of alveolar RMS, may be useful to better stratify patients; their presence identifies more precisely those patients at higher risk of treatment failure. Unfortunately, these data derive mainly from retrospective studies; therefore fusion status as a prognostic factor will be studied in ongoing and future trials.

Tumour site, size, and invasiveness

Site is a major determinant of treatment strategy and outcome: orbit, non-bladder prostate genitourinary (i.e. paratesticular and vagina/uterus), and non-parameningeal head–neck sites are associated with a better prognosis. Tumour dimension of more than 5 cm maximum diameter is the usually adopted point for identifying tumour size as an adverse factor within treatment-stratification systems, although recent evidence suggests that tumour dimension should be correlated with patient size, and the use of a fixed-size cut-off may be questioned in the future. Tumour invasiveness is difficult to assess in numerous cases, so many investigators feel it is not practical to be included in a stratification system.

Table 25.1 Prognostic factors in localized rhabdomyosarcoma

	Favourable	Unfavourable
Histology/Biology	Embryonal Spindle cell Botryoid RMS Alveolar fusion-negative	Alveolar, translocation-positive
Tumour site	Orbit Genitourinary non-bladder prostate (i.e. paratesticular and vagina/uterus) Head and neck non-parameningeal	Parameningeal Extremities Genitourinary bladder-prostate 'Other' (i.e. trunk, pelvis)
Tumour size	Maximum diameter <5 cm	>5 cm
Tumour invasiveness*	T1: tumour confined to the organ or tissue of origin	T2: tumour involving one or more contiguous organs or tissues
Lymph node involvement*	N0 = no clinical or pathological node involvement	N1 = clinical or pathological nodal involvement
Initial surgery	Complete (IRS Group I)	Incomplete (IRS Group II or III)
Patient age	1–9 years	<1 year and ≥10 years

* TNM system; although T status is a prognostic factor in many analyses, tumour invasiveness is difficult to assess in many cases and therefore is no longer part of stratification systems

Local lymph-node involvement (N1)

Local lymph-node involvement has always been regarded as a sign of tumour aggressiveness. In particular, patients N1 with alveolar histology and positive fusion status seem to present a prognosis similar to metastatic RMS.

Post-surgical status

The IRS grouping system is used:

- Group I: completely excised tumours with negative microscopic margins
- Group II: grossly resected tumours with microscopic residual disease.
- Group III: macroscopic residual disease after incomplete resection or initial biopsy
- Group IV: metastatic disease

Age

Prognosis is worse in patients over ten years of age. Young children (below one year old) generally have a worse prognosis, which may be associated with more restricted use of radiotherapy due to the higher risk of sequelae in this age group.

It is important to note that factors predictive of prognosis are often interdependent: limb tumours are generally of the alveolar type and tend to spread more frequently, both to regional nodes and to distant metastatic sites. The surgical status is also strongly determined by the site; for example, complete tumour resection is usually impossible for parameningeal RMS but easily performed for paratesticular tumour.

Metastatic disease

A pooled analysis of 788 patients treated in nine studies performed by European and American cooperative groups identified factors with an independent and significant negative impact on survival: age, unfavourable primary site (extremity and 'other' sites), presence of three or more sites of metastatic disease, and the specific presence of bone or bone-marrow involvement. Patients without any of these unfavourable characteristics showed 50% event-free survival (EFS) in comparison with 42%, 12%, and 5% in patients with one, two, or more than two adverse factors, respectively.

Treatment stratification

To take into account all the known prognostic factors, risk-adapted treatment strategies are currently based on complex staging systems. As an example, the EpSSG stratification takes into consideration six different prognostic factors leading to the identification of eight subgroups that receive different treatments according to the following four derived risk groups:

1. **Low-risk group**: includes 6–8% of the whole population of localized RMS. These children present with a small (less than 5 cm) tumour, completely resected at diagnosis (IRS group I), with favourable histology and site. Most of these patients are children with paratesticular RMS. Five-year EFS is approximately 90%, so the goal for this selected group of patients is to avoid aggressive treatment. In the current EpSSG protocol, these children are treated with a relatively short course of non-intensive chemotherapy (vincristine and actinomycin-D).
2. **Intermediate-risk group:** includes patients with favourable histology and site, with survival around 80%. The goal for this group includes to reduce treatment cautiously without compromising survival. Intensive alkylating agent-based chemotherapy is utilized, but there is an attempt to reduce cumulative dose exposure and to limit the use of radiotherapy.
3. **High-risk group**: this group includes patients with large E-RMS localized in unfavourable sites or with nodal involvement, and most A-RMS. These patients still have an unsatisfactory prognosis (survival around 70%) and are therefore the major focus of randomized trials to identify more effective strategies.
4. **Very high-risk group:** this includes mainly metastatic RMS. In this group survival is between 20% and 30%, and has not improved significantly in the past 40 years. Experimental approaches are therefore needed for these patients.

Therapeutic strategy

Surgery, radiotherapy, and chemotherapy have been combined differently over the years by international cooperative groups, in an attempt to improve outcome whilst finding the correct balance between the intensity of treatment and its possible cost in terms of late effects. In general, there is concordance on the use of intensive chemotherapy and aggressive non-mutilating surgery. Controversies relate more to the method and timing of local treatment, and, more specifically, to the place of radiotherapy in guaranteeing local control for patients who appear to achieve complete remission with chemotherapy, with or without surgery. This represented an important philosophical difference between the Société Internationale d'Oncologie Pediatrique (SIOP) malignant mesenchymal tumours (MMT) studies and those of the IRS group and, to some extent, those of the German and Italian cooperative groups. Local relapse rates are higher when radiotherapy is not systematically used, although the SIOP experience has also made it clear that, at least for RMS localized in certain sites like orbit, a significant number of patients who relapse may be cured with salvage treatment.

Surgery

Tumour resection at diagnosis should be attempted only if the tumour can be realistically excised with clear margins without danger, functional impairment, or mutilation. If this is not possible, a diagnostic biopsy is required. An attempt at surgical resection which leaves microscopic residual disease makes treatment decisions more complicated because the patient is unassessable for the efficacy of chemotherapy and may still require further local treatment. Primary re-excision (i.e. a second surgical resection before chemotherapy) may be worthwhile in cases where there is confidence that clear excision margins can be achieved without functional or cosmetic disadvantage: this may be particularly useful in limb and paratesticular tumours.

RMS usually shrinks significantly with initial chemotherapy, and secondary conservative surgery to achieve local control may become more feasible and remains an important aspect of treatment. Its implementation depends, however, on the site of disease; for example, surgery has little or no role in the primary management of orbital or parameningeal RMS. At other sites, surgery should aim to completely resect the residual tumour, although marginal resections may be acceptable provided that they are followed by radiotherapy. The efficacy and the potential morbidity of surgery and radiotherapy must be carefully assessed: in some cases, the morbidity of radiotherapy may be more acceptable than radical operations which result in important functional (e.g. total cystectomy) and/or cosmetic (e.g. amputation) consequences; in other circumstances, the morbidity of radical surgery to achieve local control may be preferred, for example to avoid pelvic or extremity irradiation in very young children.

Radiotherapy

The role of radiotherapy in the local control of RMS is unquestionable but awareness of the possible late effects, especially in young children, has led to attempts to identify groups of patients where irradiation can be withheld or modulated in its dose and target volume.

Strategies determining the use of radiotherapy require consideration of diverse factors including histological subtype, patient age, tumour size and site, response to initial chemotherapy, and presence of residual tumour after surgery. The only patients where radiotherapy can be safely withheld are those with E-RMS completely resected at diagnosis. It is also known that a certain proportion of patients with E-RMS can be cured without radiotherapy when the tumour is completely resected at secondary surgery but, as most studies suggest a survival advantage for radiotherapy, this strategy is often limited to very young children.

Studies from the European groups have attempted to relate the use of radiotherapy to the response to initial chemotherapy. The most radical approach has been used in the SIOP protocols, where radiotherapy was avoided if complete remission was achieved after initial chemotherapy, with or without second surgery (except for parameningeal RMS). This approach has proven feasible, especially in the subsets of patients with orbital embryonal RMS where up to 40% were cured without irradiation. However, the higher rate of relapse observed in this population requires consideration of the burden of second-line therapy, and the psychological impact of relapse, in the total cost of cure. There is good evidence from all groups that survival is improved when radiotherapy is given to all patients with A-RMS and to those with E-RMS with microscopic or macroscopic residual disease. The timing of radiotherapy in treatment may be important and, at least in some subgroups, such as those with parameningeal RMS, there is evidence that timely irradiation (around week 12) may improve local control.

Current guidelines for therapy within COG and EpSSG recommend doses from 40 to 55 Gy, given by conventional fractionation (single daily doses of 1.8 Gy) depending on the various clinical variables. A reduction of dose to 32–36 Gy is under exploration in children with favourable characteristics. Hyperfractionated schedules have been explored but did not show any advantage in terms of local control or survival. In adult sarcoma, preoperative radiotherapy is becoming the new standard in the case of a resectable tumour; in the next EpSSG study, pre- versus post-operative radiotherapy will be studied in a randomized trial.

The reduction of side effects can be pursued not only by avoiding or reducing the doses of radiotherapy but also through better treatment planning and the use of the most modern techniques. Radiotherapy should be performed only in a limited number of experienced centres and CT-based 3D conformal planning is mandatory to reduce irradiation of critical structures near the target volume. The target volume should be determined as the initial tumour volume plus adequate margins (1–2 cm), but after good response to chemotherapy, the residual tumour can be considered as target volume (plus margins). In large tumours, a boost can be delivered to a more limited volume with high risk of relapse. Interstitial radiotherapy (brachytherapy) using intracavitary moulds or implanted wires may be of particular relevance for small tumours at selected sites, notably in the vagina and perineum. Occasionally, this technique is utilized at other genitourinary sites, including tumours of the bladder base and prostate, and there is emerging experience of its application to head and neck sites. Although clinical studies to better understand the indications and potential advantages and disadvantages of intensity-modulated radiotherapy (IMRT) and proton therapy are still required, both are already increasingly utilized; in some countries, proton therapy is standard therapy for head and neck localizations.

Chemotherapy

Chemotherapy is an essential component of treatment for all children with RMS as the majority of patients with localized disease have micrometastases at diagnosis. Another important goal of chemotherapy is to reduce tumour volume and extension to allow for more conservative subsequent surgery or radiation therapy. Finally, it is the only available tool against metastatic lesions not otherwise amenable to local therapy (e.g. bone-marrow involvement).

Experience since the 1970s has defined the efficacy of a variety of individually active chemotherapeutic agents, subsequently combined in different multidrug regimens to increase their effect. Vincristine, actinomycin D, cyclophosphamide (or its analogue ifosfamide), and doxorubicin have been the most frequently utilized agents in the treatment of RMS. Early experience from the IRS group failed to show a convincing difference in survival when patients were treated with VAC (vincristine, actinomycin, and cyclophosphamide), with or without doxorubicin, and concern about potential cardiotoxicity justifies caution over its incorporation into primary treatment. A randomized trial recently concluded by EpSSG confirmed that the omission of doxorubicin did not impair patients' survival in high-risk localized RMS.

The substitution of cyclophosphamide by ifosfamide, in combination with vincristine and actinomycin D (with or without doxorubicin), has been the hallmark of all recent European studies. There is no evidence that an ifosfamide-based combination with vincristine and actinomycin D (IVA) is superior to VAC, although ifosfamide appears to convey some advantages over its analogue, showing a lack of cross resistance, a lower myelotoxicity profile, and (probably) a lower risk of gonadal toxicity. However, it carries a risk of renal toxicity. Currently, VAC remains the combination of choice for North American studies, while the IVA regimen is the gold standard for European groups. A recent trial coordinated by COG has compared VAC versus alternating VAC/VI (vincristine and irinotecan). The two arms produced similar results in term of progression-free survival, but the VAC/VI regimen proved to be less toxic and therefore preferable to standard VAC.

The addition of other drugs (originally, cisplatin and etoposide; later, epirubicin, carboplatin, and topotecan) has failed to demonstrate any convincing evidence for superiority over VAC or IVA, although some or all may have value in second-line therapies. The addition of temozolomide to the VI regimen is has proven beneficial for relapsed patients.

Approaches with high-dose and dose-intensified chemotherapy

The very poor prognosis of some subgroups of patients, particularly those with metastases detectable at diagnosis, has justified the search for novel strategies. The place of high-dose chemotherapy (HDCT) followed by haematopoietic stem-cell rescue (HSCR) has been explored in different trials, although there has been no direct randomized comparison with conventional-dose chemotherapy. The closest study was a non-randomized European protocol that compared 12 cycles of a six-drug regimen (CEVAIE: carboplatin, epirubicin, vincristine, actinomycin D, ifosfamide, and etoposide) to six courses of CEVAIE followed by high-dose melphalan as consolidation therapy for patients who achieved complete remission. No obvious difference in survival was identified. Similarly, unsatisfactory results were achieved with other high-dose regimens (including combinations of melphalan, etoposide, carboplatin, thiotepa, and cyclophosphamide) and with attempts to use rapid sequential HDCT with HSRC earlier in the treatment pathway. In contrast, recent data from the German group suggested a survival advantage for metastatic patients who received low-dose 'maintenance' chemotherapy with oral trofosfamide and idarubicin when compared (albeit in a non-random manner) with patients undergoing HDCT.

Nevertheless, the strategy to add a 'metronomic' (regular and frequent low-dosage) maintenance treatment after completing conventional chemotherapy is a promising alternative approach, which aims to control presumed minimal residual disease resistant to standard chemotherapy. The EpSSG RMS 2005 protocol has investigated the role of a six-month schedule of maintenance treatment using vinorelbine and low-dose oral cyclophosphamide in high-risk patients and showed a survival benefit; it is the new standard of care for this subgroup.

An alternative way to increase dose intensity is by compressing the interval between cycles of chemotherapy with granulocyte colony-stimulating growth factor (G-CSF) support. The recently completed COG trial studying this approach showed improved survival (when compared to historical controls) for patients with lower-risk metastatic E-RMS, while prognosis for those with higher-risk stage IV disease remained dismal.

Experimental approaches

A number of potentially new approaches are being investigated in preclinical and clinical studies, including the use of novel anti-neoplastic agents, immunotherapy, and molecules directed against specific biological targets. Various new anti-neoplastic agents are in current phase I and II trials (as single agents or in combination). Preclinical studies have shown that the insulin signalling pathway is frequently altered in RMS, leading to development and clinical testing of several anti-IGF-1-R antibodies. Despite responses, this approach has not been taken forward. ALK aberrations on the genomic and protein level are frequently found in RMS, and are the basis for current inclusion of RMS patients in early clinical trials testing efficacy of small-molecule inhibitors of ALK. As RAS isoforms are frequently mutated in fusion-negative RMS, intervening in the RAS–MEK–ERK pathway and PIK3CA–MTOR–AKt pathway is a policy currently being tested preclinically and clinically. Strategies to directly target the PAX3-FOXO1 fusion gene are under development but still in a preclinical phase. The observation that RMS cell lines express vascular endothelial growth factor (VEGF) and that VEGF-receptor-1 antibody inhibits VEGF signalling and delays RMS proliferation has made anti-angiogenic treatment an attractive option. A phase II randomized study on the use of bevacizumab (a humanized monoclonal antibody which blocks the binding of human VEGF to its receptors) in association with chemotherapy has recently been concluded in Europe and, unfortunately, failed to demonstrate any survival advantage.

Antibodies targeting the programmed cell-death protein 1 pathway (PD-1/PD-L1) function by removing the brakes on T cells, which can then perform active anti-tumour immune surveillance; several antibodies are currently being investigated preclinically in RMS and in early clinical basket trials.

The demonstration of a graft effect against some solid tumour cells has prompted the consideration of allogeneic bone-marrow transplantation in paediatric STS. Recent studies were however negative and, also taking into account its high toxicity, this approach is difficult to recommend.

Outcome

The advent of multidisciplinary protocols dramatically increased the overall survival (OS) of patients with RMS from around 20% in the 1970s to over 70% in the early 1990s, since which time further improvement has been slower. Treatment failures usually occur within three years from diagnosis, and are represented mostly by local or regional relapse (accounting for approximately 60% of all relapses). Survival after relapse is generally poor (below 30% at five years), but patients with favourable tumour characteristics (embryonal histology, favourable primary site) who did not receive radiotherapy during first-line treatment have a realistic chance of cure with further therapy.

Late effects of treatment

The cost of the cure is the difficult, yet essential, issue to be addressed when reviewing the outcome of survivors of all forms of cancer in childhood, particularly when survival is achieved using different philosophies and treatment modalities. The importance of accurate prognostic assessment at diagnosis is as much to ensure that patients with a good prognosis are not overtreated as to identify those with a poorer prognosis who require a more aggressive approach.

Much concern has been focused on the late sequelae of local treatment for RMS, particularly in patients with head–neck and genitourinary primaries. Chemotherapy is also associated with significant sequelae in some patients, and the concept that more intensive chemotherapy may help to reduce the use of local treatment must be balanced against the additional toxicity that the chemotherapy may bring. The more recent use of ifosfamide has raised concern about long-term renal damage, although risks seem acceptably low with cumulative doses below 60 g/m^2 as in all current European RMS protocols. The continuing use of high doses of alkylating agents (and etoposide) has been linked to an increased risk of second malignancy, and the long-term follow-up and prospective evaluation of survivors of current protocols is required in order to document the frequency and functional significance of all possible late effects of therapy.

Non-rhabdomyosarcoma soft-tissue sarcomas

The term non-rhabdomyosarcoma soft-tissue sarcoma (NRSTS) describes a very heterogeneous group of mesenchymal extra-skeletal malignant tumours, with different clinical and biological characteristics, classified on the basis of their differentiation according to the adult tissue they resemble. The term NRSTS reflects the fact that these tumours have often been treated according to the principles adopted for RMS, despite the fact they represent different entities.

Most of the NRSTS histotypes are more common in adults than in children, but the frequency of the different subtypes differs significantly according to age: infantile fibrosarcoma is a peculiar entity of young children, synovial sarcoma and malignant peripheral nerve sheath tumour (MPNST) are typical of adolescents and young adults, and liposarcoma and leiomyosarcoma occur in adults and are very rare in children (see Figure 25.1).

The pathogenesis of NRSTS is still unknown and there are no well-established risk factors. Ionizing radiation (angiosarcoma) and oncogenic viruses (leiomyosarcoma in immunocompromised patients) have been associated with the development of some NRSTS, but the aetiological relation is yet unclear. A well-known association exists between MPNST and neurofibromatosis type 1 (NF1). The lifetime risk of developing MPNST in NF1 patients has been estimated at 8–13% compared to 0.001% in the general population. Both NF1-associated and sporadic MPNST show loss or mutation of the *NF-1* gene (chromosome 17q11.2).

Tumour aggressiveness, and its propensity to local relapse and distant metastases, correlates with histological diagnosis and tumour grade and size. In general, low-grade tumours are locally aggressive, especially if they are small, but they rarely metastasize, whilst high-grade tumours are more aggressive and have a high risk of metastasis (Table 25.2).

Diagnosis

Similarly to RMS, NRSTS can arise anywhere in the soft tissues of the body, although the most common clinical presentation is a painless, growing mass localized in lower extremities; less frequent sites are the trunk or the head and neck region.

The diagnostic work-up is similar to the one used for RMS, with MRI to investigate the primary tumour and further investigations performed according to the histological subtype (i.e. lung CT is necessary in most cases, but brain MRI is necessary only in cases of rhabdoid tumour or alveolar soft-part sarcoma).

The importance of initial surgery in NRSTS is demonstrated by the fact that they are often staged according to the IRS post-surgical grouping system as used for RMS, while the TNM (tumour–node–metastasis) system seems less important, at least because nodal involvement is, in general, rare for NRSTS.

Table 25.2 Peak age of incidence, molecular findings, and clinical characteristics of the most frequent non-rhabdomyosarcoma soft-tissue sarcoma subtypes

Histotype	Peak age of incidence	Molecular findings	Clinical characteristics
Synovial sarcoma	Second to third decade	t(X;18)(p11;q11) SYT-SSX1, SYT-SSX2, SYT-SSX4	Extremity (more frequent) or axial site RR up to 60% Overall satisfactory prognosis
Malignant peripheral nerve sheath tumour (MPNST)	Third to fourth decade	Loss or rearrangement of 10p, 11q, 17q, and 22q	30% associated with NF-1 Frequently located in the trunk RR up to 50–60% in non-NF1, <10% in NF1 patients Poor prognosis
Adult-type fibrosarcoma	Fourth to fifth decade	t(2,5) and t(7,22)	Diagnosis of exclusion. Tendency to metastatic spread according to tumour grade
Epithelioid sarcoma	Third decade	-	Superficial, distant sites (fingers) Indolent course Lymph nodal spread RR <30% Intermediate prognosis
Liposarcoma	Sixth to seventh decade (earlier for the myxoid type)	Myxoid liposarcoma: t(12;16)(q13;p11) t(12;22)(q13;q12) FUS-CHOP	Different biology and clinical behaviour according to the subtype (i.e. well-differentiated, de-differentiated, or myxoid/round-cell subtype) Retroperitoneal location
Leiomyosarcoma	Sixth decade	-	Retroperitoneum Immunocompromised patients
Alveolar soft-part sarcoma	Third decade	t(X;17)(p11.2;q25) ASPSCR-TFE3	Head and neck and other unusual locations RR <20% Poor prognosis (better than adults)
Clear-cell sarcoma	Third to fourth decade	t(12;22)(q13;q12) t(9;22)(q22;q12) ATF1-EWS	Extremity site, deep-seated Poor response to chemotherapy Poor prognosis
Angiosarcoma	Fourth to sixth decade	-	Associated with lymphoedema, may occur after radiotherapy Superficial or deep Poor prognosis
Extraskeletal myxoid chondrosarcoma	Fifth to sixth decade	t(9;22)(q22;q12) t(9;17)(q22;q11.2) EWS-CHN	Slow-growing tumour of extremities
Extraskeletal mesenchymal chondrosarcoma	Second to third decade	Complex cytogenetic alteration t(11;22) (q24;q12) (as Ewing family tumours)	Head-neck region (orbit) Highly aggressive tumour
Infantile fibrosarcoma	First year of life (rare after 2 years of age)	t(12;15;)(p13;q25) ETVG(TEL)-NTRK3	Rapid growth Relatively high chemosensitivity Good prognosis
Desmoplastic small round-cell tumour	Second to third decade	t(11;22) (p13;q12) EWS-WT1	Abdominal mass widely disseminated at onset Poor prognosis
Dermatofibrosarcoma protuberans	Third to fifth decade	t(17;22) t(2;17)(p23;q23) ALK-CLTC PDGFβ-COL1A1	Subcutaneous Indolent growth Good response to ALK inhibitors
Rhabdoid tumour	Infants and young children	hSNF5/INI 1 gene mutations	Poor prognosis

RR: response rate (to chemotherapy; in most cases this also includes minor responses)
N.B. fusion transcripts are in italic

After the radiological assessment, a biopsy should be taken to define the histological diagnosis and to grade the tumour appropriately. The World Health Organization (WHO) classification of STS, last updated in 2013, classifies tumours (on the basis of their differentiation) as adipocytic, fibroblastic/myofibroblastic, fibrohistiocytic, smooth muscle, pericytic/perivascular, skeletal muscle, nerve sheath, vascular, and of uncertain differentiation. In most cases, the diagnosis of histotype requires the use of immunohistochemistry and cytogenetic/molecular investigation. A progressively increasing number of specific translocations have been identified in NRSTS (Table 25.2).

Once the histotype is defined, the grade of malignancy should be estimated. Although this usually indicates how aggressively a tumour will behave, some diagnoses (e.g. synovial sarcoma, alveolar sarcoma, angiosarcoma) should be considered high grade regardless of their morphological parameters, whereas in others (e.g. clear-cell sarcoma, extra-skeletal myxoid chondrosarcoma), biological behaviour is less predictable. Tumour grade is usually established from a combined assessment of histological features including degree of cellularity, cellular pleomorphism or anaplasia, mitotic activity, and degree of necrosis. Over the years, two different grading systems have emerged: the Paediatric Oncology Group (POG) system and the French system (FNCLCC) (developed for adult STS but also used in Europe for paediatric NRSTS).

Treatment strategy

The rarity and heterogeneity of these tumours suggest that children and adolescents with NRSTS should be referred to institutions with adequate experience and committed to enrolling patients in clinical trials. Treatment is usually based on histotype, grading, and tumour resectability. In consideration of the limited chemosensitivity, a more aggressive approach to local treatment is generally required, and surgery still represents the mainstay of treatment in adult as in paediatric NRSTS. A complete tumour resection gives the best chance of cure and may be the only treatment needed for most histotypes.

Surgery aims to be more conservative in children, preferring limb-sparing procedures and non-compartmental resections. Therefore the concept of radical surgery in children allows closer surgical margins than are generally acceptable in adults. If resection is considered unlikely at diagnosis, an incisional biopsy is required for diagnostic purposes (fine-needle biopsy does not usually provide sufficient accuracy) and other treatment modalities need to be considered before referring the child back to the surgeon for a definitive procedure. Radiotherapy is adopted when post-surgical residual disease is present (IRS III) or suspected (IRS II). Depending on the age of a child and likeliness of a sufficient margin after surgery, preoperative irradiation of the tumour may be considered, increasingly resembling the approach in adults.

NRSTS have demonstrated different chemosensitivity: from 80% in undifferentiated soft-tissue sarcoma, to 60% in synovial sarcoma, and less than 30% in other histotypes. Recent reports have suggested that the use of chemotherapy seems justified in patients with resected but large and high-grade tumours (to reduce the risk of distant relapse) and also in patients with unresectable tumours (to attempt to reduce the lesion and make it operable). As in adult NRSTS, the ifosfamide–doxorubicin combination represents the preferred regimen for paediatric NRSTS, but interesting new, more histotype-directed, drugs are under investigation.

The overall cure rate for NRSTS patients is around 70%, but it correlates with a series of prognostic variables including:

1. extent of disease at diagnosis: survival is very poor in children with disseminated disease (OS less than 20%);
2. completeness of initial surgery: five-year OS is around 90% in IRS group I, 80% in those who had marginal resection (group II), and 50% in initially unresected cases (group III);
3. tumour grade: five-year OS is 90% for Grade 1, 80% for Grade 2, and 65% for Grade 3;
4. tumour site: five-year OS is 80% for extremity tumours and 60% for axial location;
5. tumour size: five-year OS is 95% for tumours 5 cm or smaller, 55% for those larger than 5 cm.

Tumour invasiveness (T stage) and superficial/deep location are often linked to tumour size and site, and are not commonly used in risk stratification of NRSTS in children. Many of these prognostic variables are interrelated; for example, MPNST are often large, axial tumours and unresectable at diagnosis.

Synovial sarcoma

Synovial sarcoma (SS) is a malignant undifferentiated mesenchymal tumour, resembling normal synovial tissue. It represents 5–10% of all soft-tissue tumours in adults and is one of the most common NRSTS in the paediatric age range (15–25%), occurring primarily in adolescents. Histologically, two major subtypes are described: the monophasic form, characterized by spindle cells, and the more frequent biphasic form, characterized by spindle and epithelial cells organized in glandular structures. Cytogenetic studies have reported the presence of a characteristic translocation t(X;18)(p11;q11) in approximately 90% of cases. Two fusion transcripts, SYT-SSX1 and SYT-SSX2, are derived from fusion of the *SYT* and *SSX* genes localized on chromosome 18q11 and Xp11 respectively. SS usually arises in the extremities, and the lungs are by far the most common metastatic site. Prognosis is related to the presence of metastatic lesions, tumour size (larger than 5 cm) and site (extremity locations fare better than axial locations), and complete resection.

Comparative studies have highlighted that survival is lower in adults than in children, even after correction for the presence of unfavourable risk factors. This might reflect differences in the biology of the tumour at different ages and/or the different use of chemotherapy. In paediatric oncology, SS is considered as a relatively chemosensitive tumour, with a reported response rate of up to 60%. Chemotherapy has therefore been systematically used in all patients.

In 2005, EpSSG promoted a multinational study with the aims to homogenize SS treatment in Europe and collect prospective data (see **Figure 25.3**). Patients were stratified according to surgical stage, tumour size and site (extremity versus axial), and nodal involvement: low risk (IRS 1, size less than 5 cm), intermediate risk (IRS 1, size more than 5 cm, and all IRS II), and high risk (all IRS III or any N1 tumour). The study recently concluded and reported five-year EFS of 80.7% and OS of 90.7%—superior to the results reported in previous series. This study reported a 55.2% response rate to chemotherapy (including also minor responses) and demonstrated that chemotherapy can be safely omitted in low-risk patients.

Adult-type non-rhabdomyosarcoma soft-tissue sarcomas

A series of heterogeneous tumours typical of adults are collected under this definition (see **Table 25.2**). Whilst their histological appearance and biology are very different to paediatric-type NRSTS, they share the same low chemosensitivity and critical role of complete surgery to achieve cure.

For adult-type NRSTS, the possibility to resect the tumour, using a conservative approach but with adequate margins, should be considered at diagnosis. Unfortunately, this is only the case for a minority of usually large and invasive lesions. Neoadjuvant chemotherapy is therefore recommended because experience suggests that up to 40% of these patients may achieve some degree of tumour

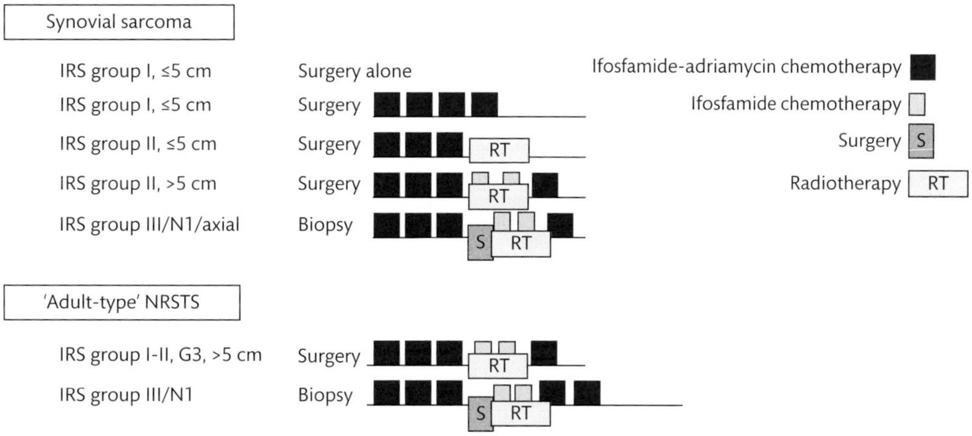

Figure 25.3 Risk-adapted treatment strategy for synovial sarcoma and 'adult-type' soft-tissue sarcoma in the European Paediatric Soft Tissue Sarcoma Study Group (EpSSG) NRSTS 2005 protocol.

IRS, Intergroup Rhabdomyosarcoma Study; G, tumour grade.

Adapted with permission from Ferrari A., et al. 'Synovial sarcoma in children and adolescents: the European Pediatric Soft Tissue Sarcoma Study Group prospective trial (EpSSG NRSTS 2005)'. *Annals of Oncology*, Volume 26, Issue 3, pp. 567–572. Copyright © 2014, Oxford University Press. DOI: https://doi.org/10.1093/annonc/mdu562

shrinkage, possibly facilitating tumour resection and giving some survival advantage.

The role of chemotherapy after complete tumour resection, to reduce the risk of distant recurrence, is controversial. There are no randomized trials in paediatric NRSTS (and probably never will be considering the limited number of patients) and the results of adult trials are clearly not in favour of chemotherapy. Survival is around 90% in patients with small, low-grade tumours after initial tumour resection alone. The scenario is completely different for patients with high-grade, large and invasive tumours: even after initial complete resection, they have a high risk of developing metastases if the treatment is limited to local therapy alone. This would suggest, in principle, the use of systemic chemotherapy to try to improve survival, despite the lack of clear evidence.

Radiotherapy plays a well-defined role in local control for adult STS but its indications are more strictly controlled in children, given the higher risk of late effects. In general, irradiation is planned when microscopic or macroscopic residuals remain after surgery or in conjunction with chemotherapy to make the tumour resectable.

In the EpSSG NRSTS 2005 protocol, ifosfamide–doxorubicin adjuvant chemotherapy is recommended for patients with large, high-grade tumours in IRS I or II group, or as neoadjuvant treatment in unresectable lesions (**Figure 25.3**). COG uses a very similar approach, but with radiotherapy concomitant to chemotherapy, in initially unresectable tumours to maximize tumour shrinkage.

In recent years, various drugs other than the ifosfamide–doxorubicin combination have shown some activity against particular STS histotypes (**Table 25.3**). The gemcitabine–docetaxel combination represents a standard second-line treatment in adult STS. Taxanes and biological agents like bevacizumab have procured responses in angiosarcoma. The peculiar vascular pattern of alveolar soft-part sarcoma (ASPS) can be affected by the use of sunitinib and cedirabinib. The extremely low response rate to chemotherapy makes the use of these agents attractive in first-line treatment.

Finally, eribulin has recently been approved on the basis of improved overall survival for patients with adipocytic sarcomas, and trabectedin is now approved for patients with leiomyosarcomas and liposarcomas. Whilst these agents have been tested mainly in adult patients and have produced only temporary responses, they also represent a promising approach for paediatric NRSTS.

Other histotypes

Other rare lesions arise from soft tissue in children, with peculiar clinical biological characteristics and different levels of aggressiveness. A brief description of the most encountered histotypes is given here.

Table 25.3 Histology-directed therapeutic options in adult-type non-rhabdomyosarcoma soft-tissue sarcoma

Hitotype	Agent
Synovial sacoma	Ifosfamide
	Taxanes
	Gemcitabine
	Vascular endothelial growth factor (VEGF) inhibitors
	Gemcitabine
	Gemcitabine and docetaxel
	Trabectedine
	Vascular endothelial growth factor (VEFG) inhibitors
	Mammalian targets of rapamycin (mTOR) inhibitors
Liposarcoma (myxoid/ round cell)	Trabectedine
Dermatofibrosarcoma protuberans	Imatinib
Alveolar soft part sarcoma	Sunitinib, cedarinibid
Clear cell sarcoma	Sunitinib

Infantile fibrosarcoma

Infantile fibrosarcoma (IFS) represents a distinct entity with peculiar characteristics and a better prognosis in comparison with adult-type fibrosarcoma. IFS is the most common sarcoma under one year of age and is rarely diagnosed after the age of two.

It is characterized by the presence of a characteristic t(12;15) translocation coding for the ETV6-NTRK3 gene fusion. Recently, transcript variants like LMNA-NTRK1 have been described, explaining, at least partially, the minor part of IFS where the ETV6-NTRK3 gene fusion is not detected. It must be kept in mind, however, that the same genetic alteration can be found in other tumours like nephroblastic nephroma.

IFS usually arises in the distal extremities, and presents as a painless, rapidly enlarging mass. Despite initial rapid growth, evolution may be indolent. It is considered an intermediate malignancy according to WHO classification because metastatic spread is rare. In addition, few cases of spontaneous regression have been described. The overall prognosis is very good (survival rates are above 90% in recent studies). Surgery is the mainstay of treatment, but chemotherapy may be needed to reduce large invasive masses in very young children. The recommended first-line chemotherapy is the combination of vincristine and actinomycin D, with the addition of alkylating agents or anthracylines in case of no response.

Despite good prognosis, mutilating surgery could not be avoided in 6% of patients in a recent EpSSG study, and toxicity due to chemotherapy was not negligible. For this reason, new agents targeting the NTRK fusion gene seem a promising alternative approach to standard chemotherapy.

Desmoplastic small round-cell tumour

DSRCT is a very aggressive neoplasm, identified by the specific translocation t(11;22)(p13;q12), with the chimeric transcript EWS-WT1. It usually arises in the abdominal cavity and is often disseminated at diagnosis, with peritoneal seeding (sometimes not clearly visible on imaging investigations) and liver metastases.

Intensive multimodality treatments (with various drug combinations and including high-dose chemotherapy with stem-cell rescue) and hyperthermic intraperitoneal chemotherapy (HIPEC) have been investigated, but prognosis remains poor. Adjuvant radiotherapy as part of multimodal treatment also seems beneficial. New tailored therapeutic approaches are urgently needed for this tumour.

Malignant rhabdoid tumour

Extracranial malignant rhabdoid tumours (MRT) are rare and often affect very young children. They may occur sporadically or as part of a cancer syndrome known as rhabdoid tumour predisposition syndrome. Although the kidney is the most common site, MRT can arise anywhere in the body. It is characterized by alterations of SMARCB1 (also known as INI1), a tumour suppressor gene located on chromosome 22. Germline mutations or deletions in one allele are the basis of the predisposition syndrome, and somatic loss or mutation of the other allele causes MRT or other tumours.

Histological diagnosis was mainly based on the recognition of rhabdoid cells, but this aspect is not always present. The diagnostic landscape changed after the discovery that the inactivation of SMARCB1 causes a loss of protein expression in the nucleus of the cells, which can be detected by immunohistochemistry. This has increased the ability to recognize MRT and probably is increasing the number of patients being diagnosed with this entity.

Despite progress in the understanding of the biological mechanisms underlying tumour development, only little progress has been made in the treatment of MRT. The outcome remains unsatisfactory, with three-year OS of 38% in the most recent study. Treating these patients is extremely difficult because a substantial proportion progress early during treatment and the use of radiotherapy is limited by their young age. An age of under one year and the presence of metastatic disease are the strongest predictors of outcome. Improved understanding of the biology and role of SMARCB1 has enabled identification of new targets for small molecules, like histone deacyetylase inhibitors, that are currently under investigation.

Fybroblastic-myofibroblastic lesions

This is a homogenous group of tumours characterized by invasive local growth but no propensity to distant dissemination. They are therefore considered intermediate malignancy lesions and need to be differentiated from more aggressive tumours. Their management is often problematic: for a long time, surgical resection has constituted the mainstay of treatment, but increased knowledge of their biological behaviour and the availability of active agents has promoted a multidisciplinary approach.

Aggressive fibromatosis (AF), also known as desmoid tumour, is a rare, deep-seated, fibroblastic tumour that arises in musculo-aponeurotic structures, mainly in extremities and deep structures in the abdomen and pelvis. Tumours usually grow fairly slowly but diffusely along muscle bundles and fascial planes, lacking a pseudocapsule, which contributes to the difficulty of obtaining clear margins when the tumour is resected. The pathogenesis of AF is most likely multifactorial: genetic predisposition, endocrine factors, and trauma all seem to play an important part. The incidence is higher in families with familial adenomatous polyposis (FAP) within which there is a particular association with intra-abdominal fibromatosis (Gardner's syndrome).

OS rates at ten years are above 90%, but many patients experience long-term morbidity due to the tumour growth or, in some cases, to the treatment (i.e. repeated aggressive resections).

Surgery retains an important role in the treatment, but microscopically or macrospically incomplete resections are of little use because AF usually rapidly regrows, probably stimulated by the tissue trauma caused by surgery. The possibility that AF can stabilize or even reduce its dimensions, spontaneously or after medical treatment, has largely diminished the use of aggressive measures like surgery or radiotherapy. However, radiotherapy can be of use in case of relapse and after second surgery, especially in older children.

Various pharmacological treatments have proved to be relatively effective: the most-used strategy is the administration of prolonged low-dose chemotherapy comprising combinations of weekly low-dose methotrexate plus a vinca alkaloid (vinblastine or vinorelbine). Other possible options include hydroxyurea, anti-inflammatory drugs, tamoxifene (although this is rarely used in children because of the side effects), or, more recently, imatinib and tyrosine kinase inhibitors like sorafenib. Studies, especially in children, are lacking. The observation that desmoid tumours may remain stable for a long time, with or without primary treatment, has prompted the suggestion that a 'wait-and-see' strategy (i.e. clinical–radiological monitoring alone) may be suitable in cases where tumour growth is slow or static. All this demonstrates the difficulty of treating AF that may become a chronic disease that often requires a personalized approach.

Inflammatory myofibroblastic tumour (IMT) generally affects the first two decades of life, can occur at any body site (with visceral tumours more frequent in children), and is often accompanied by an inflammatory syndrome characterized by fever, malaise, and raised inflammatory markers. It was considered a reactive lesion but monoclonality and the presence of a specific genetic alteration support its neoplastic nature. The finding that a substantial part of IMT presents ALK rearrangements has supported the use of ALK inhibitors like crizotinib, with good results. In the case of ALK-negative IMT, sarcoma-like regimens including intensive chemotherapy with vincristine, actinomycin D, and alkylating agents, or prolonged administration of low- dose chemotherapy with vincristine–etoposide or vinorelbine and methotrexate can be used. It is to be noted that cases of remission have been reported after anti-inflammatory or steroid therapy.

Dermatofibrosarcoma protuberans (DFP) is a rare entity (0.10 per 100,000 children aged 0–19 years) that occurs especially in the trunk and extremities. Surgery is the treatment of choice and survival is above 95%. Unfortunately, a complete conservative resection may be difficult due to tumour dimensions and localization in difficult sites. DFP is characterized by the specific translocation t(7;22) that ultimately causes tumour cell growth, activating the PDGFRbeta protein tyrosine kinase. This mechanism can be interrupted by the administration of imatinib that has demonstrated interesting activity both in adults and children with DFP

FURTHER READING

Admiraal R, et al. (2010) High-dose chemotherapy for children and young adults with stage IV rhabdomyosarcoma. Cochrane Database Syst Rev (12) CD006669. doi: 10.1002/14651858.CD006669.pub2

Alaggio R, Coffin CM (2015) The evolution of pediatric soft tissue sarcoma classification in the last 50 years. *Pediatr Dev Pathol* **18**(6), 481–94. doi: 10.2350/15-07-1666-MISC.1

Arndt CA, et al. (2009) Vincristine, actinomycin, and cyclophosphamide compared with vincristine, actinomycin, and cyclophosphamide alternating with vincristine, topotecan, and cyclophosphamide for intermediate-risk rhabdomyosarcoma: Children's Oncology Group study D9803. *J Clin Oncol* **27**, 5182–8.

Bisogno G, et al. (2009) Sequential high-dose chemotherapy for children with metastatic rhabdomyosarcoma. *Eur J Cancer* **45**, 3035–41.

Bisogno G, et al. (2018) Addition of dose-intensified doxorubicin to standard chemotherapy for rhabdomyosarcoma (EpSSG RMS 2005): a multicentre, open-label, randomised controlled, phase 3 trial. *Lancet Oncol* **19**(8), 1061–71.

Bisogno G, et al. (2019) Vinorelbine and continuous low-dose cyclophosphamide as maintenance chemotherapy in patients with high-risk rhabdomyosarcoma (RMS 2005): a multicentre, open-label, randomised, phase 3 trial. *Lancet Oncol* **20**(11), 1566–75.

Breitfeld PP, Meyer WH (2005) Rhabdomyosarcoma: new windows of opportunity. *Oncologist* **10**, 518–27.

Carli M, et al. (2005) Malignant peripheral nerve sheath tumours in pediatric age: a report from the Italian and German Soft Tissue Sarcoma Cooperative Group. *J Clin Oncol* **23**, 8422–30.

Casanova M, et al. (2004) Vinorelbine and low-dose cyclophosphamide in the treatment of pediatric sarcomas: pilot study for the upcoming European Rhabdomyosarcoma Protocol. *Cancer* **101**, 1664–71.

Chisholm JC, et al. (2017) Open-label, multicentre, randomised, phase II study of the EpSSG and the ITCC evaluating the addition of bevacizumab to chemotherapy in childhood and adolescent patients with metastatic soft tissue sarcoma (the BERNIE study). *Eur J Cancer* **83**, 177–84.

Crist WM, et al. (2001) Intergroup rhabdomyosarcoma study-IV: results for patients with nonmetastatic disease. *J Clin Oncol* **19**, 3091–102.

Davicioni E, et al. (2010) Gene expression profiling for survival prediction in pediatric rhabdomyosarcomas: a report from the Children's Oncology Group. *J Clin Oncol* **28**, 1240–6.

Ferrari A, et al. (2002) Paratesticular rhabdomyosarcoma: report from the Italian and German Cooperative Group. *J Clin Oncol* **20**, 449–55.

Ferrari A, et al.(2011) Non-metastatic unresected paediatric non-rhabdomyosarcoma soft tissue sarcomas: results of a pooled analysis from United States and European groups. *Eur J Cancer* **47**, 724–31.

Ferrari A, Casanova M (2005) New concepts for the treatment of pediatric non-rhabdomyosarcoma soft tissue sarcomas. *Expert Rev Anticancer Ther* **5**, 307–18.

Ferrari A, et al. (2013) Fibroblastic tumors of intermediate malignancy in childhood. *Expert Rev Anticancer Ther* **13**(2), 225–36.

Ferrari A, et al. (2015) Synovial sarcoma in children and adolescents: the European Pediatric Soft Tissue Sarcoma Study Group prospective trial (EpSSG NRSTS 2005). *Ann Oncol* **26**, 567–72.

Hawkins DS, et al. (2014) What is new in the biology and treatment of pediatric rhabdomyosarcoma? *Curr Opin Pediatr* **26**(1), 50–6.

Klingebiel T, et al. (2008) Treatment of children with metastatic soft tissue sarcoma with oral maintenance compared to high dose chemotherapy: report of the HD CWS-96 trial. *Pediatr Blood Cancer* **50**, 739–45.

Martelli H, et al. (1999) Conservative treatment for girls with nonmetastatic rhabdomyosarcoma of the genital tract: a report from the Study Committee of the International Society of Pediatric Oncology. *J Clin Oncol* **17**, 2117–22.

Meza JL, et al. (2006) Analysis of prognostic factors in patients with nonmetastatic rhabdomyosarcoma treated on intergroup rhabdomyosarcoma studies III and IV: the Children's Oncology Group. *J Clin Oncol* **24**, 3844–51.

Oberlin O, et al. (2008) Prognostic factors in metastatic rhabdomyosarcomas: results of a pooled analysis from United States and European cooperative groups. *J Clin Oncol* **26**, 2384–9.

Okcu MF, et al. (2003) Synovial sarcoma of childhood and adolescence: a multicenter, multivariate analysis of outcome. *J Clin Oncol* **21**, 1602–11.

Orbach D, et al. (2016) Conservative strategy in infantile fibrosarcoma is possible: the European Paediatric Soft Tissue Sarcoma Study Group experience. *Eur J Cancer* **57**,1–9.

Orbach D, et al. (2017) The EpSSG NRSTS 2005 treatment protocol for desmoid-type fibromatosis in children: an international prospective case series. *Lancet Child Adolesc Health* **1**(4), 284–92.

Pappo AS, et al. (2005) Phase II trial of neoadjuvant vincristine, ifosfamide, and doxorubicin with granulocyte colony-stimulating factor support in children and adolescents with advanced-stage nonrhabdomyosarcomatous soft tissue sarcomas: a Pediatric Oncology Group Study. *J Clin Oncol* **23**, 4031–8.

Rosenberg AR, et al. (2014) Early response as assessed by anatomic imaging does not predict failure-free survival among patients with Group III rhabdomyosarcoma: a report from the Children's Oncology Group. *Eur J Cancer* **50**(4), 816–23. doi: 10.1016/j.ejca.2013.11.031

Shern JF, et al. (2015) Pediatric rhabdomyosarcoma. *Crit Rev Oncog* **20**(3–4), 227–43.

Skapek SX, et al. (2013) PAX-FOXO1 fusion status drives unfavourable outcome for children with rhabdomyosarcoma: a children's oncology group report. *Pediatr Blood Cancer* **60**(9), 1411–17. doi: 10.1002/pbc.24532

Spalding AC, et al. (2013) The effect of radiation timing on patients with high-risk features of parameningeal rhabdomyosarcoma: an analysis of IRS-IV and D9803. *Int J Radiat Oncol Biol Phys* **87**(3), 512–16. doi: 10.1016/j.ijrobp.2013.07.003

Stevens MC (2005) Treatment for childhood rhabdomyosarcoma: the cost of cure. *Lancet Oncol* **6**, 77–84.

Stevens MC, et al. (2005) Treatment of nonmetastatic rhabdomyosarcoma in childhood and adolescence: third study of the International Society of Paediatric Oncology—SIOP Malignant Mesenchymal Tumor 89. *J Clin Oncol* **23**, 2618–28.

Sultan I, Ferrari A (2010) Selecting multimodal therapy for rhabdomyosarcoma. *Expert Rev Anticancer Ther* **10**, 1285–301.

van der Graaf WT, et al. (2017) Soft tissue sarcomas in adolescents and young adults: a comparison with their paediatric and adult counterparts. *Lancet Oncol* **18**(3), e166–75.

Van Rijn RR, et al. (2008) Imaging findings in noncraniofacial childhood rhabdomyosarcoma. *Pediatr Radiol* **38**(6), 617–34.

Wachtel M, Schäfer BW (2010) Targets for cancer therapy in childhood sarcomas. *Cancer Treat Rev* **36**, 318–27.

Weigel BJ, et al. (2016) Intensive multiagent therapy, including dose-compressed cycles of ifosfamide/etoposide and vincristine/doxorubicin/cyclophosphamide, irinotecan, and radiation, in patients with high-risk rhabdomyosarcoma: a report From the Children's Oncology Group. *J Clin Oncol* **34**(2), 117–22. doi:10.1200/JCO.2015.63.4048

Williamson D, et al. (2010) Fusion gene-negative alveolar rhabdomyosarcoma is clinically and molecularly indistinguishable from embryonal rhabdomyosarcoma. *J Clin Oncol* **28**, 2151–8.

26

Bone Tumours

Stefan Bielack, Michael Paulussen, and Lee Helman

Epidemiology

Osteosarcoma and Ewing sarcoma (ES), including peripheral neuroectodermal tumour (PNET) and Askin tumours of the chest wall, account for the majority of malignant bone tumours in children and adolescents. In both, males are affected approximately 1.5 times as often as females. The median age at presentation is around age 15 years and at least half of all diagnoses are made in the second decade of life.

Incidence

Osteosarcoma is the most frequent primary bone cancer. Its approximate annual incidence is 2–3 per million in the general population, peaking at 8–11 per million at age 15–19. A second, smaller peak in older patients is due to osteosarcoma arising in abnormal bones, such as those affected by Paget disease or prior irradiation. In paediatric and adolescent populations of Caucasian descent, Ewing sarcoma is the second most common primary malignancy of bone. Annual incidence rates are approximately 2–3 per million in children, adolescents, and young adults below the age of 25. It is exceedingly rare in African and Chinese populations.

Predisposition and genetic links

In most paediatric and adolescent patients, the aetiology remains obscure. Trauma has been implicated but little evidence exists to support this relationship. There are no known predisposing factors for ES. The predilection of osteosarcoma for the age of the pubertal growth spurt and sites of maximum growth suggest a correlation with bone growth. The incidence of osteosarcoma is increased in several disorders associated with germline alterations of tumour suppressor genes and these may account for 10% or more of all osteosarcomas. Survivors of hereditary retinoblastoma with germline mutations of the retinoblastoma gene *RB1* carry a risk that is 500–1,000 times greater than in the general population. The Li-Fraumeni cancer family syndrome, caused by germline mutations in the *p53* gene, is associated with a 15-fold increase. Radiation is another risk factor for osteosarcoma, the risk being related to the dose administered. Exposure to alkylating agents may also contribute. The use of radiation and alkylating-agent chemotherapy, together with genetic tumour predisposition, make osteosarcoma one of the more frequent secondary solid malignancies following therapy for childhood cancer.

Clinical presentation

Primary osteosarcoma is usually located in the metaphyses of long extremity bones, particularly the distal femur or the proximal tibia, followed by the proximal humerus. In total, two thirds of all paediatric osteosarcomas arise around the knee (**Figure 26.1**). Osteosarcomas of the axial skeleton or craniofacial bones generally occur in older patients. Sites most frequently affected by ES of bone are the pelvis, long bones of the extremities, ribs, scapulae, and vertebrae. Compared to osteosarcoma, involvement of flat bones of the trunk is much more common (**Figure 26.1**). If ES arises in long extremity bones, it usually does so in the diaphysis, in distinction to the typical metaphyseal presentation of osteosarcoma.

At diagnosis, accurate staging will reveal metastases in 10–30% of the patients. Without systemic therapy, however, most patients with seemingly localized bone sarcomas will develop metachronous metastases within one to two years. In osteosarcoma, primary and secondary metastases are limited to the lungs in 80% of affected individuals. The remainder have bone metastases with or without additional pulmonary involvement. Skip metastases, defined as isolated tumour foci within the same bone as the primary tumour, occur in a minority of patients. In ES, lungs and bones contain metastatic deposits at diagnosis in approximately equal proportions (around 10% of patients each), and there may be bone-marrow involvement (around 5%). In both diseases, lymph-node metastases are rare and other sites of metastatic disease are almost never involved at initial diagnosis.

Patients with bone tumours usually do not feel ill until late in the course of their disease. They typically seek medical attention because of, at first, intermittent and then continuous pain, often erroneously attributed to recent trauma. Tumour-related swelling and loss of function of adjacent joints usually develop later. In approximately 10%, the first sign of disease is a pathological fracture. Pain at bony sites other than the primary may represent metastatic involvement.

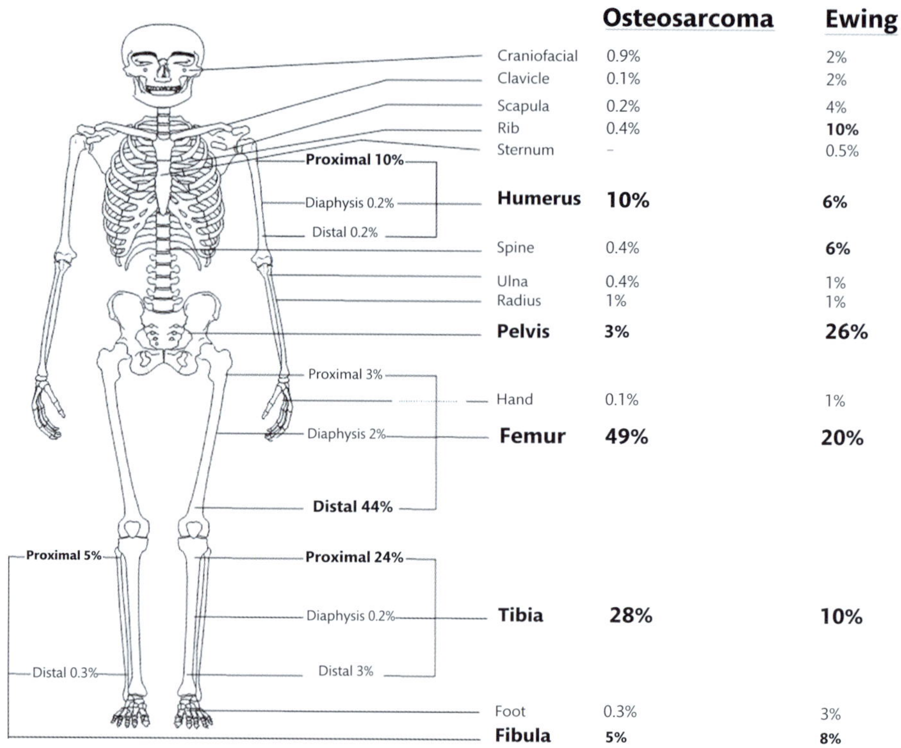

Figure 26.1 Skeletal distribution of osteosarcoma and Ewing sarcoma.

Source: data from 1,791 primary high-grade central osteosarcomas and 1,426 ES from Cooperative Osteosarcoma Study Group (COSS) and European Intergroup Cooperative Ewing's Sarcoma Study ((EI)CESS), respectively. The percentages shown for proximal, diaphyseal, and distal-extremity locations are for osteosarcoma.

Metastases in the lungs produce respiratory symptoms only with extensive involvement. Systemic symptoms, particularly fever, may be present in ES.

Diagnosis

Most patients present with a history of pain of the involved region, and physical examination is typically remarkable only for a mass at the primary site. Loss of motion of neighbouring joints, infiltration of the skin, and neurological deficits may occur, depending on the location and extent of the tumour. There are no laboratory tests that can identify patients with malignant bone tumours. Blood tests may show moderately elevated erythrocyte sedimentation rates and may reveal some degree of anaemia and leucocytosis. Elevated serum levels of lactate dehydrogenase or alkaline phosphatase may correlate with tumour burden or bone destruction, or, in osteosarcoma, with tumour phenotype, and can thus be of prognostic significance.

Imaging of the primary tumour

Plain radiographs and cross-sectional imaging, preferably by magnetic resonance imaging (MRI), are required to assess tumour size and its loco-regional extension.

Plain radiographs are used to describe the bony compartment. Osteosarcoma can present with lytic or sclerotic changes, or both. Ossification in the soft tissues in a radial or 'sunburst' pattern is typical, but neither sensitive nor specific. Periosteal bone formation with lifting of the cortex may lead to the appearance of Codman's triangle (Figure 26.2). The typical radiograph of ES shows a destructive

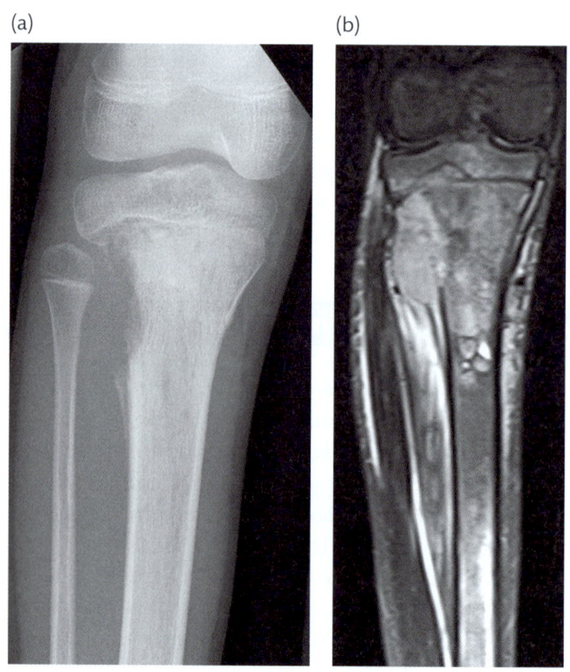

Figure 26.2 Conventional radiograph (left) and T1, gadolinium-enhanced, fat-suppressed MRI (right) of an osteosarcoma of the right proximal tibia. X-ray shows cortical destruction and Codman's triangle on the lateral aspect of the tumour.

Reproduced courtesy of T. Von Kalle, Klinikum Stuttgart, Germany osteolytic lesion of the diaphysis with destruction of the osseous cortex, elevation of the periosteum, and infiltration of surrounding soft tissue. The layered periosteal reaction may give rise to a classic 'onion-skin' appearance. MRI is the most useful tool to define the intramedullary tumour extent, its soft-tissue component, and the relation to vessels and nerves (Figure 26.2).

Serial MRIs can also be used to monitor response to induction chemotherapy. In ES, a marked shrinkage of the soft-tissue component can be used as a surrogate marker for response. In osteosarcoma, where the osteoid matrix often prevents tumour shrinkage, response can be predicted based upon the results of serial dynamic contrast-enhanced MRIs. Other methods used to predict response preoperatively include serial evaluation by angiography, quantitative bone scans, or positron emission tomography (PET).

Systemic staging

The search for metastases focuses on those sites where the majority occur: lungs and bones. The bone marrow is evaluated in ES. Plain radiographs and a computed tomography (CT) scan of the thorax must be performed to rule out pulmonary metastases. Bone metastases are searched for by a ^{99m}Tc-MDP bone scan. Skip metastases may also be visualized on the bone scan, but MRI of the whole bone is more sensitive. Whole-body MRI may lead to a higher detection rate of bone metastases, but its exact role remains to be defined. PET/CT can detect bone metastases with a higher sensitivity than bone scans, but is also less specific.

Ewing sarcoma cells may be inhomogeneously distributed within the bone marrow. It is therefore recommended that marrow samples be obtained from several sites distant from the primary. In addition to standard pathology assessment, marrow micro-metastases can be detected by reverse transcriptase polymerase chain reaction (RT-PCR) for tumour-specific ES gene (*EWS*) fusion transcripts. While involvement detectable by light microscopy carries adverse prognostic implications, assessment of micro-metastatic dissemination by RT-PCR remains investigational.

Biopsy

Imaging will often result in a high index of suspicion, but diagnosis must always be verified histologically. In order to ensure appropriate biopsy techniques and optimal evaluation of the obtained material, it is strongly recommended that biopsies should be performed in specialized paediatric bone-tumour centres. Recent years have witnessed a shift from open to tru-cut needle biopsies. Whichever technique is chosen, sufficient material must be obtained for both histological evaluation and ancillary studies. The biopsy specimen should be forwarded to the pathologist without prior fixation. Tissue is required for standard histology and immunohistochemistry, and fresh/frozen samples are required for molecular biology studies. The biopsy track and adjacent tissues must be regarded as tumour-contaminated and the approach should be planned so that these can subsequently be included into definitive local treatment. If metastases are suspected, but there is no unequivocal evidence from imaging, histological confirmation should be attempted.

Differential diagnosis

The differential diagnosis of osteosarcoma includes traumatic lesions, osteomyelitis, benign tumours such as exostosis, fibroma, osteoid osteoma, chondroma, giant-cell tumour of bone, bone cysts, as well as other primary malignant lesions of bone such as ES or lymphoma, and metastases from malignancies such as neuroblastoma or soft-tissue sarcoma. The most important clinical differential diagnosis of ES is osteomyelitis. The radiological appearance may be very similar and, on occasion, ES may be secondarily infected. On histological examination, ES must be differentiated from other small round-cell tumours, in particular embryonal rhabdomyosarcoma, neuroblastoma, small-cell osteosarcoma, and non-Hodgkin lymphoma.

Histopathology

By definition, osteosarcoma is a mesenchymal malignancy in which the malignant cell population produces osteoid, but production can vary considerably. Both abundant production, leading to hard sclerotic tumours, and very scanty production of osteoid are consistent with the diagnosis. Conventional osteosarcoma, a high-grade central malignancy of bone, accounts for 80–90% of all osteosarcomas. Its most frequent subtypes are osteoblastic, chondroblastic, and fibroblastic, but various less frequent subtypes are also considered conventional osteosarcomas. Conventional, telangiectatic, high-grade surface, and small-cell osteosarcomas all have a similar clinical course and are treated by multimodal regimens that include chemotherapy. Low-grade central, parosteal, and perisosteal osteosarcomas are treated by surgery only. Craniofacial osteosarcomas, apart from those of the skull, metastasize less frequently than conventional osteosarcomas. Never the less, the trend is to treat them by surgery plus chemotherapy. Extraskeletal osteosarcomas, usually high-grade malignancies, are exceedingly rare in young people.

ES of bone are composed of firm, grey-white soft tissue with a glistening, moist appearance on sectioning. Macroscopically, the intraosseous component of the tumour is usually firm, while the extraosseous component tends to be less firm with areas of haemorrhage and cystic degeneration secondary to tumour necrosis. All ES are high-grade malignancies. When stained with haematoxylin and eosin, they appear as a monomorphic small, blue, round, primitive-cell population, with round nuclei and scanty cytoplasm. Variable amounts of glycogen deposition stain periodic-acid-Schiff (PAS) positive. Peripheral primitive neuroectodermal tumours (pPNET)—differing from other ES by showing features of neural differentiation with prominent neurite-like cell processes containing neurosecretory granules and neurofilaments on electron microscopy, or rosettes and Homer–Wright pseudorosettes and/or expressing S-100 protein, neuron-specific enolase (NSE), or synaptophysin—were historically distinguished from ES, but share the same molecular biology and are now regarded as part of the ES family of tumours.

ES cannot be differentiated from other PAS-positive small, blue, round-cell tumours on morphological features alone, and the diagnosis must be assisted by immunocytochemistry and molecular biology (see the section 'Biology'). CD99 (Mic-2 antigen) expression is positive in more than 95% of cases but is not unique for ES. Other useful markers include vimentin, desmin, smooth-muscle actin, and CD45 (leukocyte common antigen). These help to differentiate between small round-cell tumours of myogenic, fibrogenic, and haematopoetic origin.

Biology

Biology of osteosarcoma

Although germline mutations of *p53* and *RB* are rare, these genes are altered in many osteosarcoma tumour samples. Recent data from next-generation sequencing analysis of osteosarcoma tumour specimens demonstrates that approximately 95% of these tumours have *p53* pathway alterations, with the majority of these alterations consisting of either sequence alterations or structural variants within the *p53* gene, with a much smaller number of cases having MDM2 amplifications. This data strongly suggests that *p53* alterations are the major oncogenic driver in these tumours. Intriguingly, these tumours also have the highest known rate of chromothripsis, best described as a single catastrophic event resulting in massive chromosomal rearrangements. Also common is a phenomenon known as kataegis, that is localized hypermutated chromosomal regions.

These events are no doubt the reason that the hallmarks of osteosarcoma are a chaotic-appearing karyotype and aneuploidy. Beyond *p53*, alterations are seen in *RB* in approximately 50% of tumours and there are also, frequently, alterations in *ATRX*. Consequently, loss of function of the *p53* and *RB* tumour-suppressor genes, which regulate cell-cycle progression, are believed to have important roles in osteosarcoma tumourigenesis. Rothmund–Thomson syndrome and Bloom syndrome, rare conditions caused by mutations in tumour-suppressor genes coding for helicases, are also associated with an increase in osteosarcoma, as is Werner syndrome (adult progeria).

Numerous oncogenes are also altered in osteosarcoma tumour cells. These include amplifications of the product of the murine double minute 2 gene, amplification of cyclin-dependent kinase 4, and over-expression of human epidermal growth factor receptor 2. Although it is clear that alterations in tumour-suppressor genes and oncogenes are necessary to produce osteosarcomas, it is not clear which of these events occurs first and why or how it occurs. Moreover, it is not clear which, if any, of the alterations are essential to tumour development and might therefore represent therapeutic targets.

Biology of Ewing sarcoma

The molecular key to ES is the rearrangement of the ES gene *EWS* on chromosome 22q12 with the *FLI-1* gene on 11q24. *EWS* encodes a ubiquitously expressed RNA-binding protein which appears to be involved in transcription and processing of messenger RNA. *FLI-1* codes for a protein with a carboxy-terminal DNA-binding domain that is characteristic for members of the ETS transcription factor family. As a consequence of gene fusion, the EWS RNA binding domain is replaced by the FLI-1-derived ETS DNA binding domain, resulting in a novel transcription factor with strong *in vitro* transactivation potential (Figure 26.3). The most frequent gene fusions in ES result in the type 1 (EWS exon 7 to FLI1 exon 6: 50% of cases) or type 2 (EWS 7/FLI1 5: 27%) fusions. In 10–15%, alternative *EWS* gene fusions to other *ETS* gene family members (predominantly *ERG*) can be observed (Table 26.1). While EWS, as well as its close relatives TLS (FUS) and RPB56 (hTAFII68) (FET gene family for *FUS*, EWS, TAF), and *ERG* genes are involved in several chromosomal translocations

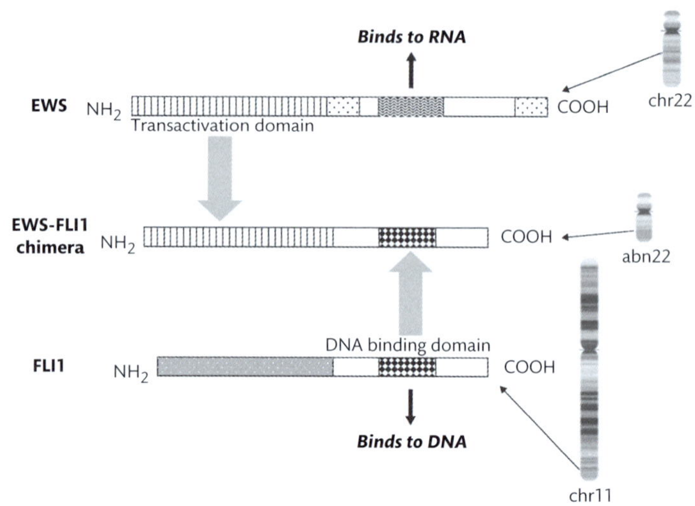

Figure 26.3 Chromosomal translocation t(11;22)(q24;q12) in Ewing sarcoma. This leads to the generation of a DNA-binding fusion protein. The gene for the RNA-binding protein EWS is located on chromosome 22 (chr22) in the region q12, the gene for the DNA- binding transcription factor FLI1 on chromosome 11 (chr11) at q24. The EWS-FLI1 chimeric protein is expressed from the abnormal chromosome 22 (abn22), while the reciprocal translocation product on chromosome 11 has no gene product.
Reproduced courtesy of Heinrich Kovar, St. Anna Kinderkrebsforschung Children's Cancer Research Institute, Vienna, Austria

in other solid tumours and in acute leukaemia, the specific combination of *EWS* with an *ETS* gene is restricted to, and therefore diagnostic of, ES. *EWS–ETS* fusion is essential for ES pathogenesis.

The classical cytogenetic demonstration of t(11;22)(q24;q12) has been largely replaced by fluorescence *in situ* hybridization (FISH) using probes flanking the *EWS* breakpoint region on chromosome 22. Using this method, even complex chromosomal rearrangements and rare *EWS* translocations with other *ETS* partner genes can be revealed. However, the most frequently used method to detect the fusion gene is RT-PCR. This requires immediate snap freezing of the biopsy since it relies on extraction of good-quality RNA. The strength of the method lies in its high sensitivity, enabling identification of single tumour cells among 10^5–10^6 normal cells.

Recently, it has become clear that at least two distinct Ewing-like tumours exist that histologically appear very similar to Ewing tumours but lack the *EWS/FUS-ETS* fusion genes. The most common entity is a tumour harbouring *CIC-DUX4/DUX4L* fusion. These are most frequently soft-tissue tumours and, clinically, appear to behave quite aggressively. Less common are the tumours associated with *BCOR-CCNB3* fusions, that appear to occur predominantly in males. To date, most of these tumours are treated with Ewing-type

Table 26.1 Gene fusions in Ewing sarcoma

Gene fusion	Cytogenetic equivalent	Observed frequency
EWS-FLI1	t(11;22)(q24;q12)	85%
EWS-ERG	t(21;22)(q22;q12)	10%
EWS-ETV1	t(7;22)(p22;q12)	<1%
EWS-ETV4	t(17;22)(q12;q12)	<1%
EWS-FEV	t(2;22)(q35;q12)	1%
FUS-ERG	t(16;26)(p11;q22)	<1%
FUS-FEV	t(2;16)(q35;p11)	<1%

therapy, although given their distinct molecular features, it is likely they should be treated and analysed separately.

Risk classification

Staging

The tumour–node–metastasis (TNM) classification for malignant bone tumours is an expansion of a staging system originally developed by the Musculoskeletal Tumor Society (MSTS). In extremity, trunk, and craniofacial locations, T1 describes a tumour 8 cm or less in dimension, T2 has the greatest dimension of more than 8 cm, while T3 is used for discontinuous tumours in the primary bone site, skip metastases. (For the first time, the eighth edition of the TNM classification provides distinct T definitions for the rarer pelvic and vertebral tumour sites, which are not elaborated upon in this chapter.) Tumour stages are categorized by grade and anatomical extent, with stage I reserved for localized low-grade sarcomas (IA T1; I B T2,3); stage II describing localized high-grade tumours (II A T1; II B T2); and stage III, high-grade sarcomas with skip metastases (T3). Stage IV A describes bone sarcomas with lung metastases (M1a); stage IV B tumours are those with lymph node (N1) or extrapulmonary distant metastases (M1b), regardless of grade.

Prognostic factors

Several prognostic factors have been identified in osteosarcoma. Primary metastases, axial or proximal extremity location, and large tumour size are of independent negative prognostic value. Factors associated with an adverse outcome in some series also include very young or older age, high levels of alkaline phosphatase or lactic dehydrogenase, and the immunohistochemical detection of p-glycoprotein (still debatable: HER2/erbB2). The relative risk associated with any presenting factor, however, is lower than that of two treatment-related variables: incomplete surgery is the most important negative prognostic indicator, and response to induction chemotherapy is the most important prognostic factor for resectable osteosarcoma. Response, however, is not all or nothing. Even a very moderate response is associated with better outcomes than none at all.

The classical factors related to poor prognosis in ES include presence of metastases, older age, large tumours, and primary site in the trunk and pelvis. Specific prognostic factors that currently influence the choice of treatment regimens include initial tumour size, the presence of pulmonary and/or extrapulmonary metastases, the presence of tumour cells at the surgical margins, and poor histological response to induction chemotherapy. The previously suggested prognostic importance of the specific *EWS–FLI1* gene fusion type has recently been refuted. As in osteosarcoma, the most clear-cut treatment-related prognostic indicator is tumour response to induction chemotherapy. Several large analyses have shown that early relapse (within two years from the time of initial diagnosis) is another predictor of death.

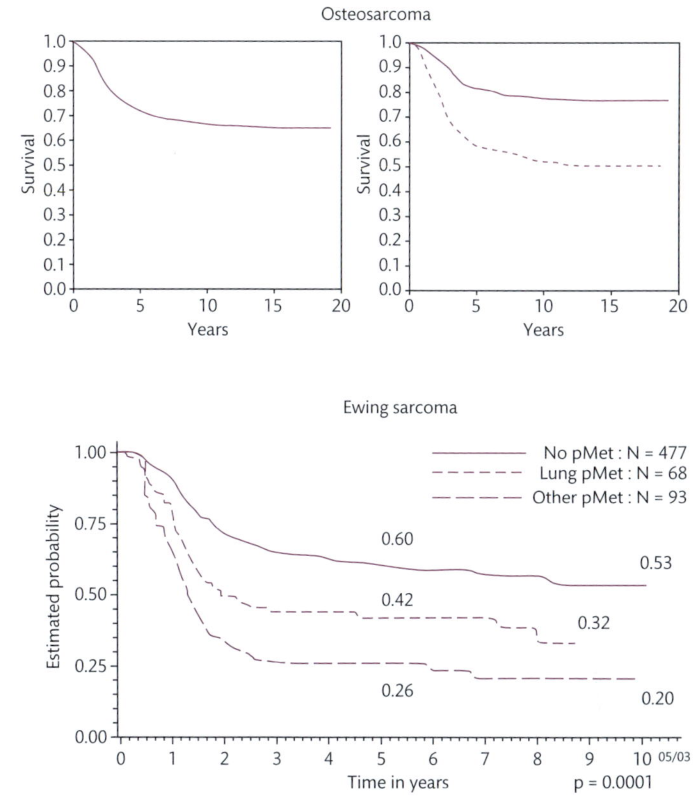

Figure 26.4 Osteosarcoma (top): left—overall survival with multimodal therapy; right—comparison of good responders (solid line) and poor responders (dashed line); good response = <10% viable tumour. Results are from 1,152 COSS patients under 20 years of age with localized extremity osteosarcoma. Ewing sarcoma (bottom): event-free survival by disease stage at initial presentation. Without primary metastases (no pMet), with lung or pleural metastases only (lung pMet), and with metastases to bones and/or bone marrow (other pMet). (CESS/EICESS data)

Treatment

Treatment principles and strategy

Many children and adolescents can be cured with appropriate therapy (Figure 26.4). Inappropriate use of diagnostic tools and suboptimal initial therapy can irrevocably compromise a patient's chances, and patients should be treated in specialized, experienced, paediatric bone-tumour centres able to provide access to the full diagnostic and therapeutic spectrum. Treatment within prospective clinical trials is considered standard clinical practice in many countries. Multinational trials such as the European and American Osteosarcoma Study EURAMOS-1 or the studies of the Children's Oncology Group (COG) and EURO-EWING groups are recent examples.

Local treatment (surgery in osteosarcoma, surgery and/or radiotherapy in ES) is an essential part of curative therapy. Most patients, however, will already have micro-metastatic disease by the time their sarcoma is detected. Prior to the 1970s, when treatment was exclusively targeted towards the primary, the outcome was extremely poor. This dismal outlook was dramatically improved when multiagent chemotherapy was added to local treatment. Many trials have since reported disease-free survival rates in the range of 50–70%. A multimodal approach has therefore emerged as the undisputed standard of care.

Currently, most institutions use an approach consisting of preoperative chemotherapy (also called neoadjuvant or induction chemotherapy), followed by definitive local therapy, and postoperative, adjuvant chemotherapy both for osteosarcoma and ES. Theoretical advantages of this approach include early treatment of micrometastatic disease and facilitation of subsequent local therapy because of shrinkage and decreased vascularity of the tumour. Furthermore, preoperative treatment permits tumour response to induction chemotherapy to be evaluated. A theoretical concern is that delayed removal of the bulk tumour could lead to the emergence of chemotherapy resistance. Only one relatively small, randomized osteosarcoma trial has prospectively compared patients treated by both pre- and postoperative chemotherapy with patients treated by primary surgery followed by the same chemotherapy. Treatment results did not differ between the two arms. Similarly, the Cooperative Osteosarcoma Study Group could not detect a survival difference between both approaches in a retrospective comparison of 157 patients undergoing primary surgery and 1,451 who received initial chemotherapy. As the delivery of initial chemotherapy also facilitates preparation for limb-salvage surgery, as well as offering the value of measuring early response, induction chemotherapy has become standard.

Local therapy

Choice of modality

In osteosarcoma, complete surgical removal of the primary tumour and, if present, all metastases is the local treatment of choice. Indications for radiotherapy are limited and basically restricted to inoperable tumours.

The radiosensitivity of ES was first recognized by James Ewing in1921 and has long played a major role. Currently, however, radiotherapy is no longer the local treatment of first choice for most ES. Increasing awareness of the risk of local recurrence has encouraged the use of surgery, and its use was associated with a survival advantage in several series. Situations in which surgery is preferable to irradiation include lesions in expendable bones, pathological fractures, distal extremity sites, bulky primary tumours, and in patients with poor response to initial chemotherapy. Preoperative radiotherapy may be indicated when there is tumour progression during chemotherapy, in emergencies such as spinal-cord compression, or when incomplete surgery is anticipated. Postoperative radiotherapy is indicated after incomplete resection or, in the opinion of some, in patients with poor histological response to induction chemotherapy. In one recent publication of the EURO-EWING consortium, postoperative radiotherapy reduced local relapse rates even in a subset of patients with good chemotherapy response.

Principles of bone-sarcoma surgery

Bone-sarcoma surgery has three aims. First and foremost, the tumour must be completely removed. Second, the patient should be left with good function. Third, it should, if possible, result in a cosmetically acceptable appearance. Complete tumour removal is of paramount importance; functional and cosmetic aspects are secondary goals. The aim should be that the tumour, including the biopsy scar and biopsy track, should be removed together with an intact cuff of the surrounding normal tissue, corresponding to the definition of 'wide' margins within the MSTS definition (Table 26.2). Wide and radical margins are considered adequate, whilst marginal or intralesional margins are associated with an increased risk of local recurrence, which in turn carry a grave prognosis.

The location, size, and regional anatomy of the tumour; its relation to nerves and vessels as well as neighbouring joints, the bones,

Table 26.2 Surgical margins in musculoskeletal oncology

Type	Resection
Intralesional	Within the lesion
Marginal	Through the pseudocapsule or reactive tissue
Wide	Lesion (including biopsy scar), pseudocapsule and/or reactive zone, and an intact cuff of normal tissue completely surrounding the mass removed as a single block
Radical	Entire anatomical compartment containing the tumour removed as one block

Source: data from Enneking WF, Spanier SS, Goodman MA, (1980). 'A system for the surgical staging of musculoskeletal sarcoma.' *Clinical Orthopaedics and Related Research*. Volume 153, Nov–Dec. pp. 106–20. Wolters Kluwer Health Inc.

soft tissues, and skin which will remain after wide resection; and the patient's growth expectancy must all be evaluated before deciding upon the type of surgery. En bloc resection with limb salvage is possible in many cases. Amputation, however, may still be the most appropriate type of surgery for selected patients with unfavourable tumour characteristics. Advantages of amputation include oncological safety, low complication rates, and a low rate of revision surgery. Disadvantages include mutilation and phantom sensations. The functional outcome is often rather poor after proximal amputations, but better with below the knee amputations.

Rotation-plasty, used for sarcomas of the distal femur and, occasionally, the proximal tibia, is the classic example of a resection-reimplantation procedure. The knee is removed en bloc together with the tumour, the only structure left *in situ* being the popliteal nerve bundle. The distal part of the tibia, together with the foot, is then rotated by 180°, the tibia is fused with the femoral stump, and anastomoses between the femoral and tibial vessels are created. The result of this reimplantation is a shortened extremity, in which the rotated foot substitutes for the knee and carries the prosthesis. Advantages of rotation-plasty include oncological safety, even in very large tumours, lack of phantom sensations, and an infrequent need for revision surgery, as well as an extremity function rivalling that of limb salvage. The highly unusual cosmetic appearance is its main disadvantage, and the procedure has therefore fallen out of favour.

Retaining the extremity requires reconstruction of bony and soft-tissue defects. Only a minority of tumours are situated in expendable bones such as the proximal fibula. Far more often, limb salvage implies replacement of a major joint. Allografts are used by some surgeons, but modular endoprosthetic systems, assembled to fit in the operating room, are employed more commonly. Autologous bones, such as vascularized fibulae bridging diaphyseal defects, can be used in selected situations. Special expandable endoprostheses are available for growing extremities. Innovative models can be lengthened non-invasively. Unfortunately, such devices still carry a high complication risk with the associated need for frequent revisions. Disadvantages of limb salvage in general already include a significant complication risk, to which infections, fractures, and prosthetic wear contribute. Several publications report local recurrence rates approximately three times higher than after ablative procedures, suggesting that resection margins may sometimes not be as wide as expected.

Principles of radiotherapy

In osteosarcoma, radiotherapy is limited to few indications. Postoperative irradiation is indicated when definitive surgery did not result in safe margins and in which revision surgery, even when mutilating, could not do so. In these cases, local control may be attempted by irradiating with very high doses, often 60 Gy and above. Both proton and heavy-ion radiotherapy are of interest and worthy of investigation in inoperable osteosarcoma.

In ES, whole-bone irradiation had traditionally been advised because the tumour was thought to arise in the bone marrow, putting the whole marrow cavity at risk. The advent of MRI, which accurately demonstrated the extent of marrow involvement, and of effective chemotherapy, questioned this approach. A randomized study undertaken by the North American Pediatric Oncology Group (POG) has demonstrated that radiotherapy to the initial tumour volume, plus a 2-cm safety margin, produced results that were equivalent to that achieved by whole-bone irradiation. Scars after biopsy or tumour resection should be included in the radiation field. To avoid constrictive fibrosis, an adequate strip of skin and subcutaneous tissue should be left when irradiating limb sites, and epiphyseal plates should be spared if possible, particularly in children.

In inoperable ES, a compartment dose of 45 Gy is recommended, with a tumour boost to at least 54–55.8 Gy: whether this can be achieved depends on the site of the tumour and the age of the patient. For preoperative radiotherapy, the standard target volume dose is 45 Gy. For postoperative radiotherapy, dosage recommendations depend on histological assessment of the resection margins and the tumour response to induction chemotherapy, and vary between 45 and 55.8 Gy.

Systemic therapy for osteosarcoma

The majority of current treatment protocols are based upon varying combinations of only four active agents: doxorubicin, cisplatin, high-dose methotrexate, and ifosfamide. Even after several decades and numerous clinical trials, the exact individual role of each of these agents and the optimal way in which they are to be combined and delivered are still being debated, as is the potential benefit of additional drugs.

Doxorubicin was introduced into osteosarcoma treatment in the 1970s and has remained an integral part ever since. A meta-analysis of trials published until 1991 concluded that doxorubicin dose intensity is an important determinant of favourable outcome and that the dose intensities of other agents do not contribute as significantly to outcome. However, the agent's cardiotoxicity remains a major issue and multiple efforts aiming to reduce the incidence and severity of this complication have been pursued. Prospective, randomized studies comparing doxorubicin-free with doxorubicin-containing regimens have produced conflicting results. Most recently, French investigators from the SFOP (Societe Francaise d'Oncologie Pediatrique) OS94 trial reported that treatment could be initiated with an anthracycline- (and cisplatin-) free preoperative regimen of high-dose ifosfamide and methotrexate, which would be continued postoperatively in the case of good response and changed to doxorubicin-based polychemotherapy only in the case of poor histological response to anthracycline-free induction. Some doxorubicin-based protocols include measures aimed towards reducing doxorubicin cardiotoxicity, with cardioprotectants such as dexrazoxane and the reduction of anthracycline peak levels by continuous doxorubicin infusions featuring most prominently. Sequential studies by American and European groups suggest that there is no major loss of efficacy with these approaches, but no controlled studies have been reported.

Methotrexate, a folate antagonist, blocks the action of dihydrofolate reductase, the enzyme responsible for reducing folate to its active form, tetrahydrofolic acid. In osteosarcoma, methotrexate is given at very high doses in the range of 8–12 g/m^2. Toxicity must be antagonized by the use of leucovorin, an activated folate. The treatment concept of high-dose methotrexate is based on the assumption that normal cells can be rescued more effectively than tumour cells, which may lack active folate transporters. Observations published in 1972 that high-dose methotrexate monotherapy was able to induce responses of pulmonary metastases led to its use as an adjuvant, first as monotherapy and, soon later, also as part of multidrug regimens. A significant survival advantage conferred by high-dose over moderate-dose methotrexate-containing combination chemotherapy was demonstrated in a randomized Italian study. However, the assumption that osteosarcoma polychemotherapy regimens which include methotrexate must necessarily be superior to other regimens has been repeatedly challenged, both in randomized settings and in uncontrolled studies.

High-dose methotrexate therapy requires meticulous attention to detail and extensive supportive measures, including hydration, alkalinization of the urine, and leucovorin administration adapted to methotrexate serum levels. Inadequate supportive care will result in severely delayed methotrexate clearance and excessive toxicity, including myelosuppression, renal toxicity, and mucositis. Some patients will experience such toxicity despite adequate supportive care, the risk apparently increasing with increasing patient age. The enzyme glucarpidase, which cleaves methotrexate, may be of benefit in selected patients with renal failure and severely delayed methotrexate clearance, but most cases of delayed methotrexate clearance can be handled by maintaining hydration and increasing leucovorin dose and frequency.

Given that, under most circumstances, patients do not experience significant myelotoxicity and given the resulting ability to schedule methotrexate at times when other agents cannot be administered, most groups incorporate high-dose methotrexate into their treatment protocols. Protocols devoid of high-dose methotrexate, but containing several of the other three 'standard' agents, can be used in healthcare settings which cannot guarantee the life-saving supportive measures without which the drug should not be prescribed.

The activity of cisplatin against osteosarcoma was proven in early phase II trials. Cisplatin therapy requires supportive hyperhydration. Ototoxicity and nephrotoxicity are dose-limiting, but both can be reduced by administering the drug as a continuous infusion. Intra-arterial administration of cisplatin into the vessel supplying the tumour was previously tried but has largely been abandoned since comparative trials failed to demonstrate enhanced anti-tumour effects compared to intravenous administration.

Following positive phase II trials, ifosfamide has been part of many osteosarcoma protocols since the mid-1980s. Its efficacy may be related to the dose administered. Supportive measures necessary to prevent haemorrhagic uropathy include hyperhydration and mesna (uromitexan). Ifosfamide may also lead to chronic renal tubular toxicity and to sterility.

Data from two European trials (by the Istituto Rizzoli and the Cooperative Osteosarcoma Study Group (COSS)) supported the use of ifosfamide, but a randomized trial by the North American POG and Children's Cancer Group (CCG) could not demonstrate that adding standard-dose ifosfamide to high-dose methotrexate, doxorubicin, and cisplatin improved outcomes. The results of the North American trial INT0133 should, however, be interpreted with caution as a second randomization of liposomal muramyl tripeptide (MTP-PE) may have interfered with the ifosfamide question. Furthermore, the ifosfamide arm contained no preoperative cisplatin. Results of a French trial, SFOP-91, which did not add, but rather substituted ifosfamide, suggest that favourable results may be obtained by regimens that rely on ifosfamide rather than on doxorubicin.

No other cytostatic agents have come close to replacing the four standard substances previously described. A combination of bleomycin, cyclophosphamide, and actinomycin D (BCD) was used in the early days of chemotherapy but was largely abandoned due to questionable efficacy. Carboplatin has some activity against osteosarcoma, but less than cisplatin. Etoposide is almost inactive when given as a single agent, but may enhance the effect of carboplatin or ifosfamide. Amongst others, negative phase II studies have been reported for paclitaxel, docetaxel, and topotecan. Gemcitabine seems to be marginally active, with stable disease achieved in some patients.

Overall, progress in the treatment of osteosarcoma has been slow and survival rates have improved little over more than two decades. Attempts to improve prognosis through treatment intensification by interval compression achieved with granulocyte colony-stimulating growth factor (G-CSF) support or by combining maximally tolerated doses of high-dose ifosfamide, high-dose methotrexate, cisplatin, and doxorubicin have failed to show benefit. High-dose chemotherapy with autologous peripheral blood stem-cell transplantation was also unsuccessful in the reported series.

Improving the prognosis for patients with poor response to induction chemotherapy remains a particular challenge. The prospective, randomized European and American Osteosarcoma Study EURAMOS-1 investigated whether the postoperative addition of high-dose ifosfamide and etoposide to a therapy backbone of methotrexate, doxorubicin, and cisplatin (MAP) was superior to MAP alone in patients whose tumours had shown a poor response to preoperative MAP. Unfortunately, this was not the case: the five-drug regimen was associated with additional morbidity and a higher risk to develop secondary leukaemias, but did not decrease the recurrence risk, and thus its use is no longer recommended. The EURAMOS-1 trial also investigated whether outcomes for good responders to induction MAP chemotherapy might be improved by adding maintenance therapy with pegylated interferonα after completing postoperative MAP. Again, no significant benefit was observed.

Whether the addition of the immunomodulator L-MTP-PE (liposomal muramyl tripeptide phenol ethanolamine) to chemotherapy improves prognosis, as evaluated in the randomized North American POG-CCG INT0133 trial, is still a matter of debate. A first analysis of INT0133 concluded that there was an interaction between L-MTP-PE and ifosfamide, which, within a rather complex factorial trial design, was evaluated in the same study. A later publication reported a survival advantage for L-MTP-PE, but could still not prove that adding L-MTP-PE improved event-free survival. It has been argued that further trials are needed before the agent might be considered for routine use.

Adding the bisphosphonate zoledronic acid to chemotherapy was investigated in a recent randomized French trial. The study was terminated early for futility.

Systemic therapy for Ewing sarcoma

ES is responsive to alkylating agents such as ifosfamide and cyclophosphamide, to doxorubicin, and to other agents such as vincristine, actinomycin D, and the topoisomerase II inhibitor etoposide. Combinations of these agents with complementary mechanisms of action have improved disease-free survival rates. Intergroup Ewing Sarcoma (IESS) studies demonstrated the superiority of a four-drug regimen using vincristine (V), actinomycin D (A), cyclophosphamide (C), and doxorubicin (D) over three-drug VAC in terms of both disease-free survival (60% versus 24%) and local control (96% versus 86%). Rosen, from the Memorial Sloan-Kettering Cancer Center (MSKCC), reported an advantage of using these drugs in combination rather than sequentially as early as 1978, but it is important to realize that a considerable number of patients in earlier series received cumulative doxorubicin doses of over 700 mg/m^2 before its use was restricted to a maximum of 400–500 mg/m^2 because of the risk of doxorubicin-related cardiomyopathy.

The IESS and MSKCC experiences led to the widespread use of similar four-drug regimens, and treatment was later extended to incorporate ifosfamide (I) and etoposide (E). In the European EICESS-92 study, patients with localized high-risk disease (tumour volume more than 200 ml) receiving VIDA benefitted from the addition of etoposide, and in the randomized POG-CCG Ewing trial (VACD versus EVADI), patients treated with EVADI appeared to have a more favourable outcome.

The incorporation of G-CSF into treatment regimens allows dose intensification by increasing the dose per cycle or by shortening the interval between treatments. The IESS-II study compared high-dose intermittent chemotherapy with moderate-dose continuous chemotherapy, resulting in a significant benefit from the more intensive regimen (68% versus 48% disease-free survival at five years). Another POG-CCG randomized study explored dose intensification (maintaining a dosing interval of 21 days) by condensing treatment duration to 30 weeks by increasing the individual doses of chemotherapy in comparison to the delivery of the same cumulative doses over 48 weeks: so far, results between the standard and the dose-intensified arms do not differ. More recently, the COG AEWS0031 trial has explored dose intensification with the use of G-CSF by decreasing the intervals between cycles (interval compression) from three to two weeks while maintaining the same dose per cycle. Published results confirm that relapse rates are lower and toxicity manageable. The role of high-dose therapy with autologous haematopoietic stem-cell rescue in certain risk groups of patients was investigated in the EURO-EWING trial. The study's results suggest that a subgroup of patients with high-risk localized disease would benefit from such a procedure.

Treatment of metastatic and recurrent disease

Primary metastases

In osteosarcoma, all detectable metastases must be removed by surgery if therapy is to be curative. As most metastases develop in the lung, this usually implies thoracotomy. There is evidence that some patients with apparently unilateral lung metastases may indeed have bilateral disease. Complete resection of osteosarcoma pulmonary metastases requires palpation of the lung. Acceptable surgical approaches include thoracotomy or median sternotomy. Approximately one quarter of all osteosarcoma patients with proven metastatic disease at diagnosis and 40% of those who achieve a complete surgical remission of both the primary and all metastases in the context of an intensive polychemotherapy regimen will go on to become long-term survivors. Solitary primary metastases may have a prognosis similar to that of localized disease.

Metastatic disease at diagnosis is the most prominent adverse prognostic factor in ES. A recently published analysis of the EURO-EWING consortium described survival rates of 10–40% at three years, with patient age, tumour size and site, and number of metastases defining distinct prognostic groups. Patients with isolated lung metastases have a better prognosis than those with extrapulmonary metastases (Figure 26.4). If pulmonary disease is present, patients also receive bilateral pulmonary irradiation at doses of 14–18 Gy. Patients with solitary or circumscribed bony lesions can receive irradiation to those sites at doses of 40–50 Gy. However, survival rates for patients with multiple bony and/or bone-marrow metastases are below 10% at two years. These discouraging results have led to more aggressive approaches utilizing high-dose chemotherapy with autologous stem-cell reinfusion. A variety of agents such as busulfan, treosulfan, melphalan, cyclophosphamide, thiotepa, etoposide, and carboplatin have been employed but without definitive evidence of improved outcome. Total body irradiation does not seem to offer benefit, but significantly contributes to toxicity. Local therapy aimed at identified metastases may improve survival.

Recurrent disease

Osteosarcoma recurrences usually involve the lung. Bone metastases and local recurrences are much less common, and other sites are rarely affected. Unfortunately, long-term survival rates remain below 20%. A short latency period and the presence of more than one or two metastases are associated with particularly poor outcomes. Complete surgery of all sites of recurrence is the only therapy with unequivocally proven impact on survival. Selected patients may be cured after multiple recurrences, provided that surgery results in a renewed complete remission. It may be prudent to irradiate suitable inoperable lesions in order to slow the progression of disease, but this is unlikely to lead to cure. Patients with inoperable recurrent osteosarcoma who receive chemotherapy may survive longer than those who do not. Recently, sorafenib (with and without everolimus) has also shown some activity in recurrent osteosarcoma. The exact role of adjuvant chemotherapy in recurrent operable osteosarcoma remains to be defined. Success has been limited, and there is no universally accepted standard regimen, although many would consider the use of a combination of ifosfamide and etoposide in patients who had not previously received those drugs.

The survival of ES patients who develop local or metastatic recurrence is poor and second remissions are usually short-lived. Patients with a longer disease-free interval represent the subset of patients most likely to survive. The role of local therapy is less clear than in osteosarcoma. Chemotherapy and radiotherapy are commonly applied in an attempt to prolong survival. Chemotherapy regimens currently used include combinations of previously used drugs, or of platinum compounds with ifosfamide and etoposide, topotecan and cyclophosphamide, irinotecan and temozolomide, or gemcitabine and docetaxel. High-dose chemotherapy with autologous haematopoietic stem-cell rescue can be considered in patients who achieved a complete remission with conventional multimodal treatment.

Unfortunately, outcomes after bone sarcoma recurrence remain poor and have not improved much over the years. Participation in studies investigating tumour biology and innovative treatment approaches should be encouraged in order to help break this stalemate.

Follow-up

Suggestions for follow-up are given in Table 26.3. Intervals between visits mirror the declining risk of relapse with time. As there is little prospectively gathered evidence, suggestions must necessarily remain somewhat arbitrary. Follow-up should, however, include regular assessments of remission as well as tests for possible late effects of treatment.

Remission status

Tumour-directed follow-up focuses on the few organ systems where relapses are likely to occur. Pulmonary metastases contribute to over 80% of recurrences of osteosarcoma and approximately half of all recurrences of ES. They will not usually cause symptoms until they have reached a very large size or penetrated the pleura. In order to

Table 26.3 Suggestions for follow-up after multimodal therapy for bone sarcoma

Time	Tumour-directed investigations	Late-effects monitoring
Baseline	Chest X-ray & CT	Echocardiogram, audiogram*, liver & kidney function
	X-ray & MRI of primary site	
Years 1 & 2	Chest X-ray q 6–12 wk	Echocardiogram q 1–2 yr, audiogram*, liver** & kidney** function
	X-ray of primary site q 4 mo	
Years 3 & 4	Chest X-ray q 2–4 mo	Echocardiogram q 1–2 yr
	X-ray of primary site q 4 mo	
Years 5–10	Chest X-ray q 6 mo***	Echocardiogram q (1–)2–4 yr****
Thereafter	A few relapses reported as late as two decades after treatment: discuss with patient whether to continue chest X-ray monitoring	Echocardiogram q (1–)2–4 yr

Every clinic visit should include detailed history and physical examination. Many institutions will add complete blood counts. Evaluate any site with unexplained pain or swelling. Chest CT scan is optional, but should always be performed if chest X-ray shows metastasis or is inconclusive. Add consultation with orthopaedic surgery and physical therapy as indicated. Offer fertility testing for males. Additional investigations may be indicated.

* If treatment included cisplatin.

** Need not be repeated if normal at one year.

*** Some groups recommend annual radiographs of the primary site until year 10.

**** Longer interval if normal function and post-pubertal at diagnosis.

Adapted with permission from Ritter J, Bielack SS, 'Osteosarcoma'. *Annals of Oncology*, Volume 21, Suppl. 7, pp. vii320–vii325. Copyright © 2010, Oxford University Press. DOI: https://doi.org/10.1093/annonc/mdq276

detect them at an earlier stage, they must be searched for by appropriate imaging, which includes serial X-rays and/or CT scans of the thorax. In ES, where bone metastases occur more frequently, technetium bone scans may be included, with other imaging methods like FDG (fluorodeoxyglucose)-PET scans or whole-body MRI used less commonly. Local recurrences are often first detected because of symptoms, most noticeably pain. Most centres still include sequential imaging of the primary site into their follow-up programme.

Late effects

Fortunately, many former bone sarcoma patients can lead relatively normal and productive lives. Nevertheless, they are more likely to suffer from chronic health conditions than survivors of most other paediatric cancers. Late complications may be caused by the tumour itself or by surgery, radiotherapy, or chemotherapy. Functional and cosmetic consequences for the musculoskeletal system depend on the location and extent of the tumour as well as the type of local treatment employed. Amputations and rotation-plasties carry the stigma of mutilation, but may lead to functional results that are similar to those after limb-salvage procedures. Revision surgery is more frequently needed after limb-salvage procedures, where periprosthetic infection, loosening, fractures, and prosthetic wear can occur. The use of expandable prostheses in skeletally immature patients is predictably associated with the need for multiple revision procedures. Radiotherapy may lead to growth reduction, functional limitations, and secondary cancers. (The late consequences of chemotherapy are more completely described in Chapter 14, 'Late Effects of Therapy and Survivorship Issues'.)

Future and remaining challenges

Osteosarcoma remains a challenging disease. It is sensitive to a small number of medications, all having significant short- and long-term toxicities. Radiation is of limited value and even sensitive tumours are incompletely eliminated by chemotherapy, mandating surgical resection and reconstruction, with their attendant morbidity. Patients with recurrent disease are difficult to cure, with a somewhat better outlook for those with resectable metastases. The role of MTP-PE (mifurmatide) therapy in osteosarcoma requires better definition.

New initiatives are required. A way to affect the osteoclastic activity important for the progression of bone lesions is to interfere with the receptor activator for nuclear factor kappa-B (RANK) pathway. RANK, RANK-Ligand, and osteoprotegrin maintain normal bone metabolism. Osteosarcoma cells express RANK-Ligand. Those resistant to chemotherapy show increased expression of genes involved in osteoclast activation. Denosumab, a humanized antibody that binds RANK-Ligand, inhibiting osteoclasts and therefore bone resorption, has been successfully used in patients with giant-cell tumour of bone, and has decreased skeletal-related events in patients with some adult cancers. A COG study is currently enrolling recurrent osteosarcoma patients.

The antibody drug conjugate, glembatumumab vedoitin, recognizes the cell-surface glycoprotein GNMB and is conjugated to the microtubule inhibitor MMAE. GNMB is highly expressed on the surface of more than 90% of primary osteosarcoma primary tumours and is currently being tested in recurrent osteosarcoma by the COG. Similarly, the chimeric anti-GD2 antibody, dinutuximab, has been approved for the treatment of neuroblastoma. Since GD2 is expressed in osteosarcomas as well as neurblastomas, the COG is currently testing this antibody in recurrent osteosarcoma.

Given the recent better characterization of osteosarcoma as a p53-driven cancer with extensive chromosomal aberrations in which multiple oncogenic pathways drive chromosomal instability during tumour evolution, clearly new approaches attempting to exploit these alterations as a potential vulnerability are needed.

In patients with ES, the addition of multi-agent chemotherapy to local control with radiation and/or surgery has improved disease-free survival from 10% to 50–70%. High-throughput microarray-based gene-expression profiling studies comparing different types of small, blue, round-cell tumours have identified a unique gene-expression pattern in ES, and gene-expression studies on large cohorts may lead to the discrimination of prognostically distinct groups, allowing better treatment stratification.

The combinations of topotecan and cyclophosphamide, and irinotecan andtemozolomide, have shown activity in patients with recurrent ES. Topotecan and cyclophosphamide combined with vincristine (VTC) has been added to the compressed vincristine, doxorubicin, cyclophosphamide, ifosfamide, etoposide (VDC-IE) schedule to study the feasibility of interval compression with that additional combination. Once the tolerable interval has been established, it is likely that a randomized study of compressed VDC-IE compared with VDC-IE-VTC will follow.

There was early excitement surrounding the use of IGF1R antibodies in the treatment of Ewing sarcoma, based upon early reports of clinical activity. The largest study, evaluating Roche IGF1R antibody R1507, assessed 115 patients with recurrent Ewing sarcoma and demonstrated a response rate of only 10%, with a median duration of response of 29 weeks. Although the single-agent activity is low, the potential to improve survival in high-risk Ewing sarcoma patients with the addition of an IGF1R antibody to standard chemotherapy is currently being tested by the COG.

Another area of interest and potential vulnerability of Ewing sarcomas is PARP inhibition. Several groups independently reported that Ewing sarcomas were highly sensitive to the inhibition of this enzyme. However, the first clinical trial with the PARP inhibitor olaparib showed zero out of twelve responses. Ongoing studies are evaluating combinations of DNA-damaging agents such as temozolamide with PARP inhibitors.

Finally, since the known oncogenic driver of Ewing sarcoma is the mutant transcription factor fusing *EWS* (or other members of the FET family) to *ETS* genes, a first-in-class inhibitor of ETS activity is currently being evaluated in a clinical trial targeting relapsed Ewing sarcoma patients.

Conclusions

The prognosis for bone-sarcoma patients is determined primarily by local treatment options, tumour dissemination, and tumour burden, as well as by the biology underlying the tumour and its response to treatment. Tumour burden can only be limited by early diagnosis, but response is subject to the impact of better therapies including the design of more effective chemotherapy combinations, increased drug intensity with improved supportive care, and surgical removal of all the tumour. In addition, more precise determination of prognostic factors should result in opportunities to better stratify treatment intensity, offering the opportunity to limit the risk of late effects from treatment in patients with favourable disease. Because of the rarity of these tumours, treatment should always be performed in centres experienced in bone-sarcoma treatment, and within the framework of controlled clinical trials where available. The evaluation of experimental approaches to treatment should be restricted to clinical trial settings.

Acknowledgements

The authors acknowledge the important contributions of Heinrich Kovar, Heribert Jürgens, and Mark Bernstein to the chapter 'Bone Tumours' in the sixth edition of *Cancer in Children*, upon which this chapter is based.

FURTHER READING

Abed R, Grimer R (2010) Surgical modalities in the treatment of bone sarcoma in children. *Cancer Treat Rev* **36**, 342–7.

Bacci G, et al. (1990) Primary chemotherapy and delayed surgery (neoadjuvant chemotherapy) for osteosarcoma of the extremities. The Istituto Rizzoli Experience in 127 patients treated preoperatively with intravenous methotrexate (high versus moderate doses) and intraarterial cisplatin. *Cancer* **65**, 2539–3.

Bielack S, et al. (2002) Prognostic factors in high-grade osteosarcoma of the extremities or trunk. An analysis of 1,702 patients treated on neoadjuvant Cooperative Osteosarcoma Study Group protocols. *J Clin Oncol* **20**, 776–90.

Bielack S, et al. (2013) Controversies in childhood osteosarcoma. *Minerva Pediatr* **65**, 125–48.

Bielack SS, et al. (2015) Methotrexate, doxorubicin, and cisplatin (MAP) plus maintenance pegylated interferon alfa-2b versus MAP alone in patients with resectable high-grade osteosarcoma and good histologic response to preoperative MAP: first results of the EURAMOS-1 good response randomized controlled trial. *J Clin Oncol* **33**, 2279–87.

Bishop MW, et al. (2016) Future directions in the treatment of osteosarcoma. *Curr Opin Pediatr* **28**, 26–33.

Brierley JD, et al. (eds.) (2016) *TNM Classification of Malignant Tumours* (8th edn). Chichester, West Sussex: Wiley-Blackwell.

Casali PG, et al. (2018) Bone sarcomas: ESMO-PaedCan-EURACAN clinical practice guidelines for diagnosis, treatment and follow-up. *Ann Oncol* **29**(Suppl_4), iv79–95.

Ciccarese F, et al. (2015) The many faces of pulmonary metastases of osteosarcoma: retrospective study on 283 lesions submitted to surgery. *Eur J Radiol* **84**, 2679–85.

Chen X, et al. (2014) Recurrent somatic structural variations contribute to tumorigenesis in pediatric osteosarcoma. *Cell Rep* **7**,104–12.

DuBois SG, et al. (2010) Angiogenesis and vascular targeting in Ewing sarcoma: a review of preclinical and clinical data. *Cancer* **116**, 749–57.

Ferrari S, et al. (2003) Postrelapse survival in osteosarcoma of the extremities: prognostic factors for long-term survival. *J Clin Oncol* **21**, 710–15.

Fletcher CDM, et al. (eds) (2013) *WHO Classification of Tumours of Soft Tissue and Bone* (4th edn), Vol. 5. Lyon: IARC.

Gaspar N, et al. (2015) Ewing sarcoma: current management and future approaches through collaboration. *J Clin Oncol* **33**, 3036–46.

Goorin AM, et al. (2003) Presurgical chemotherapy compared with immediate surgery and adjuvant chemotherapy for nonmetastatic osteosarcoma: Pediatric Oncology Group Study POG-8651. *J Clin Oncol* **21**(8), 1574–80.

Gorlick R, et al. (2013) Children's Oncology Group's 2013 blueprint for research: bone tumors. *Pediatr Blood Cancer* **60**, 1009–15.

Grier HE, et al. (2003) Addition of ifosfamide and etoposide to standard chemotherapy for Ewing's sarcoma and primitive neuroectodermal tumor of bone. *N Engl J Med* **34**, 694–701.

Isakoff MS, et al. (2015) Osteosarcoma: current treatment and a collaborative pathway to success. *J Clin Oncol* **33**, 3029–35.

Jaffe N (1972) Recent advances in the chemotherapy of metastatic osteogenic sarcoma. *Cancer* **30**, 1627–31.

Jaffe N, et al. (eds) (2009) *Pediatric and Adolescent Osteosarcoma* (*Cancer Treatment and Research series*, Vol. 152). New York: Springer.

Jiang Y, et al. (2015) Targeted therapies for advanced Ewing sarcoma family of tumors. *Cancer Treat Rev* **41**, 391–400.

Kager L, et al. (2016) The ENCCA-WP7/EuroSarc/EEC/PROVABES/EURAMOS Third European Bone Sarcoma Networking Meeting/Joint Workshop of EU Bone Sarcoma Translational Research Networks; Vienna, Austria, September 24–25, 2015. Workshop report. *Clin Sarcoma Res* **6**, 3. doi: 10.1186/s13569-016-0043-5

Kansara M, et al. (2014) Translational biology of osteosarcoma. *Nat Rev Cancer* **14**, 722–35.

Kempf-Bielack B, et al. (2005) Osteosarcoma relapse after combined modality therapy: an analysis of unselected patients in the Cooperative Osteosarcoma Study Group (COSS). *J Clin Oncol* **23**, 559–68.

Khanna C, et al. (2014) Toward a drug development path that targets metastatic progression in osteosarcoma. *Clin Cancer Res* **20**, 4200–9.

Kovac M, et al. (2015) Exome sequencing of osteosarcoma reveals mutation signatures reminiscent of BRCA deficiency. *Nat Commun* **6**, 8940. doi: 10.1038/ncomms9940

Kovar H, et al. (2016) The second European interdisciplinary Ewing sarcoma research summit—a joint effort to deconstructing the multiple layers of a complex disease. *Oncotarget* **7**(8), 8613–24. doi: 10.18632/oncotarget.6937

Ladenstein R, et al. (2010) Primary disseminated multifocal Ewing sarcoma: results of the Euro-EWING 99 trial. *J Clin Oncol* **28**, 3284–91.

Le Deley MC, et al. (2007) SFOP OS94: a randomised trial comparing preoperative high-dose methotrexate plus doxorubicin to high-dose methotrexate plus etoposide and ifosfamide in osteosarcoma patients. *Eur J Cancer* **43**, 752–61.

Machado I, et al. (2016) Ewing sarcoma and the new emerging Ewing-like sarcomas: CIC and BCOR-rearranged-sarcomas. A systematic review. *Histol Histopathol* **31**,1169–81.

Marina NM, et al. (2016) Comparison of MAPIE versus MAP in patients with a poor response to preoperative chemotherapy for newly diagnosed high-grade osteosarcoma (EURAMOS-1): an open-label, international, randomised controlled trial. *Lancet Oncol* **17**, 1396–408.

Meyers PA, et al. (2008) Osteosarcoma: the addition of muramyl tripeptide to chemotherapy improves overall survival. A report from the Children's Oncology Group. *J Clin Oncol* **26**, 633–8.

Mirabello L, et al. (2015) Germline TP53 variants and susceptibility to osteosarcoma. *J Natl Cancer Inst* **107**, pii: djv101. doi:10.1093/jnci/djv101

Oeffinger KC, et al. (2006) Chronic health conditions in adult survivors of childhood cancer. *N Engl J Med* **355**, 1572–82.

Omer N, et al. (2017) Phase-II trials in osteosarcoma recurrences: a systematic review of past experience. *Eur J Cancer* **75**, 98–108. doi: 10.1016/j.ejca.2017.01.005

Pappo AS, et al. (2014) A phase 2 trial of R1507, a monoclonal antibody to the insulin-like growth factor-1 receptor (IGF-1R), in patients with recurrent or refractory rhabdomyosarcoma, osteosarcoma, synovial sarcoma, and other soft tissue sarcomas: results of a Sarcoma Alliance for Research Through Collaboration study. *Cancer* **120**(16), 2448–56. doi: 10.1002/cncr.28728

Paulussen M, et al. (2008) Results of the EICESS-92 Study: two randomized trials of Ewing's sarcoma treatment—cyclophosphamide compared with ifosfamide in standard-risk patients and assessment of benefit of etoposide added to standard treatment in high-risk patients. *J Clin Oncol* **26**, 4385–93.

Petrilli AS, et al. (2006) Results of the Brazilian Osteosarcoma Treatment Group Studies III and IV: prognostic factors and impact on survival. *J Clin Oncol* **24**, 1161–8.

Picci P, et al. (1994) The relationship of chemotherapy- induced necrosis and surgical margins to local recurrence in osteosarcoma. *J Clin Oncol* **12**, 2699–705.

Piperno-Neumann S, et al. (2016) Zoledronate in combination with chemotherapy and surgery to treat osteosarcoma (OS2006): a randomised, multicentre, open-label, phase 3 trial. *Lancet Oncol* **17**, 1070–80.

Roth M, et al. (2016) Targeting glycoprotein NMB with antibody-drug conjugate, glembatumumab vedotin, for the treatment of osteosarcoma. *Pediatr Blood Cancer* **63**, 32–8.

Schuck A, et al. (2003) Local therapy in localized Ewing tumors: results of 1058 patients treated in the CESS 81, CESS 86, and EICESS 92 trials. *Int J Radiat Oncol Biol Phys* **55**, 168–77.

Smith MA, et al. (1991) Influence of doxorubicin dose intensity on response and outcome for patients with osteogenic sarcoma and Ewing's sarcoma. *J Natl Cancer Inst* **83**, 1460–70.

Sobin LH, et al. (2009) *UICC TNM Classification of Malignant Tumors* (7th edn). New York: Wiley.

Subbiah V, et al. (2009) Ewing's sarcoma: standard and experimental treatment options. *Cur Treat Options Oncol* **10**, 126–40.

Whelan JS, et al. (2012) Survival from high-grade localised extremity osteosarcoma: combined results and prognostic factors from three European Osteosarcoma Intergroup randomised controlled trials. *Ann Oncol* **23**, 1607–16.

Whelan J, et al. (2018) High-dose chemotherapy and blood autologous stem-cell rescue compared with standard chemotherapy in localized high-risk Ewing sarcoma: results of Euro-E.W.I.N.G.99 and Ewing-2008. *J Clin Oncol*. JCO2018782516. doi: 10.1200/JCO.2018.78.2516 [Epub ahead of print]

Winkler K, et al. (1988) Neoadjuvant chemotherapy of osteosarcoma: results of a randomized cooperative trial (COSS-82) with salvage chemotherapy based on histological tumor response. *J Clin Oncol* **6**, 329–37.

Womer RB, et al.(2012) Randomized controlled trial of interval-compressed chemotherapy for the treatment of localized Ewing sarcoma: a report from the Children's Oncology Group. *J Clin Oncol* **30**, 4148–54.

27

Wilms and Other Renal Tumours

Norbert Graf and Christophe Bergeron

Wilms tumour (nephroblastoma)

Introduction

In 1814, Rance classified Wilms Tumour (WT) or nephroblastoma for the first time as a renal neoplasia. In 1899, the surgeon Max Wilms described this tumour entity in a 90-page monograph *Die Mischgeschwülste der Niere* in much more detail. Today, this tumour is regarded as a prime example of a curable malignant disease. The improvements in the treatment of nephroblastoma are particularly based on the progress in surgery and radiotherapy, and in the development of effective chemotherapies. Interdisciplinary cooperation and prospective randomized trials have made considerable contributions to this success.

Epidemiology

The incidence of WT is seven per one million children less than 15 years of age. With 6–7% of all childhood malignancies, nephroblastoma represents the most frequent malignant renal tumour. Worldwide, WT are more common in girls than boys. The age distribution shows a peak between the second and third year of life. Children with a bilateral tumour are younger.

Aetiology and risk factors

In 1964, Miller and colleagues reported, for the first time, an association between WT and aniridia. Today, different malformations linked to WT are known and include, particularly, hemihypertrophy and urogenital malformations (cryptorchidism, hypospadias, pseudohermaphroditism, and gonadal dysgenesis). Aniridia and hemihypertrophy are very rare syndromes justifying regular checkups in children with such anomalies, for an early diagnosis. A high incidence of WT is seen in children with hemihypertrophy, WAGR syndrome (WT, aniridia, genital deformity, retardation), Beckwith–Wiedemann syndrome (BWS; hemihypertrophy, omphalocele, macrosomy, macroglossia, hypoglycaemia, and deep-rooted ears), Denys–Drash syndrome (DDS; pseudohermaphroditism, glomerulopathy, and WT), Perlman syndrome (macrocephaly, deep-rooted eyes and ears, macrosomia, and organomegalia), and von Recklinghausen's disease or neurofibromatosis type 1 (Table 27.1). Environmental factors do not play a major role in the aetiology of nephroblastoma.

Pathogenesis

Molecular biology and genetics

Nephroblastoma is a genetically heterogeneous tumour. Besides gene mutations, further mechanisms of tumour development are found as loss of heterozygosity (LOH) and loss of imprinting (LOI). Nephroblastomas mainly show an euploid set of chromosomes and the frequency of LOH is very low, in the range of less than 5%.

Several genes are known which play a crucial role in the development of nephroblastoma. WT candidate genes are on chromosomes 11p13 (*WT1*), 11p15.5 (*WT2*), 16q (*WT3*), 17q12-q21 (*WT4; FWT1*), 7p15-p11.2 (*WT5*). Deletions of *wt1* are found in 10–30% of WT. Numeric and structural changes concern particularly chromosomes 1, 6, 7, 8, 11, 12, 16, 17, and 18. LOH is mainly found on 11p (40%) and, in a lower frequency, on 1p, 7p, and 16q. Epigenetic alterations primarily affect 11p15.5 and 11p13. Further genes with documented mutations include CTNNB1, WTX (AMER1), TP53, FBXW7, MYCN, SIX1/2, DICER1, DROSHA, and DGCR8. A gain of 1q is associated with poorer event-free survival (EFS) in tumour subsets and will be validated for better stratification of postoperative treatment.

The genetics of the overgrowth syndromes are complex. As with BWS, they arise from abnormalities of imprinting in 11p15.5 with differences between BWS and hemi-hypertrophy. WAGR syndrome is caused by a complete deletion of one copy of the WTgene, *WT1*, and the adjacent aniridia gene, *PAX6* on chromosome 11p13. In patients with aniridia, this information helps to identify those at risk for developing WT, by screening them for the combined deletion of *WT1* and *PAX6*. *WT1* is also involved in DDS, caused by a germline point mutation. In familial WT, accounting for approximately 1% of patients, there is usually no associated congenital abnormality or predisposition to other tumour types. They show an autosomal dominant inheritance with a variable penetrance. Genetic linkage studies in different families have shown no association to 11p13 or 11p15.5. One gene for familial WT, *FWT1*, could be localized on chromosome 17q and another, *FWT2*, on 19q.

Nephrogenic rests and nephroblastomatosis

Nephrogenic rests can appear as preliminary stages of a nephroblastoma. Nephroblastomatosis is defined as the diffuse or multifocal occurrence of nephrogenic rests. Different forms of

Table 27.1 Syndromes and congenital anomalies with a predisposition for nephroblastoma, and its frequency

	SIOP [%]	NWTS [%]
Syndromes/anomalies with increased growth		
Beckwith-Wiedemann syndrome (BWS) • Risk for tumours 5–10% • Loss of imprinting of LIT1 1–5% • Loss of imprinting of H19 35–45% • Loss of imprinting of LIT1 and H19 (UPD 11 p15) 25–30% • Normal methylation sample 10–15%	Not known	?Not known
Isolated hemihypertrophy	3.13	2.47
Perlman syndrome	<1.00	–
Sotos syndrome	<1.00	–
Simpson-Golabi-Behmel syndrome	<1.00	–
Syndromes/anomalies without disturbances of growth		
WAGR syndrome	<1.00	–
Eye deformities	2.17	1.21
Isolated aniridia	–	0.84
Denys-Drash syndrome (DDS)	<1.00	–
Urogenital deformities	4.41	4.61
CNS deformities	1.66	0.47
Bloom syndrome	<1.00	–
Trisomy 18	<1.00	–
M. Recklinghausen	<1.00	–
Familial Wilms tumour	1.00	–

nephrogenic rests are distinguished according to their localization in the renal lobe:

- perilobar nephroblastomatosis
- intralobar nephroblastomatosis
- mixed perilobar/intralobar nephroblastomatosis
- panlobar nephroblastomatosis

Despite the histological similarity to WT, nephroblastomatosis behaves like residua of primitive embryonic tissue and does not seem to have any invasive or metastatic behaviour. The malignant potential of nephrogenic rests is justified in their high mitotic activity and the narrow association with WT. They occur in approximately 40% of all children with WT. A transformation of nephroblastomatosis to a true nephroblastoma is possible.

The histogenetic origin of other renal tumours of childhood is unclear. Clear-cell sarcoma (CCSK) possibly represents the malignant variant of mesoblastic nephroma. Malignant rhabdoid tumour of the kidney (RTK) is not exclusively located in the kidney but in many other sites including the central nervous system (CNS) (AT/RT: atypical teratoid rhabdoid tumour) and soft tissue (MRT: malignant rhabdoid tumour). In paediatric renal-cell carcinoma (RCC), the characterization of the translocation RCC is most important. Molecular biology studies have shown that the cellular subtype of congenital mesoblastic nephroma is identical with the infantile fibrosarcoma of soft tissue, both sharing histopathological features and the t(12;15) ETV6-NTRK3 gene fusion.

Pathology

Histopathology

The diagnosis of nephroblastoma is still based on the histopathological classification. In accordance with Wilms' concept, nephroblastoma is a tumour of mesodermal origin that develops in the embryonic kidney. Classic nephroblastomas (mixed type) are renal tumours with a blastemic, epithelial (tubules), and mesenchymal component (stroma). The distribution of these three components can vary, explaining epithelial, stromal, and blastemal types of nephroblastoma. Multi-centric growth of the tumour in one or both kidneys is possible. Approximately 5% are bilateral.

The histopathological classification of childhood renal tumours is dependent on the initial treatment. Patients receiving preoperative chemotherapy are classified according to the International Society of Paediatric Oncology (SIOP) Stockholm Working Classification of 2002, and patients undergoing primary surgery are classified according to the classification of the Children's Oncology Group (COG, formerly the National Wilms Tumour Study Group). According to the Stockholm classification, three risk groups can be distinguished (low, intermediate, and high), whereas in the COG classification, only 'favourable' and 'unfavourable' risk groups are defined. The tumours with a low and intermediate risk in the SIOP classification correspond largely to tumours of the group with a favourable histology according to COG. The revised SIOP classification of childhood renal tumours is given in Box 27.1.

Box 27.1 The International Society of Paediatric Oncology (SIOP) classification of childhood renal tumours for patients with a preoperative chemotherapy

A. For pre-treated cases

I. Low-risk tumours
Mesoblastic nephroma*
Cystic, partially differentiated nephroblastoma
Completely necrotic nephroblastoma

II. Intermediate-risk tumours
Nephroblastoma—epithelial type
Nephroblastoma—stromal type
Nephroblastoma—mixed type
Nephroblastoma—regressive type
Nephroblastoma—focal anaplasia

III. High-risk tumours
Nephroblastoma—blastemal type
Nephroblastoma—diffuse anaplasia
Clear-cell sarcoma of the kidney*
Rhabdoid tumour of the kidney*

B. For primary nephrectomy cases

I. Low-risk tumours
Mesoblastic nephroma*
Cystic, partially differentiated nephroblastoma

II. Intermediate-risk tumours
Non-anaplastic nephroblastoma and its variants
Nephroblastoma—focal anaplasia

III. High-risk tumours
Nephroblastoma—diffuse anaplasia
Clear-cell sarcoma of the kidney*
Rhabdoid tumour of the kidney*

* Non-Wilms tumour

Prognostic factors

As a result of preoperative chemotherapy, the distribution of the different histological subtypes changes. In particular, the percentage of the blastemal type goes down from 40% to 10%. As the remaining blastema after preoperative chemotherapy is chemoresistant, these tumours are treated as high risk in SIOP protocols. After preoperative chemotherapy, some tumours become completely necrotic or regressive in the form of necrosis, fibrosis, and a collection of xanthomatous cells. The detection of anaplasia is of prognostic importance.

The extension of the tumour (staging) must be described exactly and is essential for correct treatment stratification after surgery. Growth of the tumour beyond the tumour capsule represents the decisive feature between stage I and II. Tumour in vessels corresponds to stage II. Every incomplete operative removal, every tumour rupture or open tumour biopsy and lymph-node infiltration should be assigned to stage III. In stage IV, distant metastases are diagnosed. Bilateral tumours indicate stage V (Box 27.2).

In the European approach, the prognosis of nephroblastoma primarily depends on tumour stage, histological type, and response to preoperative chemotherapy. In addition, some molecular markers correlate with a poor prognosis (gain of 1q; LOH 1p, 11q, 16q, 22q; and p53 mutations).

Of all children with nephroblastoma, 90% can be cured today. Patients with a low- and intermediate-risk tumour, without metastasis, survive in more than 90% of cases. Patients with a tumour with diffuse anaplasia have a considerably poorer outcome. In stage IV, the prognosis of patients depends on treatment response and histology. Patients with a complete remission after preoperative chemotherapy and tumour nephrectomy have an overall survival (OS) of 80% if the histology is not high risk. The prognosis of CCSK

Box 27.2 International Society of Paediatric Oncology (SIOP) staging criteria for renal tumours of childhood

Stage I

a. The tumour limited to kidney or surrounded with fibrous pseudocapsule if outside of the normal contours of the kidney, the renal capsule, or pseudocapsule may be infiltrated with the tumour but it does not reach the outer surface, and is completely resected (resection margins 'clear')
b. The tumour may be protruding ('bulging') into the pelvic system and 'dipping' into the ureter (but it is not infiltrating their walls)
c. The vessels of the renal sinus are not involved
d. Intrarenal vessel involvement may be present

Fine-needle aspiration or percutaneous core-needle biopsy ('tru-cut') does not upstage the tumour. The presence of necrotic tumour or chemotherapy-induced changes in the renal sinus/hilus fat and/or outside of the kidney should not be regarded as a reason for upstaging a tumour.

Stage II

a. The tumour extends beyond kidney or penetrates through the renal capsule and/or fibrous pseudocapsule into perirenal fat but is completely resected (resection margins 'clear')
b. The tumour infiltrates the renal sinus and/or invades blood and lymphatic vessels outside the renal parenchyma but is completely resected
c. The tumour infiltrates adjacent organs or vena cava but is completely resected

Stage III

a. Incomplete excision of the tumour which extends beyond resection margins (gross or microscopical tumour remains postoperatively)
b. Any abdominal lymph nodes are involved
c. Tumour rupture before or intra-operatively (irrespective of other criteria for staging)
d. The tumour has penetrated through the peritoneal surface
e. Tumour implants are found on the peritoneal surface
f. The tumour thrombi present at resection margins of vessels or ureter, transsected or removed piecemeal by surgeon
g. The tumour has been surgically biopsied (wedge biopsy) prior to preoperative chemotherapy or surgery

The presence of necrotic tumour or chemotherapy-induced changes in a lymph node or at the resection margins should be regarded as stage III.

Stage IV

Haematogenous metastases (lung, liver, bone, brain, etc.) or lymph-node metastases outside the abdomino-pelvic region.

Stage V

Bilateral renal tumours at diagnosis. Each side should be substaged according to the above criteria.

has improved considerably, with OS rates of 80%, whereas the prognosis of patients with an RTK remains dismally below 20%.

Prevention and early diagnosis

Most WT appear sporadically. A general screening is not possible due to the lack of tumour markers. On the other hand, in some children having syndromes associated with nephroblastoma, the individual risk to develop a nephroblastoma can be defined by molecular genetic examinations. Ultrasound scans are recommended at three-month intervals in such children. In Germany, 10% of children with nephroblastoma are diagnosed in the context of preventive medical check-ups by paediatricians.

Clinical symptoms

The typical first sign of a WT is an asymptomatic palpable or visible abdominal mass. Pain or haematuria are rare. In addition, WT is known to present with hypertension, that is caused by an increase in renin activity and is sometimes difficult to control, or coagulopathy, caused by acquired von Willebrand syndrome. In most cases, the acquired coagulation disorder and hypertension will resolve after tumour nephrectomy. Intratumoural haemorrhage may occur, resulting in rapid abdominal enlargement that requires emergency surgery. Prenatal diagnoses by ultrasound are described (Table 27.2).

Diagnostic procedures

Besides the clinical examination, the diagnosis of nephroblastoma is primarily based on imaging studies (abdominal ultrasound, computed tomography, and/or magnetic resonance imaging) (Figure 27.1). As patients in the SIOP trials and studies are treated without histological diagnosis, all imaging studies need to be of high quality to reduce the risk of a false positive diagnosis and not indicated chemotherapy. By using abdominal ultrasound, this risk was assessed below 2% for SIOP 6 and SIOP 9. The most important criteria allowing a safe diagnosis are listed in Box 27.3.

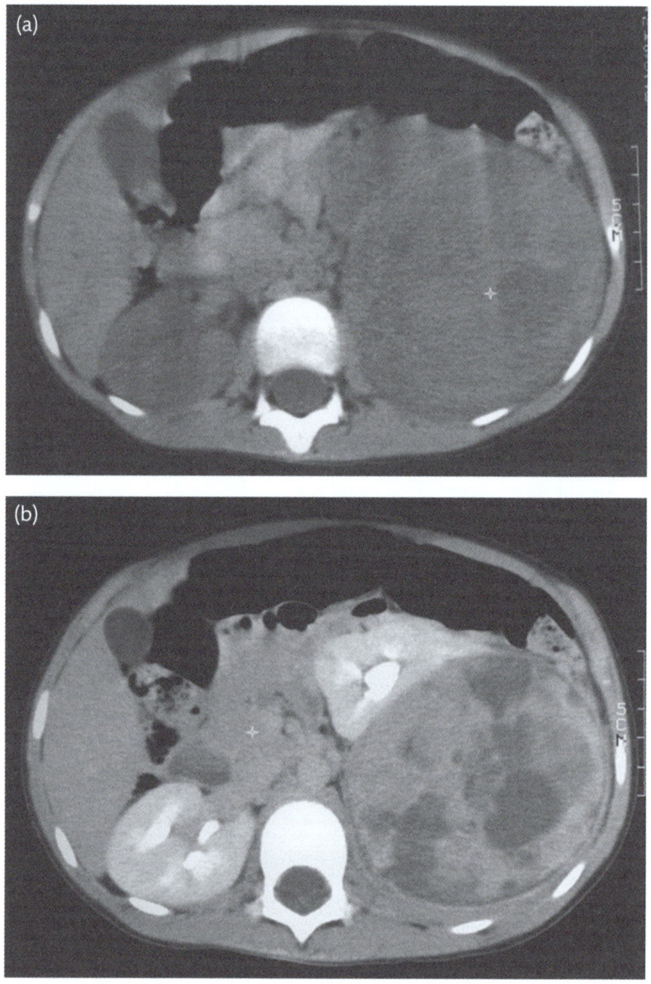

Figure 27.1 Imaging study (CT scan) of unilateral nephroblastoma: (a) with contrast enhancement; (b) without contrast enhancement.

Differential diagnoses

The following diseases need to be ruled out: neuroblastoma (but urine catecholamines are negative in nephroblastoma), lymphoma of the kidney, RCC, nephroblastomatosis, RTK, teratoma, ganglioneuroma, cystic nephroma, hamartoma, renal cysts, hematoma, renal abscess, xanthogranulomatous pyelonephritis, angiomyolipoma, and adenoma.

The diagnosis of nephroblastomatosis can only be proven by histology. It is of utmost importance that the pathologist is aware of the patient's history and of the imaging studies.

Table 27.2 First symptoms at diagnosis in children with a nephroblastoma

Symptom	Frequency [%]
Asymptomatic tumour swelling	61.6
Haematuria	15.1
Preventive medical check-up	9.2
Constipation	4.3
Weight loss	3.8
Urinary tract infection	3.2
Diarrhoea	3.2
Diagnosis at trauma	2.7
Nausea, vomiting, pain, hernia, pleural effusion, high blood pressure	Rare

Adapted with permisson from Graf N, Gutjahr P. 'Wilms-Tumoren (Nephroblastome).' In: P. Gutjahr (Ed.) *Krebs bei Kindern und Jugendlichen, 5. Überarbeitete und erweiterte Auflage*. Copyright © 2004 Deutscher Ärzteverlag.

Treatment

The treatment of this tumour should always be carried out in prospective trials in which surgery, chemotherapy, and radiotherapy are combined according to the individual risk to a patient. Today, two major study groups are treating these patients. The fundamental difference between the two groups is in their initial treatment approach: primary surgery (COG: North America) or preoperative chemotherapy (SIOP: European countries). Arguments for preoperative chemotherapy are the reduction of the tumour volume (downstaging) with the possibility to measure *in vivo* response. The number of intraoperative tumour ruptures is decreased and the number of patients with a postoperative local stage I is raised (Table 27.3 and Figure 27.2). Moreover, the chemotherapy response gives some additional prognostic factors. For more than 40 years both study groups have gained a lot of success in treating these patients.

Box 27.3 Criteria for a safe diagnosis of nephroblastoma using imaging studies

- The intrarenal tumour is solid and inhomogeneous with partly cystic areas
- The tumour has a sharp border
- The surrounding tissue is replaced rather than infiltrated
- The destruction, inclination, and replacement of calices and the renal pelvis is characteristic
- The inhomogeneity of the tumour increases after contrast enhancement
- Intratumoural bleedings are relatively frequent (27%)
- Calcifications in the tumour are rare (8%)

The most important results from their trials form the basis of today's treatment and are listed in Box 27.4.

Surgery

Surgery for a WT is almost always an elective intervention and rarely due to emergency situations after traumatic or spontaneous tumour rupture. Even if the tumour nephrectomy seems technically simple, the most experienced team of surgeons and anaesthesiologists should carry out the intervention. The tumour has to be removed radically, and tumour spread has always to be documented. Simultaneously, an adequate lymph-node dissection should be carried out. It has to be taken into account that the quality of the imaging studies has improved fundamentally and can rule out bilateral disease with great certainty. If the contralateral kidney looks normal on good-quality imaging studies, exposure of this normal kidney is not needed during surgery. If there are doubts about the diagnosis of a nephroblastoma (aspect and age) before preoperative treatment, a tru-cut biopsy of the tumour, with a posterior approach only, may be considered. On the other hand, primary complete tumour removal should always be preferred in doubt of malignancy. Renal-sparing surgery in unilateral tumours should only be done in special cases and by experienced surgeons. Surgery for thromboses of the vena cava often requires the use of the heart–lung machine. Prognosis of these patients remains good after adequate surgery. Experienced surgeons should remove primary liver metastases after preoperative chemotherapy.

Congenital mesoblastic nephromas (CMN) show an unusual growth pattern, with fine finger-shaped extensions into the adjacent kidney fat capsule. Because of these extensions, the fat capsule needs to be removed with wide excision margins.

Radiotherapy

Nephroblastoma is a radiosensitive tumour. With the development of effective chemotherapeutic combinations, its place has been restricted to patients with higher risk of local relapse and, in some cases, for the treatment of pulmonary metastases or after incomplete resection of liver metastases. Radiotherapy can also provide excellent palliation for symptomatic brain or bone metastases.

Radiotherapy is given in SIOP and COG studies in local stage III in non-high-risk or favourable histology, and in stage II in high-risk or unfavourable histology. The total dose is 14.4 Gy in intermediate-risk and 25.2 Gy in high-risk histology in the SIOP studies. For macroscopic residual disease, a local boost of 10–15 Gy is given. In COG, the irradiation dose is 10.2 Gy. Whole abdominal irradiation (15–19.5 Gy) is needed in cases of diffuse peritoneal seeding due to tumour rupture. The dose to the liver and, particularly, to the unaffected kidney should be reduced to 12 Gy. Irradiation to the lungs can be avoided if complete remission of the metastases is achieved after chemotherapy. Radiotherapy treatment planning should homogeneously include the whole width of the vertebral column, particularly at doses of more than 15 Gy, to avoid disturbances of growth and subsequent development of scoliosis. The dose to the genital organs should be below 2 Gy on at least one ovary and under 1 Gy for both testicles, if possible.

Chemotherapy

International Society of Paediatric Oncology studies

Preoperative chemotherapy is given to all patients aged over six months and under 18 years at diagnosis of a renal tumour by imaging studies. Vincristine and actinomycin D are given for four weeks in localized stages. Anthracyclines are added in case of metastatic disease and treatment is prolonged to six weeks. Patients with bilateral disease are treated individually with vincristine and actinomycin as long as there is tumour regression, but for no longer than 12 weeks. Babies less than six months of age and teenagers over 18 years are primarily operated in the context of SIOP studies, as other renal tumours (CMN, RCC) are more common in these patients.

Postoperative treatment is always carried out on the basis of the local stage and the histological type. The following guidelines apply to the individual sub-types:

- **Low-risk tumours:** in stage I, no further treatment is given. In stage II and III, vincristine and actinomycin-D (AV) are given for 26 weeks.
- **Intermediate-risk tumours:** relapse-free survival (RFS) of patients with stage 1 is 90% with only four weeks of postoperative treatment. In stage II and III, patients receive only two drugs (AV) for 26 weeks. Doxorubicin can be avoided in these patients.
- **High-risk tumours:** with RFS below 50%, treatment is intensified with carboplatin and etoposide. In the high-risk scheme, both

Table 27.3 Number of tumour ruptures at primary surgery and after preoperative treatment in SIOP (International Society of Paediatric Oncology) 1 and SIOP 2

SIOP 1	Rupture (%)		SIOP 2	Rupture (%)	
Preoperative irradiation	4	p = 0.001	Preoperative chemotherapy	5	p = 0.0025
Primary surgery	32		Primary surgery including small tumours	20	

Reproduced with permission from Graf N, et al. 'The Role of Preoperative Chemotherapy in the Management of Wilms Tumor—The SIOP Studies'. *Urologic Clinics of North America*, Volume 27, Issue 3, pp. 443–454. DOI: https://doi.org/10.1016/S0094-0143(05)70092-6.

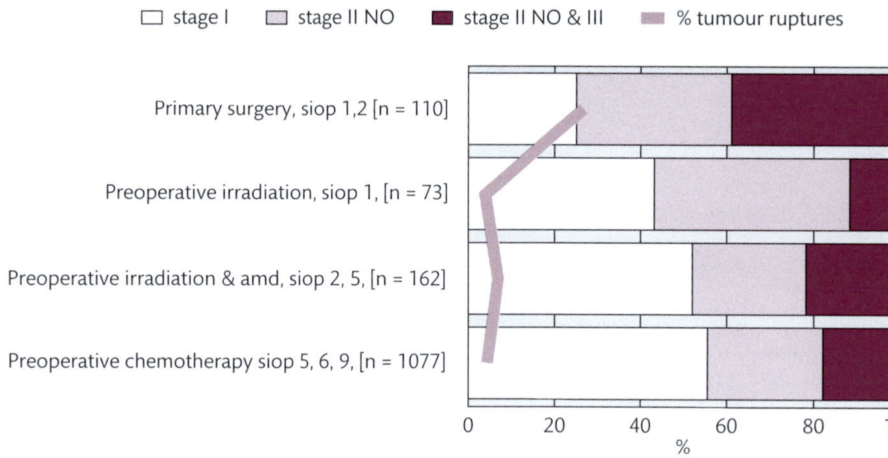

Figure 27.2 Postoperative stage distribution and rupture rate in different SIOP (International Society of Paediatric Oncology) studies.

drugs are alternately given with a combination of cyclophosphamide and doxorubicin. Patients with stage II and III need local irradiation.

- **Stage IV disease:** postoperative treatment depends on the response to preoperative chemotherapy. In case of complete remission (CR) after preoperative treatment (good responder), postoperative treatment is given according to local stage and histology as in non-metastasized tumours, but at least according to stage II. Patients with non-CR do need a more intensified treatment (VP16, cyclophosphamide, doxorubicine, carboplatin). Radiotherapy to the lungs is necessary in patients with non-CR or with high-risk tumours.

Children's Oncology Group studies

Preoperative treatment is not given. Postoperative treatment is always carried out on the basis of age, local stage, histological type, LOH 1p and 16q, and response to chemotherapy in case of stage IV. The most important drugs in the treatment are vincristine, actinomycin-D, and doxorubicine. The NWTS 4 study evaluated an early intensification of the treatment. It turned out that this so-called 'pulse intensive treatment' is equal to the standard treatment and more cost-effective by minimizing hospital visits. The duration of the treatment is shortened to six months at the longest. In the ongoing COG trial, LOH of 1p and 16q are used for stratification. Patients with LOH 1p and LOH 16q receive a more intensified treatment to improve their survival rates. There is a very low-risk arm within COG, where children below two years of age with a unilateral nephroblastoma, favourable histology, stage I, and a tumour weight of less than 550 g receive surgery only, without adjuvant chemotherapy.

Treatment of nephroblastomatosis

The treatment of nephroblastomatosis is still controversial. Initial nephrectomy should be avoided. Treatment is based on WT treatment. In cases of a simultaneous WT, treatment is given according to the histological results and the stage of the tumour. In cases of diffuse perilobar nephroblastomatosis (without WT), prolonged chemotherapy with vincristine and actinomycin-D is recommended. Impressive regressions are described. The indication for radiation treatment has to be very restrictive. During the course of the treatment, regular abdominal ultrasounds are needed, at short intervals, to recognize the development of a possible anaplastic WT as early as possible (see Figure 27.3).

Box 27.4 Major findings of NWTSG (COG), SIOP, and UK trials

- Treatment needs to be stratified according to stage and histology
- The combination of vincristine and actinomycin D is more effective than the use of a single drug (with the exception of single VCR in stage I after primary surgery)
- In stage I, no irradiation is needed
- In stage II and intermediate risk or favourable histology, no irradiation is needed
- With the addition of doxorubicin in stage III, the dose of radiation can be reduced
- Cyclophosphamide does not increase prognosis in stage IV in case of anaplasia
- Anthracyclines are decisive for the prognosis of clear-cell sarcoma
- A single bolus of actinomycin-D is as effective as a split dose
- The duration of treatment is eight weeks in stage I and up to six months in stage II and III in intermediate risk or favourable histology
- A tumour volume of more than 500 ml after preoperative chemotherapy is of prognostic significance
- The number of tumour ruptures decreases as the number of stage I increases significantly after preoperative treatment
- Preoperative chemotherapy with vincristine and actinomycin D is as effective as preoperative irradiation with 20 Gy
- After four and eight weeks of preoperative chemotherapy with vincristine and actinomycin D, the same stage distribution is achieved
- Patients with pulmonary metastases and complete remission after preoperative chemotherapy do not need lung irradiation
- Some very low-risk patients can be cured by surgery alone
- Gain 1q, LOH of 1 p and 16q are of prognostic significance
- Remaining blastema after preoperative chemotherapy is a bad prognostic feature

NWTSG: National Wilms Tumour Study Group; COG: Children's Oncology Group; SIOP: International Society of Paediatric Oncology; VCR: vincristine

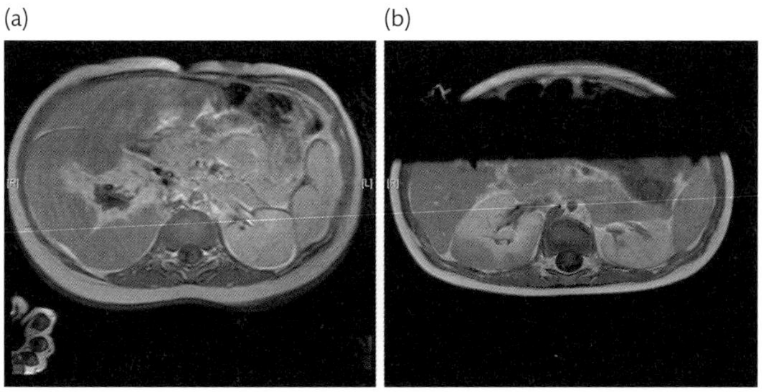

Figure 27.3 Imaging study (MRI): (a) right diffuse hyperplastic perilobar nephrogenic rests; (b) regression after two months of vincristin and actinomycine D.

Treatment of bilateral nephroblastomas

The therapeutic goal is to preserve as much healthy kidney tissue as possible. Preoperative chemotherapy is always indicated. Treatment should be individualized and given as long as it enables renal-sparing surgery, but should not exceed 12 weeks. Renal-sparing surgery on both sides is possible in more than 50% of patients. Postoperative therapy is based on the histology and the local stage, in which the highest risk group and the highest local stage of both sides are decisive for the treatment. Postoperative treatment will be given as for unilateral cases. Essential drugs in the treatment are vincristine and actinomycin-D, which might be supplemented with doxorubicine. In cases of no shrinkage of the tumour during preoperative chemotherapy, surgery is of utmost importance. The treatment of high-risk tumours is the same as for unilateral cases. The prognosis of bilateral tumours is good, with survival rates of about 70% after ten years. As a late effect, kidney malfunctions are observed that can lead to renal failure and dialysis, necessitating renal transplantation. In every case, the treatment of such a patient should be carried out in a paediatric oncology centre.

Treatment of adults with a nephroblastoma

Nephroblastoma is rarely diagnosed in adults. The treatment can be carried out according to the treatment for children. In adults, the tumour is primarily operated. The tumour is frequently more advanced than in children, with a high rate of patients with metastases at initial presentation The reasons for a poorer outcome can partially be attributed to non-standardized treatments in adulthood. Adult patients who are treated according to the guidelines for children have a better outcome. However, the increased neurotoxicity of vincristine needs to be considered in this age group.

Treatment of relapses

Approximately 15% of patients with favourable-histology WT and 50% of patients with anaplastic WT develop recurrence. Most recurrences occur within two years after diagnosis. The general profile of relapse site shows that the lungs and pleura alone account for 50–60%, abdominal recurrences make up to 30% (isolated abdomen or combined to other sites), while other sites (brain or bone) are involved in less than 10% of cases.

Treatment regimens for recurrent WT include drugs that have not been used during primary chemotherapy. Therapy of recurrent disease depends on the nature of initial treatment and of recognized prognostic factors of the primary tumour. Children having only received actinomycin and vincristine during their first treatment have a high chance of survival with conventional therapy. The chance of survival is less than 40% in all other cases. For these patients, several highly effective chemotherapy regimens, including ifosfamide, carboplatin, and etoposide (ICE), are considered as a first treatment choice. To what extent the prognosis can be improved in such patients by giving high-dose chemotherapy followed by stem-cell rescue is still unclear. International cooperation is needed to achieve better outcomes for these patients.

Follow-up

The most important acute toxicity is venous occlusive disease (VOD), currently often called sinusoid obstruction syndrome (SOS) of the liver. This is attributed to relative over-dosage of actinomycin-D in dystrophic children. Further risk factors are right-sided tumours, including the liver, treated with postoperative radiotherapy. Other acute side effects are rare and concern mainly infections, neuropathy (vincristine), and side effects on the intestine caused by the tumour. Surgical complications are lower after preoperative treatment and lie within a range of about 5%. In the long term, one needs to pay attention to skeletal growth and soft tissue which may have been affected by radiotherapy. Delayed cardiotoxicity (anthracycline) and renal failure are possible and need to be taken seriously. Second malignant neoplasms occur in about 1%. A follow-up schema for patients with nephroblastoma is given in Table 27.4.

Clear-cell sarcoma of the kidney

Clear-cell sarcoma of the kidney (CCSK) represents 3% of malignant tumours of the kidney. It occurs with a peak incidence at one to four years of age, predominantly affecting boys (in a ratio of 2:1). Four percent of CCSK have metastases at the time of diagnosis. In addition to bone and pulmonary metastases, CCSK may also spread to brain and soft tissue. The prognosis for CCSK improved after the introduction of anthracyclines to modern treatment regimens, with survival rates approaching 90% for non-metastatic tumours. Imaging studies do not allow this tumour to be distinguished from WT. Bone scintigraphy and cranial magnetic resonance imaging (MRI) have to be done in the work-up of this tumour.

A large series of 351 cases from the National Wilms Tumour Study Group (NWTSG, now part of COG) Pathology Centre has provided detailed insight into the pathology of CCSK and its microscopic and immunohistochemical features. According to the SIOP experience with chemotherapy first, 42% of patients had stage I disease, 23% had stage II, 28% had stage III, and 7% had stage IV disease. These tumours are characteristically composed of a mixture of cord cells and very clear septal cells with an extensive capillary network. CCSK is considered as a high-risk renal tumour. Gene-expression profiling studies have reported upregulation of neural markers and apparent expression of members of the sonic hedgehog signalling pathway and the AKT cell-proliferation pathway (including strong activation of *EGFR*) in CCSK. Cytogenetic studies of CCSK have reported balanced translocations t(10;17)(q22;p13) and t(10;17)(q11;p12) and del(14)(q24.1q31.1). Very recently, recurrent internal tandem duplications (ITD) of the X-linked BCL-6 co-repressor (*BCOR*) gene have been described in CCSK.

Table 27.4 Follow-up schema for children with nephroblastoma

	End of therapy	1st year	2nd year	3rd–5th year	As of 6th year
Psychosocial history	+	Every 12 m	Every 12 m	Every 12 m	Every 12 m
Clinical examination, RR	+	Every 3 m	Every 3 m	Every 6 m	Every 12 m
Imaging studies					
X-ray of the lung	+	Every 3 m	Every 3 m	Every 6 m	Every 12 m
Sonography, abdomen	+	Every 3 m	Every 3 m	Every 3 m	Every 12 m
Laboratory					
Blood picture	+	Every 4 w	Every 3 m	Every 6 m	Every 12 m
Urinalysis	+	Every 4 w	Every 3 m	Every 6 m	Every 12 m
Kidney values	+	Every 2 m	Every 3 m	Every 6 m	Every 12 m
Fanconi syndrome*	+	Every 3 m	Every 3 m	Every 6 m	Every 12 m
Vaccination status, HBV, HCV, HIV	+	End of 1st year	After vaccination	End of 5th year	
T3, T4, TSH**	+	Every 6 m	Every 12 m	Every 12 m	
Audiogram***	+	Once	Once, if path.	Once, if path.	Once, if path.
ECG/Echocardiography****	+	Every 6 m	Every 12 m	Every 12 m	Every 24 m
Bone scintigraphy*****	+	Every 6 m	Only at relapse	Only at relapse	Only at relapse

* after ifosfamide, ** after lung irradiation, ***after carboplatin, ****after anthracyclines, ***** in case of clear-cell sarcoma

Adapted with permission from Vujanić GM, et al. 'The UMBRELLA SIOP-RTSG 2016 Wilms tumour pathology and molecular biology protocol'. *Nature Reviews Urology*, Volume 15, Issue 11, pp. 693–701. Copyright © 2018 Springer Nature Publishing. DOI: 10.1038/s41585-018-0100-3

With current intensive treatment schedules, including radiotherapy and multi-agent chemotherapy regimens, outcome has significantly improved (five-year EFS ranging from 65% to 85%, five-year OS ranging from 75% to 90%). Today, NWTS/COG as well as SIOP use four drugs to treat this tumour (cyclophosphamide, VP16, vincristine, and doxorubicine). All patients with this tumour have to be referred to a centre for paediatric oncology.

Rhabdoid tumour of the kidney

Rhabdoid tumours of the kidney (RTK) are rare (2% of all renal malignancies) and extremely aggressive. Eighty percent of patients are younger than two years of age and 60% are under the age of one year. There is an overall male predominance (ratio 1.5:1). The most common location is the kidney (RTK), but brain and soft tissue can be involved. Fever and haematuria in a young patient with a renal malignancy with lung metastasis and hypercalcaemia should suggest the diagnosis of RTK. Among 639 cases of kidney tumours in the first seven months of life with specified histology and stage, nine out of eleven stage IV tumours were RTK as reported by van den Heuvel-Eibrink and colleagues in 2008. Up to 15% of patients with RTK have brain lesions. Because of the coincidence with brain metastasis, cerebral MRI is always indicated.

Common to rhabdoid tumours are deletions of the tumour-suppressor gene SMARCB1 (hSNF5/INI1) on chromosome 22. Today, mutations can be detected in at least about 80% of cases on chromosome 22q11.2. Germline mutations of SMARCB1 should be searched, especially in very young children and in those with synchronous rhabdoid tumours of the CNS and the kidney.

The diagnosis of RTK can only be made by histology. Today, the diagnosis of RTK needs to be confirmed by immunohistochemical and/or molecular genetic techniques showing the loss of INI1 protein expression resulting from SMARCB1 mutations.

The prognosis of patients with RTK remains dismal despite aggressive treatments. RTK is a very chemoresistant tumour. Common therapeutic regimens use intensive anthracycline-based polychemotherapeutic regimens and aggressive local therapy. The 142 children recruited into all NWTS studies showed an OS of 23.2% after four years. Additionally, the outcome of infants under six months of age at diagnosis was only 8% compared to 41% in patients aged two years or older ($p<0.0001$). In the UK experience of 11 patients, OS was 36% at four years. The only statistically significant prognostic factor is metastatic disease, as shown in a retrospective analysis of 70 patients in Gesellschaft fur Pädiatrische Onkologie und Hämatologie (GPOH).

In most reports, treatment is based on regimens with vincristine, dactinomycin, and doxorubicin (with or without cyclophosphamide). In today's strategies, radical nephrectomy is followed by carboplatin and etoposide alternating with cyclophosphamide and doxorubicin for half a year, including radiotherapy. The use of high-dose chemotherapy followed by autologous stem-cell transplantation is still controversial. Treatment of these patients should be centralized and given according to prospective trials. A registry for all rhabdoid tumours, independent of their primary site, is available in Europe—the so-called EURHAB protocol.

Renal-cell carcinoma

Renal-cell carcinoma (RCC) is a rare malignancy in the kidney of children and accounts for only 1.9—5% of paediatric renal tumours. The average age of children diagnosed with RCC is about ten years (range 9 to 15 years), with a male predominance. Metastases to the lungs, bone, liver, or brain are identified in about 20% of cases. Imaging is not characteristic and shows a non-specific solid intrarenal lesion with little contrast enhancement, and is often less huge than WT. Calcifications are more frequent in RCC than in Wilms tumour (25% versus 9%, respectively).

The signs and symptoms of RCC in children are most frequently abdominal pain and haematuria, sometimes accompanied by fever. Recent data suggest that paediatric RCC may be different from adult RCC, with distinct morphological characteristics and unique genetic abnormalities. Some studies have shown that most RCC can be classified according to specific genetic translocations. Such genetic translocations involve chromosome Xp11.2 resulting in *TFE3* fusions. Childhood RCC are more frequently of the papillary subtype and the Xp11 translocation type or the related t(6;11) translocation type. An association of RCC to neuroblastoma is found in children, as well as to other syndromes (tuberous sclerosis, urogenital malformations, Saethre–Chotzen, XYY syndrome). Clear-cell RCC with 3p25 abnormalities is rare in children.

Survival of children with RCC depends on the stage of disease at presentation and the possibility of complete resection, with an OS rate of 60–90%. Lymph-node (LN) involvement (N+) was found in 45% for which LNs were sampled. The five-year survival rate is 90–100% for stage I, 50–80% for stage II and III, and 10% for stage IV. Surgical resection of tumour and metastases remains the crucial mainstay of successful treatment in paediatric RCC, even in stage IV. RCC in children, as in adults, is not chemosensitive. Most localized RCC can be cured by surgery alone. In patients with distant metastasis, a combination of surgery, radiotherapy, and immunotherapy or targeted therapy (as sunitinib or sorafenib) needs to be discussed in every single case, within an adult multidisciplinary meeting.

Congenital mesoblastic nephroma

Congenital mesoblastic nephroma (CMN) is a rare paediatric tumour with a favourable clinical outcome. Although the most common renal tumour under the age of seven months is a WT, a relatively high percentage of children suffer from CMN, especially in the first two months of life.

The clinical presentation of CMN is similar to other paediatric renal neoplasms. CMN usually presents as an asymptomatic abdominal mass in an infant. CMN is a spindle-cell neoplasm with low malignant potential. Several subtypes including classical, cellular, and mixed were identified on the basis of molecular characterizations and morphological features. The cellular variant, which represents 40–60% of CMN, shows a t(12;15)(p13;q25) translocation with a resulting ETV6-NTRK3 fusion. An identical gene-fusion transcript has also been reported in congenital or infantile fibrosarcoma (IFS), which also affects the same age group and shows similar morphology, suggesting that cellular CMN represents intrarenal IFS.

As CMN patients usually have a good outcome, immediate nephrectomy is advocated and no further treatment needed. Overall EFS is more than 95%, but the occasional stage III cellular CMN in older patients has a worse prognosis. The main factors of importance as risk factors for local recurrence are cellular subtype and incomplete local excision at primary surgery. They rarely relapse within 12 months after the diagnosis, so during this period close follow-up is recommended.

FURTHER READING

Suggested reading for nephroblastoma

Chagtai T, et al. (2016) Gain of 1q as a prognostic biomarker in Wilms tumours treated with pre-operative chemotherapy in the SIOP WT 2001 trial: a SIOP Renal Tumours Biology Consortium study. *J Clin Oncol* **34**(26), 3195–203.

de Kraker J, et al. (2004) Reduction of postoperative chemotherapy in children with stage I intermediate risk and anaplasia Wilms' tumour. The SIOP 93-01 randomised trial. *Lancet* **364**(9441), 1229–35.

Dome JS, et al. (2014) Risk stratification for Wilms tumor: current approach and future directions. *Am Soc Clin Oncol Educ Book* **34**, 215–23.

Dome JS, et al. (2015) Advances in Wilms tumor treatment and biology: progress through international collaboration. *J Clin Oncol* **33**, 2999–3007.

Furtwängler R, et al. (2014) Pretreatment for bilateral nephroblastomatosis is an independent risk factor for progressive disease in patients with stage V nephroblastoma—the GPOH experience. *Klin Pädiatrie* **226**, 175–81.

Godzinski J, et al. (2014) Current concepts in surgery for Wilms tumour—the risk- and function-adapted strategy. *Eur J Pediatr Surg* **24**, 457–60.

Graf N, et al. (2000) The role of preoperative chemotherapy in the management of Wilms tumor—the SIOP studies. *Urol Clin North Am* **27**, 443–54.

Graf N, et al. (2012) Characteristics and prognosis of non-anaplastic Wilms' tumor stage II and III treated according to the SIOP trial and study 93-01. *Eur J Cancer* **48**, 3240–8.

Green DM, et al. (2001) Treatment with nephrectomy only for small, stage I/favorable histology Wilms' tumor: a report from the National Wilms' Tumor Study Group. *J Clin Oncol* **19**, 3719–24.

Grundy PE, et al. (2005) Loss of heterozygosity for chromosomes 1p and 16q is an adverse prognostic factor in favorable-histology Wilms tumor: a report from the National Wilms Tumor Study Group. *J Clin Oncol* **23**, 7312–21.

Ha TC, et al. (2013) An international strategy to determine the role of high dose therapy in recurrent Wilms' tumour. *Eur J Cancer* **49**, 194–210.

Lehnhardt A, et al. (2015) Clinical and molecular characterization of patients with heterozygous mutations in Wilms tumour suppressor Gene 1 (WT1). Report of the *WT1*-Registry of the GPN. *Clin J Am Soc Nephrol* **10**, 825–31.

Malogolowkin M, et al. (2013) Incidence and outcomes of patients with late recurrence of Wilms tumor. The international experience. *Ped Blood Cancer* **60**, 1612–15.

Mitchell C, et al. (2000) The treatment of Wilms' tumour: results of the United Kingdom Children's Cancer Study Group (UKCCSG) second Wilms' tumour study. *Br J Cancer* **83**, 602–8.

Neville HL, Ritchey ML (2000) Wilms' tumor. Overview of National Wilms' Tumor Study Group results. *Urol Clin North Am* **27**, 435–42.

Pastore G, et al. (2006) Malignant renal tumours incidence and survival in European children (1978–1997): report from the ACCIS Project. *Eur J Cancer* **42**(13), 2103–14.

Pein F, et al. (1998) High-dose melphalan, etoposide, and carboplatin followed by autologous stem-cell rescue pediatric high-risk recurrent Wilms' tumor: a French Society of Pediatric Oncology study. *J Clin Oncol* **16**, 3295–301.

Perlman EJ, et al. (2006) Hyperplastic perilobar nephroblastomatosis: long-term survival of 52 patients. *Pediatr Blood Cancer* **46**, 203–21.

Pritchard-Jones K, et al. (2015) Doxorubicin omission from the treatment of stage II/III, intermediate risk histology Wilms tumour: results of the SIOP WT 2001 randomised trial. *Lancet* **386**, 1156–64.

Pritchard-Jones K, et al. (2016) Evidence for a delay in diagnosis of Wilms' tumour in the UK compared to Germany: implications for primary care for children. *Arch Dis Child* **101**, 417–20.

Reinhard H, et al. (2004) Wilms tumor in adults—results of the SIOP 93-01/GPOH study. *J Clin Oncol* **22**, 4500–6.

Ritchey M, et al. (1992) Surgical complications after nephrectomy for Wilms' tumor. *Surg Gynecol Obstetr* **175**, 507–14.

Spreafico F, et al. (2009) Treatment of relapsed Wilms tumors: lessons learned. *Expert Rev Anticancer Ther* **12**, 1807–15.

van den Heuvel-Eibrink MM, et al. (2015) Outcome of blastemal type Wilms tumour patients treated according to intensified treatment in the SIOP WT 2001 protocol—a report of the SIOP Renal Tumor Study Group (SIOP-RTSG). *Eur J Cancer* **51**, 498–506.

Verschuur AC, et al. (2012) Treatment of pulmonary metastases in children with stage IV nephroblastoma with risk-based use of pulmonary radiotherapy. *J Clin Oncol* **30**, 3533–9.

Vujanic GM, Sandstedt (2010) The pathology of Wilms' tumour (nephroblastoma): the International Society of Paediatric Oncology approach. *J Clin Pathol* **63**, 102–9.

Wegert J, et al. (2015) Mutations in the SIX1/2 pathway and the DROSHA/DGCR8 miRNA microprocessor complex underlie high-risk blastemal type Wilms tumors. *Cancer Cell* **27**, 298–311.

Weirich A, et al. (2001) Clinical impact of histologic subtypes in localized non-anaplastic nephroblastoma treated according to the trial and study SIOP-9/GPOH. *Ann Oncol* **12**, 311–19.

Wilde JCH, et al. (2014) Nephron sparing surgery (NSS) for unilateral Wilms tumor (UWT): the SIOP 2001 experience. *Ped Blood Cancer* **61**, 2175–9.

Suggested reading for clear-cell sarcoma

Argani P, et al. (2000) Clear cell sarcoma of the kidney: a review of 351 cases from the National Wilms Tumour Study Pathology Center. *Am J Surg* **24**, 4–18.

Furtwängler R, et al. (2013) Clear cell sarcomas of the kidney registered on International Society of Pediatric Oncology (SIOP) 93-01 and SIOP 2001 protocols: a report of the SIOP Renal Tumour Study Group. *Eur J Cancer* **49**(16), 3497–506.

Gooskens S, et al. (2012) Clear cell sarcoma of the kidney: a review. *Eur J Cancer* **48**, 2219–26.

Gooskens SL, et al. (2014) Outcome of patients with relapsed clear cell sarcoma of the kidney (CCSK) registered on recent SIOP, UK-CCLG and AIEOP study. *Br J Cancer* **111**, 227–33.

Gooskens SL, et al. (2016) The clinical phenotype of the YWHAE-NUTM2B/E fusion transcript in paediatric clear cell sarcoma of the kidney. *Genes Chrom Cancer* **55**(2), 143–7.

Kenny C, et al. (2016) Mutually exclusive BCOR internal tandem duplications and YWHAE-NUTM2 fusions in clear cell sarcoma of kidney: not the full story. *J Pathol* **238**(5), 617–20.

Seibel NL, et al. (2004) Effect of duration of treatment on treatment outcome for patients with clear-cell sarcoma of the kidney: a report from the National Wilms' Tumor Study Group. *J Clin Oncol* **22**, 468–73.

Suggested reading for rhabdoid tumour

Biegel JA, et al. (1999) Germ-line and acquired mutations of INI1 in atypical teratoid and rhabdoid tumors. *Cancer Res* **59**, 74–9.

Chi SN, et al. (2008) Intensive multimodality treatment for children with newly diagnosed CNS atypical teratoid rhabdoid tumor. *J Clin Oncol* **8**, 8–14.

Furtwängler R, et al. (2014) Malignant rhabdoid tumor of the kidney: significantly improved response to preoperative treatment intensified with doxorubicin. *Cancer Genetics* **207**(9), 434–6.

Seeringer A, et al. (2014) Feasibilty of intensive multimodal therapy in infants affected by rhabdoid tumors—experience of the EU-RHAB registry. *Klin Pädiatr* **226**, 143–8.

Weeks DA, et al. (1989) Rhabdoid tumour of kidney: a report of 111 cases from the NWTS pathology center. *Am J Surg Pathol* **13**, 439–58.

Suggested reading for renal-cell carcinoma

Argani P, Ldanyi M (2006) The evolving story of renal translocation carcinomas. *Am J Clin Pathol* **126**, 332–4.

Chowdhury T, et al. (2013) Persistent complete response after single-agent sunitinib treatment in a case of TFE translocation positive relapsed metastatic pediatric renal cell carcinoma. *J Pediatr Hematol Oncol* **35**(1), e1–3.

Geller JI, et al. (2015) Characterization of adolescent and pediatric renal cell carcinoma: a report from the Children's Oncology Group study AREN03B2. *Cancer* **121**(14), 2457–64.

Moch H, et al. (2016) *World Health Organization Classification of Tumours of the Urinary System and Male Genital Organs*. Lyon: IARC Press.

Molina AM, et al. (2014) Sunitinib objective response in metastatic renal cell carcinoma: analysis of 1059 patients treated on clinical trials. *Eur J Cancer* **50**(2), 351–8.

Mourad WF, et al. (2014) State-of-the-art management of renal cell carcinoma. *Am J Clin Oncol* **37**(5), 498–505.

Selle B, et al. (2006) Population-based study of renal cell carcinoma in children in Germany, 1980–2005. More frequently localized tumors and underlying disorders compared with adult counterparts. *Cancer* **107**, 2906–14.

Suggested reading for congenital mesoblastic nephroma

Furtwaengler R, et al. (2006) Mesoblastic nephroma—a report from the Gesellschaft fur Padiatrische Onkologie und Hamatologie (GPOH). *Cancer* **106**(10), 2275–83.

Sebire NJ, Vujanic GM (2009) Paediatric renal tumours: recent developments, new entities and pathological features. *Histopathology* **54**, 516–28.

van den Heuvel-Eibrink MM, et al. (2008) Characteristics and survival of 750 children diagnosed with a renal tumor in the first seven months of life: a collaborative study by the SIOP/GPOH/SFOP, NWTSG, and UKCCSG Wilms tumor study groups. *Pediatr Blood Cancer* **50**, 1130–4.

28

Neuroblastoma

Angelika Eggert, Garrett M. Brodeur, and Gudrun Schleiermacher

Introduction

Neuroblastoma is one of the most challenging malignancies for paediatric oncologists and one of the most fascinating tumours for scientists. In 1910, Wright introduced the term 'neuroblastoma' after demonstrating its origin from embryonal neuroblasts of the sympathetic peripheral nervous system. The tumour itself was first described by Virchow, in 1864, in a child with an abdominal mass. Neuroblastoma is characterized by an extreme clinical and biological heterogeneity, ranging from low-stage, biologically favourable tumours that can spontaneously regress or differentiate to highly aggressive, metastasized tumours that progress early or relapse and cause the death of the patient.

To date, neuroblastoma serves as a paradigm for the prognostic benefit of combining molecular data with clinically defined risk factors, as well as for the potential to tailor therapy for patient subgroups according to their individual risk for recurrence. However, despite tremendous progress in understanding the pathogenesis and molecular mechanisms of neuroblastoma, prognosis of patients with advanced disease remains dismal, with long-term event-free survival (EFS) of less than 50%.

Epidemiology

Neuroblastoma accounts for 8–10% of all paediatric cancers. Its age distribution is characterized by a peak of incidence in the first year of life, followed by a rapid decline in the following years. It is rare after the age of six, and is exceptional among adults. Neuroblastoma occurs at slightly higher rates in males than in females (male:female ratio 1.1:1.2). Its mean annual incidence is 7–12 cases per million children in western countries, and its prevalence is one in 7,000 live births. However, incidence rates are rather heterogeneous, except for the extremely low rates observed in some African regions. Screening programmes were implemented in regions of several countries including Japan, Germany, France, and Canada. An increase in the prevalence of neuroblastoma has been reported in these regions, but without a significant decrease in the prevalence or mortality of neuroblastoma in patients older than one year. The increased prevalence of neuroblastoma in screened populations suggests that spontaneous regression of neuroblastoma without clinical detection is at least as prevalent as clinically detected neuroblastoma.

The aetiology of neuroblastoma is unknown, and to date there are no data supporting a major role for environmental exposures. Nonetheless, the predisposing effects of prenatal exposure to noxa or maternal food patterns during pregnancy warrant further investigation. However, the consistent incidence rates of neuroblastoma in children support the hypothesis that genetic factors play the larger role in aetiology. Recent advances in identifying neuroblastoma predisposition genes may lead to the identification of individuals who are at increased risk and would benefit from future screening efforts.

Tumour predisposition, genetics, and molecular pathogenesis

Familial neuroblastoma

A familial history of neuroblastoma is observed in 1–2% of patients. Neuroblastoma pedigrees show an autosomal dominant pattern of inheritance with incomplete penetrance. Two main neural crest-derived developmental disorders are associated with an increased risk to develop neuroblastoma: Hirschsprung's disease and Ondine's curse. Both diseases are linked to mutation of the *PHOX2B* gene, which was subsequently identified as the first predisposition mutation in neuroblastoma. *PHOX2B* encodes a transcription factor that promotes cell-cycle exit and neuronal differentiation. Perturbations of the PHOX2B-regulated differentiation pathway in the sympathoadrenal lineage may contribute to neuroblastoma tumourigenesis. Although the involvement of *PHOX2B* in familial cases of neuroblastoma is compelling, its contribution to the development of sporadic neuroblastoma is limited, with mutations detected in only 5% of cases. Associations between neuroblastic tumours and other cancer predisposition syndromes including neurofibromin 1 (*NF1*), defined by the constitutive activation of the RAS–MAPK pathway, and Costello syndrome (HRAS) have been also reported.

The discovery of a second neuroblastoma predisposition gene has represented a breakthrough in the understanding of neuroblastoma pathogenesis. Activating mutations in the anaplastic lymphoma receptor tyrosine kinase (*ALK*) gene were identified in the majority of familial neuroblastoma cases and 10% of sporadic neuroblastomas. *ALK* encodes a transmembrane receptor tyrosine kinase preferentially expressed in the developing sympathoadrenal lineage of the neural crest, where it may regulate the balance between proliferation and differentiation through multiple cellular pathways. Three types of *ALK* germline mutations with incomplete penetrance have been described in neuroblastoma families, with the R1275Q substitution being the most frequent.

Germline mutations of *ALK* and *PHOX2B* do not account for all familial neuroblastoma cases. Interestingly, various types of abnormal constitutional karyotypes have been observed in patients with neuroblastoma, including constitutional copy number anomalies, balanced and unbalanced translocations, as well as specific chromosome deletions. Further whole-genome sequencing (WGS) efforts are likely to identify additional germline mutations in patients with a family history of neuroblastoma.

Sporadic neuroblastoma

Although a few neuroblastomas occur in familial contexts, almost 98% of cases occur sporadically. In light of the developmental origins, it is likely that underlying genetic factors are at least partly responsible for the development of sporadic neuroblastomas. Genome-wide association (GWAS) studies of constitutional DNA samples have identified numerous single-nucleotide polymorphisms (SNPs) associated with different clinical features of neuroblastoma and with potential roles in the disease pathogenesis. SNPs have been identified in the *CASC15, NBAT1, BARD1, LMO1, DUSP12, HSD17B12, DDX4, IL31RA, HACE1*,and *LIN28B* genes. Neuroblastoma can demonstrate varying levels of genomic instability and harbour a wide variety of numerical and structural genetic abnormalities, reflecting the heterogenous clinical and biological behaviour of the disease.

Neuroblastoma cells frequently harbour gross cytogenetic aberrations such as double-minute (DM) chromosomes or homogeneously staining regions (HSRs) of chromosomes, which contain ectopic amplifications of the *MYCN* oncogene. Amplification of the *MYCN* oncogene, mapping to 2p24.1, is present in about 25% of all neuroblastomas and 40% of high-risk tumours. It remains one of the most important genetic abnormalities associated with advanced disease stages, a highly malignant phenotype, and poor outcome, since its discovery by M. Schwab and others in 1983. *MYCN* status is assessed in the diagnostic tumour biopsy or a sample of the resected tumour, and is routinely used in clinical practice to assign therapeutic intensity.

Several lines of evidence indicate that overexpression of MYC proteins has a major role in oncogenesis through enhancing the expression of numerous genes involved in cell proliferation, and repressing expression of genes related to differentiation and apoptosis. Ectopic MYCN expression in the neural crest is sufficient to drive neuroblastoma tumourigenesis in zebrafish and mice. As a major oncogenic driver and one of the few tumour-specific targets in paediatric cancer, MYCN deserves to be a priority of therapeutic targeting.

Other structural chromosomal alterations commonly recurring in tumours and associated with advanced disease stage and poor outcome in neuroblastoma patients include deletions on 1p, 3p, 4p, and 11q chromosome arms and gains of a consensus region from 2p and 17q. Loss of 1p36 is observed in 20–35% of cases, predicts survival in multivariate analyses, and is significantly associated with aggressive disease markers. Thus, this genomic region might contain one or more tumour-suppressor genes.

Deletions in a consensus region at 11q23 occur in about 40% of cases. Chromosome 11q loss is inversely correlated with *MYCN* amplification and, therefore, identifies a molecularly distinct high-risk patient subset. This patient subset is characterized by advanced stage, older age, and unfavourable pathology. Allelic loss at 11q is also an independent marker of reduced EFS in low- and intermediate-risk subgroups and might be a useful biomarker to improve further risk stratification of medium-risk patients.

The most common aberration in neuroblastoma is the unbalanced chromosome 17q21-qter gain occurring in around 70% of tumours. Numerous studies have reported that 17q gain is significantly associated with advanced disease stage, increased patient age, 1p LOH, 11q LOH, and *MYCN* amplification. However, the independence of 17q gain as a prognostic factor is controversial. Whether an independent prognostic factor, or merely a modifying factor, identifying the gene aberrations caused by 17q imbalance will be crucial to fully understand neuroblastoma progression.

The overall genomic profile has been shown to be of prognostic impact in neuroblastoma. Whereas numerical chromosome alterations, consisting of gains or losses of whole chromosomes, are associated with a favourable outcome, segmental chromosome alterations are associated with a higher risk of relapse.

ALK amplifications and protein overexpression have been described in sporadic neuroblastomas in addition to the activating point mutations in *ALK*. Although the most aggressive somatic *ALK* mutation, the F1174L substitution, contributes to neuroblastoma tumourigenesis in mice, this mutation has not been observed in the germline in cases of familial neuroblastoma. It appears to behave as a superactivator that is not tolerated in the germline. Co-expression of ALKF1174L and MYCN produced a synergistic effect on tumour development in mouse and zebrafish models, and *ALK* mutations are consistently correlated with aggressive neuroblastoma subtypes in patients. However, the mechanistic link between *ALK* mutations and tumour biology has not yet been fully elucidated. Nonetheless, *ALK* is a promising target for molecular therapy in clinical trials recruiting neuroblastoma patients.

Several neuroblastoma deep-sequencing studies in recent years have consistently reported a low frequency of recurrent mutations. More recent studies investigating relapsed neuroblastomas have suggested that clonal evolution is common and results in the acquisition of targetable somatic aberrations in known oncogenic pathways. Early evidence suggests that activation of the MAPK pathway and other signalling pathways inducing epithelial-mesenchymal transition (EMT) processes are contributing to treatment failure and might be promising targets for molecular targeted treatment approaches.

Inactivating mutations of the *ATRX* chromatin-remodelling gene were also recently identified in a small subset of high-risk neuroblastomas, and were mutually exclusive to *MYCN* amplifications. *ATRX* mutations are associated with activation of a telomere maintenance mechanism termed alternate lengthening of telomeres (ALT), which may be a marker of an indolent neuroblastoma course with primary chemotherapy resistance. Fischer et al. discovered recurrent genomic rearrangements of the telomerase reverse transcriptase (*TERT*) gene on chromosome 5p15.33 in 13% of neuroblastoma

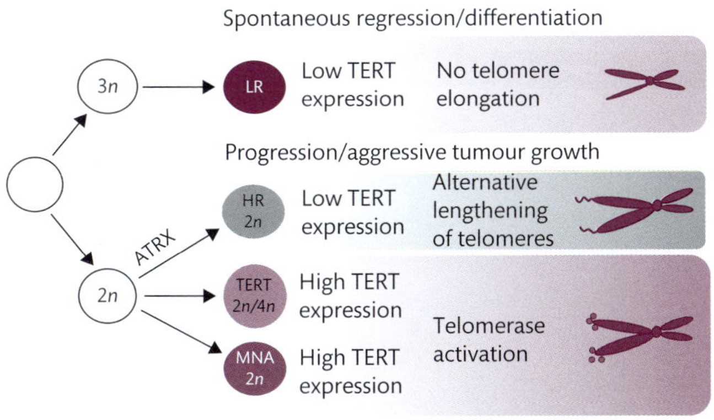

Figure 28.1 Current model of neuroblastoma evolution.

Adapted with permission from Peifer M, et al. 'Telomerase activation by genomic rearrangements in high-risk neuroblastoma', *Nature*, Volume 526, pp. 700–704. Copyright © 2015, Springer Nature. DOI: https://doi.org/10.1038/nature14980

cases. *TERT* rearrangements define a subgroup of high-risk disease and occur in mutually exclusive fashion with *MYCN* amplification and *ATRX* mutations.

These data fundamentally advance our understanding of the molecular pathogenesis of neuroblastoma (Figure 28.1). Now we know that the majority of high-risk neuroblastomas are affected by genetic alterations of *MYCN, TERT*, or *ATRX*, all of which converge on activation of telomere lengthening mechanisms. Telomeres get shortened with each cell division in somatic cells, eventually leading to replicative senescence or cell death. Cancer cells, in contrast, acquire the capability of maintaining their telomeres to provide themselves with infinite proliferative capacity. The most aggressive neuroblastoma subtypes appear to be defined by activation of telomerase, which is induced either by *TERT* rearrangements or by *MYCN* amplification. In the vast majority of the remaining high-risk tumours, the ALT pathway is activated, which is associated with *ATRX* mutations in a fraction of this subtype. Low-risk tumours appear to lack any telomere maintenance mechanisms, which may explain their inability to gain immortal proliferative capacity and consequently their potential for spontaneous regression. Advances in the development of telomerase inhibitors and their evaluation in clinical trials open up a new opportunity to establish effective treatment strategies for high-risk neuroblastoma patients.

Pathology

Peripheral neuroblastic tumours, including neuroblastoma, belong to the small, round, blue-cell neoplasms of childhood. They are derived from sympathogonia, the progenitor cells of the sympathetic nervous system in the sympathoadrenal lineage. After migrating from the neural crest, these pluripotent sympathogonia form the sympathetic ganglia, the chromaffin cells of the adrenal medulla and the paraganglia, reflecting the typical localizations of neuroblastic tumours.

The International Neuroblastoma Pathology Classification (INPC) developed by Shimada assigns peripheral neuroblastic tumours to one of four basic morphological categories:

1. **Neuroblastoma (Schwannian stroma-poor):** A tumour composed of neuroblastic cells forming groups or nests separated by stromal septa with Schwannian proliferation ranging from none to limited. This category consists of three subtypes: undifferentiated, poorly differentiated, and differentiating.
2. **Ganglioneuroblastoma, intermixed (Schwannian stroma-rich):** A tumour containing well-defined microscopic nests of neuroblastic cells intermixed or randomly distributed in the ganglioneuromatous stroma. The nests are composed of a mixture of neuroblastic cells in various stages of differentiation.
3. **Ganglioneuroblastoma, nodular (composite Schwannian stroma-rich/stroma-dominant and stroma-poor):** This lesion is characterized by the presence of grossly visible, usually haemorrhagic neuroblastic nodules (stroma-poor component, representing an aggressive clone) coexisting with intermixed ganglioneuroblastoma (stroma-rich component) or with ganglioneuroma (stroma-dominant component), both representing a non-aggressive clone. The term 'composite' implies that the tumour is composed of biologically different clones.
4. **Ganglioneuroma (Schwannian stroma-dominant):** This variant is divided into maturing and mature subtypes. The predominant ganglioneuromatous stroma of the maturing subtype contains scattered collections of differentiating neuroblasts and/or at least some maturing ganglion cells. Some fully mature ganglion cells can also be present in the maturing subtype. The mature subtype contains only mature Schwannian stroma and ganglion cells.

Morphological features used in INPC staging significantly correlate with biological properties of peripheral neuroblastic tumours, such as *MYCN* amplification or NTRK1 expression.

Biological aspects

A number of biological pathways regulating major hallmarks of cancer appear to be disrupted or at least affected in neuroblastoma. Important biological characteristics include abnormal patterns of gene or protein expression that are associated with regions of tumour differentiation, apoptosis, drug resistance, angiogenesis, invasion, or metastasis. Insight into the molecular regulation of these biological features will ultimately lead to the identification of novel drug targets.

As neurotrophin signalling has a central role in normal neuronal development and may be involved in both differentiation and regression of neuroblastoma, there has been a particular interest in alterations of these pathways. The clinical and biological roles of neurotrophin receptor tyrosine kinases 1 and 2 (*NTRK1* and *NTRK2*) and their corresponding ligands have been extensively investigated. Both *NTRK1* and *NTRK2* tumour expression are important prognostic factors influencing the clinical and biological behaviour of neuroblastoma.

Delayed activation or disruption of normal apoptotic pathways may be an important phenomenon involved in spontaneous regression of neuroblastoma as well as therapy resistance. Abnormal expression or activation patterns occur in major proteins in the apoptotic signalling cascade, including the BCL2 family, BIRC5, and *caspase 8*. *Caspase 8* inactivation mainly occurs via epigenetic silencing. Alterations in DNA methylation represent one of the most common molecular events in neoplasia, and CpG-island hypermethylation of

Table 28.1 Tumour site and clinical characteristics

Tumour site	Main symptoms and signs	Incidence (%)	Metastases (%)	Outcome
Neck	Mass mimicking lymphadenopathy, Horner syndrome	4	2	Good
Thorax: Upper	Respiratory symptoms	6	5	Good
Thorax: Lower	Incidental X-ray detection	6	2	Good
Abdomen	Central or lateral mass, symptoms related to metastatic disease (fever, pallor, anorexia, bone pain, irritability)	70	75	Poor
Pelvis	Lower abdominal mass, dysuria, constipation	5	5	Good
Not identified	Fever, pallor, anorexia, bone pain, irritability	1	100	Very Poor

gene promoters is a frequent mechanism for functional inactivation of relevant tumour-associated genes.

Acquired resistance to chemotherapeutic agents may also be conferred by enhanced drug efflux via overexpression of classical multidrug resistance proteins, including the ATP-binding cassette subfamily B member 1 (ABCB1), and ATP-binding cassette subfamily C member 1 (ABCC1) proteins. The ATP-binding cassette subfamily G member 2 (ABCG2) is another important contributor to a drug-resistance phenotype in neuroblastomas, especially immature and stem-like cell populations. Their potential clinical significance in neuroblastoma has been addressed in several studies.

Enhanced tumour angiogenesis and elevated expression of proangiogenic factors, such as vascular endothelial growth factor A (VEGFA), both correlate with an aggressive neuroblastoma phenotype. Inhibitors of angiogenesis are currently being evaluated in clinical trials as a potential treatment option. Deep-sequencing approaches for comprehensive molecular characterization of neuroblastoma are currently doing a great deal to advance our understanding of neuroblastoma biology. A detailed molecular profile from the tumour, metastases, and/or circulating tumour cells or tumour-associated DNA in the peripheral bloodstream could allow patient-tailored precise prognostication, while also identifying key targets that could be therapeutically exploited.

It is likely that immune factors and interactions with the tumour microenvironment contribute to the variation in neuroblastoma biology. These can also strongly influence the efficacy and application of immunotherapies, which currently hold high potential for high-risk patients. Since age at diagnosis is of strong prognostic impact in patients with neuroblastoma, it could be suggested that stage- and age-related differences in the host reaction to a developing tumour might influence outcome. Further evidence for the involvement of the immune system in neuroblastoma control derives from observations of the neuroblastoma-associated paraneoplastic syndrome, opsoclonus-myoclonus syndrome (OMS). Lymphoid infiltrates are frequently observed in the tumours in OMS patients, and these patients typically have an excellent oncological prognosis. Higher levels of CD163+ M2 macrophages have also been detected in tumour tissue from patients with INSS (International Neuroblastoma Staging System) stage 3 or 4S neuroblastoma compared with tumour tissue from patients with INSS stage 4 metastatic disease, a finding associated with outcome in several other cancers. Age-dependent differential expression of inflammatory genes associated with tumour-associated macrophages has been demonstrated in neuroblastomas. Cancer-associated fibroblasts in the neuroblastoma microenvironment have been suggested to contribute to immunosuppression, which could consequentially favour tumour development.

Altogether, neuroblastoma infiltration with suppressive myeloid cells can decrease anti-tumour immune responses and favour tumour growth in high-risk disease. Both active and passive immunotherapies, including antibody-based therapies, are now being explored for neuroblastoma patients.

Clinical presentation, diagnosis, and staging

Neuroblastoma can arise at any site along the sympathetic nervous system chain, but the distribution varies across the sites with age. About 70% of primary tumours occur within the abdomen, and more than half of these arise in the adrenal gland. Infants more frequently present with adrenal, thoracic, and cervical primary tumours. The clinical presentation of neuroblastoma reflects the site of tumour origin, the extent of regional and metastatic disease, and the presence of paraneoplastic syndromes (Table 28.1).

Cervical neuroblastomas (4% of cases) mimic adenopathies and often include Horner syndrome (ptosis, miosis, anhydrosis) and heterochromia. Thoracic neuroblastomas represent 15% of all cases. Tumours in the upper mediastinum cause respiratory distress as well as Horner syndrome, while tumours arising in the middle and lower mediastinum are usually asymptomatic and discovered on routine chest X-ray. The typical neuroblastoma patient is a toddler, failing to grow, with abdominal distension and a palpable lateral or central hard, fixed mass. Pelvic tumours are uncommon and present as suprapubic masses causing constipation and urinary disturbances.

Approximately half of all patients have disseminated disease at the time of diagnosis. The most commonly involved organs are the bone marrow, skeleton, liver, and lymph nodes, with less common involvement of the lung and central nervous system. Disseminated disease is usually associated with non-specific symptoms, including fever, pallor, anorexia, and bone pain, with consequent refusal to walk and mood changes. Retro-orbital and orbital metastases are rather frequent, and produce a typical appearance of proptosis and periorbital ecchymoses (Figure 28.2). In infants, stage 4S or MS is characterized by massive liver involvement with or without the presence of bluish nodules in the subcutaneous tissue and bone-marrow infiltration. Infants with stage 4S can present with significant respiratory distress due to a massively enlarged liver. By definition, stage 4S patients do not have bone lesions. Neuroblastoma in adolescents and adults has a slow, indolent clinical course with a worse overall outcome compared to that in children, although the primary tumour and site distributions and metastatic patterns are similar.

The anatomical connection between the sympathetic nervous system and the spinal cord accounts for the propensity of

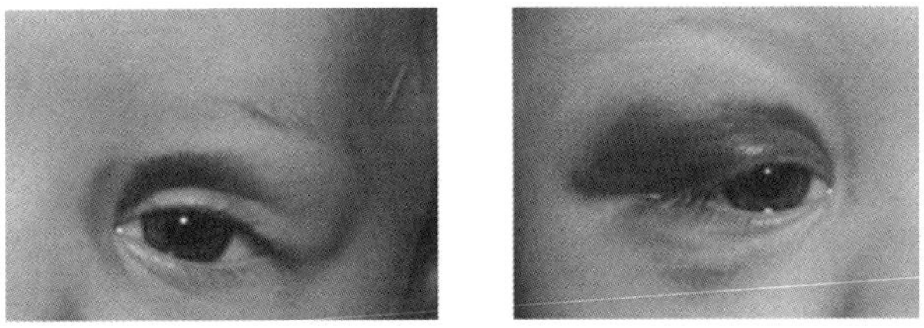

Figure 28.2 Retro-orbital and orbital metastases with a typical appearance of proptosis and periorbital ecchymoses in a child with stage 4 neuroblastoma.

neuroblastoma to infiltrate the intervertebral foramina. Paraspinal tumours tend to grow through the neural foramina of the vertebral bodies, causing spinal-cord compression as a presenting sign of the tumour. Motor deficits are the most frequent symptoms experienced by patients with paraspinal tumours, followed by radicular or back pain, bladder or bowel dysfunction, and, rarely, sensorial manifestations. Only 5% of patients have clinical evidence of epidural compression. Early detection of this phenomenon is crucial because symptoms may rapidly worsen, leading to irreversible paraplegia.

Ganglioneuroblastomas are well-differentiated locoregional tumours, and may occasionally cause symptoms either directly related to effects of the tumour mass or related to paracrine secretion of various substances. Ganglioneuromas can entrap and impinge on vessels, nerves, vessels, gastrointestinal (GI) track, or other tissues. Vasoactive intestinal peptide (VIP) causes watery diarrhoea, which may require treatment with somatostatin. Antineuronal antibodies can trigger an autoimmune reaction that may occur as a cerebellar syndrome or OMS. OMS occurs in 2% of neuroblastoma patients and is characterized by multidirectional rapid eye movement (opsoclonus), myoclonus, and brainstem ataxia. These symptoms may precede the detection of a tumoural mass by several months and improve if the primary tumour is removed, but in many cases patients require specific immunosuppressive treatment. Symptoms may reappear during infectious episodes and the majority of these children appear to have long-term neurological deficits.

Increased catecholamine levels may cause high blood pressure, in particular when elevated epinephrine or norepinephrine levels are present, although hypertensive crises are very rare in patients with neuroblastoma. Hypertension may also be caused by stimulation of the renin-angiotensin system from pressure by the retroperitoneal mass on the renal artery.

Tumour markers

Urinary metabolites produced by catecholamine degradation, namely vanillylmandelic acid (VMA) and homovanillic acid (HVA), are the most sensitive (90% positive cases) and specific disease markers. Plasma-free and total normetanephrine, metanephrine, and methoxytyramine represent a convenient alternative to urine markers. Overall levels and the ratio of VMA to HVA in the urine have prognostic value, and are related to age, histology, stage, and *MYCN* amplification. Screening for neuroblastoma using a urinary assay for catecholamines at six months of age was pioneered in Japan in the early 1970s. Two large population-based studies in Quebec and Germany showed that screening at 12 months of age detected many neuroblastomas that would never have been diagnosed clinically, but observed no reduction in the incidence of advanced-stage neuroblastoma. Cumulative mortality was not different from concurrent or retrospective mortality. As a result, routine screening was ceased because of the low clinical impact for treating neuroblastoma. However, a great deal of biological information on favourable neuroblastoma subtypes has been derived from these studies. Lactate dehydrogenase (LDH), ferritin, and enolase 2 (formerly neuron-specific enolase (NSE)) have been identified as markers for neuroblastoma in patient serum, and correlate with tumour stage, extension, and prognosis. New serum tumour markers and useful molecular markers to monitor minimal residual disease might be identified by ongoing liquid-biopsy studies.

Diagnostic criteria

The following examinations are required for accurate diagnosis and staging according to the INSS:

- Magnetic resonance imaging (MRI) or computed tomography (CT) of the primary tumour site.
- Biopsy of the primary tumour or metastatic site for histological examination and determination of biological prognostic factors (*MYCN* amplification).
- Bone-marrow aspirate and trephine biopsy at two different sites.
- ^{123}I Metaiodobenzylguanidine (MIBG) scintigraphy before tumour excision to evaluate the primary tumour site and detect metastatic sites (**Figure 28.3**). Detection of a single equivocal lesion requires confirmation by another imaging modality.
- Bone scintigraphy or 18-fluorodeoxyglucose (FDG)-positron emission tomography (PET)/CT is required only in exceptional cases when MIBG cannot confirm a primary tumour. An isolated bone uptake should be confirmed by another imaging modality and/or a biopsy.
- Assay of urinary catecholamine levels (HVA and VMA). Additional assays should include serum ferritin, LDH, and NSE levels.

Staging

Disease staging is necessary to define prognosis and select appropriate treatment intensity. The INSS definitions are based on local and distant extension as well as tumour resectability (**Table 28.2**).

The INSS stage of locoregional tumours is dependent on the degree of surgical resection, which is subjectively assessed and prone to variation between surgeons. The International Neuroblastoma Risk Group (INRG) classification system was developed to facilitate comparison of risk-based clinical trials conducted in different world regions by defining homogeneous pretreatment patient cohorts. The premise is that a staging system based on preoperative, diagnostic images will be more robust and reproducible than one based on operative findings and approaches. Since the surgical risk factors are

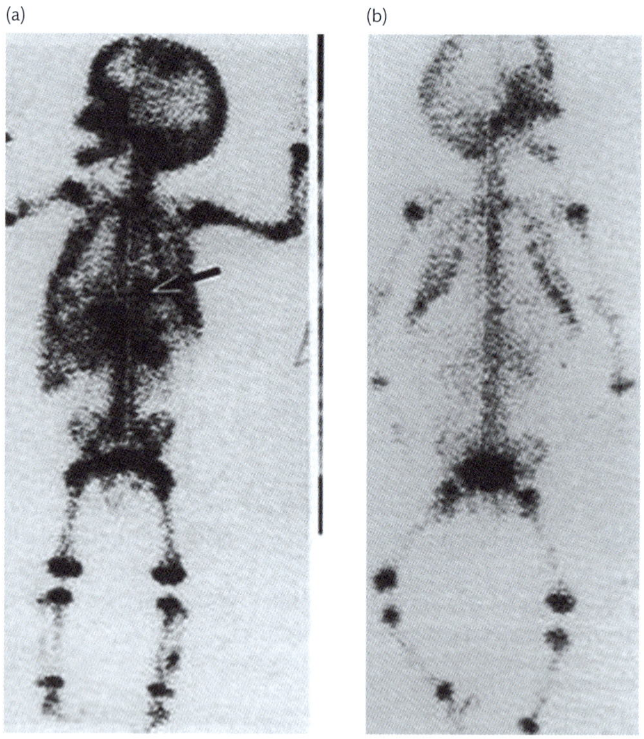

Figure 28.3 MIBG scan: (a) uptake by the primary tumour (right adrenal gland) as well as bone and bone-marrow metastases are visualized; (b) normal uptake after chemotherapy.

Table 28.2 The International Neuroblastoma Staging System (INSS)

Stage	Description
Stage 1	Localized tumour with complete gross excision, with or without microscopic residual disease. Representative ipsilateral lymph node microscopically negative for tumour.
Stage 2A	Localized tumour with incomplete gross excision. Representative ipsilateral non-adherent lymph nodes microscopically negative for tumour.
Stage 2B	Localized tumour with or without complete gross excision, with ipsilateral non-adherent lymph nodes positive for tumour. Enlarged contralateral lymph nodes must be microscopically negative for tumour.
Stage 3	Unresectable unilateral tumour, infiltrating across the midline, with or without regional lymph-node involvement; or localized unilateral tumour with contralateral lymph-node involvement; or midline tumour with bilateral extension by infiltration or lymph-node involvement.
Stage 4	Any primary tumour with dissemination to distant lymph nodes, bone, bone marrow, liver, and/or other organs (except as defined for Stage 4S).
Stage 4S	Localized primary tumour (as defined for Stage 1, 2A, or 2B), with dissemination limited to liver, skin, and/or bone marrow*. Limited to infants <18 months of age.

** Marrow involvement in stage 4S should be minimal (<10% nucleated cells in bone-marrow biopsy). More extensive marrow involvement should be considered stage 4. The MIBG scan should be negative in the marrow for stage 4S.

based on radiographic images, the term 'image-defined risk factors' (IDRFs) was chosen, and a consensus was reached for the IDRFs listed in Table 28.3.

These criteria, based on the relation of the tumour with the adjacent structures and vasculature (Figure 28.4) predict severe surgical complications and are the basis for the new INRG Staging System (INRGSS; Table 28.4).

Several international groups have developed models of clinical-risk stratification to facilitate the delivery of risk-adapted treatments. Various biological features were added to the different clinical characteristics, but the most important prognostic factors remain patient age, tumour stage, and *MYCN* amplification. Two extremely different clinical courses of disease can easily be discriminated. The favourable subtype of neuroblastoma arises in the first months of life, with many patients showing spontaneous regression of the disease and most having excellent survival with minimal or no treatment, provided the tumour is not *MYCN* amplified. The aggressive, unfavourable neuroblastoma subtype occurs in children older than 18 months and is associated with a poor outcome. It presents with metastatic disease at the time of diagnosis, and tumours often harbour a *MYCN* amplification. Between these two extremes there are less well-defined subgroups with intermediate characteristics.

The INRG Task Force has developed the INRG Consensus Pretreatment Classification Schema to establish a consensus approach for current pretreatment risk stratification. The prognostic effect of 13 variables in an 8,800-patient cohort was analysed, and a schema with four main prognostic groups (Table 28.5) and 16 pretreatment designations was developed (Table 28.6). This approach greatly facilitates the comparison of risk-based clinical trials conducted in different regions of the world.

The assessment of more complex molecular patterns and the recent establishment of mRNA-based molecular risk classifiers will allow more refined and precise risk-stratification approaches in the near future, and will consequently enable physicians to tailor appropriate treatment strategies to individual patients.

Treatment

The treatment of children with neuroblastoma primarily depends on patient age, disease extension, and some features of tumour histology and biology. The currently employed treatment modalities include surgery, chemotherapy, radiotherapy, immunotherapy, and biological response modifiers. Major clinical phase 3 randomized trials from the European International Society of Paediatric Oncology European Neuroblastoma Network (SIOPEN), the Children's Oncology Group (COG), the German Society for Paediatric Oncology and Haematology (GPOH), and the Japanese Neuroblastoma Study Group (JNBSG) are currently being performed, have completed inclusion, or are in preparation.

Surgery

Surgery plays a key role for both diagnosis and treatment. The goals of primary surgery are to confirm the diagnosis, acquire tissue samples for classification as well as for histological and biological studies, and to resect the tumour with minimal morbidity. When the anatomical characteristics (site, size, and relationship with the surrounding structures) indicate that surgical resection is feasible, surgery is the treatment of choice for patients presenting with localized disease. An international panel of surgeons and

Table 28.3 Image-defined risk factors (IDRFs) in neuroblastic tumours

Ipsilateral tumour extension within two body compartments
Neck
• Tumour encasing carotid and/or vertebral artery and/or internal jugular vein
• Tumour extending to base of the skull
• Tumour compressing the trachea
• Cervico-thoracic junction
• Tumour encasing brachial plexus roots
• Tumour encasing subclavian vessels and/or vertebral and/or carotid artery
• Tumour compressing the trachea
Thorax
• Tumour encasing the aorta and/or major branches
• Tumour compressing the trachea and/or principal bronchi
• Lower mediastinal tumour, infiltrating the costo-vertebral junction between T9 and T12
Thoraco-abdominal
• Tumour encasing the aorta and/or the vena cava
• Abdomen/pelvis
• Tumour infiltrating the porta hepatis and/or the hepatoduodenal ligament
• Tumour encasing branches of the superior mesenteric artery and the mesenteric root
• Tumour encasing the origin of celiac axis and/or of the superior mesenteric artery
• Tumour invading one or both renal pedicles
• Tumour encasing the aorta and/or the vena cava
• Tumour encasing the iliac vessels
• Pelvic tumour across the sciatic notch
Intraspinal tumour
• Extension, regardless of location, provided that more than one third of the spinal canal in the axial plane is invaded and/or the perimedullary leptomeningeal spaces are not visible and/or the spinal cord signal is abnormal
Infiltration of adjacent organs/structures
• Pericardium, diaphragm, kidney, liver, duodeno-pancreatic block and mesentery
Conditions to be recorded, but not considered as IDRFs
• Multifocal primary tumours
• Pleural effusion, with or without malignant cells
• Ascites, with or without malignant cells

Adapted with permission from Monclair T, et al. 'The International Neuroblastoma Risk Group (INRG) Staging System: An INRG Task Force Report', *Journal of Clinical Oncology*, Volume 27, Issue 2, pp. 298–303. Copyright © 2009 American Society of Clinical Oncology. DOI: 10.1200/JCO.2008.16.6876

radiologists identified surgical risk factors detectable by imaging and established radiological criteria for a safe resection. Surgery is the only treatment necessary to cure the majority of patients with localized disease, even if macroscopic remnants of the tumour are left behind. If surgical risk factors are detected, presurgical chemotherapy is necessary to shrink the tumour prior to resection. However, frequently IDRFs persist after neoadjuvant chemotherapy. Since neuroblastoma has an elevated tropism towards lymphatic vessels, it is important to perform a surgical exploration of the locoregional lymph nodes, especially in abdominal and pelvic sites. In paravertebral sites with infiltration through the intervertebral foramina, laminectomy is indicated only in selected cases with acute, severe neurological symptoms. In fact, chemotherapy can rapidly reduce both tumour size and the impact of spinal-cord compression in these cases.

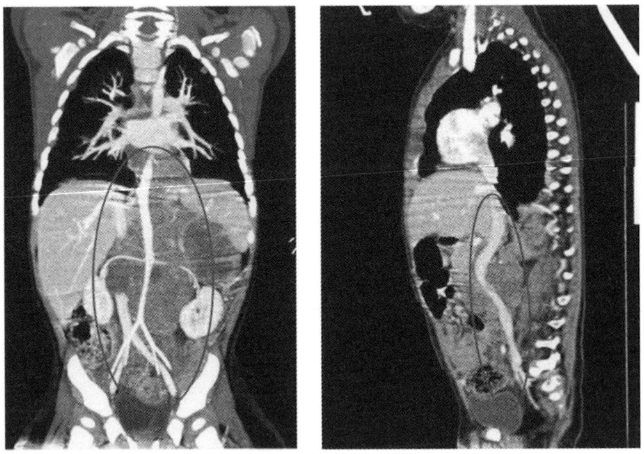

Figure 28.4 Angio-CT, coronal view, showing a large abdominal neuroblastoma encasing the major retroperitoneal vessels.

In contrast to its pivotal role in treating localized disease, the function of aggressive surgery remains controversial for metastatic disease. Meta-analyses in large patient cohorts are hampered by fragmented and inconsistent documentation of surgical approaches and a lack of immediate postoperative imaging results. Both limitations should be addressed in upcoming trial protocols. However, considering the high incidence of local relapse, the current strategy in most treatment protocols is to resect the primary tumour after inducing remission of the metastases. In delayed primary or second-look surgery, the surgeon evaluates therapy response and removes the residual tumour to a maximum extent, whenever possible.

Radiotherapy

Neuroblastoma is a radiosensitive tumour, and tumouricidal doses range from 15 to 36 Gy (with fraction doses ranging from 150 to 400 cGy) depending on tumour site, volume, and patient age. Definition of the role of external-beam radiotherapy (EBRT) and the optimal mode of its application are under continuous refinement. The lack of randomized trials addressing the contribution of radiotherapy hampers proper evaluation of the impact of this treatment modality on clinical outcome to date. EBRT is also successfully used as palliative treatment on painful sites.

Radiometabolic salvage therapy is used for high-risk neuroblastomas with active residual tumour prior to myeloablative chemotherapy. It utilizes ^{131}I carried by ^{131}I-MIBG, a noradrenalin analogue that is actively taken up by tumour cells via the norepinephrine transporter and incorporated into the neurosecretory granules of neuroblastoma cells. Dosimetry problems, together with the non-homogeneous uptake of ^{131}I-MIBG throughout the tumour and toxicity have limited the use of this therapeutic approach to selected treatment centres. Some groups have used radiometabolic therapy as first-line treatment, but the results from long-term patient follow-up were not favourable in these cases. Other approaches have included general radiometabolic therapy using ^{131}I-MIBG in the conditioning

Table 28.4 International Neuroblastoma Risk Group Staging System (INRGSS)

Stage	Description
Stage L1	Radiological risk factors absent. Localized tumour not involving vital structures as defined by the list of image-defined risk factors and confined to one body compartment.
Stage L2	Locoregional tumour with presence of one or more image-defined risk factors.
Stage M	Distant metastatic disease (in contrast to stage MS).
Stage MS	Metastatic disease in children <18 months with metastases confined to the skin, liver, and/or bone marrow (bone-marrow involvement should be limited to <10% of total nucleated cells on smears or biopsy).

phase prior to haematopoietic stem-cell transplantation. Its use as salvage treatment in relapsed disease is under investigation.

Chemotherapy

Chemotherapy has an important role in treating neuroblastoma, since the majority of patients present with metastatic or locally advanced disease at diagnosis and require systemic treatment. Alkylating agents (cyclophosphamide, ifosfamide, busulfan, melphalan), platinum analogues (cisplatin and carboplatin), vinca alkaloids (vincristine), epipodophyllotoxins (VP16, VM26), and anthracyclines (doxorubicin) have well-established activity and efficacy against neuroblastoma, and are considered standard options. Only a few new drugs have been introduced into first-line therapy in recent years. Topotecan, irinotecan, and temozolomide are expected to slightly improve response in high-risk neuroblastoma patients. High-dose chemotherapy with various combinations of busulfan, melphalan, carboplatin, and etoposide, followed by autologous peripheral blood stem-cell (PBSC) rescue, is currently used as consolidation treatment in high-risk patients.

Risk-adapted treatment

Low- and very low-risk groups

This group includes children with INSS stage 1 and 2, infants with stage 3 (L2) and 4S neuroblastomas without unfavourable biological markers. Since these patients have an excellent prognosis, the goal is to reduce the risk of side effects while maintaining high survival rates. The predicted survival is almost 100%, both for patients who are treated with a moderate dose of chemotherapy (COG and SIOPEN groups) and patients who are treated without cytotoxic agents (Memorial Sloan–Kettering Cancer Center (MSKCC) and German groups). German studies have shown that infants with radiologically diagnosed neuroblastoma may safely be observed over time without obtaining a definitive surgical histological diagnosis, thus avoiding the potential complications of surgery. Chemotherapy is mandatory if severe symptoms (especially neurological symptoms) are present or if tumour progression occurs. Neuroblastomas lacking *MYCN* amplification or in the stage 4S/MS group undergo spontaneous regression in the majority of cases. Chemotherapy or low-dose radiotherapy should be reserved for patients with large tumours or massive hepatomegaly causing mechanical obstruction, respiratory insufficiency, or liver dysfunction.

Table 28.5 The four main prognostic neuroblastoma subgroups

Pretreatment risk group	5-year EFS (%)	Proportion of patients (%)
Very low	>85	28.2
Low	>75 to ≤85	26.8
Intermediate	≥50 to ≤75	9.0
High	<50	36.1

Intermediate-risk group

The intermediate-risk group encompasses a wide spectrum of conditions, including patients with stage 3 (L2) disease with tumours lacking *MYCN* amplification who are more than 18 months of age, and patients with stage 4 (M) disease who are under 18 months old. Stage 1 (L1) *MYCN*-amplified tumours have also recently been included in this group by SIOPEN. Survival is nearly 90% in this group, but may be poorer in some subgroups, and so the challenge is to identify patients for whom therapy may be further reduced as opposed to those who require more treatment. Surgical resection and moderate-dose, multi-agent chemotherapy are the backbone of therapy. High-dose chemotherapy with PBSC rescue is not proposed, and the role of radiotherapy is less well-defined.

High-risk group

This group includes all stage 4 (M) patients more than 18 months of age and stage 2, 3, and 4S patients with *MYCN*-amplified tumours. These patients are generally treated with dose-intensive, multi-agent chemotherapy in the induction phase that consists of high-dose cisplatin with etoposide, vincristine, doxorubicin, and cyclophosphamide or ifosfamide, and, more recently, topotecan. Current treatment regimens for induction chemotherapy employed by the SIOPEN, GPOH, and COG trial groups will be compared in a randomized fashion in the near future to identify the most beneficial approach.

Induction chemotherapy is followed, where possible, by primary tumour resection, then myeloablative chemotherapy with PBSC rescue in the consolidation phase. The idea of eliminating resistant tumour clones with supralethal chemotherapy has been studied in neuroblastoma since the early 1980s, and the results of several randomized phase III cooperative trials (COG 4 and GPOH NB 1997) have shown improved EFS. Current international evidence points to a superiority of busulphan/melphalan in comparison to carboplatin, etoposide, and melphalan as the conditioning regimen prior to PBSC. Recent data also suggest that tandem intensification is feasibile and may be of benefit for certain patients.

Irradiation of the tumour bed or residual primary tumour is performed after myeloablative therapy. Most protocols usually employ a dose of 21 Gy to the primary site as consolidation therapy (SIOPEN) or 36 Gy to MIBG-active residual tumour at the primary site (GPOH). The indication for irradiating metastatic lesions is less clear, other than for palliation. Randomized trials and implementation of quality-assured radiotherapy are now being set up since

Table 28.6 International Neuroblastoma Risk Group (INRG) Treatment Classification System

INRG stage	Age (months)	Histological classification	Grade of tumour differentiation	MYCN	11q aberration	Ploidy	Pretreatment risk group
L1/L2	Any	GN maturing GNB intermixed					A Very low
L1	Any	Any except GN maturing or GNB intermixed		NA			B Very low
				Amp			K High
L2	<18	Any except GN maturing or GNB intermixed			No		D Low
				NA	Yes		G Intermediate
	≥18	GNB nodular; neuroblastoma	Differentiating	NA	No		E Low
			Poorly differentiating or undifferentiating	NA	Yes		H Intermediate
L2	Any			NA			High risk
M	<18			NA		Hyperdiploid	F Low
	<12			NA		Diploid	I Intermediate
	12 to <18			NA		Diploid	J Intermediate
	<18			Amp			O High
	≥18						P High
MS	<18			NA	No		C Very low
					Yes		Q High
				Amp			R High

Amp = amplified; GN = ganglioneuroma; GNB = ganglioneuroblastoma; NA = not aftablemplified

Reproduced with permission from Susan L. Cohn, et al. 'The International Neuroblastoma Risk Group (INRG) Classification System: An INRG Task Force Report.' *Journal of Clinical Oncology*, Volume 27, Issue 2, pp. 289–97. Copyright © 2009 American Society of Clinical Oncology. DOI: 10.1200/JCO.2008.16.6785.

current irradiation protocols, including fractionation protocols, are rather heterogeneous.

Most high-risk neuroblastomas initially respond to therapy but subsequently relapse. Therefore, much attention has been given to biological therapies including differentiation-inducing agents such as retinoid derivatives or immunotherapy with monoclonal antibodies (MoAbs) targeting the disialoganglioside GD2. Retinoids are a class of compounds that can induce terminal differentiation of neuroblastoma cells *in vitro*. Current international evidence for a clinical benefit of retinoic-acid therapy in high-risk neuroblastoma patients is very limited and does not necessarily warrant further implementation of this approach in first-line treatment.

Although the profound immunosuppression produced by high-dose chemotherapy regimens provides unfavourable conditions for the application of active immunotherapy, the use of passive antibody-based immunotherapy is feasible. GD2 is a surface glycolipid antigen present on neuroblastoma cells. It is expressed only weakly in the normal tissues of the central and peripheral nervous systems. Therapies using various MoAbs have been assessed in phase I and II settings, and their safety profile has been established. Anti-GD2 therapies have been studied, with or without cytokines, in phase III trials for neuroblastoma patients in first response. A COG randomized phase III trial of the anti-GD2 ch14.18 MoAb plus cytokines after PBSC rescue demonstrated a clear survival advantage in patients receiving immunotherapy compared to untreated controls. Application of the anti-GD2 ch14.18 MoAb without immune-modulating cytokines is still under investigation. Future trials will mostly likely assess the effect of ch14.18 chimeric antibodies in parallel to induction chemotherapy.

Treatment of spinal-cord compression

The routine use of MRI has increased the number of cases with documented infiltration of neural foramina or the spinal canal. In the majority of cases, no neurological symptoms arise and no specific treatment is required. There is very little evidence that an asymptomatic intraspinal tumour will continue to grow after resection of the extraspinal component. Some cases suggest that intraspinal neuroblastoma in patients with no neurological symptoms might remain stable or even regress without specific treatment. If more than 50% of the spinal canal is taken by the tumour or in case of clinical symptoms of spinal-cord compression, dexamethasone should be administered in addition to chemotherapy.

Patients with neuroblastoma who present with signs of spinal-cord compression require urgent, specific treatment. Rapid therapeutic decisions must be made within a few hours if neurological deficits and clinical progression are detected. The decision whether to administer emergency chemotherapy should be made immediately after detailed conference between the oncologist and neurosurgeon, and the start of treatment should never be delayed. Laminectomy should be considered only in infants showing very rapid neurological deterioration due to the long-term consequences of this procedure. If chemotherapy has been started, the tumour should be biopsied when the patient is stable a few days after chemotherapy.

Treatment of relapse

Survival of children with recurrent or refractory neuroblastoma remains very poor, and very few can be salvaged. A small cohort of patients, mainly represented by children with stages 1 and 2 who developed local recurrence or late relapse, may still benefit from further conventional treatment including aggressive surgery, external or metabolic radiotherapy, and chemotherapy. However, experimental therapies are proposed for the majority of patients. An umbrella trial incorporating all promising current options for relapsed neuroblastoma treatment is currently being developed by the SIOPEN trial group.

New drugs

To best confront the heterogenous nature of neuroblastoma, comprehensive molecular profiling must be utilized to tailor treatment and identify novel therapeutic targets. The major hope is now focused on new drugs directed against these molecular targets. Here, we concentrate on the most promising ones close to clinical exploitation. Current established collaborative networks, such as Innovative Therapies for Children with Cancer (ITCC) in Europe, are testing an increasing number of targeted agents in paediatric cell lines and animal models, providing strong evidence supporting its biology-driven use, and testing feasible and effective combinations with chemotherapy or other targeted agents. The inclusion of robust predictive biomarkers in phase I/II clinical trials will enhance the success in drug development and reduce exposures and toxicity for populations unlikely to benefit from a particular therapy. These approaches will also help determine the indication for inclusion of novel therapeutic strategies in first-line treatment, in particular of high-risk neuroblastoma patients.

Targeting ALK

Targeting mutated and activated ALK in neuroblastoma is likely to produce clinical benefit since:

1. activating point mutations or amplification occurs in 10% of primary neuroblastomas and up to 30% of relapse tumours;
2. normal ALK expression is confined to developing neural tissues;
3. cells expressing mutated ALK exhibit oncogene addiction with ALK inhibition leading to cell death;
4. ALK mutations can be inhibited by small molecules; and
5. ALK can be activated by mechanisms other than mutation and amplification, suggesting that ALK inhibition might be useful for a larger patient subset.

Crizotinib (PF-02341066) was the first ALK inhibitor evaluated for neuroblastoma. While excellent clinical responses have been achieved in patients with non-small-cell lung cancer and adult anaplastic large-cell lymphoma (ALCL), only very limited responses were achieved in neuroblastoma patients. The ALK F1174L mutation confers primary as well as acquired crizotinib resistance, since this mutant protein does not directly interact with the crizotinib-binding site within the ATP-binding pocket. Several structurally distinct, third-generation ALK inhibitors with enhanced potency and specificity are currently in early-phase clinical trials, including ceritinib (LDK378) and lorlatinib (PF-06463922), a dual-specificity ALK/ROS inhibitor.

Targeting MYCN

In light of the frequency and importance of *MYCN* amplification in the pathogenesis of high-risk neuroblastoma, blocking MYCN signalling represents an important approach for developing new therapeutics. Efforts are limited by difficulties associated with selective pharmacological inhibition of nuclear transcription factors, but various strategies aimed at counteracting MYCN activity more indirectly are actively being pursued:

Targeting MYCN binding to DNA. Development of small molecules directly targeting MYC family members has focused on blocking the interaction between MYCN and MAX, which is necessary for DNA binding.

Targeting MYCN transcription. Bromodomain and extra-terminal (BET) family adaptor proteins localize to MYC/MYCN promoters. The prototypic BET inhibitor, JQ1, disrupts BET recruitment to chromatin and has been shown to downregulate the MYC/MYCN transcriptional programme and suppress transcription of *MYCN* itself. The orally bioavailable OTX015 is currently the only BET inhibitor in early-phase clinical trials.

Targeting synthetic lethal interactions of MYCN. Genes that are synthetically lethal with MYCN expression include *AURKA*, *CDK1*, *CDK2*, and *CHEK1*. Several CDK inhibitors with excellent selectivity and potency are under development.

Targeting oncogenic stabilization of MYCN. MYC family proteins bind to a proteasomal degradation complex that includes AURKA and E3 ubiquitin ligases. An attractive strategy to target oncogenic stabilization of MYCN is to promote dissociation of the AURKA:MYCN complex to trigger rapid proteasomal degradation of MYCN. AURKA inhibitors, such as alisertinib (MLN8237), induce a conformational change in the kinase that actively reinitiates MYCN degradation, independent of any requirement for enzymatic inhibition of the kinase itself.

Targeting MYCN expression. A novel mechanism regulating MYCN expression involves the modulation of the let-7 family of miRNAs by LIN28B, which negatively regulate *MYCN* expression.

Targeting RTKs and PI3K. Aberrant PI3K/mTOR activity in neuroblastoma correlates with poor outcome, drives oncogenic stabilization of MYCN, and can be targeted using clinical PI3K/mTOR inhibitors. Early-phase trials of compounds active against PI3K, mTOR, or AKT are underway.

Targeting histone deacetylases

Histone deacetylase (HDAC) inhibitors are an emerging class of promising novel anti-cancer drugs. Neuroblastoma is the first tumour entity in which expression of all classical HDAC family members have been systematically investigated. All 11 classical HDAC family members are expressed, but HDAC8 is the only isozyme that significantly correlates with advanced disease stage, age, unfavourable tumour histology, 11q aberration, and poor survival. Since HDAC8-selective inhibitors are available, HDAC8 may be a promising target for neuroblastoma differentiation therapy.

Targeting MDM2/TP53

Another appealing approach for molecular therapy of neuroblastoma is provided by a crucial protein–protein interaction that regulates the cellular decision between life and death: the physical association between the TP53 tumour-suppressor protein and its major negative regulator, MDM2. Escape from the TP53-orchestrated failsafe programme is a necessary event for tumourigenesis, and is achieved in neuroblastoma cells by inappropriately increased activity of MDM2 to keep TP53 in check. Consequently, targeted disruption of the TP53-MDM2 interaction may be a powerful means to unleash the potent anti-tumour capacities of wild-type TP53 in neuroblastoma cells without inflicting the collateral genotoxic damage associated with conventional chemotherapeutic drugs.

Conclusion

Neuroblastoma has remained a challenging disease for both clinicians and researchers for many decades. Advances in our understanding of the genetics genomics, epigenetics, and biology of neuroblastoma have provided molecular markers that predict tumour behaviour and patient outcome with very high accuracy. Together with recent information on altered signalling pathways in aggressively growing tumours, this knowledge will help to establish therapeutic strategies specifically targeting key molecular factors of neuroblastoma tumour progression.

Risk classification continues to be optimized, and future approaches will need to integrate profiling of mRNA and microRNA expression, epigenetic modifications, and whole-genome copy number variations with the current INRG system. The remaining challenges will be to bridge the gap between characterizing the molecular properties of neuroblastoma and understanding the precursor cells giving rise to the disease, focusing on those features that make the cells susceptible to malignant transformation and on determining how to combine targeted agents with standard cytotoxic agents, and when to introduce them during therapy. Furthermore, interactions between neuroblastoma and the host will need to be more clearly defined, in terms of the role of the immune response and other host-dependent factors.

It is imperative that new agents or therapeutic strategies be moved into frontline therapy to enhance induction response or maximize treatment of minimal residual disease. The focus must now shift towards multidisciplinary translational research teams using validated preclinical models to select the most promising combinations of molecularly targeted therapies, broad-spectrum chemotherapy, and immunotherapy to cure patients who currently have a poor prognosis and to reduce therapy for those with more favourable outcomes.

FURTHER READING

Acosta S, et al. (2009) Comprehensive characterization of neuroblastoma cell line subtypes reveals bilineage potential similar to neural crest stem cells. *BMC Dev Biol* **9**, 12.

Barone G, et al (2013) New strategies in neuroblastoma: therapeutic targeting of MYCN and ALK. *Clin Cancer Res* **19**, 5814–21.

Bourdeaut F, et al. (2005) Germline mutations of the paired-like homeobox 2B (PHOX2B) gene in neuroblastoma. *Cancer Lett* **228**, 51–8.

Brockmann M, et al. (2016) Small molecule inhibitors of aurora-A induce proteasomal degradation of N-Myc in childhood neuroblastoma. *Cancer Cell* **30**, 357–8.

Brodeur GM (2003) Neuroblastoma: biological insights into a clinical enigma. *Nat Rev Cancer* **3**, 203–16.

Cohn SL, et al. (2004) The International Neuroblastoma Risk Group (INRG) Classification System: an INRG Task Force. *J Clin Oncol* **27**, 289–97.

De Grandis E, et al. (2009) Long-term follow-up neuroblastoma-associated opsoclonus-myoclonus-ataxia syndrome. *Neuropediatrics* **40**, 103–11.

DuBois SG, Matthay KK (2008) Radiolabeled metaiodobenzylguanidine for the treatment of neuroblastoma *Nucl Med Biol* **35**(S1), S35–48.

DuBois SG, et al. (2016) Phase I study of the aurora A kinase inhibitor alisertib in combination with irinotecan and temozolomide for patients with relapsed or refractory neuroblastoma: a NANT (New Approaches to Neuroblastoma Therapy) trial. *J Clin Oncol* **34**, 1368–75.

Eleveld TF, et al. (2015) Relapsed neuroblastomas show frequent RAS-MAPK pathway mutations. *Nat Genet* **47**, 864–71.

Fulda S (2009) The PI3K/Akt/mTOR pathway as therapeutic target in neuroblastoma. *Curr Cancer Drug Targets* **9**, 729–37.

Gripp KW (2005) Tumor predisposition in Costello syndrome. *Am J Med Genet C Semin Med Genet* **137C**(1), 72–7.

Haas-Kogan DA, et al. (2003) Impact of radiotherapy for high-risk neuroblastoma: a Children's Cancer Group study. *Int J Radiat Oncol Biol Phys* **56**, 28–39.

Hart LS, et al. (2016) Preclinical therapeutic synergy of MEK1/2 and CDK4/6 inhibition in neuroblastoma. *Clin Cancer Res* **23**(7), 1785–96.

Henssen A, et al. (2016) Targeting MYCN-driven transcription by BET-bromodomain inhibition. *Clin Cancer Res* **22**, 2470–81.

Hirschmann-Jax C, et al. (2004) A distinct 'side population' of cells with high drug efflux capacity in human tumor cells. *Proc Natl Acad Sci USA* **101**(39), 14228–33.

Janoueix-Lerosey I, et al. (2008) Somatic and germline activating mutations of the ALK kinase receptor in neuroblastoma. *Nature* **455**, 967–70.

Maris JM (2010) Recent advances in neuroblastoma. *N Engl J Med* **362**, 2202–11.

Matthay KK, et al. (2016) Neuroblastoma. *Nat Rev Dis Primers* **2**, 16078.

Matthay K, et al. (2009) Long-term results for children with high-risk neuroblastoma treated on a randomized trial of myeloablative therapy followed by 13-cis-retinoic acid: a Children's Oncology Group study. *J Clin Oncol* **7**, 1007–13.

Monclair T, et al. (2009) The International Neuroblastoma Risk Group Staging System: an INRG task force report. *J Clin Oncol* **27**, 298–303.

Oberthuer A, et al. (2015) Revised risk estimation and treatment stratification of low- and intermediate-risk neuroblastoma patients by integrating clinical and molecular prognostic markers. *Clin Cancer Res* **21**, 1904–15.

Ohira M, Nakagawara A (2010) Global genomic and RNA profiles for novel risk stratification of neuroblastoma. *Cancer Sci* **101**, 2295–301.

Parodi S, et al. (2007) The prognostic role of urinary catecholamines in infants with disseminated neuroblastoma may be mediated by MYCN amplification. *Ped Blood Cancer* **48**, 593.

Peifer M, et al. (2015) Telomerase activation by genomic rearrangements in high-risk neuroblastoma. *Nature* **526,** 700–4.

Pinto NR, et al. (2015) Advances in risk classification and treatment strategies for neuroblastoma. *J Clin Oncol* **33**, 3008–17.

Pugh TJ, et al. (2013) The genetic landscape of high-risk neuroblastoma. *Nat Genet* **45**, 279–84.

Schleiermacher G, et al. (2014) Recent insights into the biology of neuroblastoma. *Int J Cancer* **135**, 2249–61.

Schramm A, et al. (2015) Mutational dynamics between primary and relapse neuroblastomas. *Nat Genet* **47**, 872–7.

Schramm A, et al. (2005) Biological effects of TrkA and TrkB receptor signaling in neuroblastoma. *Cancer Lett* **228**, 143–53.

Schulte JH, Eggert A (2015) Neuroblastoma. *Crit Rev Oncog* **20**, 245–70.

Schwab M, et al. (1983) Amplified DNA with limited homology to myc cellular oncogene is shared by human neuroblastoma cell lines and a neuroblastoma tumour. *Nature* **305**, 245–8.

Shimada H, et al. (1999) Terminology and morphologic criteria of neuroblastic tumors: recommendations by the International Neuroblastoma Pathology Committee. *Cancer* **86**, 349–63.

Villani A, et al. (2017) Recommendations for cancer surveillance in individuals with RASopathies and other rare genetic conditions with increased cancer risk. *Clin Cancer Res* **23**(12), e83–90.

Weiss WA, et al. (1997) Targeted expression of MYCN causes neuroblastoma in transgenic mice. *EMBO J* **16**, 2985–95.

Witt O, et al. (2009) Targeting histone deacetylases in neuroblastoma. *Curr Pharm Des* **15**, 436–47.

Yalçin B, et al. (2010) High-dose chemotherapy and autologous haematopoietic stem cell rescue for children with high-risk neuroblastoma. *Cochrane Database Syst Rev* **5**, cd 006301.

Yu AL, et al. (2010) Anti-GD2 antibody with GM-CSF, interleukin-2, and isotretinoin for neuroblastoma. *N Engl J Med* **363**, 1324–34.

29

Germ-Cell Tumours

Gabriele Calaminus and James C. Nicholson

Introduction

Germ-cell tumours (GCT) constitute a highly heterogeneous group of tumours characterized by a wide range of histologies, benign and malignant, and clinical presentation at many different anatomical sites. In adolescents and adults, over 90% of cases develop within the gonads, mostly in males, whilst around half of childhood GCT occur at extra-gonadal midline sites such as the sacrococcygeal region, central nervous system (CNS), and mediastinum. The diverse nature of GCT necessitates cooperation between paediatric oncologists and surgeons (according to tumour site) and radiation oncologists, as well as related disciplines of endocrinology and neurology. Coordination of this multidisciplinary care is critical in the success of treatment.

During the past three decades, a dramatic improvement in prognosis of malignant GCT (MGCT) has been achieved. This progress can mainly be attributed to national and international cooperative therapeutic protocols using platinum-based combination chemotherapy as part of a multimodal therapeutic approach. Identification of risk groups relating to age, histology, primary site, and stage have led to stratification of chemotherapy.

Epidemiology and biology

GCT can occur in all age groups, ranging from the fetal period to adulthood. The annual incidence is approximately 0.5 per 100,000 in children under 15. However, the overall incidence of teratomas is likely to be underestimated because of under-reporting to registries.

Registry and trial data show a distinct distribution pattern with regard to site and tumour histology of GCT. The histological subtypes of GCT in neonates are almost exclusively mature and immature teratomas (0.9 per 100,000 in girls; 2.6 per 100,000 in boys), sometimes admixed with subtle foci of yolk-sac tumours (YST). YST predominate later in infancy and during early childhood. Whilst the incidence of GCT drops steadily during childhood to below 0.1 per 100,000, a significant increase is observed after the onset of puberty (**Figure 29.1**).

In children, the most frequent primary sites of GCT are the testes (25%), ovaries (25%), sacrococcygeal region (20%), and the CNS (20%); they may also arise in the head–neck region, anterior mediastinum, retroperitoneum, and urogenital system (10%). In adolescence and young adulthood, testicular GCT are the most frequent cancer in males and females.

Sacrococcygeal, vaginal, and head and neck GCT develop during the neonatal period and infancy/early childhood. Histologically, they present as teratomas and YST (**Table 29.1**). Testicular GCT may also develop during infancy and childhood; however, they show a bimodal age distribution with a second incidence peak during adolescence and adulthood. In this age group, GCT present as seminomas and malignant non-seminomatous GCT, which may include embryonal carcinoma (EC), YST, and choriocarcinoma, often with mixed histology. In contrast, ovarian and CNS GCT predominantly develop after the onset of puberty and during the second (and third) decade of life. The remainder of this chapter will focus on the management of extracranial GCT as management of intracranial (CNS) GCT is addressed elsewhere.

Conditions predisposing to germ-cell tumours

In adolescents, there is an association between testicular GCT and testicular dysgenesis, resulting from inadequately treated undescended testes. GCT are also associated with constitutional disturbances of sex chromosomes such as Klinefelter syndrome. The risk of developing GCT is increased in phenotypic females with testicular feminization and streak gonads (frequently associated with ambiguous sexual differentiation, Swyer syndrome) and in Turner's syndrome; in these patients, Y-chromosome fragments are often detected and dysgerminoma can occur in association with gonadoblastoma. Maternal exposure to oestrogen may influence the appearance of testicular GCT in young men, an association not seen for GCT in infants and childhood.

Embryology and histological classification

GCT are believed to arise from primordial germ cells (PGC), which are totipotent and capable of differentiating into all GCT subtypes. During normal development, PGC migrate from the extra-embryonic yolk sac to the gonads; the occurrence of GCT at midline extra-gonadal sites is thought to result from aberrant migration. Despite their common origin, GCT are characterized by marked heterogeneity, impacting on their behaviour and management. Their complex classification reflects their degree of differentiation,

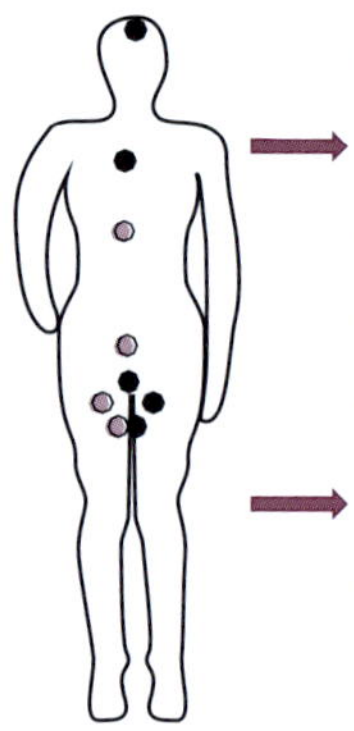

	< 18 years[1])	> 18 years[2])
Brain	20 %	3%
Mediastinum	4 %	10% (male)
Abdomen	4 %	2%
Coccyx	18 %	
Ovary	27 %	10%
Testis	25 %	85%
Other	2 %	?

Figure 29.1 Distribution of germ-cell tumours.

Source: data from: (1) Kaatsch P, et al. (2015) Pediatric germ cell tumours from 1997–2011. Incidence rates, time trends and survival. Pediatrics. 135(1), 136. doi: 10.1542/peds.2014-1989 and (2) Siegel R, et al. (2014) Cancer Statistics 2014. CA Cancer J Clin. 64(1), 9. doi: 10.3322/caac.21208.

and is based on the 2006 World Health Organization (WHO) classification of testicular cancer (Table 29.1).

Germinomatous tumours (also known as seminomas (testis), dysgerminomas (ovary), and germinomas (extragonadal)) arise from cells that remain in the pluripotent undifferentiated state with morphological features of undifferentiated germ-cell epithelium. YST and choriocarcinoma (CHC) follow an extra-embryonic differentiation pattern and are characterized by secretion of alpha-1-fetoprotein (AFP) or human chorionic gonadotropin (HCG or ß-HCG), respectively. EC consists of immature totipotent cells resulting from embryonic differentiation. Somatic differentiation results in the formation of teratomas, mature or immature, and mimicking structures of all germ layers. The histological grade of immaturity is defined by the extent of immature (predominantly neuroepithelial) elements (Table 29.2). This correlates with the risk of loco-regional relapse, particularly after incomplete resection, and is therefore essential in risk assessment of pure teratomas. Gonadoblastoma is a benign but premalignant condition, with stromal components associated with dysgenetic gonads, occurring

Table 29.1 Revised World Health Organization (WHO) classification for germ-cell tumours

	Group	Histology	Epigenetics	Genetics
Prepubertal	Germ-cell tumours of infancy and childhood	Teratoma	Premeiotic Loss of imprinting	Normal
		Yolk sac tumour		-1p,+1q, -6q,+20
Postpubertal	Germ-cell tumours of adolescence and adulthood	Teratoma	Meiosis I Loss of imprinting	+12p
		Seminoma		
		Malignant non-seminoma		
	Spermatocytic seminoma (testis)		Meiosis II Gametal imprinting	+9
	Cystic teratoma (ovary)		Meiosis II Gametal imprinting	(23,X)x2

Reproduced with permission from Stark DP, et al. 'Tumors in Adolescents and Young Adults'. *Prog Tumor Res*, Volume 43, pp. 115–127. Copyright © 2016 Basel, Karger. DOI: https://doi.org/10.1159/000447081

Table 29.2 Histological summary of paediatric germ-cell tumours

I	Germinoma[1]	A. Intratubular	
		B. Invasive	
II	Teratoma	A. Mature	
		B. Immature[2,4]	Grade 1. Immature tissue <10% of the sample surface Grade 2. Immature tissue 10–50% of the sample surface Grade 3. Immature tissue 50% of the sample surface
		C. Malignant teratoma (teratoma with non-germ-cell malignant component)	
III	Embryonal carcinoma		
IV	Yolk sac tumour[3]		
V	Choriocarcinoma		
VI	Gonadoblastoma		
VII	Mixed malignant germ-cell tumour (each component to be listed)		

1. Synonyms: dysgerminoma (ovary), seminoma (testis), germinoma (extragonadal).
2. Degree of immaturity is sometimes expressed according to Gonzalez-Crussi in terms of % of sampled surface (grade 1, <10%; grade 2, 10–50%; grade 3, >50%).
3. Yolk sac tumour is also known as endodermal sinus tumour.
4. Common to each of these: +/– microfoci of probable yolk sac tumour.

only in the presence of the Y chromosome. Left untreated it may become malignant, typically as a germinoma. In contrast to testicular GCT of adult patients, there is no evidence to suggest that paediatric GCT develop from carcinoma *in situ*.

In most patients, response to different treatment modalities can be predicted from histology and tumour-marker profile. Paediatric GCT often present with more than one histological subtype; in this situation selection of therapy is based on the strategy employed for the most aggressive malignant component.

Tumour markers

The secretion of AFP and HCG by some subtypes of GCT is well recognized and can be exploited in diagnosis and monitoring, on and off treatment. AFP, an α-globulin, has very high levels at birth as it is the main fetal serum-binding protein, but falls to adult levels of less than 12 ng/ml (less than 10 kU/l; 1 ng/ml ≡ 0.84 kU/l) between one and two years of age. Therefore, isolated AFP levels should be interpreted cautiously in children under two. AFP is produced by YST and, at low levels, by some EC and immature teratomas.

HCG is a glycoprotein produced by the placenta and made up of α and β subunits. The α subunit is structurally similar to other hormones including luteinizing hormone (LH) and follicle-stimulating hormone (FSH). So the more specific β subunit is used in assays to avoid cross reactivity with other hormones. βHCG secretion by tumour is seen typically in the presence of choriocarcinoma, with lower levels produced by some germinomas, indicating the presence of syncytiotrophoblastic giant cells. Since relative levels of 'free β' and intact dimer (α + β) vary between different tumour subtypes, measurement of 'total HCG' (both free β and dimer) is recommended.

Lactate dehydrogenase (LDH) and placental alkaline phosphatase (PLAP) are sometimes measured in GCT. LDH is a non-specific marker of malignancy of limited value in the assessment of paediatric tumours, and PLAP is raised in only around 20% of germinomas and may therefore be used as an additional diagnostic tool if elevated.

Molecular biology

The rarity of GCT and their subtypes has hampered progress in understanding their biology, although patterns are now emerging in terms of genomic changes and gene expression. The group of Ichimura et al. described similar mutations of the MTOR pathway in intracranial and testicular GCT, which underlines the common origin of the disease and the possibility to develop diagnostic and therapeutic targets for the disease regardless of the location.

Gain of the short arm of chromosome 12 (12p) is a well-recognized abnormality found almost universally in adult testicular GCT, usually arising by isochromosome formation. It has also been observed in ovarian and mediastinal GCT but is relatively rare in children. The incidence of 12p gain increases through childhood, and the pattern of imbalances seen on chromosomes 1, 6, 13, and 20 differs between pre- and postpubertal patients with mediastinal GCT. No consistent correlation between cytogenetic imbalance and primary site has been observed, and teratomas are associated with complete absence of chromosome imbalance. Pediatric GCT commonly arise at extragonadal sites. It has been proposed that non-gonadal GCT arise from ectopic primordial germ cells that have aberrantly migrated during embryogenesis. During a time between their migration and development to mature gametes, primordial germ cells are characterized by their lack of imprinting, which can be assessed by the evaluation of allelic gene expression and DNA methylation in differentially methylated control regions. Gonadal and non-gonadal GCT are derived from primordial germ cells that have consistently lost the imprinting of SNRPN and partly lost imprinting of H19 and IGF-2. More recent work has also suggested an association between global-methylation patterns and resistance to treatment.In addition, paediatric and adult MGCT differ significantly in their protein-coding gene-expression profiles (messenger RNA, mRNA), supporting the suggestion that they differ biologically, segregating by both histology and age. In contrast, and in keeping with their presumed primordial germ-cell origin, it has also been shown that MGCT all overexpress two microRNA clusters (miR 371-373 and miR 302-367), regardless of patient age, histological subtype, and anatomical site of the tumour. These are not only detectable in tumours but also in the serum and in cerebrospinal fluid (CSF) in intracranial sites. These circulating microRNAs have been found to be both sensitive and specific for the diagnosis of MGCT, with potential use in diagnosis, disease monitoring, and prognostication (**Figure 29.2**).

Diagnosis

Clinical presentation

GCT tend to occur as relatively indolent masses, with clinical symptoms determined by their site of origin. Gonadal GCT comprise around half of childhood GCT. Ovarian tumours typically occur in girls over the age of five years; they are usually teratomas or dysgerminomas, more complex mixed tumours being seen during adolescence. They present as palpable abdominal masses, often with visible distension, and there may be pain associated with torsion or rupture. Symptoms associated with hormonal disturbances such as virilization and menstrual disturbance may be seen in postpubertal patients with ovarian primaries. Testicular GCT present as painless scrotal swellings, either in the first years of life when YST and teratomas predominate, or in adolescence, when seminomas and mixed MGCT are seen.

The most common sites for extragonadal GCT are the CNS (discussed in Chapter 24, 'Other Central Nervous System Tumours of Childhood'), sacrococcygeal region, mediastinum, retroperitoneum, and head and neck, typically in the midline. Most sacrococcygeal tumours are teratomas (mature or immature) and occur more commonly in girls than boys. They may be diagnosed antenatally, by routine scanning, or as a visible mass on neonatal examination. Cases

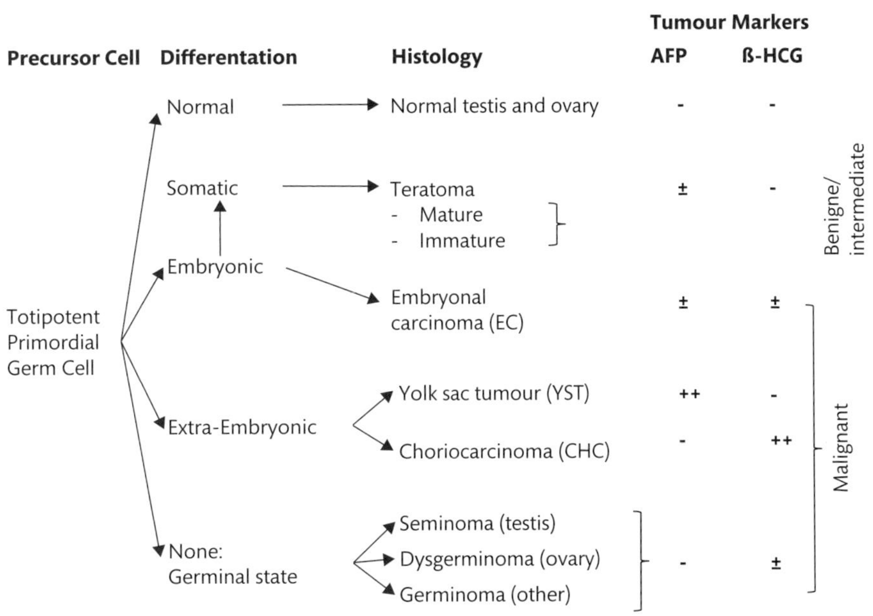

Figure 29.2 Biological characteristics of germ-cell tumours.

that present later, with partly or exclusively internal tumours, are more likely to have malignant components, typically YST, and to present with functional disturbances resulting from the effects of tumour bulk or nerve damage. Mediastinal GCT are more common in boys than girls and the majority occur from adolescence onwards, almost exclusively in the anterior mediastinum. Symptoms may result from airway compression, superior vena cava obstruction, and, occasionally, aberrant hormone production.

Approximately 20% of MGCT have metastases at the time of diagnosis, although they are rarely associated with presenting symptoms, and mostly identified as a result of staging investigations. GCT most commonly spread to the lungs, but occasionally to liver, bone, or bone marrow. Metastasis to the CNS is associated with CHC, and may be seen in approximately 4% of young males with malignant testicular GCT, but in less than 1% of cases in younger children. This possibility should therefore be borne in mind in patients with very high levels of HCG.

Investigations

Radiology and staging

In many patients with extracranial GCT, initial assessment will be made with ultrasound of the abdomen and pelvis, and should include assessment of tumour position and size, as well as the presence of lymphatic spread or peritoneal seeding. This is followed by detailed three-dimensional imaging with computed tomography (CT) or magnetic resonance imaging (MRI) scan. CT scan is required for assessment of lung metastases and extent of abdominal disease. MRI is the investigation of choice for sacrococcygeal GCT, in order to define extension into the sacral and spinal canal. Plain X-rays have limited value in initial assessment, except for mediastinal tumours, but are valuable in follow-up, particularly chest X-ray. Skeletal metastases and bone-marrow involvement are seen in less than 10% of patients overall, and are rare in the absence of pulmonary metastases, but are particularly associated with malignant sacrococcygeal GCT. Technetium bone scan should therefore be considered in the presence of organ metastases. CNS imaging only needs to be considered in patients (mainly adolescent males) in which CHC is identified histologically or by markers. The use of positron emission tomography (PET) scans is controversial but might add important information for patients with bulky disease after chemotherapy and with negative markers under treatment, to evaluate response other than by reduction of tumour volume.

Laboratory investigations

AFP and total HCG should be measured in all cases of suspected GCT, as raised tumour markers may be of value in diagnosis and monitoring of GCT, both on and off treatment: caution should be exercised in interpretation of AFP levels in infants. GCT may be treated without tissue diagnosis on the basis of radiological findings and raised tumour markers, although histological confirmation is usually available at diagnosis in gonadal tumours, for which primary excision is part of treatment. Neoadjuvant chemotherapy with delayed surgery may be the treatment of choice for some extragonadal GCT, in which case raised markers may obviate the need for potentially hazardous biopsy. However, in equivocal cases (non-diagnostic markers, hepatic or upper retroperitoneal tumours), a diagnostic biopsy should be performed, and should include storage of fresh tumour tissue for genetic and biological studies. Where a biopsy is performed in a mixed tumour, the GCT components in the tissue diagnosis may differ from the subtype suggested by marker estimation, or may under-report the range of histologies present as a result of sampling error. This is unlikely to influence treatment, provided that the tumour is fully staged.

Thresholds above which marker levels can be considered diagnostic are controversial. For AFP, moderately elevated levels may be consistent with the presence of microfoci of YST or immature hepatic/intestinal elements in immature teratomas. HCG may be moderately elevated in germinomas, and levels up to 50 IU/l are usually considered consistent with this diagnosis, although caution should be exercised in labelling levels any higher than this as CHC, given that CHC are rare in young people and typically associated with HCG levels over 1,000 IU/l.

In female patients with ovarian GCT and in male patients with mediastinal GCT, constitutional karyotyping is also recommended.

In addition to routine blood tests before chemotherapy, special consideration should be given to assessment of renal function as most regimens used for treatment of GCT incorporate nephrotoxic agents including platinum compounds and ifosfamide.

Treatment

Surgery

Most extracranial GCT are amenable to primary resection, and this is the treatment of first choice for localized tumours. If the diagnosis of an MGCT has been made histologically or with raised markers, and the initial radiological assessment shows infiltration or metastatic spread, preoperative chemotherapy will increase the likelihood of microscopically complete resection. In general, there is no role for debulking surgery in pediatric GCT. In patients with tumour residual after initial resection, second-look surgery is essential. Surgical removal of metastases is not indicated unless they show insufficient response to chemotherapy. Close attention to surgical recommendations for GCT is essential to optimize outcomes whilst minimizing morbidity.

Testis

The resection of testicular tumours is performed as unilateral orchidectomy after high inguinal incision, to avoid scrotal contamination; transscrotal surgery will lead to upstaging of tumours which might otherwise be stage 1, with the result that patients may receive chemotherapy that could have been avoided. There is no evidence that retroperitoneal lymph-node dissection improves prognosis in children, and it leads to increased morbidity including risk to future sexual function.

Ovary

Primary surgical resection (salpingo-oopherectomy) is standard management in ovarian GCT. Ascitic fluid or peritoneal washings should be collected for cytological examination, and biopsies of any suspicious area on peritoneal surfaces, lymph nodes, omentum, or contralateral ovary performed. Unresectable or bilateral tumours should be biopsied with a view to fertility-preserving surgery where possible, following neoadjuvant chemotherapy, except in the presence of gonadoblastoma or XY gonadal dysgenesis, when bilateral gonadectomy is recommended. Whilst oophorectomy remains standard practice for mature teratomas of the ovary, there is a trend towards more conservative fertility preservation surgery. This kind of surgery should be done in experienced centres to avoid tumour-cell spillage and to deliver the balance between maximal resection of the tumour and preservation of ovarian tissue.

Coccyx

A dorsal approach to sacrococcygeal tumours is appropriate for most cases in view of their predominantly external components. Some have substantial internal components deep in the pelvis for which an additional anterior approach via laparotomy is required. The coccyx should be resected en bloc to avoid tumour rupture, and infiltrated skin areas should also be removed en bloc with the tumour. Separation of tumour and rectum is mostly possible with digital control, and bowel and bladder function recover postoperatively in the majority of patients.

Other sites

MGCT at other extragonadal sites such as the mediastinum, retroperitoneum, and genitourinary tract are less likely to be amenable to complete resection, and the surgical approach should be individualized.

Evolution of chemotherapeutic strategies—balancing efficacy and toxicity

Until 1980, the prognosis of children with MGCT was poor. The modern era of GCT chemotherapy began in the mid-1970s with the identification of the efficacy of cisplatin in testicular GCT, given in combination with vinblastine and bleomycin (PVB) following tumour resection. With this regimen, the overall good response rate was also translated into durable remissions. Nevertheless, the challenge of relapsed or refractory tumours established the need for second-line therapies. Etoposide soon emerged as an active drug with a single-agent efficacy superior to vinblastine. The resulting combination of cisplatin, etoposide, and bleomycin (BEP) is now standard chemotherapy for GCT in adult patients. The efficacy of ifosfamide in cisplatin-refractory GCT has since been demonstrated, and combinations of cisplatin with ifosfamide and either etoposide or vinblastine for recurrent testicular GCT are considered standard relapse treatment. These observations led to studies incorporating ifosfamide into the first-line treatment of GCT, and although the inclusion of ifosfamide with cisplatin and etoposide (PEI) did not result in significantly improved outcome, this demonstrated that MGCT could be treated successfully with combination chemotherapy from which bleomycin is excluded.

Selection of suitable chemotherapeutic regimes is based on a balance between efficacy and adverse effects. Cisplatin has been retained in the majority of first-line treatment approaches for GCT but it is associated with a risk of toxicity to kidneys and hearing. For this reason, strategies employing carboplatin instead of cisplatin have been explored. However, although the auditory and renal toxicity of carboplatin-based regimens are less than for cisplatin, carboplatin is more myelotoxic at therapeutically equivalent doses. Whilst this has not been found to be a dose-limiting effect in children, adult patients may tolerate this less well and there has been some reluctance to pursue a carboplatin-based approach in adult protocols. Pulmonary toxicity is the main concern associated with the use of bleomycin, particularly in older patients and the very young, and in the presence of renal impairment. These concerns have led to the development of regimens omitting bleomycin or using it at a reduced dose. The cisplatin, etoposide, and ifosfamide (PEI) combination is associated with a higher degree of myelosuppression and also carries a risk of tubular nephropathy, particularly in small children. Etoposide, used in the majority of GCT strategies in both adults and children, carries the risk of secondary leukaemia, estimated to be in the region of 1% over ten years of follow-up.

Development of cooperative protocols

Prospective trials for gonadal and non-gonadal GCT in children and adolescents were initiated by national groups in the 1980s. Early experience from North American (Children's Cancer Group; CCG) studies showed that patients with ovarian GCT had a better prognosis than children with non-gonadal GCT due to the higher rate of incomplete tumour resections in non-gonadal tumours. A subsequent American Intergroup protocol adopted the 'watch and wait' policy for stage I testicular GCT and achieved good results for intermediate-risk patients (testicular stage II, ovarian and non-gonadal stages I and II) with four cycles of cisplatin, etoposide, and bleomycin. In high-risk patients (stages III and IV), the therapeutic impact of cisplatin-dose intensification (200 mg/m^2/cycle) was evaluated, indicating that higher doses of cisplatin may result in higher response and complete remission rates, but without improvement in overall survival (OS)OS. Furthermore, high-dose cisplatin was also associated with higher rates of renal and auditory toxicity. A subsequent report from this study group failed to demonstrate a protective benefit of amifostine against hearing loss during cisplatin therapy at escalated doses.

UK experience with the UKCCSG GC I and GC II protocols also demonstrated the high therapeutic efficacy of platinum-based regimens and promoted the use of carboplatin-based chemotherapy (JEB (carboplatin–etoposide–bleomycin) utilizing carboplatin at 600 mg/m^2/cycle) in preference to cisplatin (BEP). Results of 184 patients treated between 1989 and 1997 confirmed the high efficacy of the JEB regimen, with five-year event-free survival (EFS) of 88% and OS of 93%, comparable to outcomes with cisplatin-based strategies from other national groups and with a favourable toxicity profile.

The French cooperative protocol TGM 85 used a similar chemotherapeutic approach, and in the consecutive TGM 90 protocol, cisplatin was replaced by carboplatin (400 mg/m^2/cycle). The results were less favourable than with the UKCCSG JEB regimen, the difference attributed mainly to the lower dose of carboplatin. In both the French TGM 90 and the UK GC II studies, the analysis of prognostic factors revealed the prognostic impact of high serum AFP levels at diagnosis, a finding that was not reproduced by other studies that used a cisplatin-based regimen.The German protocols for testicular (MAHO) and non-testicular (MAKEI) GCT included cisplatin and etoposide-based chemotherapy regimens, with recommendations for delayed tumour resection after neoadjuvant chemotherapy. Even from the beginning of the 1980s, EFS rates above 80% were achieved with the first MAKEI and MAHO protocols, resulting in a step-wise reduction in duration of chemotherapy from a maximum of eight cycles to six and, currently, four or five. As with strategies used by other national groups, an expectant 'watch and wait' strategy was introduced in the MAKEI 96 protocol for patients with completely resected low-stage tumours. This resulted in sparing of chemotherapy for almost 75% of patients with stage Ia MGCT. A neoadjuvant approach to locally invasive and/or metastatic tumours was shown to facilitate complete tumour resection.

Current therapeutic approaches

In general, current paediatric GCT strategies stratify therapy according to initial diagnostic parameters, and only in cases of insufficient response to treatment is therapy further intensified. Although there is some variation between protocols in the application of risk factors, there are common themes, summarized in Table 29.3.

Gonadal tumours are considered lower risk than extragonadal, but this is largely because they are more likely to be completely resected. Increasing age is generally associated with increased risk, and often associated in older teenagers with higher-risk adult-type histology. The impact of metastases on risk and the need for treatment intensity varies according to the type of tumour, and the risk associated with high levels of AFP is of uncertain significance. Complete control of disease at primary and metastatic sites is essential in all cases, and residual disease following treatment confers a relatively adverse prognosis. A collaboration between the UK's Children's Cancer

Table 29.3 Standard chemotherapy regimens for paediatric extracranial germ-cell tumours

PEI	**MAKEI 96, MAHO 98**		
Cisplatin[1]	20 mg/m²	Over 1 h	Day 1,2,3,4,5
Etoposide	100 mg/m²	Over 3 h	Day 1,2,3
Ifosfamide[2]	1500 mg/m²	Over 3 or 20 h	Day 1,2,3,4,5
Two to four cycles			
PVB	**MAHO 98**		
Cisplatin[1]	20 mg/m²	Over 1h	Day 4,5,6,7,8
Vinblastin	3 mg/m² or 0.15 mg/kg	IV bolus	Day 1,2
Bleomycin[3]	15 mg/m²	Over 24 h	Day 1,2,3
Three cycles			
BEP	**MAHO 98**		
Bleomycin[3]	15 mg/m²	Over 24 h	Day 1,2,3
Etoposide	80 mg/m²	Over 3 h	Day 1,2,3
Cisplatin[1]	20 mg/m²	Over 1 h	Day 4,5,6,7,8
Three cycles			
BEP	**USA: Children's Oncology Group**		
Bleomycin	15 mg/m²	Over 24 h	Day 1
Etoposide	100 mg/m²	Over 3 h	Day 1,2,3,4,5
Cisplatin[1]	20 mg/m²	Over 1 h	Day 1,2,3,4,5
Four cycles			
High-dose BEP	**USA: Children's Oncology Group**		
Bleomycin	15 mg/m²	Over 24 h	Day 1
Etoposide	100 mg/m²	Over 3 h	Day 1,2,3,4,5
Cisplatin[1]	40 mg/m²	Over 1 h	Day 1,2,3,4,5
Four cycles			
JEB	**UKCCSG/CCLG GC3**		
Carboplatin	600 mg/m²	Over 1 h	Day 2
Etoposide	120 mg/m²	Over 1 h	Day 1,2,3
Bleomycin[3]	15 mg/m²	Over 15 min	Day 3
Four or six cycles			
PE	**Brazilian GCT group**		
Cisplatin	20/30 mg/m²	Over 1 h	Day 1,2,3,
Etoposide	100/120 mg/m²	Over 1 h	Day 1,2,3,4,5
Five cycles			

1. Given with mannitol-forced diuresis.
2. Given with mesna uroprotection.
3. Omitted in children <1 year, and at reduced dose (7.5 mg/m²) in children <2 years.

and Leukaemia Group (CCLG) and the USA's Children's Oncology Group (COG), with pooling of trial data, helped to refine risk factors further, with age and stage being the most important predictors; the greater risk often attributed to extragonadal tumours is more likely to be a consequence of age and stage than site in itself, as shown also in publications by other groups.The approach to treatment of MGCT can be summarized as follows:

- Surgical resection at diagnosis, where possible, with inguinal approach for testicular tumours, and sampling of ascites and nodules for ovarian tumours.
- Biopsy or marker diagnosis in unresectable tumours.
- 'Watch and wait' for completely resected stage 1 gonadal primaries avoids chemotherapy in over 70% of cases, and effective salvage is available for the remainder.
- Platinum-based chemotherapy for all stage II–IV patients; ranging from two cycles of a two-drug regimen for completely resected stage II (MAKEI) to four to six cycles of a three-drug regimen for highest risk (stage IV extragonadal).
- Surgery following chemotherapy for residual tumour.
- There is no place for radiotherapy in the first-line treatment of extracranial GCT.

Approach to treatment of teratomas

Mature teratomas are considered benign and are cured by surgical excision which should be complete in order to avoid recurrence. Sacroccoccygeal teratomas may recur as malignant tumours in around 10% of cases, underlining the need to aim for complete excision and also to monitor AFP closely for recurrence. Surgical excision is also the mainstay of treatment for immature teratomas and although they may show clinical features of malignancy, a role for chemotherapy has not been established. The risk of recurrence can be estimated from the primary site of the tumour, histological grade of immaturity, and completeness of the tumour resection. Pure immature teratomas of the ovary may be associated with secondary peritoneal deposits for which surgery remains the treatment of choice. The significance of small foci of YST and/or mildly raised AFP in immature teratomas is uncertain and management subject to controversy. If small YST foci are present and an incomplete resection has been obtained, a close 'watch and wait' procedure with tumour-marker follow-up (AFP) is mandatory.

Follow-up

Most relapses occur within the first two years after diagnosis, although much later recurrences have been observed. Most groups would therefore recommend close monitoring of markers for secreting GCT and imaging, at least for marker-negative GCT, for three to five years from the end of treatment. AFP and ß-HCG are usually monitored weekly until they reach the normal range, then at reduced frequency (every one to three months) for the remaining period of follow-up. In 'watch and wait' patients, the decline of AFP level should be evaluated with respect to its serum half-life of approximately six to seven days. The interpretation of AFP may be difficult in infants but a slowing of the rate of decline or a secondary rise in AFP level strongly suggests the presence of residual or recurrent YST.

Imaging of the primary site of tumour should be undertaken at the end of treatment. In the case of residual abnormalities after chemotherapy, further surgery is indicated, even in a secreting tumour with normalized markers, since mature teratomas may remain after successful treatment of the malignant component of a mixed tumour, imposing a risk of tumour progression. PET scans have not been proven useful in this situation, as they cannot readily distinguish between mature teratomas and residual necrosis or fibrosis.

Monitoring for late effects of treatment needs to be tailored to the treatment received. Audiometry should be performed during and at the end of treatment in patients who have received cisplatin therapy. Patients who have received bleomycin require lung-function testing. Although routine monitoring of blood counts is not indicated, the risk of treatment-related secondary leukaemia should be considered as part of routine follow-up, in patients who have received etoposide.

Relapse treatment

There is no international consensus on strategies for treatment of recurrent GCT. In patients previously treated with a carboplatin-based or non-platinum-based therapy, cisplatin-based regimens such as PEI or VIP (vinblastine, ifosfamide, cisplatin) have been used successfully. Failure following primary treatment with cisplatin may be treated with carboplatin and etoposide. Newer relapse strategies are increasingly exploiting the efficacy of gemcitabine, oxaliplatin, and taxol in combination.

In Germany, a standardized strategy is used for patients with local recurrent extracranial MGCT in the abdomen. This is a combination of local deep hyperthermia with platinorientatated chemotherapy (HyperPEI). Results are promising and reveal a salvage rate of about 70%. Aggressive local therapy is central to the strategy because most relapse occurs at the primary site. Local radiotherapy, at doses above 45 Gy, has shown some benefit after incomplete resection of the recurrent tumour. Radiotherapy may also be useful in the treatment of brain metastases.

The therapeutic value of high-dose chemotherapy with autologous stem-cell transplantation has been investigated in a small number of patients with relapsed or refractory disease, but further clinical trial evidence is needed to establish the role of high-dose therapy more clearly. Long-term survival is likely to be achieved only in those patients in whom clinical complete remission can be achieved by other treatment prior to high-dose chemotherapy.

Future perspectives

In view of the high cure rates achieved by current protocols for standard-risk GCT, research should now focus on the better identification of patients more likely to fail first-line treatment, the intensification of treatment in high-risk patients, and the reduction of therapy with its associated toxicities in low-risk cases.

As insufficient local tumour control at the primary site represents the main problem in most relapsing patients, further advances in outcomes for relapsed GCT may depend on improvements in local therapy. Novel approaches need to be explored for high-risk GCT. Locoregional hyperthermia combined with platinum-based chemotherapy offers a therapeutic concept in locally recurrent extracranial tumours. The augmentation of standard treatment with the development of targeted therapies to oncogenes, growth factors, and receptors should also be a goal for the future.

Timely progress in these areas for such a rare tumour group requires multinational cooperation in both biological studies and clinical trials. A strong focus is also needed on the rehabilitation and quality of life of the survivors of GCT, and such outcomes should be taken into consideration when planning treatment.

FURTHER READING

Baranzelli MC, et al. (1999) Prognostic factors in children with localized malignant nonseminomatous germ cell tumors. *J Clin Oncol* **17**(4), 1212.

Billmire D, et al. (2004) Outcome and staging evaluation in malignant germ cell tumors of the ovary in children and adolescents: an intergroup study. *J Pediatr Surg* **39**(3), 424–9.

Blohm ME, et al. (1998) Alpha 1-fetoprotein (AFP) reference values in infants up to 2 years of age. *Pediatr Hematol Oncol* **15**(2), 135–42.

Bokemeyer C (2002) Extragonadal germ cell tumors of the mediastinum and retroperitoneum. Results from an international analysis. *J Clin Oncol* **20**(7), 1864–73.

Calaminus G, et al. (2003) Prognostic value of tumor size, metastases, extension into bone, and increased tumor marker in children with malignant sacrococcygeal germ cell tumors. A prospective evaluation of 71 patients treated in the German cooperative protocols Maligne Keimzelltumoren (MAKEI) 83/86 and MAKEI 89. *J Clin Oncol* **21**(5), 781–6.

Cushing B, et al. (2004) Randomized comparison of combination chemotherapy with etoposide, bleomycin, and either high-dose or standard-dose cisplatin in children and adolescents with high-risk malignant germ cell tumors. A pediatric intergroup study—Pediatric Oncology Group 9049 and Children's Cancer Group 8882. *J Clin Oncol* **22**(13), 2691–700.

De Giorgi U, et al. (2005) Salvage high-dose chemotherapy for children with extragonadal germ-cell tumours. *Br J Cancer* **93**(4), 412–17.

Eble JN, et al. (eds) (2004) *World Health Organization Classification of Tumours. Pathology and Genetics of the Urinary System and Male Genital Organs*. Lyon: IARC.

Einhorn LH, Donohue JP (1977) Improved chemotherapy in disseminated testicular cancer. *J Urol* **117**(1), 65–9.

Frazier AL, et al. (2015) Revised risk classification for pediatric extracranial germ cell tumors based on 25 years of clinical trial data from the United Kingdom and United States. *J Clin Oncol* **33**(2), 195–201.

Fukushima S, et al. (2014) Mutually exclusive mutations of KIT and RAS are associated with KIT mRNA expression and chromosomal instability in primary intracranial pure germinomas. *Acta Neuropathol* **127**(6), 911–25.

Göbel U, et al. (2001) Multimodal treatment of malignant sacrococcygeal germ cell tumors. A prospective analysis of 66 patients of the German cooperative protocols MAKEI 83/86 and 89. *J Clin Oncol* **19**(7), 1943–50.

Göbel U, et al. (2010) Brain metastases in children and adolescents with extracranial germ cell tumor—data of the MAHO/MAKEI-registry. *Klin Pädiatrie* **222**(3), 140–4.

Göbel U, et al. (2014) Testicular germ cell tumors in adolescents—results of the protocol MAHO 98 and the identification of good risk patients. *Klin Padiatrie* **226**(6–7), 316–22.

Heifetz SA, et al. (1998) Immature teratomas in children: pathologic considerations. A report from the combined Pediatric Oncology Group/Children's Cancer Group. *Am J Surg Pathol* **22**(9), 1115–24.

Kaatsch P, et al. (2015) Pediatric germ cell tumours from 1997–2011. Incidence rates, time trends and survival. *Pediatrics* **135**(1), 136.

Lopes LF, et al. (2009) Cisplatin and etoposide in childhood germ cell tumor: Brazilian Pediatric Oncology Society protocol GCT-91. *J Clin Oncol* **27**(8), 1297–303.

Mann JR, et al. (1998) UKCCSG's germ cell tumour (GCT) studies: improving outcome for children with malignant extracranial non-gonadal tumours—carboplatin, etoposide, and bleomycin are effective and less toxic than previous regimens. United Kingdom Children's Cancer Study Group. *Med Pediatr Oncol* **30**(4), 217–27.

Mann JR, et al. (2000) The United Kingdom Children's Cancer Study Group's second germ cell tumor study: carboplatin, etoposide, and bleomycin are effective treatment for children with malignant extracranial germ cell tumors, with acceptable toxicity. *J Clin Oncol* **18**(22), 3809–18.

Marina N, et al. (2005) Amifostine does not protect against the ototoxicity of high-dose cisplatin combined with etoposide and bleomycin in pediatric germ-cell tumors: a Children's Oncology Group study. *Cancer* **104**(4), 841–7.

Murray MJ, et al. (2016) A pipeline to quantify serum and cerebrospinal fluid microRNAs for diagnosis and detection of relapse in paediatric malignant germ-cell tumours. *Br J Cancer* **114**(2), 151–62.

Murray MJ, et al. (2016) The present and future of serum diagnostic tests for testicular germ cell tumours. *Nat Rev Urol* **13**(12), 715–25.

Palmer RD, et al. (2007) Malignant germ cell tumours of childhood: new associations of genomic imbalance. *Br J Cancer* **96**(4), 667–76.

Palmer RD, et al. (2010) Malignant germ cell tumors display common microRNA profiles resulting in global changes in expression of messenger RNA targets. *Cancer research* **70**(7), 2911–23.

Pashankar F, et al. (2016) Is adjuvant chemotherapy indicated in ovarian immature teratomas? A combined data analysis from the Malignant Germ Cell Tumor International Collaborative. *Cancer* **122**(2), 230–7.

Perlman EJ, et al. (2000) Genetic analysis of childhood endodermal sinus tumors by comparative genomic hybridization. *J Pediatr Hematol Oncol* **22**(2), 100.

Poynter JN, et al. (2010) Trends in incidence and survival of pediatric and adolescent patients with germ cell tumors in the United States, 1975 to 2006. *Cancer* **116**, 4882–91.

Schmoll H-J, et al. (2003) Long-term results of first-line sequential high-dose etoposide, ifosfamide, and cisplatin chemotherapy plus autologous stem cell support for patients with advanced metastatic germ cell cancer: an extended phase I/II study of the German Testicular Cancer Study Group. *J Clin Oncol* **21**(22), 4083–91.

Schneider DT, et al. (1999) Acute myelogenous leukemia after treatment for malignant germ cell tumors in children. *J Clin Oncol* **17**(10), 3226–33.

Schneider DT, et al. (2000) Primary mediastinal germ cell tumors in children and adolescents: results of the German cooperative protocols MAKEI 83/86, 89, and 96. *J Clin Oncol* **18**(4), 832–9.

Schneider DT, et al. (2001) Genetic analysis of childhood germ cell tumors with comparative genomic hybridization. *Klin Padiatrie* **213**(4), 204–11.

Schneider DT, et al. (2001) Multipoint imprinting analysis indicates a common precursor cell for gonadal and nongonadal pediatric germ cell tumors. *Cancer Res* **61**(19), 7268–76.

Schneider DT, et al. (2002) Genetic analysis of mediastinal nonseminomatous germ cell tumors in children and adolescents. *Genes Chromosomes Cancer* **34**(1), 115–25.

Schneider DT, et al. (2004) Epidemiologic analysis of 1,442 children and adolescents registered in the German germ cell tumor protocols. *Pediatr Blood Cancer* **42**(2), 169–75.

Siegel R, et al. (2014) Cancer Statistics 2014. *CA Cancer J Clin.* **64**(1), 9.

Veltman I, et al. (2005) Identification of recurrent chromosomal aberrations in germ cell tumors of neonates and infants using genomewide array-based comparative genomic hybridization. *Genes Chromosomes Cancer* 43(4), 367–76.

Wermann H, et al. (2010) Global DNA methylation in fetal human germ cells and germ cell tumours: association with differentiation and cisplatin resistance. *J Pathol* **221**(4), 433–42.

Wessalowski R, et al. (2013) Regional deep hyperthermia for salvage treatment of children and adolescents with refractory or recurrent non-testicular malignant germ-cell tumours: an open-label, non-randomised, single-institution, phase 2 study. *Lancet Oncol* **14**(9), 843–52.

30

Childhood Liver Tumours

Giorgio Perilongo and József Zsiros

Introduction

Childhood liver tumours are a heterogeneous group of neoplasms encompassing individually rare histological varieties. Hepatoblastoma and hepatocellular carcinoma are the two most frequent subtypes; undifferentiated sarcoma of the liver, atypical teratoid/rhabdoid tumour, primary hepatic germ-cell tumour, lymphoma, angiosarcoma are examples of other, very rare primary liver tumours in childhood. This chapter will focus only on hepatoblastoma and hepatocellular carcinoma.

Hepatoblastoma

Biology

Hepatoblastoma is an embryonal tumour of the liver. The term 'embryonal' implies that its origin is related to a derangement in the mechanisms regulating normal hepatic organogenesis. Various hypotheses have already linked the different histological subtypes of hepatoblastoma to specific stages of the arrest of normal hepatic organogenesis. It is hypothesized that hepatoblastoma arises from undifferentiated hepatic stem cells or human fetal liver multipotent progenitor cells (hFLMPC) capable of differentiation into a variety of tissues. This phenomenon could explain why there are histological differences between the various hepatoblastomas and why almost 40% of them have mixed histological components including both epithelial and mesenchymal elements. Further investigation is required to clarify which developmental signalling, and transcriptional pathways are affected and at what level, and for what reason such changes occur. Nevertheless, different genetic abnormalities have been described in association with hepatoblastoma.

Hepatoblastoma, as most of paediatric tumours do, presents with a limited number of cytogenetic alterations and genetic mutations (average 2.9 mutations per case). Mutation of the β-catenin (*CTNNB1*) gene, the key molecule of the Wnt signalling pathway, represents the only recurrent alteration found in two thirds of hepatoblastoma. Hepatoblastoma is the tumour with the most interstitial deletions or missense mutations in the *CTNNB1* gene (reported in 60–70% of the cases). Mutations in other components of the β-catenin degradation complex, including those affecting the APC and AXIN2, have also been reported. Thus, overall, the Wnt pathway is involved in about 90% of the genetic abnormalities documented in hepatoblastoma. Due to mutations in β-catenin it bypasses the proteasomal degradation pathway and is translocated into the nucleus where it acts as a transcriptional activator and can be detected by immunohistochemistry. Potential prognostic relevance of this finding has been proposed. It has been recently shown that the Hippo pathway (YAP) most likely cooperates with β-catenin in the pathogenesis of hepatoblastoma. The mechanism of YAP activation and its cooperation with β-catenin remain to be discovered.

Microarray analysis shows that the glypican 3 (*GPC3*) gene, mutated in Simpson–Golabi–Behmel tissue overgrowth syndrome, in which an association with an increased risk of hepatoblastoma development has been hypothesized, is one of the most overexpressed genes in hepatoblastoma.

Growth regulation of hepatoblastoma involves the insulin-like growth factor II (IGF2) signalling pathway. IGF2 is a maternally imprinted gene and encodes a fetal peptide hormone that regulates cell proliferation, differentiation, and cell migration. IGF2 is expressed in hepatoblastoma, inversely correlated with the degree of differentiation: it is lacking in fetal-type cells and high in embryonal-type cells. High expression of IGF2 is the hallmark of the Beckwith–Wiedemann syndrome—an overgrowth syndrome characterized by hemihypertrophy and organomegaly—and this finding could explain the higher incidence of hepatoblastoma in children affected by this condition.

Epidemiology

The estimated incidence of hepatoblastoma is 1.2 per million, with a male prevalence, but no geographical variations have been reported. Little is know about the risk factors for hepatoblastoma development. A consistent association appears to exist between risk of hepatoblastoma and very low birthweight; duration of oxygen therapy has been identified as a significant factor associated with that risk. The International Agency for Research on Cancer has recently classified tobacco smoke (via parental smoking) as a human carcinogen for childhood hepatoblastoma.

Most cases of hepatoblastoma are sporadic but at least three congenital conditions have been linked to an excess risk: trisomy 18, Beckwith–Wiedemann syndrome, and familial adenomatous polyposis (FAP). For patients with Beckwith–Wiedemann syndrome, the risk of developing hepatoblastoma in those children presenting uniparental disomy on chromosome 15.5 is increased to 4.7%. For this reason, routine screening with ultrasound and serum AFP is recommended at least during the first years of life. Children with a positive family history of FAP have a 750- to 7,500-fold increased risk of developing hepatoblastoma. An accurate family history aiming to identify the presence of a positive history of FAP is part of the diagnostic work-up of all children with hepatoblastoma.

The suggestion that hepatoblastoma is a developmental aberration is supported by the fact that a wide spectrum of congenital malformation syndromes and isolated anomalies have been reported in cases of hepatoblastoma. The overall frequency of anomalies among children with hepatoblastoma appears to be higher than for any paediatric tumour other than Wilms.

Clinical presentation

Hepatoblastoma is a tumour of early childhood, with more than 80% of the patients being diagnosed under the age of two years. An asymptomatic abdominal mass in an otherwise healthy young child is the classical presenting feature of hepatoblastoma, and systemic symptoms are rarely present. The presence of clinical signs of associated syndromes, such as Beckwith–Wiedemann syndrome, should always be sought and may dominate the clinical picture. The hallmark of hepatoblastoma is an elevated serum level of alpha fetoprotein (AFP), although tumours associated with normal or low (less than 100 ng/ml) levels of AFP do occur, but are very rare (less than 2%). Levels may be more difficult to interpret in very young infants because of the high physiological production of AFP, and should always be interpreted in relation to the normal range for age. Extremely high levels of AFP in some patients can generate erroneously low results on standard laboratory testing and require appropriate serum dilution for a reliable assessment. Paraneoplastic abnormalities of calcium metabolism can occur with a picture of pseudo-osteoporosis and spontaneous fractures. Rarely, hepatoblastoma can also secrete β-human chorionic gonadotropin (β-HCG) which may result in pseudo-precocious puberty in males. Thrombocytosis, related to the hyperproduction of thrombopoietin by tumour cells, is frequently documented at presentation. Infrequently, a child with hepatoblastoma will present with an acute abdomen due to tumour rupture or intra-tumoural haemorrhage.

Diagnosis

Whilst the presence of a hepatic mass in a young child, associated with elevated AFP, is extremely suggestive of the diagnosis of hepatoblastoma, surgical biopsy is required to establish histological diagnosis.

Radiological investigation is required to define the extent of the primary disease and confirm or exclude the possibility of metastases. Abdominal ultrasound and computed tomography (CT) and/or magnetic resonance imaging (MRI) scans are the conventional tools to document the presence, extension, and characteristics of a hepatic mass. As slightly more than 20% of patients present with lung metastases, contrast-enhanced CT of the lung is part of the diagnostic work-up for any child presenting with hepatoblastoma.

Laboratory investigations should include a full blood count and serum AFP and β-HCG. In most children with hepatoblastoma, liver-function tests are within normal limits.

Histological classification

In order to reach a consensus on the histopathology and classification of paediatric liver tumours, and hepatoblastoma in particular, an International Pathology Symposium was organized in 2011. Pathologists expert in paediatric liver tumors, including those serving as central reviewers of the major cooperative clinical trials, convened together. The histological classification of malignant paediatric liver tumours that they elaborated is reported in **Box 30.1**.

Box 30.1 SIOPEL classification of primary malignant paediatric liver tumours

Epithelial tumours

Hepatocellular

Hepatoblastoma

- Epithelial variants
  - Pure fetal with low mitotic activity
  - Fetal, mitotically active
  - Pleomorphic, poorly differentiated
  - Embryonal
  - Small-cell undifferentiated
  - INI1-negative
  - INI1-positive
  - Epithelial mixed (any/all of above)
  - Cholangioblastic
  - Epithelial macrotrabecular pattern

Mixed epithelial and mesenchymal

- Without teratoid features
- With teratoid features

Hepatocellular carcinoma (HCC)

- Classic HCC
- Fibrolamellar HCC
- Hepatocellular neoplasm not otherwise specified (NOS)

Biliary

Cholangiocarcinoma

Combined (hepatocellular cholangioca)

Mesenchymal tumours

Malignant

Embryonal sarcoma

Rhabdomyosarcoma

Vascular tumours

Epithelioid haemangioendothelioma

Angiosarcoma

Other malignancies/tumours of uncertain origin

Malignant rhabdoid tumour INI1-negative (documented INI1 mutation or INI1-positive)

Nested epithelial stromal tumour

Other

Germ-cell tumour

Teratoma

Yolk sac tumour

Reproduced with permission from López-Terrada et al. 'Towards an international pediatric liver tumor consensus classification: proceedings of the Los Angeles COG Liver Tumors Symposium'. *Modern Pathology*, Volume 27, pp. 472–491. DOI: https://doi.org/10.1038/modpathol.2013.80

About 55% of hepatoblastomas are epithelial (30% fetal, 20% fetal-embryonal, 3% macrotrabecular, 2% small-cell undifferentiated), and 45% are mixed epithelial and mesenchymal. However, when all types are considered, around 85% contain both fetal and embryonal components in variable proportions. Evidence is accumulating that small-cell undifferentiated hepatoblastoma is associated with unfavourable outcome, whilst pure fetal hepatoblastoma with a low mitotic index (less than 2 mitoses per 10 HPF (high-power fields)), if completely resected, has an excellent outcome even without adjuvant treatment.

Staging and risk stratification

Two different systems to describe tumour extension or stage are presently in use: one used by the North American Cooperative Group on Childhood Hepatic Tumors, and another one used by the International Childhood Liver Tumour Strategy Group (SIOPEL group), consisting mainly of European investigators. The American system is based on the results of the initial surgical procedure (postsurgical system). It encompasses four stages:

- Stage I—complete tumour resection without microscopical residual
- Stage II— tumour grossly resected with evidence of microscopical residual
- Stage III— tumour unresectable or resected with gross residual tumour or positive lymph nodes
- Stage IV— tumours presenting with metastases.

A progressive decline in the survival rate with evolution of stage in this system has been firmly documented.

The SIOPEL group developed an alternative system that describes tumour extension before any surgery (presurgical system); this is known as the PRETEXT system (*pre*treatment *ext*ension of the disease). It has been developed in accordance with the surgical anatomy of the liver, based on the vascular structures. This identifies four sectors, two in each lobe. The PRETEXT category is defined by the number of sectors involved by the tumour (see **Table 30.3**). The presence of distant metastases is identified by the addition of the letter 'M'; extension of tumour into portal vein is indicated by the letter 'P'; extension into the vena cava and/or hepatic veins by the letter 'V'; and the presence of intra-abdominal extrahepatic disease by the letter 'E'. The prognostic relevance of the PRETEXT system has also been well documented.

In 2011, a global coalition, the Children's Hepatic Tumours International Collaboration (CHIC), was constituted with the main aim of creating a common approach to staging and risk stratification in hepatoblastoma. The data derived from the prospective randomized trials conducted by the North American, European, German, and Japanese cooperative trials on hepatobalstoma were merged in a single large database. A total of 1,650 children were entered into that database. The patient risk-stratification system they elaborated is reported in **Figure 30.1**

In summary, within the backbone of the PRETEXT system it clearly emerged that the completeness of surgical resection still remains the most important single prognostic factor for hepatoblastoma, and only those children in whom complete tumour resection is achieved can hope for cure. The second most important, negative prognostic factor is the presence of metastases at diagnosis. Furthermore, the analysis of the data so far collected confirms the fact that a normal (for age) or low level (less than 100 ng/ml) of AFP is a hallmark of a poorer prognosis: in the SIOPEL group experience, three-year overall survival (OS) of children presenting with low or normal AFP was around 15%. An association between small-cell undifferentiated hepatoblastoma and low or normal for age AFP has been proposed. Finally, the age of the patients also emerged as a potential prognostic factor, with a different cut-off within each PRETEXT category.

The biological meaning of this risk stratification is still to be investigated. Similarly, the impact of the different histological subtypes of hepatoblastoma is a matter of current analysis. However, solid evidence supports the concept that hepatoblastoma with pure fetal histology and low mitotic activity is associated with a very good outcome whilst, alternatively, small-cell undifferentiated tumours carry a dismal prognosis.

Treatment strategies

The goal of any therapeutic strategy directed at the cure of children with hepatoblastoma is to achieve complete tumour resection, although surgery alone is not sufficient and the best chance of cure can only be realized with a multidisciplinary treatment strategy that also includes systemic chemotherapy. The two major cooperative groups offer different approaches to primary treatment. The North American Children's Oncology Group (COG) utilizes a strategy based on an initial attempt at surgical resection (primary surgery) regardless of the tumour extension within and/or outside the liver. In contrast, the SIOPEL group takes an approach based on the use of primary chemotherapy before definitive surgery (neoadjuvant chemotherapy) regardless of the initial tumour extension. The rationale for using primary chemotherapy is to reduce the tumour volume and to make the tumour more solid, less prone to bleed, and better demarcated from the surrounding healthy liver parenchyma and, ultimately, more easily resected. The results of these two strategies have been comparable, both achieving five-year OS and event-free survival (EFS) rates of over 70%.

Historically, the most significant step in improving the prognosis of hepatoblastoma was the introduction of cisplatin-based chemotherapy, after which resection rate and three-year OS improved from historical rates of 44% and 30% to more than 80% and 70%, respectively. COG conducted a trial that compared cisplatin (90 mg/m^2 as an infusion over six hours) followed by doxorubicin (80 mg/m^2 as a continuous infusion over 96 hours) with the combination of cisplatin (delivered as per above) on day one, and vincristine (1.5 mg/m^2) and 5-fluorouracil (600 mg/m^2) on day two (C5V). They subsequently chose C5V as their standard chemotherapy, not because there was a significant difference between the two regimens but because of a difference in toxicity profiles. It should be noted, however, that while tumour progression accounted for 86% of all reported events for patients treated with C5V, it represented only 56% of all events observed in those patients treated with cisplatin/doxorubicin. The SIOPEL group has adopted the combination cisplatin (90 mg/m^2 as an infusion over 24 hours) followed by doxorubicin (60 mg/m^2 infusion over 48 hours) as its therapeutic gold standard. The COG recently conducted an upfront window vincristine /irinotecan (VI) treatment of high-risk hepatoblastoma. In the 32 children they enrolled, three-year EFS and OS rates were 49% (95% CI, 30–65%) and 62% (95% CI, 42–77%), respectively. These data allowed them to conclude that the VI combination appears to have substantial activity against high-risk hepatoblastoma.

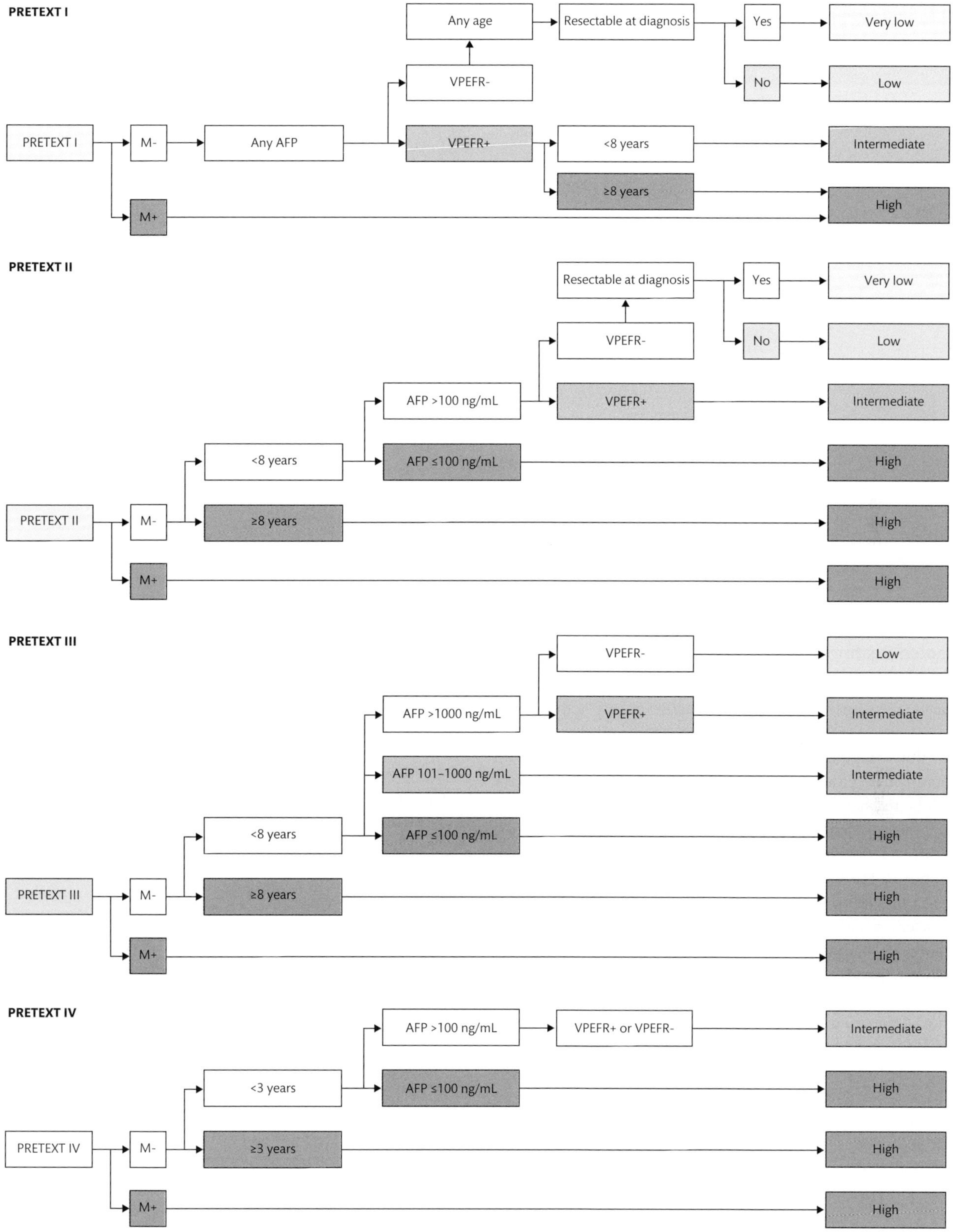

Figure 30.1 Risk-stratification trees from the Children's Hepatic Tumors International Collaboration

AFP = α-fetoprotein; M = metastases; PRETEXT = PRETreatment EXTent of disease group; VPEFR = macro-vascular involvement of hepatic veins (V) or portal bifurcation (P), contiguous extrahepatic tumour (E), multifocal tumour (F), and spontaneous rupture (R).

Reproduced with permission from Meyers RL, et al. 'Risk-stratified staging in paediatric hepatoblastoma: a unified analysis from the Children's Hepatic Tumors International Collaboration'. *Lancet Oncology*, Volume 18, Issue 1, pp. 122–131. Copyright © 2017 Elsevier Ltd. DOI: 10.1016/S1470-2045(16)30598-8

Table 30.1 Results of the North American trials for childhood hepatoblastoma

Trial	Type of trial/inclusion criteria	Regimen	Outcome
CCG 862	Single arm All patients	Vincristine + cyclophosphamide/doxorubicin alternating with vincristine, cyclophosphamide, 5-fluorouracil	3-year OS: Stage I = 94% Stage II = 57% Stage III = 20% Stage IV = 14%
CCG 823F	Single arm	Cisplatin/doxorubicin	2-year OS: Stage II = 86% Stage III = 58% Stage IV = 32%
POG 8697	Single arm	Cisplatin/vincristine/5-fluorouracil	4-year OS: Stage I/PFH = 100% Stage I/II = 90% Stage III = 67% Stage IV = 12%
INT 0089	Prospective randomized trial	Cisplatin/vincristine/5-fluorouracil vs cisplatin/doxorubicn	4-year OS: Stage I/II 100% vs 96% Stage III 66% vs 71% Stage IV 33% vs 42%
POG 9345	Single arm Stage III/IV	Carboplatin followed by carboplatin/vincristine/ 5-fluorouracil	4-year OS: Stage III =73% Stage IV = 27%
COG P9645	Prospective randomized Stage III/IV	Cisplatin/vincristine/5-fluorouracil vs cisplatin/carboplatin	3-year OS: All patients = 75% vs 56%

Stage I = microscopic complete resection; Stage II = microscopical residuals; Stage III = macroscopical residual; Stage IV = presence of metastases; OS = overall survival.

Risk-adapted treatment

In the course of subsequent clinical trials, these two principal regimens have been further refined. COG achieved 100% three-year survival in children with pure fetal hepatoblastoma after gross complete resection (Stage I and II, favourable histology) with adjuvant chemotherapy using four cycles of C5V. These excellent results have prompted the further reduction of chemotherapy to only two cycles for most of these patients and, for children with completely resected (Stage I) pure fetal hepatoblastoma and low mitotic index (less than 2 mitoses per 10 HPF), omission of all adjuvant chemotherapy. On the other hand, children with unresectable and metastatic tumour still do not enjoy satisfactory long-term outcome and have OS of approximately 50% and 30% respectively. The current COG strategy is to explore whether the addition of doxorubicin will benefit patients with unresectable localized disease, whilst the very poor results achieved in patients with metastases at diagnosis has prompted a search for new agents using a therapeutic 'window approach'.

The SIOPEL group have been able to show that cisplatin alone is as effective as combination cisplatin/doxorubicin in children with standard-risk hepatoblastoma (data from SIOPEL 3 SR study—see Table 30.2). For children with high-risk hepatoblastoma, the SIOPEL group undertook a trial (SIOPEL 3) exploring the use of alternating courses of cisplatin and the combination of carboplatin/doxorubicin. The results were encouraging, with improved EFS and OS estimates at three years of 65% (95% CI, 57–73%) and 69% (95% CI, 62–77%) for the whole group, 75% and 77% for patients with PRETEXT-IV tumours, and 57% and 63% for those with lung metastases.

In the subsequent generation of clinical trials directed at children with advanced hepatoblastoma, the SIOPEL group looked into a further intensification in the use of cisplatin, based on the weekly administration. Three-year OS and EFS of the whole cohort of high-risk hepatoblastoma were 79% (95% CI, 66–87%) and 83% (73–93%) respectively. Particularly significant were the results achieved in the group of children presenting with metastases, whose corresponding figures were 77% (95% CI, 63–90%) and 79% (95% CI, 66–92%) respectively

Concerns about the ototoxicity and nephrotoxicity of cisplatin have stimulated both the COG and the SIOPEL group to investigate the possibility of integrating the use of toxicity-protective agents within their standard regimens. The SIOPEL group has recently closed a prospective randomized controlled trial in low-risk hepatoblastoma that tested the role of sodium thiosulfate (STS), an otoprotective agent, in preventing hearing loss in children treated with cisplatin alone. The preliminary data indicate that STS does not jeopardize the prognosis of these children and significantly reduces the hearing loss that these children may suffer.

The results of the series of trials so far run by the North American Study Group and by SIOPEL are reported in Tables 30.1 and 30.2, while their present therapeutic recommendations are summarized in Table 30.3.

Following the earlier cooperation between the SIOPEL group and COG, large cooperative trials on childhood hepatoblastoma will be launched in the near future. The therapeutic recommendations of these trials are reported in Table 30.3.

Orthotopic liver transplantation

In the past two decades, the role of orthotopic liver transplantation for children with hepatoblastoma has been quite clearly delineated. In summary, children with hepatoblastoma eligible for transplant should meet the following criteria:

Table 30.2 Results of the International Childhood Liver Tumor Strategy Group (SIOPEL) trials for childhood hepatoblastoma

Trial	Type of trial/inclusion criteria	Regimen	Outcomes
SIOPEL 1	Single arm/all patients	Cisplatin/doxorubicin	5-year OS 66% 3-year EFS 75%
SIOPEL 2 SR	Single arm SR-HB	Cisplatin alone	3-year OS 91% (±7%) 3-year PFS 89% (±7%)
SIOPEL 2 HR	Single arm HR-HB	Cisplatin and carboplatin/doxorubicin	3-year OS 53% (±13%) 3-year PFS 48% (±13%)
SIOPEL 3 SR	Prospective randomized trial SR-HB	Cisplatin/doxorubicin vs cisplatin alone	Cisplatin/doxorubicin: 3-year OS 93% (±5%) 3-year EFS 85% (±7%) Cisplatin alone: 3-year OS 95% (±4%) 3-year EFS 83% (±7%)
SIOPEL 3 HR	Single arm HR-HB	Cisplatin and carboplatin/doxorubicn	3-year OS 69(±7)% 3-year EFS 65(±8)%
SIOPEL 4 HR	Single arm HR-HB	Weekly cisplatin with doxorubicin and carboplatin	3-year OS 83% (±10%) 3-year EFS 79% (±8%)

SR = standard risk; HR = high risk; SR-HB = standard-risk hepatoblastoma: tumour confined to the liver, involving at the most three hepatic sectors associated with alpha fetoprotein >100 ng/ml; HR-HB = high-risk hepatoblastoma: tumour involving the entire liver, and/or presenting with metastases, and/or with vascular invasion, and/or with extrahepatic abdominal disease, and/or with alpha fetoprotein <100 ng/ml; EFS = event-free survival; OS= overall survival; PFS = progression-free survival.

- They have had a response to chemotherapy—a criterion which implies that any child with hepatoblastoma should be treated with chemotherapy regardless of the type of resection which is envisaged.
- They have a tumour completely confined to the liver but deemed unresectable. Usually these are those clearly involving all four sectors of the liver as judged by magnetic resonance imaging (MRI) scan and/or angiography, or which lie so close to the main vessels at the hilum of the liver and/or to the hepatic veins to make a tumour-free excision margin highly unlikely.

The presence of metastases at diagnosis is not an absolute contra-indication to transplant but requires complete clearing of the lungs with chemotherapy. In managing a child who may be a potential candidate for transplantation, it is important to ensure early assessment by a transplant team, so that the treatment strategy can be carefully timed.

Table 30.3 Hepatoblastoma: summary of the therapeutic recommendations of the Children's Oncology Group and of the SIOPEL group, according to the PRETEXT system

PRETEXT	Therapeutic recommendation
Small I/M−	Surgery at diagnosis (primary surgery) Completely resected UH-CDDP x 2 If complete resection and pure fetal histology, no further therapy
II/M−	Upfront chemotherapy CDDP x 2 Surgery CDDP x 2 vs CDDP x 4
III and IV/M−	Three-arm randomization: Historical COG regimen—CV5D vs SIOPEL 3 High-risk regime—CDDP alternating with carbo/DOXO vs SIOPEL 3 Standard-risk regimen—CDDP alone
M+	Upfront chemotherapy as per SIOPEL 4 regimen—weekly CDDP/DOXO and, based on clearing of the metastases, CDDP/DOXO vs I/V or CDDP/DOXO vs CDDP/DOXO alternating I/V

C5VD = cisplatin, vincristine, 5-fluorouracil, doxorubicin; CDDP = cisplatin; DOXO = doxorubicin; I = irinotecan; V = vincristine; M− or M+ = absence or presence of metastases; S = surgery; UH = unfavourable histology, meaning no pure fetal hepatoblastoma with low mitotic index.

Hepatocellular carcinoma

Hepatocellular carcinoma is an even rarer tumour than hepatoblastoma. Among the 213 liver tumour cases diagnosed in the UK National Registry of Childhood Tumours between 1995 and 2006, there were 154 (72.3%) cases of hepatoblastoma and 22 of hepatocellular carcinoma, including five fibrolamellar tumours (10.3%). All other diagnoses represented a heterogeneous group of even rarer primary liver tumours. Hepatoblastoma dominated the under one year and one to four years age groups, with low rates for other tumours. In 5–9 and 10–14 year olds there was a more even distribution of rates between the tumour groups, but hepatocellular carcinoma had a higher incidence than other tumours in 10–14 year olds, albeit still very low in absolute terms.

The majority of hepatocellular carcinoma cases across all ages seen in developing countries are due to hepatitis B virus infection (HBV) and to aflatoxin exposure, while in developed countries, the more common aetiological links are to alcohol abuse and smoking. Hepatitis C virus (HCV) is also a factor, especially in Japan. The incidence of hepatocellular carcinoma in HBV hyperendemic areas in China and Thailand appears to have fallen. Hepatocellular carcinoma may also arise in children with various inherited metabolic disorders.

Similar to hepatoblastoma, a hard abdominal mass is the classical presenting symptom of hepatocellular carcinoma, but is more commonly associated with systemic symptoms such as fatigue, anorexia, and abdominal pain. Jaundice is rare but has been reported. In cases that arise in the context of pre-existing liver conditions, the clinical features of the underlying disease may dominate the clinical picture. Seventy per cent of patients with hepatocellular carcinoma presented with elevated AFP. In patients with a fibrolamellar carcinoma,

AFP level is normal but high-serum vitamin B12-binding capacity (transcobalamin) has been shown to be elevated and may be used as a tumour marker. Finally, the serological evidence of pre-existing infection or of metabolic conditions may be present in affected patients.

The diagnostic strategy is similar to that described for hepatoblastoma. Abdominal ultrasound and contrast-enhanced CT or MRI scans serve to delineate tumour extension within the liver and abdomen, chest CT is recommended to rule out lung metastases, and the definitive diagnosis relies on the histological assessment of a biopsy.

The prognosis of children with hepatocellular carcinoma is unsatisfactory. Results from the use of cisplatin and doxorubicin, with surgery, in the first SIOPEL study gave five-year EFS and OS of 17% and 28%, respectively. No improvement in the prognosis was observed in the subsequent study, where an alternating regimen with cisplatin, carboplatin, and doxorubicin was used, and long-term survival is reported only among the group of patients who achieve complete resection. The experience of the North American group is comparable: 46 patients were enrolled in the INT-0098 trial which compared treatment with cisplatin/doxorubicin with the C5V regimen. EFS at five years was 19% for the whole cohort, but ranged from 88% for children with completely resected (Stage I) tumour to 0% for those with metastatic disease.

There is still some uncertainty about the role of chemotherapy in hepatocellular carcinoma and the place of liver transplantation is less well established than for hepatoblastoma. However, the introduction of biological agents, specifically sorafenib, a small-molecule multikinase inhibitor, is opening new approaches to the treatment of this challenging tumour.

FURTHER READING

Alkhouri N, et al. (2010) Familial adenomatous polyposis in children and adolescents. *J Pediatr Gastroenterol Nutr* **51**, 727–32.

Aronson DC, et al. (2005) Predictive value of the pretreatment extent of disease system in hepatoblastoma: results from the International Society of Paediatric Oncology Liver Tumour Study Group SIOPEL-1 study. *J Clin Oncol* **23**, 1245–52.

Brown J, et al. (2000) Pretreatment prognostic factors for children with hepatoblastoma—results from the International Society of Paediatric Oncology (SIOP) study SIOPEL 1. *Eur J Cancer* **36**, 1418–25.

Bell A, et al. (2017) Novel advances in understanding of molecular pathogenesis of hepatoblastoma: a Wnt/βcatenin prospective. *Gene Expr* **17**(2), 141–54.

Bulterys M, et al. (1999) Hepatic tumors. In: LAG Ries, et al. (eds) *Cancer Incidence and Survival among Children and Adolescents: United States SEER Program 1975–1995*, pp. 91–7. NIH Pub. No. 99-4649. Bethesda, MD: National Cancer Institute, SEER Program.

Czauderna P, et al. (2002) Hepatocellular carcinoma in children; results of the first prospective study of the International Society of Pediatric Oncology. *J Clin Oncol* **20**, 2798–804.

Czauderna P, et al. (2016) The Children's Hepatic Tumors International Collaboration (CHIC): novel global rare tumor database yields new prognostic factors in hepatoblastoma and becomes a research model. *Eur J Cancer* **52**, 92–101.

De Ioris M, et al. (2008) Hepatoblastoma with a low serum alpha-fetoprotein level at diagnosis: the SIOPEL group experience. *Eur J Cancer* **44**, 545–50.

Eichenmüller M, et al. (2014) The genomic landscape of hepatoblastoma and their progenies with HCC-like features. *J Hepatol* **61**, 1312–20.

Katzenstein HM, et al. (2002) Treatment of unresectable and metastatic hepatobalstoma: a Pediatric Oncology Group Phase II Study. *J Clin Oncol* **20**, 3438–44.

Katzenstein HM, et al. (2002) Hepatocellular carcinoma in children and adolescents: results from the Pediatric Oncology Group and the Children's Cancer Group Intergroup Study. *J Clin Oncol* **20**, 2789–97.

Kitanovski L, et al. (2009) Multifocal hepatoblastoma in a 6-month-old girl with trisomy 18: a case report. *J Med Case Reports* **3**, 8319.

Li J, et al. (2008) Cancer incidence among children and adolescents in the United States, 2001–2003. *Pediatrics* **121**, e1470–77.

López-Terrada D, et al. (2014) Towards an international pediatric liver tumor consensus classification: proceedings of the Los Angeles COG Liver Tumors Symposium. *Mod Pathol* **27**(3), 472–91.

Malogolowkin MH, et al. (2006) Intensified platinum therapy is an ineffective strategy for improving outcome in pediatric patients with advanced hepatoblastoma. *J Clin Oncol* **24**, 2879–84.

Malogolowkin MH, et al. (2008) Redefining the role of doxorubicin for the treatment of children with hepatoblastoma. *J Clin Oncol* **26**, 2379–83.

Meyers RL, et al. (2017) Risk-stratified staging in paediatric hepatoblastoma: a unified analysis from the Children's Hepatic Tumors International Collaboration. *Lancet Oncol* **18**(1), 122–31.

O'Neill AF, et al. (2017) Characterization of pulmonary metastases in children with hepatoblastoma treated on Children's Oncology Group Protocol AHEP0731 (the treatment of children with all stages of hepatoblastoma): a report from the Children's Oncology Group. *J Clin Oncol* 35(30), 3465–73.

Ortega JA, et al. (1991) Effective treatment of unresectable or metastatic hepatoblastoma with cisplatin and continuous infusion doxorubicin chemotherapy: a report from the Children's Cancer Study Group. *J Clin Oncol* **9**, 2167–76.

Ortega JA, et al. (2000) Randomized comparison of cisplatin/vincristine/fluorouracil and cisplatin/continuous infusion doxorubicin for treatment of pediatric hepatoblastoma: a report from the Children's Cancer Group and the Pediatric Oncology Group. *J Clin Oncol* **18**, 2665–75.

Otte JB, et al. (2004) Liver transplantation for hepatoblastoma: results from the International Society of Pediatric Oncology (SIOP) Study SIOPEL-1 and review of the world experience. *Pediatr Blood Cancer* **42**, 74–83.

Perilongo G, et al. (2000) Hepatoblastoma presenting with lung metastases: treatment results of the first cooperative, prospective study of the International Society of Paediatric Oncology on childhood liver tumors. *Cancer* **89**, 1845–53.

Perilongo G, et al. (2004) Risk-adapted treatment for childhood hepatoblastoma. Final report of the second study of the International Society of Paediatric Oncology—SIOPEL 2. *Eur J Cancer* **40**, 411–21.

Perilongo G, et al. (2009) Cisplatin versus cisplatin plus doxorubicin for standard risk hepatoblastoma. *N Engl J Med* **361**, 1662–70.

Pritchard J, et al. (2000) Cisplatin, doxorubicin, and delayed surgery for childhood hepatoblastoma: a successful approach—results of the first prospective study of the International Society of Pediatric Oncology. *J Clin Oncol* **18**, 3819–28.

Roebuck DJ, et al. (2007) 2005 PRETEXT: a revised staging system for primary malignant liver tumours of childhood developed by the SIOPEL Group International Childhood Liver Tumor Strategy Group. *Pediatr Radiol* **37**, 123–32.

Roebuck DJ, et al. (2007) Assessment of extrahepatic abdominal extension in primary malignant liver tumours of childhood. *Pediatr Radiol* **37**, 1096–100.

Trobaugh-Lotrario AD, et al. (2009) Small cell undifferentiated variant of hepatoblastoma: adverse clinical and molecular features similar to rhabdoid tumors. *Pediatr Blood Cancer* **52**(3), 328–34.

Zimmermann A (2005) The emerging family of hepatoblastoma tumours: from ontogenesis to oncogenesis. *Eur J Cancer* **41**, 1503–14.

Zsíros J, et al. (2010) Successful treatment of childhood high risk hepatoblastoma with dose intensive multiagent chemotherapy and surgery—final results of the SIOPEL-3HR study of the Childhood Liver Tumor Strategy Group. *J Clin Oncol* **28**, 2584–90.

Zsiros J, et al. (2013) Dose-dense cisplatin-based chemotherapy and surgery for children with high-risk hepatoblastoma (SIOPEL-4): a prospective, single-arm, feasibility study. *Lancet Oncol* **14**(9), 834–42.

31

Retinoblastoma

Guillermo Chantada and Carlos Rodríguez-Galindo

Introduction

Retinoblastoma is a malignant tumour arising from the embryonic neural retina and occurs in about one in 14,000–18,000 live births. Thus, an estimated 8,000 children develop retinoblastoma each year worldwide. In some less developed countries, an increased incidence of retinoblastoma has been reported; however, in others, a similar pattern to developed nations was found. The reason for this is not known; environmental or genetic factors may play a role. When retinoblastoma is diagnosed in the intraocular stage (as it usually occurs in the most affluent countries), disease-free survival has been over 90% for the past decades. However, in less developed countries, retinoblastoma is diagnosed later, when the disease has disseminated to extraocular sites. Consequently, survival in these countries is lower than 50% for most affected children.

Presenting signs and symptoms

Retinoblastoma presents in two distinct clinical forms:

1. The bilateral or multifocal, hereditary form (30–35% of cases) is characterized by the presence of germline mutations of the *RB1* gene. These may be the result of a new germline mutation (in 75% of cases) or may be inherited from an affected survivor (accounting for the remaining 25% of cases). In less developed countries, familial cases are less common.
2. The unilateral form (65–70% of cases) is mainly sporadic (in about 90% of cases); the remaining 10% have germline mutations. However, in the absence of a positive family history, it is not possible, without performing a mutational analysis, to determine which unilateral cases are inheritable (Figure 31.1).

Patients with bilateral retinoblastoma tend to present before one year of age, and those with unilateral disease often present in the second or third year of life. However, there are wide variations in the age of diagnosis in different countries, according to the degree of socioeconomical development; children in less developed countries are diagnosed at a later age. It is uncommon for retinoblastoma to be diagnosed during the first month of life, except in familial cases where screening is performed. However, regardless of the family history, more than 90% of neonatal cases have either bilateral disease at presentation or will develop asynchronous bilateral retinoblastoma.

The presenting features of retinoblastoma vary according to the level of socioeconomic development. In developing countries, late diagnosis is common and patients usually present with proptosis and an orbital mass, often with pre-auricular adenopathy (Figure 31.2). In developed countries, the most common presenting signs are the presence of a white reflex in the child's eye (leukocoria; Figure 31.2), which occurs in two thirds of cases, or, less frequently, strabismus. Less common presenting signs include a painful red eye, glaucoma, poor vision, orbital cellulitis, hyphema, or unilateral mydriasis. Even though leukocoria is frequently present, it may be overlooked since it may be only seen when the child looks sideways. It may also be noticeable in a flash photograph. Whilst leukocoria is a relatively specific sign with few differential diagnoses, strabismus is very common in children and often due to a benign cause. However, the occurrence of strabismus in a young child calls for a dilated examination of the retina, with special attention given to the macula.

A syndrome associated with deletion of the long arm of chromosome 13 (the 13q deletion syndrome) has been reported, with mental retardation and dysmorphic features. Identification of these anomalies may precede the recognition of concomitant retinoblastoma. Such children require karyotype analysis and retinal examination.

Trilateral retinoblastoma refers to the association of bilateral retinoblastoma with an asynchronous intracranial embryonal tumour. This association can occur in about 3% of patients with the genetic form, and appears to be more common in familial cases. The prognosis has until recently been almost uniformly fatal, but with current therapies results may be more encouraging. Even though it can be detected concomitantly with intraocular retinoblastoma, the interval between the diagnosis of bilateral retinoblastoma and the diagnosis of the brain tumour is usually around 20 months.

Biology

Retinoblastoma was the first cancer to be described as a genetic disease. In 1971, Knudson proposed the 'two-hit hypothesis', in

If parent was ...

	Bilateral	Unilateral	Unaffected
Chance of offspring having retinoblastoma	45% affected; 55% unaffected	7-5% affected; 85-93% unaffected	<<1% affected; 99% unaffected
Laterality	85% bilateral; 15% unilateral; 0%	85% bilateral; 15% unilateral; 0%	33% bilateral; 67% unilateral; 0%
Focality	100% multifocal; 96% multifocal; 4% unifocal; 0%	100% multifocal; 96% multifocal; 4% unifocal; 0%	100% multifocal; 15% multifocal; 85% unifocal; 0%
Chance of next sibling having retinoblastoma	45%; 45%; 45%; 45%	45%; 45%; 45%; 7-15%	5%*; <1%*; <1%*; <1%

*If parent is a carrier, then 45%

Figure 31.1 Card for genetic counselling of retinoblastoma.
Reproduced courtesy of David H. Abramson, Chief, Ophthalmic Oncology Service, Memorial Sloan-Kettering Cancer Center, New York, USA

which two mutational events in a developing retinal cell lead to the development of retinoblastoma. This hypothesis was subsequently extended to suggest that the two events could be mutations of both alleles of the *RB1* gene. *RB1* is located within chromosome 13q14. Its product, pRb, is a key substrate for G1 cyclin-cdk complexes, which phosphorylate target gene products required for the transition of the cell through the G1 phase of the cell cycle. pRb is the major gatekeeper controlling growth regulation, and its lack or inactivation removes the constraint on cell-cycle control. The *RB1* is a large gene, and mutations have been described in almost every exon. There are no mutational hot spots, although new germline mutations have an overwhelming preference for the paternal allele. This second hit occurs at a much higher frequency than the first hit, and it is more sensitive to environmental factors such as ionizing irradiation, thus explaining the increased risk of irradiation-induced malignancies in survivors of retinoblastoma.

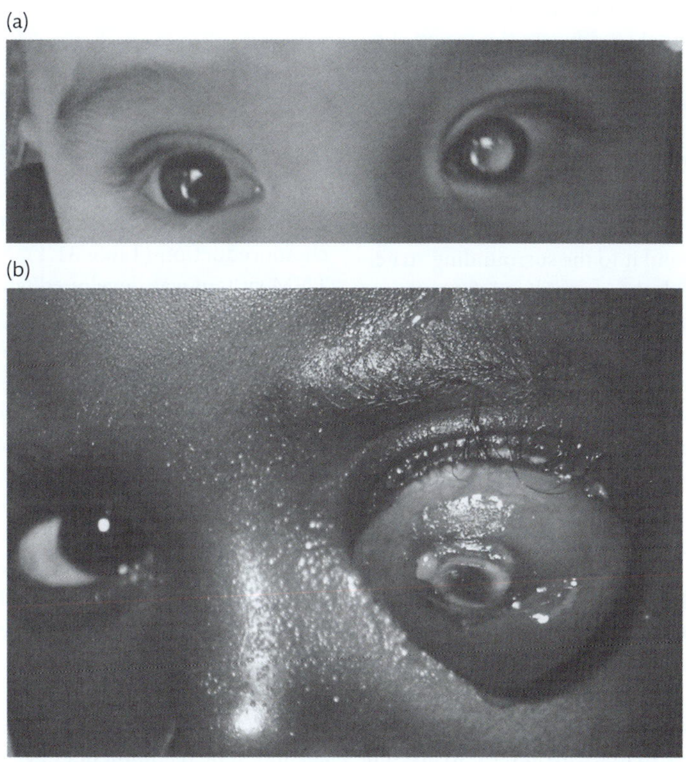

Figure 31.2 Clinical presentation of retinoblastoma: (top) massive orbital dissemination; (bottom) leukocoria.
Reproduced courtesy of Kahaki Kimani, Senior Lecturer, Department of Ophthalmology, University of Nairobi, Kenya.

Recently, cases of retinoblastoma with no RB1 mutation but MYCN amplification in small children with unilateral involvement were reported.

Identification of the cell of origin of retinoblastoma remains elusive. Recent studies suggested that it derives from cone precursors, but other reports suggest that more than one cell can be implicated.

Histology

Retinoblastoma is a tumour of neuro-epithelial origin consisting of small, undifferentiated, anaplastic cells with scanty cytoplasm and large nuclei that stain deeply with haematoxylin, arising from the nucleated layer of the retina. Calcification usually occurs in necrotic areas. Retinoblastoma cells often express photoreceptor-differentiation antigens, neuron-specific enolase and the ganglioside GD2 (but not CD99), glial fibrillary acidic protein, or S-100. Retinoblastoma cells may show features of photoreceptor differentiation and Flexner–Wintersteiner rosettes, which are characteristic of retinoblastoma but may be present in other ophthalmic tumours (medulloepithelioma). Alternatively, it may present with highly undifferentiated retinoblasts or a mixed pattern.

The tumour may grow either in an endophytic pattern seeding the vitreous or in an exophytic form into the subretinal space. The active seeds of retinoblastoma can remain viable for long periods following chemotherapy or radiation. When the tumour grows from the retina outwards into the subretinal space (exophytic pattern), it produces retinal detachment, sometimes with no clear view of the mass, and can resemble Coats disease or other forms of exudative retinal detachment. Both vitreous and subretinal seeding are the major obstacles to curing intraocular tumours with chemotherapy, because of the difficulty of chemotherapy to reach these areas with low vascular supply.

Retinoblastoma can disseminate outside the eye, through the optic nerve and/or the subarachnoid space to the chiasm, the brain, and the meninges. It can also escape from the eyeball, through the sclera, and invade the orbit and beyond it to the surrounding structures. The tumour cells can also reach the choroid and, from there, may gain access to the systemic circulation, giving rise to haematogenous metastasis involving the bone, bone marrow, or any other organ. Metastatic retinoblastoma usually involves the central nervous system (CNS), either as a solitary mass or multiple lesions, or with leptomeningeal dissemination. It can also invade facial structures such as the pre-auricular lymph nodes and the bones of the skull.

Diagnostics and extent of disease evaluation

Grouping and staging

A grouping system for intraocular disease, generated by international experts, has been in use for the past 15 years (Box 31.1), and recently data were incorporated into the tumour–node–metastasis (TNM) system. For staging of extraocular disease, a group of international retinoblastoma experts developed, by consensus, a staging system that articulates with the intraocular grouping system proposed for the eye-conserving therapies with chemoreduction (Table 31.1). More recently, a new version of the TNM system was developed which also incorporates imaging and heredity data.

Box 31.1 International Grouping System for intraocular disease

Group A

Small tumours away from foveola and disc
- Tumours <3 mm in greatest dimension confined to the retina, and
- Located at least 3 mm from the foveola and 1.5 mm from the optic disc

Group B

All remaining tumours confined to the retina
- All other tumours confined to the retina not in Group A
- Subretinal fluid (without subretinal seeding) <3 mm from the base of the tumour

Group C

Local subretinal fluid or seeding
- Local subretinal fluid alone >3 mm to <6 mm from the tumour
- Vitreous seeding or subretinal seeding <3 mm from the tumour

Group D

Diffuse subretinal fluid or seeding
- Subretinal fluid alone >6 mm from the tumour
- Vitreous seeding or subretinal seeding >3 mm from the tumour

Group E

Presence of one or more of these poor prognosis features
- More than two thirds of globe filled with the tumour
- Tumour in anterior segment
- Tumour in or on the ciliary body
- Iris neovascularization
- Neovascular glaucoma
- Opaque media from haemorrhage
- Tumour necrosis with aseptic orbital cellulitis
- Phthisis bulbi

Imaging studies

All children with retinoblastoma should undergo gadolinium-enhanced magnetic resonance imaging (MRI) of the orbits and brain. MRI is preferred to computed tomography (CT) scan because it allows for a better estimation of the invasion to the optic nerve, it evaluates accurately the pineal area. and it avoids the exposure to radiation in these susceptible patients. MRI is also helpful in the differential diagnosis with Coats disease and other inflammatory conditions, and with persistent hyperplastic primary vitreous (PHPV). Given the short interval between the diagnosis of retinoblastoma and the occurrence of trilateral retinoblastoma, routine screening with MRI every six months until five years of age might be recommended, yet it is not clear whether earlier diagnosis can impact survival. Benign pineal cysts may be encountered in these children, causing occasional diagnostic and management dilemmas.

Table 31.1 International Staging for Retinoblastoma

Stage	Description
Stage 0	Patients treated conservatively (subject to presurgical ophthalmological classifications)
Stage I	Eye enucleated, completely resected histologically
Stage II	Eye enucleated, microscopic residual tumour
Stage III	Regional extension a) Overt orbital disease b) Preauricular or cervical lymph-node extension
Stage IV	Metastatic disease a) Haematogenous metastasis—1. Single lesion; 2. Multiple lesions b) CNS extension—1. Prechiasmatic lesion; 2. CNS mass; 3. Leptomeningeal disease

Ancillary studies

Additional evaluation of metastatic disease needs to be considered only in patients with International Retinoblastoma Staging System (IRSS) stage I and high-risk features, and all patients with IRSS stage II onwards. These investigations include bilateral bone-marrow aspirates and biopsies, and lumbar puncture with examination of the cytospin. Since retinoblastoma cells may adhere to the tube, the examination of the cytocentrifugate should be done to improve the yield of this procedure. Bone scintigraphy is only recommended in children with confirmed metastatic disease or those with bone pain.

Treatment

Retinoblastoma is special among paediatric tumours in that two different treatments goals are sought by treating physicians: patient survival, usually led by a paediatric oncologist, and eye survival, usually led by a paediatric ophthalmologist. Each need different parameters to be considered for treatment in the context of a multidisciplinary team. So, the treatment of retinoblastoma includes surgical procedures, local therapies, radiotherapy, and chemotherapy that can be given systemically or locally. Conservative therapies should be used with caution in less developed countries where patient compliance is poor or uncertain. Deaths after refusal of enucleation or toxicity have been published.

Surgery

Enucleation is the simplest and safest therapy for retinoblastoma. A prosthetic implant is fitted after the procedure to minimize cosmetic deficits. Enucleation should be performed by an experienced paediatric ophthalmologist in order to obtain a long optic-nerve stump. Initial enucleation is indicated in all eyes with secondary glaucoma, invasion of anterior segment (anterior chamber, iris), rubeosis iridis, impossibility of close follow-up or limitations for using local therapies, and group E eyes in most unilateral non-hereditary patients. Secondary enucleation is indicated after failure of conservative approaches and after neoadjuvant chemotherapy in extraocular disease. Even though enucleation is a curative treatment for retinoblastoma and may be performed in most settings, regardless of their complexity, it is not always accepted by the families, especially in less developed countries. In some countries, up to 50% of affected families opt out of enucleation as initial treatment; these children die of a potentially curable disease. Therefore, in these problematic settings, comprehensive strategies, including psychosocial support, should be implemented to improve survival. Some surgical procedures, such as pars plana vitrectomy, are contraindicated in children with retinoblastoma, and other aggressive surgeries, like orbital exenteration, are currently seldom performed.

Focal therapies

Focal treatments are used for small tumours (less than 3–6 mm), usually in patients with bilateral disease, and in combination with chemotherapy. These treatments include photocoagulation with an argon laser (for the treatment of tumours posterior to the equator), transpupillary thermotherapy (which applies focused heat, usually with a diode laser, at subphotocoagulation levels), and cryotherapy (for the treatment of small anterior lesions).

Radiotherapy

Radiotherapy, in combination with focal treatments, can provide excellent tumour control. However, radiation therapy increases the risk of second malignancies in heritable retinoblastoma survivors, and so contemporary management of intraocular retinoblastoma is designed to avoid or delay its use; the role of external-beam radiation (EBRT) is currently very limited in developed countries. Radiation therapy continues to have a major role in the treatment of patients with extraocular disease.

Several techniques can be used, usually through lateral or anterior fields. Recommended total doses are 4000–4500 cGy, although doses of 3600 cGy, in conjunction with other techniques, are under investigation. The use of modern radiotherapy techniques like intensity-modulated radiotherapy (IMRT) and proton therapy may lower the risk of long-term toxicity, especially by reducing the dose to the brain and other non-ocular structures.

Radioactive plaque technique is useful when treating localized tumours, both because the procedure time is short and also because a high dose of irradiation is delivered to the areas of interest while minimizing radiation effects to the extraocular structures. The radioactive implant is placed on the sclera over the base of the tumour, and is kept there for two to four days—the time needed to deliver approximately 4000 cGy to the apex of the tumour. Different radioactive episcleral plaques can be used, although ^{125}I and ^{106}Ru are the most widely used. Control rates of 85–90% can be achieved. This treatment has not been associated with an increased risk of secondary tumours when used in children with germline mutations.

Chemotherapy

The uses of chemotherapy for the treatment of retinoblastoma include three different scenarios.

Tumour chemoreduction for conservative treatment

Chemoreduction using systemic chemotherapy has been used as primary treatment for intraocular disease not amenable for local therapy, in order to decrease tumour size and make the tumours suitable for local therapy, for the past two decades. Carboplatin in combination with vincristine or etoposide, given intravenously, have been the most frequently used agents. A recent randomized study showed that the combination of carboplatin and etoposide yielded marginally better results than carboplatin and vincristine. Topotecan in combination with periocular carboplatin, alternating with the carboplatin–etoposide–vincristine regimen, proved to be effective in advanced intraocular retinoblastoma.

The effectiveness and short-term toxicity of systemic chemoreduction were reported by many groups. With this treatment, most intraocular tumours usually show dramatic shrinkage. However, consolidation with local treatment is needed in most cases to prevent relapse. Tumour location and size correlate with responsiveness to chemotherapy. Systemic chemoreduction followed by local therapy is still the standard therapy for patients with less advanced disease, such as groups A to C (see Box 31.1), in whom up to 90% of the eyes can be salvaged without using EBRT. For patients with advanced intraocular tumours, belonging to group D (see Box 31.1), and especially those with vitreous seeds, ocular salvage rates are not so encouraging with this therapy. Most of these patients have been traditionally considered for initial enucleation. However, single-institution experiences using superselective intra-arterial chemotherapy administration in the ophthalmic artery have shown improved salvage rates. Melphalan has been the most commonly used agent for intra-arterial chemotherapy, but carboplatin and topotecan have also been employed. This treatment was reported to be highly effective in eyes with retinal detachment and subretinal seeds, which were considered for enucleation in the past. Tandem administration of intra-arterial chemotherapy to both eyes in the same procedure is feasible. This strategy is usually recommended in children older than six months, weighing more than 6 kg, and it has also been effective as salvage therapy after failure of systemic chemoreduction and EBRT, with a salvage rate of 58% in results of single-referral institutions. However, intra-arterial chemotherapy is being used in middle-income countries as well, with encouraging results.

Intra-arterial chemotherapy has a favourable systemic toxicity profile compared to systemic chemotherapy. However, ocular toxicity, including severe choroidal damage leading to reduced vision has been reported. Long-term effects of intra-arterial chemotherapy are less known, but reports from Japan failed to find evidence of increased risk of secondary malignancies. Intra-arterial chemotherapy as a frontline eye-salvage procedure for unilateral group D and selected E patients is increasingly used by some treatment groups, with ocular survival higher than 80%. Even though no toxic mortality associated to this treatment was reported, occasional events of metastatic relapse were reported in this population. So, this modality should be used with caution for unilateral group D and E disease in areas where high-risk pathology is more prevalent and a higher risk of extraocular relapse is seen, since enucleation yields excellent survival outcome and is usually well tolerated.

More recently, intravitreous injection of melphalan became an effective therapy for children with vitreous seeds. Though contraindicated for decades because of the fear of accidental orbital seeding of the tumour, an improved technique, reported recently, has made it a safe and relatively inexpensive treatment. However, it needs to be administered by experienced ophthalmologists. The combined sequential use of intra-arterial chemotherapy and intravitreous chemotherapy appears to be a promising strategy for eyes with vitreous seeds. The optimal dose and schedule of intravitreous melphalan are still not known. According to the current classification of vitreous seeds, those presenting as clouds would need more prolonged and intensive therapy for tumour control.

Even though chemoreduction followed by local treatment has become the standard therapy for intraocular retinoblastoma, there are several limitations to this approach. Systemic chemotherapy may increase the risk of secondary malignancies, certainly as far as their potential induction is concerned, and especially treatment-induced leukaemia. Finally, this treatment is tedious and needs meticulous management; resources are only available in specialized centres.

Adjuvant chemotherapy for high-risk stage I and II disease

After enucleation, the eye should be comprehensively evaluated by an experienced ocular pathologist: histopathological microstaging using standardized criteria for risk assessment is essential to define groups with a different risk of extraocular relapse. Invasion to the choroid, sclera, and optic nerve are considered as significant risk factors for extraocular relapse. The role of adjuvant chemotherapy for some of these patients, to reduce the relapse rate, is a matter of controversy. Because these factors are infrequent in developed countries, there have been no randomized studies published in the literature as for other malignancies. There is almost universal agreement that there is no need of adjuvant chemotherapy for patients with intraretinal disease and in those with prelaminar optic-nerve invasion. The role of chemotherapy in isolated choroidal invasion is controversial because the relapse rate, when there is no concomitant postlaminar optic-nerve involvement, is only about 3%. Different degrees of choroidal invasion may have different prognostic implications and some subgroups, such as those with massive invasion (defined as greater than 3 mm), might benefit from adjuvant chemotherapy. However, since the overall survival of these children is in the range of 95% with no other therapy than enucleation, it is unlikely that a benefit from adjuvant chemotherapy will be unequivocally proven.

Invasion to the optic nerve beyond the lamina cribrosa is a major risk factor for relapse, and adjuvant therapy is recommended by most groups. When the resection margin is free of tumour, most treatment groups recommend adjuvant chemotherapy alone. With the use of current high-resolution MRI, postlaminar optic-nerve invasion may be presumed preoperatively by detecting contrast enhancement in the distal portion of the nerve. Some of these patients have received neoadjuvant chemotherapy in an attempt to avoid tumour residue at the resection margin. However, identifying postlaminar optic-nerve invasion through imaging studies is a challenge and the sensitivity of MRI when the optic nerve is not enlarged is about 60% in centres with extensive experience. Patients with invasion of the resection margin of the optic nerve are classified as IRSS stage II because microscopic tumour residue is left behind after enucleation, and they are uniformly considered for adjuvant therapy with chemotherapy and orbital radiotherapy. In recent series, about 70% of these patients survive, albeit with important cosmetic and neuroendocrinological sequelae because of radiation.

The importance of microscopic scleral invasion as a risk factor for relapse is less clear because it usually occurs with other concomitant factors. When there is evidence of microscopic transscleral invasion, these children should be considered as stage II, but patients with only intrascleral invasion (stage I) need adjuvant chemotherapy as well. The chemotherapy regimens used for the adjuvant therapy of children with stage I disease and pathology risk factors include the combination of carboplatin and etoposide, or more intensive regimens including the same agents at higher doses together with alkylating agents such as cyclophosphamide or ifosfamide and an anthracycline, as it is used in other centres. The use of more intensive regimens is warranted for children with stage II disease such as those with postlaminar optic-nerve and tumor at the resection margin or microscopical scleral invasion. However, there is no consensus on the adequate treatment intensity for these children.

Treatment of overt extraocular retinoblastoma (stages III and IV)

In all these cases, neoadjuvant chemotherapy is warranted. Extensive and mutilating surgeries such as orbital exenteration are of no use. About 70% of patients with stage III disease are curable with an aggressive approach using neoadjuvant chemotherapy, enucleation of the residual mass, and adjuvant chemo- and radiotherapy. The agents used are the same as those used for high-risk stage I and II disease. Orbital relapse after enucleation is also curable with the same approach.

Although a complete remission is usually achieved with conventional chemotherapy in patients with stage IV disease, it is usually short-lived and ultimate survival is infrequent. However, recent series report that a high proportion of metastatic retinoblastoma outside the CNS (stage IVa) may be cured using high-dose chemotherapy and autologous stem-cell rescue. Patients usually receive four to six cycles of conventional induction chemotherapy, followed by high-dose chemotherapy and autologous stem-cell rescue. Different preparative regimens have been used, but thiotepa-containing regimens appear to be effective because of its high penetration to the CNS. This modality has also been explored for children with CNS metastasis (stage IVb), but very few patients survive, even with this treatment. Recent reports suggest that this strategy may also be effective for trilateral retinoblastoma.

Second malignancies in retinoblastoma survivors

The cumulative incidence of second cancers in patients with germline mutations of the *RB1* gene is greatly increased with the use and dose of radiation therapy and, to a lesser extent, chemotherapy. This incidence is reported to increase steadily with age, to up to 40–60% at 40–50 years of age, although more recent studies estimate a considerably lower risk for patients irradiated with more modern techniques. Patients with non-hereditary retinoblastoma are not inherently at an increased risk.

Almost any neoplasm has been described in survivors of retinoblastoma and 60–70% of the tumours occur in the head and neck areas. The most common second tumours are osteogenic sarcoma (arising both inside and outside the irradiation field), soft-tissue sarcomas, and melanomas. Uterine leiomyosarcomas are more frequent in women surviving hereditary retinoblastoma. Survivors of bilateral retinoblastoma are also at risk of developing epithelial cancers late in adulthood, particularly in the lung. There is an ongoing debate about the use of whole-body MRI for screening of second malignancies, but no formal recommendation besides frequent medical follow-up, avoidance of sun exposure, and healthy life habits is currently issued.

FURTHER READING

Abramson DH, et al. (2008) A phase I/II study of direct intraarterial (ophthalmic artery) chemotherapy with melphalan for intraocular retinoblastoma initial results. *Ophthalmology* **115**, 1398–404.

Aerts I, et al. (2013) Results of a multicenter prospective study on the postoperative treatment of unilateral retinoblastoma after primary enucleation. *J Clin Oncol* **31**, 1458–63.

Antoneli CB, et al. (2003) Extraocular retinoblastoma: a 13-year experience. *Cancer* **98**, 1292–8.

Canturk S, et al. (2010) Survival of retinoblastoma in less-developed countries: impact of socioeconomic and health-related indicators. *Br J Ophthalmol* **94**, 1432–6.

Chantada GL, et al. (2010) Results of a prospective study for the treatment of unilateral retinoblastoma. *Pediatr Blood Cancer* **55**, 60–6.

Corson TW, Gallie BL (2007) One hit, two hits, three hits, more? Genomic changes in the development of retinoblastoma. *Genes Chromosomes Cancer* **46**, 617–34.

De Camargo B, et al. (2010) Cancer incidence among children and adolescents in Brazil: first report of 14 population-based cancer registries. *Int J Cancer* **126**, 715–20.

De Graaf P, et al. (2012) Guidelines for imaging retinoblastoma: imaging principles and MRI standardization. *Pediatr Radiol* **42**, 2–14.

De Jong MC, et al. (2014) Trilateral retinoblastoma: a systematic review and meta-analysis. *Lancet Oncol* **15**, 1157–67.

Dunkel IJ, et al. (2010) Intensive multimodality therapy for patients with stage 4a metastatic retinoblastoma. *Pediatr Blood Cancer* **55**, 55–9.

Francis JH, et al. (2015) The classification of vitreous seeds in retinoblastoma and response to intravitreal melphalan. *Ophthalmology* **122**, 1173–9.

Kleinerman RA, et al. (2005) Risk of new cancers after radiotherapy in long-term survivors of retinoblastoma: an extended follow-up. *J Clin Oncol* **23**, 2272–9.

Laurie NA, et al. (2006) Inactivation of the p53 pathway in retinoblastoma. *Nature* **444**, 61–6.

Leal-Leal CA, et al. (2006) Survival in extra-orbital metastatic retinoblastoma: treatment results. *Clin Transl Oncol* **8**, 39–44.

Lumbroso-LeRouic L, et al. (2016) Conservative treatment of retinoblastoma: a prospective phase II randomized trial of neoadjuvant chemotherapy followed by local treatments and chemothermotherapy. *Eye (Lond)* **30**, 46–52.

Munier FL, et al. (2008) New developments in external beam radiotherapy for retinoblastoma: from lens to normal tissue-sparing techniques. *Clin Exp Ophthalmol* **36**, 78–89.

Qaddoumi I, et al. (2012) Topotecan and vincristine combination is effective against advanced bilateral intraocular retinoblastoma and has manageable toxicity. *Cancer* **118**, 5663–70.

Rushlow DE, et al. (2013) Characterisation of retinoblastomas without RB1 mutations: genomic, gene expression, and clinical studies. *Lancet Oncol* **14**, 327–34.

Sastre X, et al. (2009) Proceedings of the consensus meetings from the International Retinoblastoma Staging Working Group on the pathology guidelines for the examination of enucleated eyes and evaluation of prognostic risk factors in retinoblastoma. *Arch Pathol Lab Med* **133**, 1199–202.

Shields CL, et al. (2014) Intra-arterial chemotherapy for retinoblastoma in 70 eyes: outcomes based on the international classification of retinoblastoma. *Ophthalmology* **121**, 1453–60.

Xu XL, et al. (2009) Retinoblastoma has properties of a cone precursor tumor and depends upon cone-specific MDM2 signaling. *Cell* **137**, 1018–31.

Index

Notes
Abbreviations used in subentries can be found on pages (ix) to (xiii)
Tables, figures and boxes are indicated by an italic *t*, *f* and *b* following the page number
vs. indicates a comparison or differential diagnosis